ANATOMIC AND CLINICAL PATHOLOGY

REVIEW

ANATOMIC AND CLINICAL PATHOLOGY

REVIEW

MEGHAN HUPP, MD

Great Lakes Pathologists, SC
West Allis, Wisconsin

ELSEVIER

Elsevier
1600 John F. Kennedy Blvd.
Ste 1800
Philadelphia, PA 19103-2899

ANATOMIC AND CLINICAL PATHOLOGY REVIEW

ISBN: 978-0-323-87113-6

Library of Congress Control Number: 2021947604

Content Strategist: Michael Houston
Content Development Manager: Somodatta Roy Choudhary
Content Development Specialist: Akanksha Marwah
Publishing Services Manager: Deepthi Unni
Project Manager: Janish Ashwin Paul
Design Direction: Amy Buxton

Printed in India

Last digit is the print number: 9 8 7 6 5 4 3 2 1

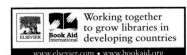

This book is for the trainees in the University of Minnesota Anatomic and Clinical Pathology program.

It's also dedicated to my biggest supporter—my husband, Lyric. Thank you for being you.

ACKNOWLEDGMENTS

Many people have contributed indirectly to the creation of this book by teaching me throughout my training, including the Laboratory Medicine and Pathology Department at the University of Minnesota. Most of all, I'd like to thank Dr. Michael Linden for teaching me not only hematopathology, but also interpersonal, professional, and leadership skills. This would not have been possible without your tireless support.

This work grew out of my incessant note-taking during medical school and residency. I realized early in my Pathology training that there was a need for a "broad picture" guide for residency, similar to those ubiquitous handbooks that are always tucked under the arms of anxious medical students. The following text is the result of my effort to provide both scaffolding for training and a review text for the Anatomic and Clinical Pathology board exams.

This text is not and was not intended to be a stand-alone resource for rotations or board exams. It's simply a guide to make the process easier.

I hope you find this text useful in your training, board studying, and as a refresher for in-practice pathologists.

CONTENTS

CHAPTER 1

General Pathology

Basic Cell Biology

APOPTOSIS

- Regulated by increased TNF, p. 53 activity, down-regulation of Bcl-2
- Can be blocked (but not reversed) by survivin (apoptosis inhibitor)
- T-lymphocytes first bind and activate TNF receptors (FAS and TRAIL) → activation of caspase 8 or 9 → activation of caspase 3 (always a late event)

PD-1 AND PD-L1

See Fig. 1.1.

RNA TRANSCRIPTION

RNA POL 1—in nucleolus—rRNA only
- RNA POL 2—main polymerase—protein-coding genes and some noncoding
- Recognizes TATA box, GC box, and CAAT box
- RNA POL 3—a few others

Basic Histology/Pathobiology

MICROSCOPY TUTORIAL

- **A.** Kohler illumination
  1. Adjust interpupillary distance
  2. Focus slide at 10×
  3. Close field diaphragm (bottom)
  4. Center circle of light using screws
  5. Raise/lower condenser to obtain sharp outline
  6. Open field diaphragm
  7. Adjust iris diaphragm (>75%)
- **B.** Parfocal adjustment
  1. Focus on slide on highest dry objective with coarse/fine knobs
  2. Change to lowest objective
  3. Use diopter adjustment to refocus, one eye at a time
- **C.** Turn light all the way down before turning off

COLLAGENS

- Fibrillar
  - I—hard and soft tissues—osteogenesis imperfecta

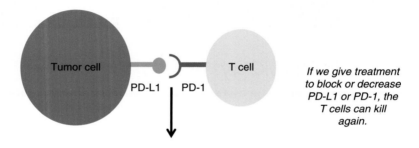

Fig. 1.1   Programmed death-1 (PD-1) and programmed death-ligand 1 (PD-L1) interaction prevents T-cell-mediated cytotoxicity.

- II—cartilage, vertebral disks—achondrogenesis type II, spondyloepiphyseal dysplasia syndrome
- III—hollow organs and soft tissues—vascular Ehlers-Danlos
- V—soft tissues, blood vessels—classic Ehlers-Danlos
- IX, XI—cartilage and vitreous—Stickler syndrome
- Nonfibrillar
  - IV—basement membrane—Alport syndrome

AMYLOIDOSIS

- Types
  - AL amyloid—usually lambda—monoclonal gammopathy or plasma cell myeloma
  - AA amyloid—secondary amyloidosis (rheumatoid arthritis, hepatitis C, intravenous drug abuse), familial Mediterranean fever, apoSAA, and so on
  - AH amyloid—IgG_1—systemic heavy chain amyloidosis
  - Beta-2 amyloid—beta-protein precursor—Alzheimer
  - Mutated transthyretin—familial neuropathy (hereditary)
  - Normal transthyretin—senile cardiac amyloidosis (causes cardiomyopathy)
  - Beta-2 microglobulin—carpal tunnel, found after long-term dialysis in joint capsules and ligaments
  - AGel amyloid—gelsolin—Finnish familial amyloidosis
- Amyloid versus collagen—10 nm versus 50 nm
- Congo red stain requires thick sections (10 μm)

IGG₄-RELATED ENTITIES

- Lymphadenopathy
- Autoimmune pancreatitis
- Lymphoplasmacytic sclerosing cholangitis
- Chronic sclerosing dacryoadenitis
- Chronic sclerosing sialoadenitis
- Eosinophilic angiocentric fibrosis
- Reidel thyroiditis

ROSETTES AND PSEUDOROSETTES

- Pseudorosettes surround vessel (nontumor tissue)
  - Common in ependymomas, medulloblastomas, primitive neuroectodermal tumors (PNETs), glioblastoma multiformes, and so on
- Rosettes surround neuropil, stroma, or a tumor lumen
  - Homer-Wright true rosettes surround neuropil in neuroblastomas, medulloblastomas, and PNETs
- Flexner-Wintersteiner true rosettes surround lumen containing cytoplasmic projections of tumor cells in retinoblastomas
- True ependymal rosettes surround empty lumen in well-differentiated ependymomas

GIANT CELL TYPES

- Langhans—ring/horseshoe-shape at cell periphery
  - TB, syphilis, sarcoidosis, fungi
  - *Not Langerhans*
- Touton—nuclei form a ring surround by foamy cytoplasm
  - Fibrous histiocytoma (dermatofibroma), juvenile xanthogranuloma
- Osteoclast-like—giant cell malignant fibrous histiocytoma, leiomyosarcoma, osteosarcoma, tumoral calcinosis
- Foreign body—haphazard, overlapped, centrally placed nuclei

MUCIN TYPES

- Hyaluronic acid (nonsulfated mucopolysaccharide)
  - Increased in dermatoses
  - Positive for Alcian blue at pH 2.5
  - Hyaluronidase sensitive
- Chondroitin/heparan sulfate (sulfated mucopolysaccharide)
  - Positive for Alcian blue at pH 2.5 and pH 0.5
  - PAS-positive, diastase-resistant

COMMON MORPHOLOGIC FEATURES

- Cherry red nucleoli
  - Melanoma
  - Prostate
  - Epithelioid angiosarcoma
  - Poorly differentiated adenocarcinoma
- Intranuclear pseudoinclusions
  - PEComa
    - "Clear cell sugar tumor"
  - Angiomyolipoma
  - Lymphangioleiomyoma
  - Chromophobe renal cell carcinoma
  - Papillary thyroid carcinoma
  - Melanoma
  - Hepatocellular carcinoma

- Oncocytes—very pink, lots of mitochondria
  - Warthin tumor
  - Hashimoto
  - Elderly salivary glands
  - Salivary retention cysts
  - Oncocytoma of salivary gland
  - Oncocytoma of kidney
  - Hurthle cell tumor of thyroid
  - Bronchial carcinoids
  - Mucoepidermoid carcinoma of the lung
- Hemangiopericytoma-like vessels (staghorn vessels)
  - Solitary fibrous tumor
  - Myofibroma/myopericytoma
  - GIST
  - Synovial sarcoma
  - Extraskeletal myxoid chondrosarcoma
  - Ovarian sclerosing stromal tumor
- Nuclear grooves
  - Papillary thyroid carcinoma
  - Solid pseudopapillary tumor of pancreas
  - Chondroblastoma
  - Pulmonary adenocarcinoma in situ
  - Thyroid oncocytes
- Cytoplasmic tails on fine needle aspiration
  - Sarcoma
  - Melanoma
  - Squamous cell carcinoma (tadpole cells)
- Rosettes
  - Follicular thyroid carcinoma
  - Neuroendocrine
  - Ependymal central nervous system lesions

Cytology Basics

- Signs of malignancy
  - Dirty background
    - "Tigroid" background suggestive of germ cell tumors (seminoma or dysgerminoma), Ewing sarcoma, and rhabdosarcoma
  - 3D clusters
  - Isolated cells
  - Necrotic ghost cells without inflammatory cells
  - Haphazard cellular arrangement
  - Irregular size and shape
  - Irregular chromatin patterns
  - Variable numbers of nucleoli
- Signs of benignity
  - Clean background
  - Sheets of cells
  - Inflammatory cells

- Mesothelial cells versus adenocarcinoma
  - Adenocarcinoma
    - Smooth community border
    - Express MOC31 and BerEP4
  - Mesothelial cells
    - Mesothelial cells have windows and lacy skirts
    - Express WT1 and calretinin
    - Mesothelioma
      - Knobby, scalloped community border
      - EMA positive (while *reactive* mesothelial cells are not)

Immunophenotypes and Differentiating Neoplasms

NEOPLASM OF UNKNOWN ORIGIN

- By cell shape
  - Spindle cell
    - Sarcomatoid carcinoma
    - Sarcoma
    - Melanoma
    - Panel: Pankeratin, p40, SMSA, desmin, SOX10
  - Anaplastic
    - Anything
    - Panel: Pankeratin, CD45, SOX10
  - Round cell
    - Round cell sarcoma
    - Lymphoma
    - Small cell carcinoma
    - Panel: CD99, NKX2.2, desmin, myogenin, CD45, TdT, INSM1, pankeratin, SOX10
  - Epithelioid
    - Carcinoma
    - Melanoma
    - Large cell lymphoma
    - Panel: Pankeratin, CD45, SOX10
- By degree of pleomorphism
  - Monomorphic
    - Clear cell sarcoma
    - Burkitt lymphoma
    - Mesothelioma
    - Prostate cancer
    - Gastrointestinal stromal tumor
    - Ewing sarcoma
    - Synovial sarcoma
    - INI-1–deficient tumors
    - Follicular dendritic cell tumors
  - Pleomorphism
    - Melanoma
    - Diffuse large B-cell lymphoma
    - Adenocarcinoma (especially serous and pancreatic)

- Urothelial carcinoma
- Sarcomatoid carcinoma
- CIC and BCOR rearranged sarcomas

IMPORTANT IMMUNOPHENOTYPES AND EXPRESSION

- See Table 1.1
- S100—Schwann cells (not actual neurons), melanocytes, Langhans cells, cartilage, some myoepithelium, skin adnexa
  - SOX10 is more specific for melanoma than S100
- ER/PR—luminal cells in ducts and lobules of breast
- CD31, Factor 8—vascular endothelium
- c-Kit/CD117—mast cells
- Smooth muscle alpha actin—blood vessel walls, myoepithelium in breast
- Vimentin
  - Stains a lot of things—not helpful in most spindle cell tumors
  - Uses
    - Renal cell carcinoma (not chromophobe)
    - Endometrioid (not endocervical) adenocarcinoma
- D2-40 stains lymphatic endothelial cells, not venous
  - CD31 is opposite
- High-molecular-weight keratin (CK5/6)—squamous epithelium
- Low-molecular-weight keratin (CK7, CK20)—glandular epithelium
- CD15—neutrophils
- Myofibroblasts −/+AE1/AE3; −HMWK (like CK5/6)
- Neurons—NSE, neurofilament, synaptophysin
- Leiomyoma −/+SMA and desmin; −S100, CD34, C117
- GIST—−/+S100, CD34, CD117; −SMA and desmin
- Chordoma—brachyury

TABLE 1.1 ■ **Distribution of Cytokeratin (CK) 20 and CK7 Expression Across Neoplasm Type and Cell of Origin**

	CK7+	CK7−
CK20+	Cholangiocarcinoma/ biliary duct carcinoma Gastric adenocarcinoma Ovarian mucinous adenocarcinoma Pancreatic adenocarcinoma Urothelial cell carcinoma	Colorectal adenocarcinoma Gastric adenocarcinoma Merkel cell carcinoma
CK20−	Ductal and lobular breast carcinoma Malignant mesothelioma Endometrial adenocarcinoma Ovarian serous & endometrioid carcinoma Pulmonary adenocarcinoma	Hepatocellular carcinoma Prostatic carcinoma Renal cell carcinoma Small cell carcinoma of lung SCC of esophagus, lung, skin Thyroid carcinoma (follicular and papillary) Adrenocortical Mesothelial Gastric Seminoma

SCC, Squamous cell carcinoma.

SPECIAL STAINS

- Sudan black or oil red O—fat
- Van Gieson—collagen
- Trichrome—muscle (red) and collagen (blue-green)
- Reticulin—reticulin fibers (black) and collagen (brown)
- Congo red—amyloid
- PAS—glycogen, fungi, basement membrane, mucin, hyaline casts (magenta)
  - With diastase—glycogen does *not* stain, everything else does
- Prussian blue—iron
- Fontana-Masson—melanin and capsule-deficient cryptococcus

SMALL ROUND BLUE CELL TUMORS

"Mr. Sleep"

- Melanoma
- Rhabdomyosarcoma
- Sinonasal undifferentiated carcinoma (SNUC)
- Synovial sarcoma
- Lymphoma
- Esthesioneuroblastoma
- Ewing sarcoma
- Peripheral neuroectodermal tumor (PNET)
- (and small cell carcinoma, Merkel cell carcinoma, Wilms tumor, desmoplastic small round cell tumor)

MORPHOLOGIC FINDINGS OF IMPORTANT INFECTIOUS ORGANISMS

- Pneumocystis pneumonia
  - Soap bubble clusters—foamy proteinaceous cast of alveoli
  - Calcofluor white, toluidine blue, GMS
  - Cup with a dark spot (crushed ping pong ball/flat basketball)
- CMV
  - Viral inclusions
  - One of the most common opportunistic infections
  - Cytomegaly, large basophilic nuclear inclusions, small basophilic cytoplasmic inclusions
  - Mostly in alveolar macrophages
  - Must confirm with viral culture, IHC, or PCR/ISH
- Aspergillus
  - Fruiting bodies (conidiophores) form in cavitary lesions
  - Charcot-Leyden or calcium oxalate crystals may form
  - Squamous atypia may occur (reactive, not malignant)
- Blastomycosis
  - Broad-based budding yeast
  - Woody terrain, lumber industry
  - In immunocompetent, neutrophilic/granulomatous response
- Mucormycosis
  - Life-threatening
  - Broad ribbons, aseptate

- Cryptococcus
  - Abundant mucicarmine + capsule
  - Opportunistic
  - Marked by productive cough

Gross Pathology

- Head and neck
  - If depth of invasion (DOI) is >5 mm, do a neck dissection or obtain a frozen section
  - Microscopic DOI is important in staging
- Lymph nodes
  - Extranodal extension is important
  - Also measurement of metastasis within the lymph node
- Melanoma
  - Frozen sections not advised
  - Surface ulceration is added to staging, but do not confuse previous biopsy/Mohs/resection changes
- Gastrointestinal junction (GEJ)
  - Obtain frozen sections on esophageal margin
  - Open stomach along greater curvature
  - Masses that cross GEJ will be staged as esophageal/GEJ *unless* the epicenter of the mass is >2 cm into stomach
  - Staged by DOI
- Whipple specimens
  - Usually distal duodenum becomes dusky from surgeon tying off vessels, useful to help orient yourself
  - Important vessels—superior mesenteric artery (SMA) and vein (SMV)
  - Margins = proximal stomach, distal duodenum, vascular groove (may have SMV), pancreatic neck, bile duct, uncinate (dissected off SMA)
  - Cannot really tell posttreatment tumor bed versus tumor
  - Staging based on *size* for exocrine tumor
    - Neuroendocrine tumors staged differently
    - Ampullary/duodenal masses are staged by depth of invasion (not size)
  - Frozen sections—bile duct and pancreatic neck margins
  - Extrapancreatic extension no longer included in staging

Odds and Ends

- Viral receptors
  - CD4—HIV and HTLV (retroviruses), T-cells
  - CD21—EBV, B-cells
- HPV—E6-p53, E7-Rb
- Sarcoidosis hypercalcemia mechanism
  - Increased 1-alpha-hydroxylase expression
  - Increased vitamin D expression
  - Hypercalcemia
- Calcium oxalate crystals are clear on H&E
  - Mainly found in cysts
  - Polarizable and refractile
  - Radio-opaque

CHAPTER 2

Breast Pathology

Basic Pathology

- Abbreviations
    - ADH—atypical ductal hyperplasia
    - DCIS—ductal carcinoma in situ
    - IDC—invasive ductal carcinoma (of no special type)
    - ALH—atypical lobular hyperplasia
    - LCIS—lobular carcinoma in situ
    - ILC—invasive lobular carcinoma
    - CCC—columnar cell change
    - CCH—columnar cell hyperplasia
    - FEA—flat epithelial atypia
    - TDLU—terminal ductal lobular unit
    - Functional unit of breast tissue
        - ER—estrogen receptor
        - PR—progesterone receptor
        - AR—androgen receptor
- Embryology
    - Thickening of the epidermis with formation of milk line at 5 weeks
        - Milk line = mammary ridge; runs axilla to groin bilaterally
- Subsequent involution of mammary region except at normal breast location
    - Failure—supernumerary nipple (2.4% of babies) or ectopic breast tissue
- Nottingham grading for invasive carcinoma
    - Ductal formation (1—>75% duct formation, 2—10–75%, 3—<10%)
    - Pleomorphism/nuclear atypia (1, 2, 3)
    - Mitotic activity (counting depends on microscope)
    - Grades (based on sum of 1–3)
        - 1 = 3, 4, 5
        - 2 = 6, 7
        - 3 = 8, 9
- Stains
    - Myoepithelial layer = +SMM-HC, calponin, CD10, p63
    - D2-40 stains lymphatic endothelial cells, not venous (CD31 is opposite)
    - E-cadherin—+ in IDC, – in ILC
    - Some high-grade lesions express p63
- Radiologic-pathologic correlation is key
    - Must explain radiologic findings (including calcifications) or contact the radiologist
- Microinvasive carcinoma (pT1mi)—≤1 mm
- Margins <1 mm are inadequate
    - 2-mm margin for DCIS or DCIS with microinvasion (>1 mm of invasion)
    - Report all margins that are <5 mm from invasive or DCIS

- 6–72 hours of fixation in 10% buffered formalin for HER2 analysis
  - Cold ischemia time <1 hour
- Be careful not to classify as weakly ER or PR+ if <1% positive
  - Could exclude patients from trials
  - Under 10% tend to respond like triple-negative cancers

Benign Breast Pathology

- Apocrine change
  - Eosinophilic cytoplasm
- Clear cell change
  - Myoepithelial cells are prominent
- Mastitis
  - Acute
    - First month of breast feeding
  - Periductal
    - Marked acute and chronic inflammation
    - Associated with smoking
  - Fat necrosis
    - Trauma/surgery
  - Lymphocytic
    - Hard mass(es), type 1 diabetes, autoimmune thyroid disease
  - Granulomatous
    - Sarcoidosis, fungal infection, foreign body
- Squamous metaplasia of lactiferous ducts (SMOLD)
  - Most commonly seen in older women who smoke
- Classic mammary duct ectasia
  - Lots of foamy macrophages
  - Postmenopause, multiparous
  - Thick, white nipple discharge and nipple retraction
- Nodular fasciitis
  - SMA+
- Fibromatosis
  - Infiltrative margins, nuclear beta-catenin+

BENIGN MIMICS AND PITFALLS

- Involuting breast tissue
  - Can look like multiple small intracanalicular fibroadenomas
  - "Fibroadenomatoid change"
- Mammary hamartoma
  - Ducts, lobules, stroma, and fat all jumbled up
  - Altered TDLUs separated by dissecting bands of fibrosis
  - Hard to diagnose on core biopsy
  - Differential diagnosis (DDx): fibroadenoma (FA) next to fat; FAs should not have fat in them
- Microglandular adenosis (MGA)
  - Mimic tubular carcinoma and is negative for myoepithelial markers
  - Negative for ER/PR–, SMA–, EMA–, GCDFP-15–
    - ER/PR negativity is a handy clue. The morphology mimics a low-grade carcinoma, which is typically ER/PR+. Stop and take a step back

- Positive for S100, laminin (no myoepithelial cells, but there is a basal lamina), type IV collagen
- No atypia, equal-sized *round* glands everywhere, infiltrates fat and normal TDLUs
- Luminal secretions are densely eosinophilic and PAS+ diastase resistant
- Differential diagnosis
  - Tubular carcinoma has teardrop glands
  - Secretory adenosis—MGA but *with* myoepithelial cells around tubules
  - Sclerosing adenosis has myoepithelial cells, lobulocentric
  - Collagenous spherulosis is p63+
  - Acinic cell carcinoma—significant morphologic and immunophenotypic overlap BUT acinic cell carcinoma has cytoplasmic granules
- Fibrocystic change classifications
  - Nonproliferative fibrocystic change
    - Cysts
    - Papillary apocrine change and apocrine cysts
    - Epithelial-related calcifications
    - Mild epithelial hyperplasia
    - Ductal ectasia
    - Nonsclerosing adenosis
    - Periductal fibrosis
  - Proliferative fibrocystic change without atypia
    - Moderate or florid usual ductal hyperplasia
    - Sclerosing adenosis
    - Radial scar
    - Intraductal papilloma or papillomatosis
  - Proliferative lesions with atypia
    - ADH
    - ALH
- Lactational change
  - Most common during pregnancy and lactational period, but can be sporadic
  - May present as mass—lactational adenoma
  - Considered hyperplastic process
  - May present as incidental clustered calcifications
  - May wax and wane
- Nipple adenoma or florid papillomatosis of the nipple
  - Clinically similar to Paget's disease of the nipple
  - Circumscribed, proliferative changes just below skin
  - Florid usual ductal hyperplasia, sclerosing adenosis, papillary lesions, apocrine metaplasia
  - *ADH/DCIS may occur within lesion*
  - May locally recur if not excised completely

CORE BIOPSY NONMALIGNANT RESULTS IN WHICH EXCISION IS RECOMMENDED PRUDENT

- Lesions associated with an "upgrade"
  - ADH (to DCIS)
  - Lobular neoplasia (to DCIS or invasive cancer)
  - FEA (to DCIS or invasive cancer)
- Heterogeneous lesions
  - Papillary lesions (may hide DCIS in papilloma or papillary carcinoma)

- Radial scars
  - Central star-like sclerosis, peripheral cysts, trapped tubules, +/− elastosis
  - Not *always* excised
- Mucocele-like lesion
- Spindle cell lesion
- Fibroepithelial lesions (not clear-cut fibroadenoma)

Radiologically Suspicious Lesions

- Mammogram
  - Margins
    - Indistinct
    - Spiculated
    - Microlobulated
  - Calcifications
    - ~80% of breast calcifications are benign
    - Benign
      - Larger, fewer, widely dispersed, round
      - Diffuse and bilateral
      - Apocrine cyst, fibrocystic change, fibroadenoma, sclerosing adenosis, fat necrosis
      - Vascular or skin
      - Dystrophic
    - Indeterminate
      - Amorphous
        - Fibrocystic change > milk of calcium > ADH > lobular neoplasia > low-grade DCIS
      - Coarse
      - Regional
    - Malignant
      - Fine, smaller
      - More numerous
      - Clustered
      - Pleomorphic
      - Linear and segmental, shaped like rod/branch/teardrop
        - DCIS, IDC
    - Magnification views on diagnostic mammogram allow for higher definition views of small, fine calcifications
- Ultrasound
  - Echogenicity
    - Hypoechoic—benign or malignant
    - Hyperechoic—benign
    - Isoechoic—hamartoma
  - Acoustic shadowing
    - Darker behind, malignant
    - Can also be from densely sclerotic tissue
  - Acoustic enhancement
    - Lighter behind, benign
  - Malignant features
    - Irregular hypoechoic mass
    - Nonparallel orientation (taller than wide)
    - Shadowing

- MRI
  - Spiculated or lobulated enhancing mass with fast initial phase kinetics and plateau/washout delayed phase kinetics
  - Non–mass-like enhancement (NMLE)
    - Area of increased blood flow
    - Not a mass
    - Lobular or in situ process

BI-RADS CATEGORIES

- 0—incomplete evaluation
- 1—normal
  - Risk for cancer—5 in 10,000—continue annual screening
- 2—typically benign (normal follow-up)
  - Risk: 5 in 10,000—continue annual screening
- 3—probably benign
  - Risk: <2%—6-month follow-up
- 4—suspicious abnormality
  - 4a—low suspicion of malignancy
    - Benign biopsy not necessarily discordant
    - 6-month follow-up if benign biopsy
  - 4b—intermediate suspicion of malignancy
    - If benign biopsy result, follow-up dependent on radiologic-pathologic correlation
  - 4c—moderate concern but not classic for malignancy
  - Malignant biopsy result is expected
  - Risk: 2%–95%
- 5—highly suggestive of malignancy
  - Risk ≥95%—biopsy or excision
- 6—biopsy-confirmed malignancy

Breast Cytology

- Sheets
  - Fibrocystic change
  - Fibroadenoma
  - LCIS
- Tight three-dimensional clusters
  - Fibroadenoma/phyllodes
  - Intraductal papilloma
  - LCIS
  - Ductal proliferation (hyperplasia through DCIS)
  - Well-differentiated IDC
  - Mucinous carcinoma
- Loose three-dimensional clusters
  - Phyllodes
  - DCIS
  - IDC
- Branching papillary clusters
  - Fibroadenoma
  - Intraductal papilloma

- Papillary carcinoma
- Isolated cells
  - Carcinoma
  - Pregnancy
- Microacinar formation
  - Slight rosetting of nuclei within solid LCIS/DCIS without lumens

Ductal Neoplasia

ADH VS. UDH

- UDH
  - Features
    - Hill-shaped proliferations
    - Polymorphic, heterogeneous
    - Slit-like lumens
    - Swirling/streaming
    - Intranuclear pseudoinclusions and grooves
    - No distinct cell borders
    - Anisonucleosis
    - Overlapping nuclei
    - Intermixed apocrine change
  - If florid in fibrocystic change, call it "proliferative change"
    - Must be extensive and expanding ducts
- ADH
  - "Proliferation of monomorphic evenly placed epithelial cells involving TDLUs"
  - <2 mm for each lesion
  - Features
    - Mushroom-shaped proliferations
    - Monomorphic
    - Micropapillary, solid, or cribriform
    - Punched-out lumens with smooth contours
    - Bridging
    - Distinct cell borders
    - No swirling/streaming
    - Necrosis
    - Epithelium-associated calcifications
  - If found on breast core → lumpectomy
    - 5%–10% have IDC
    - See Table 2.1

DCIS

- Complete involvement of 1+ ducts with ADH features >2 mm in aggregate diameter
  - Low-grade—need size, cytology, and architecture criteria
    - Monomorphic cells completely involving ducts/lobules
    - 1.5–2× size of normal RBC (or normal duct cells)
    - Chromatin usually diffuse/finely dispersed
    - Occasional nucleoli
    - Occasional mitoses
    - Cells polarized toward lumen

TABLE 2.1 ■ **Differentiating Atypical Ductal Hyperplasia vs. Usual Ductal Hyperplasia Using Immunohistochemistry**

	ADH/DCIS	**UDH**
ER	(+)	Mosaic (+)
CK5/6	(−)	Mosaic (+)

Note: Cannot use for lesions with apocrine features; does not stain reliably. ER, Estrogen receptor; ADH, atypical ductal hyperplasia; DCIS, ductal carcinoma in situ; UDH, usual ductal hyperplasia.

- Strong diffuse ER (PR is redundant for DCIS), −CK5/6 (but + in myoepithelial cells)
  - Also ADH
    - Only low-to-intermediate grade
  - Grows discontinuously, jumps around
- Intermediate grade = features between low and high
- High-grade—cytology criteria only
  - Pleomorphic
  - High-grade nuclei
  - Does not need to be >2 mm
  - Does not have rigid spaces and monotony like low-grade
  - Grows continuously
- Architectural patterns—comedo, micropapillary, solid, cribriform, apocrine, papillary, spindled
- Imaging
  - Can be picked up on screening mammogram
    - Linear, comma-, or rod-shaped crystals in a segmental distribution toward the nipple
  - Not usually picked up with ultrasound (cannot see calcifications)
  - MRI—"clumped segmental enhancement"
  - DCIS retains myoepithelial layers, IDC does not
  - No clinical role for testing HER2 in DCIS (but there is an ongoing study)
  - DCIS is more frequently HER2+ than the invasive
- Van Nuys Prognostic Index
  - Score 1–3 in four categories
    - Size—≤15 mm, 16–40 mm, >40 mm
    - Nuclear grade
    - Distance from margin—≥10 mm, 1–9 mm, <1 mm
    - Age—over 60 years, 40–60 years, <40 years
  - Risk for recurrence
    - Low risk (4–6 points)
    - Lumpectomy only
    - Intermediate risk (7–9 points)
    - Lumpectomy and radiation
    - High risk (10–12 points)
- Mastectomy

INVASIVE DUCTAL CARCINOMA

- DCIS with microinvasion (<2 mm) is treated like DCIS
  - No chemotherapy, no Herceptin

- High-grade lesions tend to be better circumscribed than low-grade
- *If it does not meet criteria for any variants, it is called "IDC of no special type"*
- Variants
  - Tubular
    - Apical snouts, always open lumina, naked glands infiltrating fat
  - Cribriform
  - Medullary
  - Adenoid cystic
  - Inflammatory
  - Micropapillary
  - Mucinous
    - Pure mucinous carcinomas
      - Pools of extracellular
      - Present at an older age
      - Type A tumors—low cellularity, favorable prognosis
      - Type B tumors—greater cellularity, may be + for neuroendocrine markers, ER+, usually older
    - Mucinous micropapillary carcinoma
      - Micropapillary architectural pattern
      - Greater incidence of HER2 positivity, lymph node positivity and distant metastasis)
  - Metaplastic spindle cell
    - Negative for nuclear beta-catenin, triple negative
    - Rarely nuclear beta-catenin+ but should have some p63 and pankeratin (even if focal)
    - Differential diagnosis
      - Fibromatosis (nuclear beta-catenin+)
      - Nodular fasciitis (SMA+ and keratin−)
      - Phyllodes tumors (usually ER+ and keratin−)
  - Cannot be definitively diagnosed on core biopsy
  - Should not have architecture other than 90% tubular/cribriform/mucinous in the invasive component
  - Prognosis (with relation to IDC of no special type)
    - More favorable prognosis: mucinous, tubular, medullary, cribriform, adenoid cystic
    - Poorer prognosis: inflammatory, invasive micropapillary, central fibrotic focus, basal phenotype
- Extensive intraductal component (EIC)
- 25% of primary tumor is DCIS
- Paget disease of the nipple
  - Often associated with underlying in situ or invasive carcinoma
  - Often HER2+, intermediate-to-high-grade nuclei
  - Direct dermal invasion is rare and does not change outcome
  - Tumor cells in the epidermis can contain melanin pigment (melanotic Paget)
  - Paget vs. melanoma requires IHC panel!
- Multifocal = multiple tumors in the same quadrant
  - Multicentric = multiple tumors in different quadrants
- Enlarged, unfolded, partially cystic lobules
- Spectrum: columnar cell change → columnar hyperplasia → flat epithelial atypia

- *All are ER+, HER2–, HMWK– ; "low-grade breast neoplasia family"*
  - Includes CCC, CCH, FEA, ALH, ADH, LCIS, low-grade DCIS
  - Recurrent genetic aberrations
    - LOH in 1q, 16q, 17p
    - Losses of 16q, 17p; gain of 1q
      - High-grade 11q13 and 17q1 amplification
  - Frequently coexisting with low-grade invasive cancer (tubular or classic ILC)
    - Rosen's triad—tubular carcinoma, lobular neoplasia (LCIS/ILC), columnar cell lesions
- Columnar cell change (CCC)
  - 1–2 layers, uniform pattern with minimal pleomorphism, irregular contours, prominent myoepithelial layer, apical snouts, secretions, +/– dense calcifications
  - Stains like ADH—PITFALL
  - Frequently associated with sclerosing adenosis
- Columnar cell hyperplasia (CCH)
  - >2 layers, increased nuclear hyperchromasia, tufting/mounds, stratification, irregular contours, prominent myoepithelial layer
- Flat epithelial atypia (FEA)
  - CCC or CCH with atypia, neoplastic
  - AKA "clinging-type DCIS"
  - *Cytologic atypia without architectural atypia*
  - Morphology:
    - Acini and terminal ductules are enlarged and dilated, regular "rigid" contours
    - Myoepithelial cells are often attenuated
    - Round nuclei, monomorphic
    - Can have apical snouting
    - Occasional tufts but NO arcades, bridges, or micropapillae
      - Nuclear ER/PR+, cytoplasmic Bcl-2+, LMWK+ (CK8, CK18, CK19)
      - CCC and FEA have loss of HMWK and gain ER +
  - Differential diagnosis
    - Tubular carcinoma (which is identical to FEA but *without* myoepithelium and can be insidious)
    - Blunt duct adenosis
- Obtain multiple levels—20% will have ADH
- Should be excised and treated, behaves like ADH

Papillary Lesions

- Differential diagnosis
  - Benign intraductal papilloma, papilloma with atypia (atypical papilloma), encapsulated papillary neoplasm, solid papillary carcinoma
  - Nipple discharge (bloody) differential—papilloma vs. DCIS
  - Pink at low power → likely benign
  - Blue at low power → likely malignant
- Intraductal papilloma (IDP)
  - Sclerotic stroma (pink on low power) helps indicate benign
  - Central
    - Single, large
    - Postmenopausal
    - Presents as mass

- Peripheral
  - Multiple, usually smaller
  - Can occur at the periphery of radial scars
  - Present as mammogram abnormality
- Traditionally excised, 0%–29% upgraded on excision
- Atypical intraductal papilloma
  - IDP with ADH of epithelium
  - Can use CK5/6 to distinguish between UDH and ADH
  - 10%–59% upgraded on excision
- Papillary DCIS
  - Subtype of DCIS, no preexisting papilloma
  - Cellular with little stroma (blue on low power)
  - Expands ducts, usually extensively involved
  - No myoepithelial cells on fibrovascular cores but still present on duct lining
- Papilloma with DCIS
  - DCIS focus engrafted onto scaffolding of normal background papilloma
- Encapsulated papillary carcinoma (EPC)
  - Papillary carcinoma within an apparent cystically dilated duct surrounded by THICK FIBROUS CAPSULE
    - Usually only one duct involved
    - Expansive growth
  - Can look like IDP on core biopsy, low-grade features
  - No myoepithelial cells on papillary cores *or* outside lining of duct
  - Large central lesion in postmenopausal women, close to nipple
  - Can get high-grade EPC but VERY rare
    - Mitotically active, necrosis, high-grade nuclei
    - More frequently associated with conventional IDC
  - Classified as in situ carcinoma (Tis), acts like DCIS
    - Excise!
    - Perform sentinel node biopsy too
    - 27% have IDC on excision (higher than conventional DCIS)
- Solid papillary carcinoma (SPC)
  - Variant of DCIS, staged and acts like carcinoma in situ
  - Young patients, subareolar, well-circumscribed (fibroadenoma clinically)
  - Morphology
    - Nearly or completely solid
    - Inconspicuous fibrovascular cores
    - Jigsaw nests that form acini and rounded microcysts
      - PAS+ diastase-resistant secretions
    - Spindled cells, neuroendocrine differentiation, or mucinous differentiation in a significant subset
      - Fibroepithelial cores may be myxoid, intra- or extracellular
    - No myoepithelial cells
  - ER/PR+, HER2–
  - Chromogranin/synaptophysin+, CK5/6–
  - If it has conventional invasion, just use "invasive ductal carcinoma"
    - Typically is associated with invasive mucinous carcinomas
    - Usually jagged, unlike round noninvasive nests
    - Coexisting IDC in 63%
  - "Invasive SPC" large nests going into the fat

- EPC vs. SPC
  - Both low-grade
  - EPC—one big lesion
  - SPC—many lesions
- Juvenile papillomatosis
  - Benign localized proliferative cystic disease with intraductal epithelial hyperplasia
  - 15% have necrosis, ~30% have atypia
  - 10%–15% will develop breast cancer, but usually have family history too

Lobular Neoplasia

ALH AND LCIS

- LCIS is when >50% to 75% of the lobules are involved and distended by monomorphic lobular cells (that have lost e-cadherin expression)
  - Low-grade have dark, low-grade nuclei; plasmacytoid; evenly spaced and not overlapping
  - When not quite ALH, can use "indeterminate epithelial proliferation"
- Vacuolated ductal/lobular cells are concerning for lobular neoplasia
  - Cytoplasmic lumens/vacuoles, plasmacytoid, histiocytoid, signet ring, dyscohesion
  - Indistinct cell borders
- Classic LCIS vs. variants
  - Pleomorphic, with necrosis, apocrine, with signet rings
  - LCIS-N (with necrosis) has a high frequency of associated ILC on excision
  - LCIS-P (pleomorphic) nuclei are 3.5–4× size of lymphocyte positive moderate/marked pleomorphism, more frequently ER– and HER2+
  - Variants (except apocrine) require complete excision (more likely to be upgraded on excision, microinvasion is common)
    - Also classic DCIS with
      - Mass lesions
      - Discordant radiology and pathology
      - LN associated with high-risk lesion (e.g., ADH, DCIS)
      - High-risk patient (e.g., family history, exposures, genetic markers)
    - Everyone needs lifetime follow-up and tamoxifen
- LCIS undermines ductal epithelium (pagetoid) and creates outpouchings into the periductal spaces
  - Has flattened nonneoplastic epithelium over the neoplastic
- Do not need to quantify or evaluate margins for LCIS as you do for DCIS
  - Unless pleomorphic!
- 1q+, 16q–, 11q+/–
  - E-cadherin *(CDH1)* gene is on 16q22.1
    - Mutation or inactivation
    - Germline mutation = hereditary diffuse gastric cancer (HDGC), autosomal dominant with variable penetrance, ~40% risk for ILC
- Radiation not used for ILC or LCIS
- LCIS is no longer pTis
  - Pleomorphic LCIS does not change stage anymore

Invasive Lobular Carcinoma

- Variants: solid, alveolar, pleomorphic, signet-ring, histiocytoid
  - Pleomorphic arises from classic ILC, unlike high-grade IDC (which typically arises independent of low-grade)

- Usually ER/PR+ unless pleomorphic
- Loss of ≥ 8 genes at 16q22.1 and includes e-cadherin and beta-catenin
  - Well-to-moderately differentiated—diploid, ↑ ER/PR, ↓ HER2
  - Poorly differentiated—aneuploid, ↓ ER/PR, ↑ HER2

Types of Breast Cancer by Gene Expression

- Overall, chemotherapy and novel targeted therapies are indicated in all groups
  - Luminal A and B are not as mitotically active, so not quite as responsive to chemo
    - High Ki67 does better with chemo
  - Luminal disease: hard to optimize therapy (undertreatment or overtreatment)
- Most powerful prognostic marker is nodal status still
- HER2 membranous stain interpretation
  - No staining—0+
  - Barely perceptible—1+
  - Weak or partial—2+
  - Moderate to strong—3+
- Luminal A
  - ER/PR+, HER2–, low proliferation rates, CK8/18+
    - Sometimes PR–
  - Continuous spectrum, arbitrarily put into two groups
  - Lobular, tubular, mucinous, cribriform
  - Most heterogeneous gene expression, copy number
  - Excellent prognosis, use endocrine therapy (+/– chemo)
  - Distant metastases in luminal A tumors often appear more than 10 years after initial primary breast diagnosis
- Luminal B
  - Triple positive (usually, not always)
    - PR+/–, HER2+/–
    - Increased expression of ER gene, luminal cytokeratin genes, and proliferation genes
  - Higher histologic grade
  - Poor prognosis, high ki67
  - Endocrine therapy and chemo
- HER-2 enriched
  - ER/PR–, HER2 overexpressed
    - Can be ER+ (30%)
  - 17q, *ERBB2*
  - 60% HER2+ tumors fall clinically into this group
  - Neoadjuvant chemo → pretty good prognosis
  - *Not* usually estrogen-dependent
- Basal-like
  - Triple negative (ER, PR, HER2/neu)
  - + for CK5/6 (CK17, CK19—all basal keratins), EGFR (basal markers!)
  - Often form a well-circumscribed mass
  - BRCA-1 associated, younger patients, higher incidence in Western African descendants
  - p53 mutated
  - High-grade histology and high proliferation rate
    - Histologically heterogeneous
    - Can have large central acellular zone (necrosis or fibrosis occupying >30% of mass), peripheral/predominant lymphocytic infiltrate

- True gland formation is rare
- Medullary-like (not used anymore) and metaplastic types fit here
- Adenoid cystic and secretory will stain basal-like but have good prognosis
  - AGGRESSIVE! Median survival—24 months (rarely live beyond 4 years, way worse than other tumor types)
    - Independent prognostic indicator in LN+ and LN– disease
    - More likely to metastasize to brain and lung; liver and bone less likely
    - Paradoxically, has highest complete remission rate
  - No targeted therapy now, may try PARP inhibitors (especially *BRCA1*-mutated)
    - Sensitive to chemo
  - Being further characterized now into subgroups
    - Basal 1
    - Basal 2
    - Mesenchymal
    - Luminal androgen receptor (AR)
      - Apocrine
      - *PIK3CA* mutations
      - Use antiandrogen therapy
- Other
  - Molecular apocrine
    - Based on growth factor receptor rather than cell of origin
    - ER/PR–, HER2+ or HER2–, AR+
  - Claudin low
    - Triple negative, poor survival
    - High frequency of metaplastic differentiation
    - Response rate to neoadjuvant therapy is between basal and luminal
- Normal breast like
  - Not real, likely caused by contamination with normal breast

Treatment for Ductal and Lobular Neoplasia

- Miller-Payne Grading for neoadjuvant chemotherapy response
  - MPG 1—worse (no response to chemotherapy)
  - MPG 2—minimal reduction
  - MPG 3—wide range from 30%–90% reduction
  - MPG 4—"almost complete response"
  - Prior core biopsy necessary for comparison
  - No consideration of lymph node status
  - Can also use "residual cancer burden calculator"
- ER+ *and* PR+ disease has a better response to hormone therapy (and a more favorable prognosis) than disease that is +/– or –/+
- Triple negative cancer responds well to cytotoxic chemotherapy
  - ↑ cell synthesis and turnover
- Effects of irradiation ("radiation-associated atypia/epithelial abnormality")
  - Atrophy of glands
  - Spotty atypia of luminal cells
  - Dominant involvement of lobules
  - Cellular proliferation
  - Cellular necrosis
- Carcinoma usually looks similar to original before radiation

- Lymph node metastases
  - Isolated tumor cells (ITCs) in nodes
    - ≤0.2 mm and ≤200 cells by H&E or IHC
  - Micrometastases
    - 0.2 mm but <2.0 mm
  - Do not need axillary dissection for patients with positive sentinel nodes and only T1/T2
    - Postneoadjuvant chemo
  - Stage on current specimen except metastases and inflammatory carcinoma
  - Can get *new* degenerative calcifications filling ducts (especially in HER2 overexpressed)
  - Do NOT call ITCs negative in lymph nodes
    - → micrometastases = positive!
  - Calculate residual cancer burden (MD Anderson calculator)
    - Go over whole tumor bed at 20×, estimate tumor cellularity for each field, average out
    - Also need two largest dimensions of residual cancer for calculation
- Myoid metaplasia of myoepithelial cells is common after neoadjuvant chemo
- PDL1 IHCs are specific for each anti-PD1/PDL1 drug
- Most surgeons will reexcise DCIS ≤2 mm from margin, less likely to excise IDC
  - IDC invades with a broad front
- Goal of systemic therapy is to prevent distant metastases
- Almost everyone with invasive carcinoma who gets lumpectomy gets adjuvant radiation
  - Recurrence or second cancer after that → mastectomy

Other Malignant Tumors

- Inflammatory breast cancer is a clinical diagnosis (peau d'orange) that can be caused by any mammary carcinoma

INVASIVE BREAST CARCINOMA WITH NEUROENDOCRINE FEATURES

- Positive for neuroendocrine markers
- Most common histologic types: ductal, mucinous, solid papillary
- Majority are ER/PR+, HER2–
  - Secretory breast cancer—t(12;15)(p13;q25) *(ETV6-NTRK3)*
- Childhood, rare, favorable prognosis
- Remember "mammary analog secretory carcinoma" in salivary glands
  - Adenoid cystic carcinoma
- Two cell populations: epithelial (CD117) and myoepithelial (actin)
- Versus polymorphous low-grade adenocarcinoma (all one population)
- t(6;9) *(MYB-NFIB)*
- ER–

POSTRADIATION ANGIOSARCOMA OF THE SKIN/SUBQ/BREAST

- Primarily high-grade but low-grade can occur
- History of radiation to breast, short latency period of a few years
  - 0.2–1% of patients who received radiation
- Spindle cell mass forming vascular structures
- CD31+, CD34+, ERG+, MYC+ (due to gene amplification)

- DDx
  - Kaposi sarcoma—HHV-8+, HIV history
  - Primary leiomyosarcoma—extremely rare, desmin+, SMA+
  - Pseudoangiomatous stromal hyperplasia (PASH)—benign stromal proliferation, negative for vasculature markers CD31 and ERG
    - Can be CD34+
- Other vascular lesions in the breast
  - Angiolipomas
  - Perilobular hemangiomas
  - Angiomatosis
  - Postmastectomy lymphangiosarcoma of the arm (Stewart-Treves syndrome)
  - Papillary endothelial hyperplasia (Masson's lesion, Masson vegetant intravascular hemangioendothelioma)—abnormal thrombus organization
  - Atypical vascular lesion (aka benign lymphangiomatous papules of the skin)—seen after radiation too
    - Dilated anastomosing vascular channels, circumscribed, may contain prominent endothelial cells
    - 2–5 years after radiation, <1 cm

Fibrous AND Fibroepithelial Lesions

- Report size, grade, and margins
  - No synoptic report
- Fibroadenomas and phyllodes have somatic *MED12* mutations
- Fibroadenoma—stroma compressing glands into slit-like spaces
  - Complex fibroadenoma = FA + sclerosing adenosis, cysts >3 mm, papillary apocrine metaplasia, and/or epithelial/luminal calcifications
    - Higher risk for malignancy
  - Tubular adenoma = variant
    - Well-circumscribed, closely packed glands with some intervening stroma
    - Young women
- Phyllodes vs. fibroadenoma
  - Mitoses (>3/10 hpf), stromal overgrowth (no epithelium in one 4× field), stromal fragmentation, fat infiltration, heterogeneity, subepithelial stromal condensation, nuclear pleomorphism
  - "Stromal overgrowth" for borderline phyllodes = no epithelial component in one 4× field
  - If malignant heterologous elements are present in a Phyllodes tumor, it's enough to call it malignant
    - Hematogenous spread
  - If unable to differentiate fibroadenoma vs. phyllodes, call it "fibroepithelial lesion"
- Pseudoangiomatous stromal hyperplasia (PASH)
  - ↑ collagenous stroma with anastomosing slit-like channels with myofibroblasts resembling endothelium (CD34+)
    - Can form fascicles and resemble myofibroblastoma
    - vimentin+, CK–, F8–, PR–/+, ER–, CD34+, desmin+, SMA+
  - Can be mistaken for angiosarcoma
  - Myofibroblastic proliferation
  - Common incidental finding in gynecomastia
  - Can be seen in fibroadenomas and phyllodes tumors. May have gynecomastoid hyperplasia (micropapillary UDH) (in women)

- May be secondary to cyclosporine use
- May be tumor-forming (mistaken for fibroadenoma clinically/radiologically)
- Median age = mid-to-late 30 s
- Myofibroblastoma
  - Men and postmenopausal women
  - Mobile, palpable, solid
  - Benign tumor of myofibroblasts
  - Short fascicles, lobulated
  - Positive for actin, CD34, SMMS, desmin, ER/PR, AR
  - Loss of 13q14
- Fibromatosis
  - Abundant collagen, stellate
- Nodular fasciitis
  - t(17;22) *(MYH9-USP6)*

Male Breast Disease

- Gynecomastia
  - Can rarely have lobules, usually just ducts
  - No increase in breast cancer risk
- Male breast cancer
  - Risk factors: Western countries, older age, obesity, estrogen exposure, radiation, Klinefelter syndrome
  - More likely to be ER+ than female breast cancer
  - When stage-corrected, prognosis is similar to female
  - *CHEK2, PTEN, CYP17, BRCA2* mutations; Lynch syndrome
  - Presents at later stage than in female
  - Ductal is *much* more common than lobular
  - Paget disease is more common

Molecular/Cytogenetics

- Sporadic cancer genetics
  - Grade 1 IDC and classic ILC have loss of 16q and gain of 1q
- Prognostic utility of any tests is weaker in node-positive disease
  - Oncotype is the best with 1–3 positive nodes (TransATAC study)
- Oncotype Dx
  - In official NCCN guidelines and AJCC staging manual
  - 21 genes, reports a score of 0–100
  - ER+, HER2–
  - **Must be ER+, node negative or 1–3 positive nodes**
    - Needs 2 mm of invasion
    - Stay away from biopsy site (increased proliferative/healing)
  - Separates into low-, intermediate-, and high-risk groups (for distant recurrence risk)
    - HR gets adjuvant chemotherapy
  - TAILORx study (*NEJM*, Sparano et al., 2015) showed intermediate risk do as well with hormone therapy as with hormone and chemotherapy (RS <25 without other significant risk, do not use chemo)
  - Selective estrogen receptor modulators for premenopausal, aromatase inhibitor for post-menopausal

- Mammoprint
  - 70 genes
  - ER+, HER2+/−
  - Prognostic and predictive
  - Separates into low- and high-risk groups for distant recurrence
    - Can save clinically high-risk patients from chemo if in low-risk group
  - Node negative and node positive
  - Need more invasive, stay away from bx site
  - MINDACT
- IHC4 assay (historical)
- Prosigna
  - Can be done in-house
  - Node positive → high, intermediate, low
    - Node negative → high, low
  - Useful for really late recurrence (5–10 years)
- Breast cancer index (BCI)
  - Predicts risk for distant recurrence
    - Early and late
    - Outperforms others for late recurrence
  - Novel genes (*HOXB13* and *IL17BR* ratio)
  - Expensive
  - Also reports likely benefit from extended endocrine therapy
- EndoPredict assay
- Genetic predispositions for breast cancer
  - Family history
  - *BRCA1* or *BRCA2* (17q21 and 13q12)
    - Tumor suppressor gene
    - Breast cancer in 40 s or 50 s
    - Poorly differentiated carcinomas
    - ER/PR−, HER2/neu−
    - Ovarian, colonic, pancreatic cancers too
  - Li Fraumeni (p53 mutations)
  - Cowden (10q)
  - Ataxia telangiectasia (*ATM* on chromosome 11)

CHAPTER 3

Dermatopathology

Definitions and Associations

- Acantholysis—dyscohesion of keratinocytes
  - Massive acantholysis differential diagnosis (DDx): Hailey-Hailey, Darier (more parakeratosis), Grover (spongiosis and corp ronds), pemphigus vulgaris
- Acanthosis—diffuse epidermal hyperplasia
- Anthracotic—black pigment
- Epidermolytic hyperkeratosis—ballooning, falling apart, with keratohyaline granules
- Chilblains/perniosis—purple acral macules sometimes associated with frostbite
  - Normal epidermis, dermal edema, perivascular lymphocytes, +/− thrombi
- Acute dermatitis—epithelial spongiosis
- Chronic dermatitis—acanthosis > spongiosis
- Pilar cyst—very dense pink (visible at 1×)
- DRESS—drug reaction with eosinophilia and systemic symptoms
- Lichenified—thickened as a result of mechanical irritation
- Impetiginized—dermatosis with secondary impetigo (subcorneal pustules with gram-positive cocci)
- Ruptured cyst—cholesterol/keratin clefts + granulomatous inflammation
- Blue nevus—darkly pigmented dendritic melanocytes, clinically looks blue-black
- Dysplastic nevus—asymmetric, shouldering, stromal response around rete
- Dermal-epiderma interface vacuolization—drug reaction or connective tissue disease or lichenoid dermatoses
- Intertrigo—vacuolization of the epidermis
- Spongiotic dermatitis—allergic contact dermatitis
  - Eczema, wet, crust, pale pink serum with dead keratinocytes
- Urticarial change—superficial and deep perivascular and interstitial inflammation with neutrophils and eosinophils, sparse, no epidermal involvement
  - Neutrophilic urticarial dermatosis—patient has systemic lupus erythematosus (SLE), is very sick, increased neutrophils around eccrine glands
- Myofibroblasts—corkscrew nuclei and cytoplasm, easier to see with condenser down
- Smooth muscle nuclei are spindled with perinuclear glycogen "snacks"
- Touton giant cell (GC)—dense cytoplasm inside ring, foamy outside
- Ballooning—intracellular edema, dying cells
  - Interface dermatitis (erythema migrans, Stevens-Johnson syndrome, nutritional deficiency) vs. viral infection

Congenital/Inherited Conditions

- Gorlin (nevoid basal cell carcinoma) syndrome—*PTCH1* gene (>*PTCH2*)
  - Multiple basal cell carcinomas (BCCs), odontogenic keratocysts, palmar/plantar pits
- Birt-Hogg-Dube—*FLCN* (folliculin)
  - Trichodiscoma and fibrofolliculoma

- Tuberous sclerosis—*TSC1* or *TSC2*
  - Facial angiofibromas and PEComas
- Cowden—*PTEN*
  - Trichilemmoma
- Hereditary leiomyomatosis and renal cell carcinoma (HLRCC)—*FH* (fumarate hydratase)
  - Multiple cutaneous leiomyomatosis
- Brooke-Spiegler—*CYLD* gene (16q)
  - Cylindromas
- Goltz syndrome
  - Widespread skin abnormalities, focal dermal hypoplasia, focal hair loss, abnormal nails, skeletal abnormalities
    - Slightly papillated epidermis overlying adipose tissue with no dermis
- Maffucci syndrome
  - Multiple chondromas and hemangiomas
- Darier disease
  - *ATP2A2*
  - Diffuse and dyskeratotic
  - Numerous greasy papules on a seborrheic area after puberty
  - Hyperkeratosis, acantholytic dyskeratosis in the upper epidermis, papillomatosis, acanthosis
- Grover disease
  - Indistinguishable from Darier disease histologically
  - Not associated with *ATP2A2* mutation and occurs at an older age
  - Very tiny papules on chest/back of older males
- Hailey-Hailey disease
  - Isolated/focal and without dyskeratosis
  - Acantholysis, intertriginous areas
  - Involves all layers with individual cells falling off
  - Dilapidated brick wall
- Bart syndrome
  - Congenital absence of skin
- Gardner syndrome
  - Multiple pilomatricomas, usually ruptured and/or calcified
  - Beta-catenin mutation

Non neoplastic

PATTERNS TO REMEMBER

- Busy dermis pattern
  - Increased normal dermal constituents
  - "Busy dermis can kill grandma's sweet niece"
    - Blue nevus
    - Dermatofibroma and dermal spitz nevus
    - Cutaneous metastases
    - Kaposi sarcoma
      - Increased vessels around eccrine glands, endothelial cells, and superficial spindled cells
      - Dissecting, ill-formed vessels
      - Promontory sign (new vessels around old)
      - HHV-8+
    - Granuloma annulare (and variations)

- Scleromyxedema
- Neurofibroma
- "Invisible dermatoses"
  - Not much seen on biopsy
  - Urticaria
  - Mastocytosis
  - Tinea versicolor
  - Vitiligo
  - Macular amyloidosis
  - Viral exanthema
  - Ichthyosis
  - Scleroderma
  - Postinflammatory hyperpigmentation
- Shelled-out pattern
  - Angioleiomyoma
  - Glomangioma
  - Leiomyoma
  - Schwannoma
  - Mycetoma
- Acantholysis
  - Congenital absence or problem with desmosomes
    - Grover—back, older males
    - Hailey-Hailey—temperature-mediated, axilla
    - Darier—all over but less striking microscopically
  - Antibodies to desmoglein—pemphigus
  - Chemical
  - Infection
- Dermal mucin
  - Granuloma annulare
  - Lupus erythematosus
  - Papular mucinosis
  - Basal cell carcinoma
  - Pretibial myxedema
- Inflammatory
  - Perivascular and interstitial pattern—not likely to be lymphocytes
  - Neutrophilic dermatosis
    - Most common—nearby folliculitis
    - Bowel-loop associated
    - Sweet syndrome
    - Pyoderma gangrenosum
    - Bechet
  - 6 Ls of lymphocytic perivascular infiltrate (superficial and deep) DDx
    - So robust that you cannot see vessels, nodules coalesce
    - Lupus—increased periadnexal inflammation (and pernio)
    - Lymphoma (and pseudolymphoma)
    - Light—polymorphous light eruption
    - Lue (secondary syphilis)
    - Lyme
    - Lymphocytosis of Gerstner
    - (And perniosis/chilblains)

- Perivascular and lichenoid inflammation with eosinophils
  - Bug
  - Drug
  - Urticaria
  - Pemphigus vulgaris, urticarial stage
  - Pregnancy
  - Bullous pemphigoid
- Vacuolar interface dermatitis with lymphocytes
  - Clinically appears bullous
  - Lymphocytes attack keratinocytes
  - Prototype—erythema multiforme (EM), Stevens-Johnson syndrome (SJS), toxic epidermal necrolysis (TEN)
- Eczematous dermatoses
  - Distinguished from each other by clinical presentation
  - Hallmark = spongiosis
    - Irregular acanthosis, hyperkeratosis, superficial perivascular lymphs
  - Contact dermatitis, nummular dermatitis, photoallergic dermatosis, atopic dermatosis
- Wedge-shaped lymphocytic inflammation
  - Pityriasis lichenoides et varioliformis acuta (PLEVA)
  - Lymphomatoid papulosis
  - Bug

HAIR LOSS

- Lichen planopilaris (a scarring alopecia)
  - Free hair shafts
  - Gray fibrosis around follicles that are grouped in 2s and 3s, fewer sebaceous glands
  - Follicular asymmetry
  - DDx—lupus, folliculotropic mycosis fungoides (MF), scar tracks in drop-out areas
- Alopecia areata (a scarring alopecia)
  - Lymphocytes swarming bulb
  - Miniaturization
  - Nonanagen (not regular circle outlines or a ton of dead keratinocytes)
  - Dilated ostia with tiny hair
  - Peribulbar lymphocytic inflammation
  - Catagen/telogen shift (irregular outline)
  - Infundibular dilation (yellow dots clinically)
  - "Exclamation point" hairs
- Decalvans alopecia
  - Neutrophilic scarring alopecia

INFECTIOUS

- General patterns
  - Panniculitis = subcutaneous inflammation
    - Lobular = lupus; septal = erythema nodosum
    - Vasculitis present?
      - Yes → erythema induratum (tuberculid)
      - Id reaction = inflammation to antigen elsewhere

- ▪ Touton GCs with granulomas
- ▪ Panniculitis with spill-over into deep dermis (nodular and diffuse)
- ● Folliculitis—acneiform, infectious (bacterial, viral)
  - ▪ Sebaceous necrosis and dense follicular necrosis → herpes!
    - ▫ Can have reactive vasculitis
- ● Viral
  - ▪ See "blistering disorders" for herpes simplex virus (HSV) and varicella zoster virus (VZV)
  - ▪ Molluscum—Henderson-Patterson (molluscum) bodies, pox virus
  - ▪ Orf-pox virus (get from cows)
    - ▫ Hugely acanthotic, oozy, vascular proliferation, viral inclusions
- ● Bacterial
  - ▪ Scale crust, can have secondary bacterial colonies
  - ▪ Impetigo
    - ▫ *S. aureus*, honey-colored crust
    - ▫ Bullous with some neutrophils = localized form of staphylococcal scalded skin syndrome (SSSS)
      - ▫ NOT a direct infection, reaction to toxin (antidesmoglein-1)
    - ▫ Nonbullous—subcorneal neutrophils, spongiosis, bacteria must be present
  - ▪ Ecthyma
    - ▫ Staph pyogenes
    - ▫ Deeper than impetigo
    - ▫ Ecthyma gangrenosum = severe form
  - ▪ Cellulitis
    - ▫ Infection of deep dermis/subcutaneous
    - ▫ Adults—group A streptococcus
    - ▫ Children—*S. aureus*
    - ▫ Erysipelas—St. Anthony's Fire, group A streptococcus, superficial and involving lymphatics
  - ▪ Botryomycosis
    - ▫ Rare chronic granulomatous disease
    - ▫ Secondary to bacteria (usually *S. aureus*)
    - ▫ Granular bodies
    - ▫ Splendore–Hoeppli (SH) reaction
      - ▫ Strongly eosinophilic amorphous material with radiating star-like or club-shaped-like configurations
    - ▫ Erythrasma—wood lamp, filamentous bacteria
- ▪ Tuberculosis—See Table 3.1.
- ▪ Fungal
  - ▪ General
    - ▫ Neutrophils in corneum
    - ▫ Parakeratosis
      - ▫ Sandwich sign—orthokeratosis, fungal elements, parakeratosis or compact orthokeratosis, then granular layer

TABLE 3.1 ▪ **Tuberculosis in the Skin**

	Direct	Blood	Local
Good immunity	Prosector wart	Lupus vulgaris	Scrofuloderma
Bad immunity	Chancre	Military	Lupus orificialis cutis

- +/– "holes"
- Needs PAS
- Tinea surfs, candida dives
- Chromoblastomycosis and phaeohyphomycosis
  - Traumatically implanted (classically by a splinter)
  - Pseudoepitheliomatous hyperplasia, acanthosis, parakeratosis, large purulent pustule extending into dermis, many neutrophils, brown spherules ("copper pennies") throughout perilesional tissue, hypergranulosis
  - Dematiaceous fungi
- Angioinvasive fungal
- Rhizopus, aspergillus, fusarium, candida
- Cryptococcus
  - Can cause panniculitis
- Superficial fungal infection with subcorneal pustule
- Follicular pustule = staphylococcus, candida
  - Nonfollicular pustule = acute generalized exanthematous pustulosis (AGEP), psoriasis, reactive arthritis, infections
  - Tinea versicolor does not have a lot of inflammation
- Fungal angioinvasion—aspergillus, fusarium, mucor family, candida
- Parasites
  - Leishmaniasis
    - Incomplete marquee sign—organisms lining vacuoles in histiocytes look like light bulbs on a marquee sign
    - Dense dermal histiocytic infiltrate with lymphocytes and plasma cells
    - Basophilic intracellular organisms with an eccentric kinetoplast and lacking a capsule
    - Major DDx = histoplasmosis (GMS stain will be positive)
- Insects
  - Arthropod bite
    - Superficial and deep perivascular infiltrate of lymphocytes and rare eosinophils
    - May see insect parts
- Pustular urticaria
  - Id reaction to arthropod bite
- Scabies—one of the only intraepidermal parasites with minimal mixed inflammation
  - Also tungiasis (sand flea—pustules with black dots) and bot fly
  - Sometimes Strongyloides

GRANULOMAS

- Suppurative
  - Infection, ruptured hair follicles, iodine ingestions
  - Looks like BCC clinically
- Noncaseating
  - Sarcoidal—compact, confluent, naked
  - Palisading
    - Rheumatoid arthritis
    - Granuloma annulare
      - Blue—mucin
      - Red—fibrinoid necrosis
  - Tuberculoid—cuffs of lymphocytes

- TB, rosacea, leishmaniasis
- Necrobiosis lipoidica (NLD)
  - Hyperplastic and spongiotic epidermis
  - LARGE area of pink necrobiotic collagen with necrotic vessels, fibrinoid, some neutrophilic debris
    - Surrounded by palisading necrosis
  - Layers of cake involving whole dermis
  - Yellow plaques on dorsal hands and feet, translucent skin with telangiectatic vessels
- Necrobiotic xanthogranuloma (NXG)
  - Necrobiotic collagen, tons of histiocytes with Touton giant cells
  - "Peppered bacon," collagen clefts, X-shaped in dermis
  - Usually have monoclonal gammopathy!
    - Treat paraprotein to treat NXG
  - Deforming yellow plaques on face
  - Deeper than NLD
- Granuloma faciale
  - Smoldering granulocytic vasculitis and fibrosis
  - Nodules with peau d'orange
- (Juvenile) xanthogranuloma (JXG)
  - Fibrohistiocytic lesion, non Langerhans cell, derived from dermal dendritic cells
  - Children, nodules in dermis elevating skin
  - Touton giant cells, lots of eosinophils, foamy histiocytes
  - Collarette = papillae reach around and "hug" lesion
    - Sign of benignity
    - Also seen in pyogenic granuloma, poroma, angiokeratoma
  - Multiple? Consider neurofibromatosis type 1 or juvenile myelomonocytic leukemia

LICHEN/LICHENOID LESIONS

- Lichenoid inflammation—lichen planus, drug eruption, lichenoid dermatitis, syphilis, lichenoid pigmented purpura, lichenoid reaction in a tattoo
  - "Lichenified" = thickened as a result of mechanical irritation
- Lichen planus
  - Pruritic purple polygonal papules
  - Wedge-shaped hypergranulosis
  - Compact hyperkeratosis
  - Mild spongiosis
  - Vacuolization of loss of basal layer
  - Lichenoid lymphocytic infiltrate
  - Sawtooth rete ridges
  - Some necrotic cells in basal layer (Civatte bodies)
  - Colloid bodies in papillary dermis
  - Does not involve eccrine ducts
- Hypertrophic lichen planus
  - Acanthotic, hyperkeratotic, lichenoid infiltrate with associated interface changes (basal layer vacuolation, cytoid bodies)
  - Clinical—multiple lesions, shin/wrists
  - Unlike classic lichen planus, eosinophils are present
- Lichenoid AK
  - See squamous neoplasms

- Lichen striatus
  - Linear eruption on a child
  - Acanthosis and atrophy, no orthokeratosis "basket weave" keratin (was probably itched)
  - Lichenoid infiltrate extending to epidermis and eccrine ducts
  - Lichen striatus
    - This and lupus are the only entities that look like lichen planus with deep eccrine involvement
    - Can get spongiosis (clinically wet and oozy)
- Lichen nitidus
  - Aggregate of histiocytes, very focal
  - Drug reaction with mogamulizumab and tremelimumab
- Lichen simplex chronicus
  - Caused by chronic rubbing/friction—itchy plaque increasing in size
  - Superficial perivascular lymphoplasmacytic infiltrate
  - Acanthosis, hyperkeratosis, focal parakeratosis, hypergranulosis
  - Vertical orientation of dermal collagen ("streaking fibrosis")
  - Plaque version of prurigo nodule
- Pityriasis lichenoides (PLEVA) (see "Pityriasis" section)
- Lichen sclerosus
  - Elastin stain shows dropout of fibers in sclerosis
  - Only one with atrophic epithelium

BLISTERING DISORDERS

- Subepidermal
  - Autoimmune
  - Dermatitis herpetiformis
    - Granular direct immunofluorescence (DIF) for IgA
    - In dermal papillae and basement membrane
  - All epidermolysis bullosa variants (except EBA) are inherited and present in childhood
    - Skin fragility, milia, scarring
    - Cell-poor subepidermal blisters with negative DIF
  - Epidermolysis bullosa acquisita
    - DIF stains floor of blister
    - No eosinophils
  - Bullous pemphigoid
    - Subepidermal blister with eosinophils inside
    - DIF stains roof of blister, linear IgG and/or C3
    - Antibodies against *COL17A1* gene product - collagen 17
  - Erythema multiforme
    - Target-shaped wheals
    - Most common cause—herpes or drug
    - Necrotic keratinocytes, spongiosis, basal liquefaction, papillary edema, interface lymphocytes
    - Early lesion of SJS/TEN
  - Porphyrias
    - Porphyria cutanea tarda
      - Subepidermal blister, festooning, cell-poor, caterpillar bodies on roof, IgG+ and C3+, DIF around papillary vessels

- Most common cause—uroporphyrin decarboxylase deficiencies
  - Acute intermittent porphyria
    - No skin lesions
    - Porphobilinogen deaminase (hydroxymethylbilane synthase) deficiency
    - Abdominal pain and psychosis
  - Pseudoporphyria
    - Hemodialysis or drugs (NSAIDS, tetracyclines, furosemide)
- Others
  - Lichen planus
  - Mastocytosis
  - Bullous lupus erythematosus
    - Antibodies against collagen VII
  - Lichen sclerosus
  - Graft-vs.-host disease (GVHD)
    - After hematopoietic transplant, should always have interface dermatitis
- Intraepidermal
  - Contact dermatitis
  - Infections
    - Bullous impetigo
    - SSSS
    - HSV
    - VZV—necrotic follicles or sebaceous cells, Tzanck cells
  - Pemphigus vulgaris
    - Suprabasilar cleft, normal stratum corneum, acantholysis around cleft
      - "Tombstone row"
    - Not a lot of inflammation
    - Autoimmune disorder against desmoglein-3 component of desmosomes
    - Very diffuse (Nikolsky sign)
    - Flaccid vesicles with mouth involvement
    - Intracellular IgG
  - Hailey-Hailey (see "Congenital/Inherited Conditions")
  - Darier (see "Congenital/Inherited Conditions")
  - Grover (see "Congenital/Inherited Conditions")
- Friction blister
  - Granular layer
  - Pallor and degenerative changes of epidermis
- Pustular erosive dermatitis
  - Ulcerative atrophic *or* hypertrophic epidermis, parakeratosis, chronic inflammation, no hair follicles, subcorneal pustules
- Pemphigus
  - All pemphigus stains positive for IgG and complement
  - Pemphigus vulgaris (see "Intraepidermal Blister" section)
  - Bullous pemphigus (see "Subepidermal Blister" section)
  - Pemphigus vegetans
    - Intertriginous area
    - Pseudoepitheliomatous hyperplasia, intraepithelial pustules with neutrophils and eosinophils
  - Pemphigus foliaceus
    - Desmoglein-1 antibodies
    - Chickenwire but more superficial than paraneoplastic

- "Crusted cornflake plaques" on trunk with mouth involvement
- Paraneoplastic pemphigus
  - Castleman, acute lymphoblastic leukemia/lymphoma, thymoma, Waldenstrom
  - Stomatitis/mucositis
  - Lichenoid with spongiosis and suprabasal acantholysis
  - DIF—chicken-wire and on basal—lots of the antibodies are positive
- Pityriasis
  - Pityriasis rosea
    - Viral
    - Herald patch, then many patches on chest and back
    - Erythema, induration, scale
    - Subacute dermatitis with focal hyperkeratosis and angulated parakeratosis and absent granular layer
  - Pityriasis rubra pilaris
    - Group of disorders with scaling patches with well-defined borders
    - Entire body *or* knees and elbows *or* hands and feet
      - Islands of sparing
      - When involving palms and soles, called *keratoderma*
    - Morphology
      - Regular stubby psoriasiform acanthosis
      - Follicular plugging, hyperkeratosis (especially over follicles), telangiectasia, alternating parakeratosis
      - Sparse mixed inflammation
  - PLEVA (Mucha-Habermann)
    - Crops of papules with necrotic central areas, wedge-shaped
    - Vacuolar interface dermatitis with a lymphocyte in almost every hole
    - Compact stratum corneum with/without ulcer or crust
    - Red blood cell (RBC) extravasation, transepidermal elimination of RBCs
    - Marginated neutrophils in dermal vessels
    - DDx—lymphomatoid papulosis
  - Pityriasis lichenoides chronica
    - Vacuolar interface dermatitis with a lymphocyte in almost every hole
    - Transepidermal elimination of RBCs
  - Pityriasis versicolor
    - Mild superficial perivascular inflammation
    - Mild hyperkeratosis and acanthosis
    - May have hyperpigmentation of the basal layer
    - "Spaghetti and meatballs" in corneum—Malassezia

VASCULAR DISORDERS AND VASCULITIS

- Levamisole-induced vasculitis
  - Mixed with cocaine
  - Retiform purpura and eschars on ears, nose tip, and fingertips
  - Necrotizing vasculitis and thrombotic vasculopathy
- Calciphylaxis
  - Look for clots and calcifications in interstitium
  - Necrotic epidermis secondary to thrombosed vessels
    - Eschar-like lesion on fatty area

- Multiple calcified small vessels in the subcutaneous fat lobules
- Calcinosis cutis
    - Idiopathic—elbows
    - Dystrophic—damaged connective tissue
        - CREST syndrome (calcinosis, Raynaud phenomenon, esophageal dysmotility, sclerodactyly, telangiectasia), dermatomyositis, lupus
    - Iatrogenic—line with calcium citrate
        - Metastatic—calciphylaxis, caused by deranged calcium metabolism
- See Chapter 18 "Immunology" for vasculitides Vasculitis with thrombosis—neutrophils in vessel wall
- Lymphocytic vasculitides
    - Purpura pigmentosa vasculitis
    - Erythema multiforme
    - Pityriasis lichenoides
    - Drug eruptions
    - Sjogren viral exanthems
    - Rickettsial infection
    - Lymphomatoid papulosis

OTHER INFLAMMATORY/NONNEOPLASTIC CONDITIONS

- Perniosis
    - Painful purple papules on finger tips in cold
    - Periadnexal/perivascular (superficial and deep) lymphocytic inflammation, acral skin
    - Epidermis is spared
- Psoriasis
    - Time of epidermal turnover is too fast, Th_{17}
    - Diffuse parakeratotic scale, hyperkeratosis, Munro microabscesses (neutrophils in corneum), decreased or absent granular layer, club-shaped rete, tortuous/dilated papillary vessels (cause Auspitz sign)
    - Hypogranulosis
- Sarcoidosis—noncaseating, well-demarcated, "naked" granulomas in dermis or subcutaneous
    - Schaumann bodies (calcifications) or asteroid bodies; Langerhans giant cells (horseshoe-shaped collection of nuclei)
- Scleroderma—increased hyaline, decreased adnexa, squared off punch biopsy, perivascular lymphocytes
    - Morphea—localized sclerotic plaques on trunk
    - Linear scleroderma
- Sjogren—lymphocytes in salivary gland
- Nutritional deficiency
    - Parakeratosis and hypogranulosis
    - Psoriasiform epidermal hyperplasia
    - Intermittent outer epidermal pallor and ballooning
    - Basal necrotic keratinocytes with sharp demarcation
    - Superficial vascular inflammation
    - Zinc, essential fatty acids, niacin, glucagonoma
    - Perform PAS if there are neutrophils in the cornified layer to rule out fungus
- Lupus erythematosus
    - Features
        - Vacuolar change of basal layer

- ▪ Thickened basement membrane
- ▪ Dermal mucin
- ▪ Periadnexal lymphocytes
- ▪ Types
  - ▪ Discoid
    - ▫ Atrophic, dyspigmented, scarred areas on sun-exposed skin
    - ▫ Follicular plugging and fibrosis
  - ▪ Subacute
    - ▫ Annular scaly plaques and papules on sun-exposed skin
  - ▪ Acute
    - ▫ Malar rash and erythematous papules
- ▪ Lupus panniculitis
  - ▪ Do not need to have SLE
  - ▪ DDx—lymphoma
  - ▪ Clinically/grossly depressed areas
- ▪ Spongiotic dermatitis
  - ▪ Subcorneal Langerhans cell aggregates favor allergic contact dermatitis
  - ▪ Large vesicle with granular fluid and occasional Langerhans cells
- ▪ Rheumatoid nodules
  - ▪ Sharply demarcated fibrinoid necrosis surrounded by palisading histiocytes
  - ▪ Extensor surfaces
  - ▪ Usually first 2 years of disease
  - ▪ Treatment—conservative excision

Neoplasms

FOLLICULAR/ADNEXAL TUMORS

Normal Anatomy

- ▪ Hair follicle—infundibulum (has granular double layer), isthmus (no granular layer), matrix/bulb
- ▪ Apocrine—empty into follicles
- ▪ Sebaceous
- ▪ Eccrine—empty onto skin (palms and soles)
- ▪ Pacinian corpuscles—pressure on fingers/toes

Syringoma

- ▪ Numerous duct structures lined by double-layer of cuboidal cells, not apocrine
- ▪ Can get multiple on face, small papules
- ▪ Paisley tie, tadpoles
- ▪ DDx
  - ▪ Microcystic adnexal carcinoma—bland, large and infiltrating into subcutis (may be difficult to diagnose on shave biopsy), clinically a large plaque
  - ▪ Infiltrating BCC
  - ▪ Desmoplastic trichoepithelioma

Hidrocystoma

- ▪ Tiny irregular cyst that looks collapsed
- ▪ Two cell layers with apical snouts
- ▪ On face

Steatocystoma

- Cyst lined by "shark-tooth"/sawtooth epidermis
- No granular layer, no keratinization
- Looks like EIC (epidermal inclusion cyst, infundibular cyst) but with sawtooth epidermis
- Derived from sebaceous duct (and usually located next to sebaceous gland), oily, treat with isotretinoin
- Syndromes—steatocystoma multiplex, other genetic
- Can coexist with vellus hair cysts (which have granular layers and keratinization)

Vellus Hair Cyst

- Cyst lined by similar epi as steatocystoma or epidermal inclusion cyst
    - In middle = multiple vellus hairs
- Can occur with statocysts
- Infundibular portion of vellus follicles
- Can be eruptive

Pilar Cyst

- Cyst with isthmus-like epithelium, lots of keratin (dense pink), scalp
- Can calcify

Pilomatricoma (also called *pilomatrixoma*)

- Ghost cells and calcifications
- Tumor of basaloid keratinizing cell
- Multiple pilomatricomas? Consider Gardner syndrome (beta-catenin mutation)

Dermoid Cyst

- Lateral angle of eye or midline of forehead or neck
- Keratinized squamous epithelium with attached pilosebaceous structures (sweat glands and smooth muscles may be present)

Irritated Seborrheic Keratosis

- Squamous proliferation, piled up, squamous eddies, solar elastosis
- Rounded, smooth bottom
- Careful about squamous cell carcinoma in situ!

Trichoblastoma

- Trichoblastomas, trichoepitheliomas, and other benign infundibular tumors do not have mucin or desmoplasia in mucin and are not on face of elderly/sun-damaged skin
- Large blue islands of cells in superficial dermis with nodular stroma; clefting around stroma (not around nests)
- Looks like BCC (very blue), well-defined basal layer
- From bulb of hair follicle
- Likely pigmented
- Adamantoid trichoblastoma has lots of infiltrating lymphocytes (or lymphadenoma)

Trichoepithelioma

- Papillary mesenchymal body (epithelium in claw-like form "grabbing" mesenchyme), more hair differentiation

- Stromal-stromal clefting
  - BCC has stromal-epithelial clefting
- Otherwise similar to trichoblastoma

Trichodiscoma

- Sun-damaged skin → solar elastosis disappears, replaced by myxoid stroma with wisps of epithelium, surrounded by proliferating sebaceous glands (catchers mitts)
- Birt-Hogg-Dube syndrome (also associated with chromophobe renal cell carcinoma and oncocytomas)

Tricholemmoma

- CD34+ BerEP–

Basal Cell Carcinoma (BCC)

- BerEP4+ CD34–, stromal epithelial clefting
- Has follicular differentiation and may be of follicular origin
- May have dermal mucin
- Histologic subtypes
  - Superficial spreading
    - Treated topically (and can skip around—hard to surgically clear)
  - Nodular
  - Micronodular
  - Infiltrative/morpheaform
    - Small infiltrative nests, usually angled
    - Keloidal collagen
  - Basosquamous
- BCC of Pinkus
  - Not sun-exposed skin (lower back or axilla)
  - Fenestrated/reticulated

Sebaceous Tumors

- Spectrum
  - Sebaceous hyperplasia (pink on low-power)
  - Sebaceous adenoma (<50% basaloid cells)
  - Sebaceoma (>50% basaloid cells)
  - Sebaceous carcinoma (pleomorphic)
- Sebaceous adenoma and sebaceoma are both associated with Muir-Torre syndrome (they tend to be cystic in this setting), which has a colorectal carcinoma risk
  - Differentiation between these two is not really important
  - Could do mismatch repair testing
- Sebaceous gland hyperplasia and pseudobasal cell carcinoma-like hyperplasia can happen over a dermatofibroma

Poroma

- Eccrine or apocrine
  - Ductal cells differentiate
- Red ulcerated nodules, usually on hands and feet
- Littler keratinized ducts with large nests of bland cells
  - looks like seborrheic keratosis with anastomosing cords without hyperkeratosis and with small CK7+ ducts scattered throughout

- DDx
  - Hidroacanthoma simplex is *in* the epidermis
  - Poroma comes off the epithelium
  - Dermal ductal tumor is completely dermal

Microcystic Adnexal Carcinoma

- Poorly circumscribed, numerous infiltrative small ducts and cords in dermis and subcutis
- Bland tumor cells
- No peripheral palisading or stroma retraction
- Nasolabial fold or scalp

Endocrine Mucin-Producing Sweat Gland Carcinoma

- Face of elderly
- CK7+, ER+, synaptophysin+
- May progress to mucinous carcinoma

Jigsaw Puzzle Differential

- Cylindroma (children/easy = big pieces), spiradenoma (adult/hard = little pieces)
- Trabecular with hyaline droplets of basement membranes, three types of cells
- Syndrome—Brooke Spiegler (turban tumor syndrome)
  - Cylindromas, spiradenomas, and trichoepitheliomas
- Cannonball, paisley tie

SQUAMOUS AND WARTY LESIONS

Condylomas and Similar Lesions

- Condylomas
  - If no obvious cytopathic effect or koilocytic change, look for parakeratosis in the dells
- Verruca plana
  - Plantar wart
  - Granular layer has holes, koilocytes, hypergranulosis, minimally papillated surface
  - HPV 3 and 10
- Verruciform xanthoma
  - Genital skin
  - Verruca with foamy/xanthoma cells in dermis
    - Foam cells derived from dermal dendritic cells, CD68+
  - Very pink and dyskeratotic-appearing
- Warty dyskeratoma
  - Acantholysis with dyskeratosis (corp ronds), hyperkeratosis, acanthosis
- Porokeratosis
  - Cornoid lamellae
    - Diagonal parakeratosis, parakeratosis, dyskeratotic cells dripping like wax directly under tier
  - Clinically annular
    - If multiple, consider disseminated superficial actinic porokeratosis (widespread, shows abnormal UV sensitivity → cancer)
  - if biopsied in the center of the lesion, may miss diagnosis (patchy lichenoid changes only)

Epidermolytic Acanthoma

- AKA epidermolytic hyperkeratosis
- Not a wart
- Single neoplasm on genital skin
- Eosinophilic globular degeneration of cytoplasm

Clear Cell (Pale Cell) Acanthoma

- Abrupt transition to clear/pale cells
- May have epidermal neutrophils
- Deficient in glycogen phosphorylase
  - PAS+, diastase sensitive

Seborrheic Keratoses (SK)

- Base is flat, epidermis and stratum corneum thickened (acanthosis and hyperkeratosis, respectively), keratin horns
  - Sticks up, no budding
- Inverted follicular keratosis (IFK)
  - Looks like irritated SK with endophytic growth
  - Tons of squamous eddies
- Clonal seborrheic keratosis
  - Nests of clonal cells that do not reach top of epithelium
  - DDx—melanocytic lesion, squamous cell carcinoma in situ
- If suprabasal cells blend with basal cells, consider condyloma diagnosis

Benign Lichenoid Keratosis (BLK) or Lichenoid AK or Lichenoid Keratosis

- Clinical features—erythematous plaque +/− pigment
  - Single lesion
  - Rare on head and neck, never on face
- Proposed etiology—chronically irritated/inflamed solar lentigo that has involuted
  - May have a lentigo at the edge
- Acanthosis (usually), lichenoid infiltrate, and interface dermatosis
- *Change* in orthokeratin but not to "malignant" corneum
- Papillated surface
- May have *V*-shaped hypergranulosis

Actinic Keratoses *(AK)*

- Budding of basal cells, not full thickness, follicular sparing, basal cells most atypical
  - Dives down, budding present
- Flag sign—return of orthokeratosis (blue) over follicles in cutaneous horn (pink)

Squamous Cell Carcinoma in Situ

- Full thickness, basal sparing (eyeliner sign)
  - "Bowen disease"
- Pagetoid spread of necrotic keratinocytes
- Can spread around (AK does not)

Squamous Cell Carcinoma

- Squamous cell carcinoma in situ + invasion

PIGMENTED LESIONS

General

- Normal number of melanocytes per keratinocytes
  - Sun-exposed—1 in 4
  - Sun-protected—1 in 10
- Best way to tell neoplastic melanocytes—pleomorphic and large pink nucleoli
- Stains
  - Melan-A/MART = most specific
  - SOX10 is better for melanoma screening than S100
  - p16 (CDKN2A) is retained in nevi and lost in melanoma (nuclear and cytoplasmic)
  - PRAME stains 90% to 98% of primary and metastatic melanoma, not desmoplastic melanoma
- Melanophages—macrophages that have eaten lots of melanin after melanin incontinence, chunky and dark
- Fibrosis above dermal melanocyte nests
  - Special site nevus (back or thigh)
  - Regression in melanoma
  - Prior biopsy or trauma
- Pigmented lesion in a scar
  - Recurrent nevus if contained within the bounds of scar
  - Melanoma if spreading past the scar
- Furrows are friends
  - Pigment in cornified layer above furrows suggests benign melanocytic lesion

Nonmelanocytic

- Dirty socks → *SOLAR LENTIGO*, not a melanocytic lesion; miniature SK
  - Lentigo simplex = nevus precursor, melanocytic
  - Solar lentigo → reticulated SK → SK (on a spectrum)
  - Clinically, may be asymmetrically pigmented secondary to melanophages
  - use SOX10 if needed (Melan-A, MART, MiTF, S100)
    - SOX10 and S100 stain desmoplastic/spindled melanocytes
- Benign lichenoid keratosis (see "Actinic Keratoses" section)

Benign Nevi

- Junctional—at epidermis-dermis face (benign melanocytes HMB45+)
- Compound—junctional and dermal, should mature (get smaller) as they go deep
- Intradermal—just in dermis, should mature (melanocytes *not* HMB45+)
- Signs of chronicity in dermal nevi (ancient change)
  - Pseudovascular channels
  - Multinucleated rosettes
- Blue nevi
  - Heavily pigmented in deep dermis, no nests or junctional component, clustered around adnexa, sclerotic stroma, no maturation
  - *GNAQ* or *GNA11* mutations
- Spitz nevus
  - Finely melanized, grungy gray cytoplasm
  - Spindled nests

- Matures as it goes deeper
- Pigmented spindle cell nevus of Reed
  - Variant of Spitz nevus
  - Clinically and histologically mimics melanoma
  - On the thigh of a woman in her thirties
    - If in a child, call *pigmented Spitz nevus*
  - Spindled junctional nests and single cells, epidermal hyperplasia, parakeratosis, hypergranulosis
    - Melanophages in a ribbon-like band
- Dermal melanocytosis (Mongolian spot)
  - DDx is blue nevus (which also has sclerotic dermal)
    - This is like a sparse version of blue nevus
    - Nevus of Ito
  - Nevus of Ota is a "dermal melanocytosis" of the lateral sclera
    - Can get glaucoma
- Polypoid nevus of pregnancy
- Pigmented epithelioid melanocytoma (PEM)
  - Wedge-shaped (means good)
  - Lots of pigment with nests of small epithelioid blue cells
  - Blue nevus family
    - Cellular, atypical, epithelioid, deep penetrating, regular
  - Low grade
    - FISH or CGH
  - Loss of 5-hydroxymethylcytosine (HMC) is hallmark
- Myerson nevus
  - Spongiotic nevus with superficial crust
- Deep penetrating nevus
  - Cyclin D1+, nuclear beta-catenin+
    - Beta-catenin pathway is altered

Borderline Nevi

- Dysplastic nevus
  - Epidermal hyperplasia
  - Increased single cell melanocytes at the dermal-epidermal junction, architecturally atypia, concentric/lamellar fibrosis, melanocytic bridging
  - Junctional component extends beyond the dermal component (shoulders)
  - Does not extend into the reticular dermis
  - Lymphocytic inflammation
- Atypical junctional melanocytic hyperplasia
  - Single cells with mild to moderate atypia
  - On sun-damaged skin
  - Skip areas are common
  - Not quite melanoma in situ but too much for nevus
- Melanocytic lesions with mild (nuclei are smaller than keratinocytic nuclei, uniform hyperchromasia) or moderate atypia (larger than keratinocytic nuclei) are just observed
  - Severe atypia is reexcised

Melanoma

- 20% of melanomas arise in preexisting nevus

- On acral sites, most melanomas are lentiginous (single sites) and are permitted to have some pagetoid spread
- Clark level (in melanoma)
  - I—Melanoma in situ
  - II—Papillary dermis
  - III—Expanding papillary dermis
  - IV—Reticular dermis
  - V—Fat
- Lentigo maligna
- Melanoma in situ (MIS) on sun-damaged face/neck
- Clues—cannot fit in a 4× field, *any* nesting, skip areas
- Melanoma in situ
  - Large confluent junctional nests but single cells predominate
  - Hypercellular lesion
  - Adnexal involvement
  - Prominent pagetoid spread
  - Atypical nevus giant cells at dermal-epidermal junction
  - Host inflammatory response (evidence of regression)
  - High-grade cytologic atypia
  - Dyscohesion at the junction (may have clefting)
  - Clinically large (almost always >6 mm)
- Signs arguing against melanoma
  - Benign nested junctional component
    - Junction always goes bad before dermis
- Regression
  - Asymmetric inflammation
  - Flattening of papillae
  - Superficial dermal fibrosis
    - Has compressed elastin + fibers, scars do not
- Melanomas are always entire submitted (even huge reexcisions)
- Grossing considerations
  - Frozen sections not advised
  - Surface ulceration is added to staging, but do not confuse previous biopsy/Mohs/resection changes
    - Mention it in gross description
  - Important measurements—0.8, 1.0, 2.0, 4.0 cm

Melanoma Subtypes

- Desmoplastic melanoma
  - Head and neck of elderly
  - May not have identifiable intraepidermal component
  - S100+, SOX10+, HMB45–, MART-1–
  - Lymphocytic aggregates (help differentiate between neural lesion and melanoma)
- Uveal melanoma
  - Sporadic—*GNAQ1, GNA11, BAP1*
  - Inherited—*BAP1*
    - Autosomal dominant syndrome
    - Uveal and cutaneous melanoma, astrocytoma, mesothelioma, clear cell renal cell carcinoma

OTHER NEOPLASMS

Vascular Neoplasms

- Atypical vascular lesion of the breast
  - Look like lymphangiomas but occur in breast after radiation
  - Benign—usually submitted as "rule out angiosarcoma"
  - Can do MYC stain or FISH (radiation-induced angiosarcoma is positive)
- Epithelioid hemangioma—eosinophils and lymphocytes, increased vessels with large "blister" endothelial cells, pulsatile plaque/nodule on scalp near ear
  - Rule out kimura (epithelioid hemangioma is the skin version of kimura disease)
  - "Angiolymphoid hyperplasia with peripheral eosinophilia"
- MYC stain is positive in radiation-induced angiosarcoma, not in atypical superficial vascular proliferation
- Aggressive angiomyxoma
  - Vulvar region in young female
  - Myxoid and hypocellular
  - Lots of thick-walled vessels (+/− hyalinization)
  - Stellate/spindled fibroblasts
- Kaposi sarcoma
  - Associated with HIV and HHV-8
  - Mild cellular atypia
  - Cutaneous is classic but can involve gastrointestinal system, lymph nodes, and organs
  - LANA stain is specific

Hematolymphoid Neoplasms

- Langerhans cell histiocytosis
  - Clinical
    - Peak in childhood and again in 7th to 8th decade
    - Skull, long bones, spleen, liver, lung, ear, eye
  - Morphology
    - Eosinophils, epidermotropism, large oval cells in dermis with reniform nuclei
    - Reniform nuclei
  - CD1a+, S100+ (CD68+ in normal histiocytes, variable in LCH)
    - Langerin (CD207) = most specific for Langerhans cells
- Rosai Dorfman or "sinus histiocytosis with massive lymphadenopathy"
  - Diffuse dermatitis with histiocytes and lymphocytes
  - Emperipolesis of plasma cells through histiocytes
  - Dark and light areas
  - 10% have skin involvement—dermal nodule
  - S100+ (although Langerhans cells also stain), CD207− (langerin)
- Grenz zone → B-cell lymphoma or dermatofibroma
  - Nodular lymphocytic infiltrate = lymphoma or pseudolymphoma
  - B-cell lymphomas primary to skin
    - Primary cutaneous marginal zone lymphoma
    - Primary cutaneous follicular lymphoma
    - Primary cutaneous diffuse large B-cell lymphoma
  - Mantle cell lymphoma can be secondary to skin
- Blastic plasmacytoid dendritic cell neoplasm—BPDCN, CD123+
- Urticaria pigmentosa
  - = Cutaneous mastocytosis + classic clinical picture (multiple lesions in a child)

- Primary cutaneous anaplastic large-cell lymphoma
  - ALK–, but favorable prognosis (like ALK+ ALCL), CD30+
  - Rule out lymphomatoid papulosis (LyP), which is like a precursor lesion
  - Has atrophic epithelium, gren zone, and dense nodular lymphocytic infiltrate
- Mycosis fungoides
  - Patch → plaque → tumor
  - Atypical morphology, deeply cleaved, cerebriform
  - Epidermotropism with halos, Pautrier morphology
  - CD4+ typically, loss of CD7 and/or CD26
- Sezary syndrome
  - Erythroderma + blood involvement

Lesions Associated with Hematolymphoid Neoplasms

- Erythema elevatum diutinum
  - Nodules on dorsal hand, over joints, on extensor surfaces
  - Associated with IgA monoclonal gammopathy
  - Moderately dense perivascular neutrophilic infiltrate + lymphocytes, histiocytes, and eosinophils
  - Fibrinoid vessel change
    - Essentially a "fibrosing vasculitis"
  - With time, becomes fibrotic (concentric fibrosis of inflamed vessels)
- Necrobiotic xanthogranuloma
  - Rare multisystem histiocytic disease in older adults
    - Typically a yellowish plaque near the eye
    - 80% associated with paraproteinemia (like monoclonal gammopathy of undetermined significance)
- Palisading xanthogranulomas and necrobiosis in deep dermis and subcutaneous fat (septal)
  - Amorphous eosinophilic debris, cholesterol clefts
  - Multinucleated GCs, histiocytes, cholesterol clefts in tiered arrangement
- Scleromyxedema—generalized form of lichen myxedematosus or papular mucinosis
  - Associated with monoclonal gammopathy (IgG lambda) in 80%
  - Graves disease—pretibial myxedema
  - Carney syndrome—myxoma
- Juvenile myelomonocytic leukemia and JXG (see earlier)

Miscellaneous Neoplasms

- Tuberous xanthoma
  - Elbows, knees, buttocks secondary to hyperlipidemia
  - Large aggregates of foam cells in dermis without Touton cells or other inflammation
  - DDx
    - Xanthelasma and eruptive xanthomas—small, yellow papules
    - Verruciform xanthomas—not associated with hyperlipidemia, verruciform
    - Xanthoma disseminatum—normolipemic histiocytic proliferation with Touton giant cells and moderate lymphoplasmacytic inflammation
- Merkel cell carcinoma
  - Caused by UV exposure or Merkel cell carcinoma polyoma virus (MCPyV)
  - CK20
- Angiomyofibroblastoma of the vulva
  - Benign myofibroblastic neoplasm composed of bland spindle cells
  - Desmin+, S100–

- Pagetoid cells in epidermis
  - DDx—acral nevus (a little pagetoid is okay), actinic keratosis, squamous cell carcinoma in situ, extramammary Paget; Paget (always from breast)
  - Extra-mammary Paget disease
    - Primary cutaneous apocrine (GCDFP-15+ CK7+)
    - Secondary involvement of visceral adenocarcinoma (CK20+, lineage-specific markers like CDX-2)
- Glomus tumor
  - Painful nodule on finger/toe
  - Hemorrhagic
  - Masses of modified smooth muscle cells around vascular channels
- Multinucleated cell angiohistiocytoma
- Dermatofibroma → dermatofibrosarcoma protuberans → fibrosarcoma
  - DF—CD34−, Factor VIII+
  - DFSP—CD34+, Factor VIII−
  - As it transforms to frank fibrosarcoma...
    - CD34 expression decreases
    - Ki67 increases
    - Storiform pattern turns into herringbone
    - Plump nuclei and increased mitotic rate
- Fibrous papule/angiofibroma
  - Fibrotic stroma that pushes elastosis down and out
  - Concentric follicular fibrosis, telangiectatic vessels
  - Classically on nose
  - Benign, associated with sebaceous hyperplasia
- Acral fibrokeratoma
  - Looks like tiny extra digit
  - Vertically oriented collagen, hyperkeratosis
- Pleomorphic adenoma
  - Similar to fibroadenoma but with significant squamous epithelial component
  - Chondroid syringoma in skin
- Neurofibroma
  - Neural spindle cells, admixed mast cells, entrapped adnexa
- Epidermolytic acanthoma
  - Shredded wheat
  - Verrucous and hypergranulosis
  - Found in vulva, not HPV-associated
- Neurothekeoma
  - Nested, grayish, myxoid
  - NKIC3

Odds and Ends

- Favoring primary cutaneous lesion versus metastasis
  - p63+
  - D240+
  - CK5/6+
- Chondrodermatitis nodularis helicis
  - Lesion on ear caused by positional ischemia
- Cholesteatoma (in ear)
  - Granulation tissue, bone frags, expanding keratin cysts

- Mast cells can pick up nonspecific IHC (like for VZV)
- Argyrosis
  - Deposition of metallic silver and silver sulfide
  - Intensified by sunlight exposure (reduction of silver) and increased melanin synthesis
  - Silver granules in vascular and adnexal basement membrane and dermal elastic figures (brown-black on H&E)
  - Confirm with darkfield microscopy
- CD34 expression
  - Positive in solitary fibrous tumor, superficial acral fibromyxoma, epithelioid sarcoma, intradermal spindle cell lipoma
  - Negative in neurothekeoma
- Aggressive digital papillary adenocarcinoma and epithelioid sarcomas
  - ACRAL BADDIES
- Acral soft tissue lesions with similar histology
  - Superficial acral fibromyxoma—hypercellular
  - Digital myxoid cyst—collarette of epithelium, increased mucin but no significant increase in cellularity
  - Perineurioma—whorled
- Clues to benign vs. malignant
  - Undermining of the epithelium is only okay in cysts
    - Otherwise it suggests malignancy
  - Epidermal collarette (hugging lesion) → almost always benign
- Progressive macular hypomelanosis requires Fontana-Masson confirmation
- Pigment in the … clinically appears … resulting from Tyndall effect
  - Corneum—black
  - Basal—brown
  - Papillary dermis—gray
  - Deep dermis—blue
- Pyoderma gangrenosum
  - Tons of neutrophils without vasculitis, diagnosis of exclusion (perform bug stains and culture)
- Lupus miliaris disseminatus faciei
  - Caseating granulomas in the superficial dermis
  - Present as multiple papules on face
- Melanoma in lymph node without a primary can be due to capsular nevus or (more likely) regressed primary
- Vertically oriented vessels are suggestive of trauma
- Dilated pore of Winer (DPOW)
  - Plugged-up follicle with filiform peripheral silhouette
- Acne rosacea
  - Tuberculoid granulomas with lymphocytic cuff near follicles, plasma cells

CHAPTER 4

Gynecologic Pathology

Vagina and Vulva

- Granular cell layer of squamous epithelium disappears around the vaginal introitus
- Differentiated vulvar intraepithelial neoplasia (dVIN)
  - Acts like VIN3, but there is only dysplasia in basal layer and dyskeratosis
  - Loss of orientation
  - Lichen sclerosus (white and thin clinically) → dVIN → keratinizing squamous cell carcinoma (no HPV)
    - LS = flattened atrophic epithelium, dermal thick scar (homogenization of collagen) with loss of rete
      - Earlier lesions have lichenoid inflammation
      - If not perfect, call it *lichenoid dermatitis*
  - Pitfall—can be missed on low power
  - Clues to dVIN
    - Premature keratinization
    - Dyskeratosis
    - Large cells with vesicular chromatin and macronucleoli
    - Binucleation
    - Prominent desmosomes/cell borders
    - History of lichen sclerosus in elderly patient
- Verrucous carcinoma
  - Condylomatous lesion with lichenoid inflammation
  - Little to no atypia
  - Invades with broad pushing border
  - *PIK3CA* mutations
- Get fungal stains on vulvar biopsies if itching/burning/parakeratosis
- Condyloma
  - Hypergranulosis
  - Parakeratosis on edges
  - High mitotic figures
- "Benign keratosis" if clinical impression is concerning for condyloma but has no viral cytopathic changes
- Angiomyofibroblastoma (angiofibroma) of vulva
  - Benign
  - Morphology
    - Nests of epithelioid/spindled fibroblastic cells
    - Richly vascularized myxocollagenous stroma
    - Mast cells
  - ER+, PR+, desmin+, and SMA+
- One-third of DES daughters develop vaginal adenosis

Cervix

NON NEOPLASTIC

- Pink stroma with mucinous glands, round nuclei all lined up at base
  - Versus endometrial—blue stroma with nonmucin-producing glands, elongated nuclei that can be jumbled
- Can have neutrophils
  - Do not call chronic cervicitis unless you see polypoid change with tons of lymphocytes and plasma cells
- Tunnel cluster
  - Benign cervical cluster of small cysts
- Squamous metaplasia can look thickened on colposcopy
- Benign pitfalls mistaken for carcinoma
  - Microglandular hyperplasia
    - Commonly has subnuclear vacuoles, rarely may have mucinous or hyaline stroma
  - Papillary syncytial metaplasia
- Tubo-endometrioid metaplasia of endocervical glands can get myxoid stroma (mimicking desmoplasia)

NEOPLASTIC

- For squamous dysplasia and malignancies, see the "Cytology" section
- Endocervical dysplasia
  - Elongated nuclei (like tubular adenoma)
- Endocervical adenocarcinoma features
  - HPV-driven (p16+), apically oriented, hyperchromatic pencillate nuclei with floating mitoses and basal karyorrhectic debris
    - Adenocarcinoma in situ (AIS) if superficial (only to the depth that benign glands go to) and no desmoplasia
      - Keep an eye out for *surface-only* AIS
    - Adenoma malignum = minimal deviation adenocarcinoma
      - Strongly associated with lobular endocervical glandular hyperplasia (LEGH)
  - Patterns of invasion
    - Expansile ("AIS-like"—looks like AIS but goes way too deep)
      - Silva A pattern
      - Does not have convincing desmoplasia
      - Nondestructive
      - No lymph node metastasis risk
    - Infiltrative
    - Polypoid
  - Treatment
    - Low-grade—radical hysterectomy
    - High-grade—chemoradiation (leave pelvic organs in place)
- Features that favor adenocarcinoma over AIS in tough cases
  - Malignant glands deep in stroma
  - Confluent growth
  - Incomplete gland formation
  - Single cells
  - Less lobular architecture, more cribriform formation

- Primary endocervical adenocarcinoma can look like well-differentiated endometrial
  - Endocervical = no secretory changes, p16+, ER/PR–, vimentin–, CEA+
    - Mucinous morphology is by far the most common but can also get clear cell and gastric type
  - Endometrial = secretory changes, p16 wild-type, ER/PR+, vimentin+
- SMILE
  - Stratified mucin-producing intraepithelial lesion
  - "AIS-stratified type"
  - Like HSIL but more distinct nuclei due to increased cytoplasmic mucin
  - May transform to adenocarcinoma or adenosquamous carcinoma
- Tubal metaplasia is p16+ (possible pitfall)
- Small cell carcinoma of the cervix is associated with HPV 18

Gynecologic Cytology

GENERAL NOTES

- Reactive changes
  - Inflammation
  - Atrophy
    - Small blue cells, monomorphic
  - Radiation changes
    - Smudgy big nuclei
    - Bizarre cells
    - History!
  - Intrauterine device (IUD)
    - Looks atrophic, may have reactive changes
    - History!
  - Nucleoli in squamous cells
  - Not seen in squamous dysplasia
  - Only reactive changes OR invasive squamous cell carcinoma (SCC)
- Robin's egg blue = keratin
- Immunosuppressed females
  - Pap 2× per year for the first year, and then annually
- ASCUS and negative high-risk HPV → repeat cotesting in 1 year
- ASCUS and positive high-risk HPV → colposcopy

BETHESDA SYSTEM

- Unsatisfactory
  - ≥75% of squamous cells are obscured by WBCs or blood
- Negative for intraepithelial lesion or malignancy
- Atypical squamous cells of unknown significance (ASCUS)
  - Includes atypical parakeratosis
    - Orangeophilic
    - Pyknotic nuclei
    - Arrow-shaped clump of blue cells is a form
- Low-grade squamous intraepithelial lesion (LSIL)
  - Includes koilocytic changes

- If 21 to 24 years, follow-up in 1 year with repeat pap
- 18% have intraepithelial lesion (HSIL)
- High-grade squamous (HSIL)
- Invasive squamous cell carcinoma
- Atypical glandular cells of unknown significance (AGUS)
  - Follow-up—colposcopy + biopsy of any lesions, endocervical curettage, endometrial sampling
- Adenocarcinoma in situ (AIS)
  - Most commonly associated with HPV18
  - Follow-up—colposcopy + biopsy, endocervical curettage
- Adenocarcinoma
  - Endocervical
  - Endometrial
    - Intracytoplasmic neutrophils
  - Extrauterine
  - NOS
  - Other

INFECTION

- Trichomonas
  - Acute inflammation with neutrophil balls, perinuclear halos, reactive epithelial changes
  - Frothy, yellow-green discharge and punctate cervical hemorrhages
  - May be concomitant with Leptothrix (filamentous bacteria)
- Bacterial vaginosis
  - Can only diagnose if there is no lactobacillus
  - Fishy/ammonia odor
- Candidiasis
  - Shish kebab squamous cells on hyphae, neutrophils
  - Only treat if symptomatic or pregnant
  - Thick, white discharge with vaginal irritation
- *Haemophilus ducreyi* chancroid
  - "Raised papular lesions that undergo ulceration and subsequent accumulation of granulation tissue"
  - Painful deep ulcers
- Actinomyces
- Herpes simplex virus

Uterus

NON NEOPLASTIC

Polyps

- Thickened vessels, dilated glands, squamous/tubular metaplasia, fibrous stroma, gaping lymphatics
- Watch out for endometrial intraepithelial carcinoma (EIC, minimal volume serous carcinoma) on surface of polyps in women in late 60s
- If a pathologist diagnoses a polyp on an endometrial biopsy in a woman with abnormal uterine bleeding, it triggers a dilation and curettage

Dating

- Proliferative
  - Features
    - Mitoses in glands or stroma
    - Test-tube or small donut glands
    - Pseudostratified nuclei
    - Can have irregular glands, but they will be tighter than secretory
  - Cannot date proliferative
  - Disordered proliferative phase
    - Not quite atypical
    - Cystic and budding "animal-shaped" glands, barely increased crowding
    - Must have mitoses (in a proliferative setting)
    - Suggests anovulatory cycles
    - MORE of this = simple hyperplasia
- Interval endometrium = days 16 to 17
  - Subnuclear vacuoles and rare mitoses, stromal edema with round (seemingly bare) nuclei
  - Late proliferative/early secretory
- Secretory
  - Gland changes first (d6d20)
    - Subnuclear vacuoles (d18) → both sides of nucleus → supranuclear → luminal secretions
    - Glands become tortuous and look more packed together
    - Rarely becomes atypical/hyperplastic (need higher threshold)
  - Then stroma changes (d21–28)
    - Pale and edematous (d21) → predecidual changes around spiral arteries (d24) → decidual under surface → coalesces → stroma condenses → stromal breakdown → menstruation
  - Inactive endometrium
  - Looks like proliferative without mitoses (just less than 1:1 gland-to-stroma ratio), blue donuts, dark blue stroma
  - Compared with atrophy, which has a much lower gland-to-stroma ratio and very attenuated thin epithelium (strips)
  - Cannot date a polyp, cycles differently than background
  - Luteal phase defect
  - Disparity of >3 days between calendar date and histologic date on two consecutive biopsies

Other Non neoplastic

- Lower uterine segment (LUS)
  - Polyp-like fibrous stroma, no thick vessels, mucinous/endocervical epithelium (+/− tubal metaplasia), fewer glands
  - Polyps arising here can be mixed endometrial (p53) and endocervical
  - Endocervical glands have closed lumens; LUS glands have open lumens
- Elevated FSH is seen in the perimenopausal period as the ovaries become less responsive
- Atrophy
  - Number-one cause of postmenopausal bleeding (PMB)
  - Tiny strips of simple cuboidal epithelium on endometrial biopsy (EMB) or endometrial curettage (EMC)
  - 60s to 70s → worry about serous adeno arising in background of atrophy

- If it looks like atrophy but in younger woman and/or woman on progestins, call it *inactive* (+/− with exogenous progestin effect if decidual stromal change)
  - <1 mitotic figure in whole atrophy case, usually
- If more, call *weakly proliferative* and suggest that there is some reason for increased estrogenic stimulation (obese, polycystic ovarian syndrome, tumor, hormone replacement therapy)
- Endometrial stromal breakdown
  - Stromal condensation into "blue balls" with oncocytic surface epithelium
    - +/−: tufting, metaplasia, fibrin thrombi, neutrophils
    - Background endometrium
      - End-secretory: normal menses
      - Proliferative: dysfunctional uterine bleeding
  - Can be a cause for bleeding, suggests anovulatory cycles
- Chronic endometritis—PLASMA CELLS
  - Treatable cause for bleeding
  - Spindled stroma with lymphoid aggregates, look for PCs at aggregate periphery
    - Unopposed progestins
  - Very decidualized bubblegum-pink stroma
  - Tiny round glands without mitotic activity
  - In pregnancy, caused by progesterone from corpus luteum
- Unopposed estrogen (and tamoxifen)
  - Proliferative!

HYPERPLASIA AND ATYPIA

- Simple—too many glands with stroma between
- Complex—less stroma between
- +/− atypia—ROUNDED nuclei
  - Pale/vesicular chromatin (nuclear margination) +/− prominent nucleoli, loss of polarity, larger nuclei, more pleomorphism
  - Eosinophilic cytoplasm
    - Atypical polypoid adenomyoma
  - Squamous morules and/or atypical hyperplasia involving a polyp, considered a clonal process
  - Squamous morules have central necrosis occasionally frequently

ENDOMETRIAL CARCINOMA

See Fig. 4.1.

General

- FIGO grading
  - Applies to endometrioid/mucinous only
  - Grade 1: <5% solid
  - Grade 2: 5% to 50% solid
  - Grade 3: >50% solid
  - Not including morule/squamous areas
    - Squamous morular metaplasia occurs almost exclusively in complex hyperplasia and more malignant
  - Grades 2 and 3 are considered high grade (HG) and need nodes taken
  - If SEVERE cytologic atypia, bump-up one FIGO level

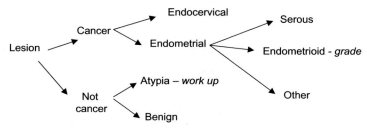

Fig. 4.1 Algorithm for diagnosing glandular lesions of the endometrium.

TABLE 4.1 ■ **Endometrial Adenocarcinoma Types**

Feature	Type 1	Type 2
Histologic subtype	Endometrioid	Serous and clear cell
Unopposed estrogen	Present	Absent
Menopausal status	Pre- and peri-	Post-
Precursor lesion	Atypical hyperplasia	Carcinoma in situ
Tumor grade	Low	High
Myometrial invasion	Variable, often minimal	Variable, often deep
Behavior	Indolent	Aggressive
Genetic alterations	*PTEN*, microsatellite instability, *K-RAS*	*TP 53*

- Immunophenotype
  - CK7+, CK20– CA125+, BerEP4+, B72-3+
  - Grades 1 and 2 = ER/PR+
- Syndromic associations
  - Lynch syndrome (hereditary non-polyposis colorectal carcinoma, HNPCC)
    - Autosomal dominant
    - Mismatch repair, microsatellite instability
      - MLH1, PMS2, MSH2, MSH6 proteins
    - Causes colorectal, endometrial, stomach, ovarian cancers
      - Endometrial carcinoma is the first cancer in 50% of women with Lynch
      - MMR testing is done on all endometrial carcinomas
    - Pathologic features
    - Tumor-infiltrating lymphocytes
    - LUS tumors
    - Undifferentiated histology
    - Synchronous ovarian tumor
  - Cowden
    - *PTEN* mutation
  - Muir-Torre syndrome
  - *BRCA1/BRCA2* mutations
  - See Table 4.1
- Staging notes
  - Adnexal involvement
    - Direct extension or metastasis = pT3a

- Free-floating tumor does not count
- Metastasis versus synchronous primary
  - Synchronous primary has a more favorable prognosis and is more common in microsatellite instable tumors
- Lymph node involvement
  - 10% to 15% of endometrial carcinomas have nodal metastases
  - Important note for hysterectomy frozen sections
    - Your findings will determine whether the surgeon performs a pelvic lymph node dissection or closes.
    - Criteria to take nodes:
      - >50% depth of invasion
    - When measuring depth of invasion—invisible line at normal myometrium
    - Cutoff at ½ of full depth (< ½ = 1a, > ½ = 1b)
      - LUS involvement
      - >2 cm in size
      - FIGO 2 or 3
  - Sentinel lymph node definitions
    - Isolated tumor cells—isolated clusters not larger than 0.2 mm
    - Micrometastasis—more than 0.2 mm but not larger than 2 mm
      - Single focus
    - Metastases—larger than 2 mm
- *POLE* tumors
  - Ultramutated
  - Very good prognosis, even though one-half have high-grade histology
  - Usually low stage
  - Possibly able to be more conservative with therapy

Histologic Pitfalls

- Cancer involving adenomyosis has dark stroma around a very round gland and may have associated benign glands
  - True invasion has lighter desmoplasia and jagged glands
- Confusing endocervical for endometrial
  - Endocervical
    - Younger patients
    - Apoptotic debris, floating mitotic activities, AIS in adjacent glands, goblet cells
    - p16+ (diffuse), CEA+, PR−, ER+/−, vimentin -
  - Endometrial
    - Older obese patients
    - Squamous differentiation, stromal foamy histiocytes, second tumor type (e.g., serous, mucinous)
    - p16 patchy +/−, ER/PR+, vimentin+ (stromal), CEA−, loss of PTEN, p53 wild-type
- Menstrual blood!
  - Big reactive glands, stromal balls, fibrin, neutrophils

Serous

- Nuclear atypia and papillary architecture, slit-like spaces, exophytic growths, frequently develops in polyps; scalloped luminal borders, hobnailing (or ruffled luminal border)
- High mitoses, papillary epithelial tufts (floating)
- Gaping/staghorn glands invading myometrium, very HG cytology, red macronucleoli
- Atrophic adjacent epithelium

- ↑ Ki-67, ↑ nuclear p53 (strong and diffuse or null), ↑ p16, ↓ER/PR, no PTEN loss
- Can have minimal volume on surface of polyps
- Can have glandular appearance without papillae
  - Well-formed glands with UGLY cells
- *No low-grade version*
- Serous endometrial intraepithelial carcinoma
  - SEIC or EIC—precursor to serous carcinoma
  - Single layer with cytologic changes consistent with serous
  - Can metastasize

Clear Cell

- Classically arise in a background of endometrioid carcinoma
- Grossly yellow
- High-grade nuclei (cleared out chromatin but not as bad as serous), hyalinized stroma (sometimes myxoid), papillary/tubulocystic/solid, hobnailing, eosinophilic or clear cytoplasm
  - Can look like serous with occasional clear cells
- Very rare, poor prognosis
- Immunophenotype
  - Positive for: napsin A, HNF1 beta, focal racemase
  - Negative for: ER, p16, WT-1
  - P53 wild-type (positive in all is correlated with poor prognosis)

Endometrioid

- Morphology
  - Back-to-back glands without stroma between
  - Cribriform
  - Expansive
  - Labyrinthine pattern
- Immunophenotype
  - ER/PR + (hormonally driven)
    - Stains gland but not squamous component
    - CEA stains squamous and not glands
    - CEA stains glands AND squamous in endocervical
  - p53 wild-type
    - Very high-grade endometrioid acquires *p53* mutation
  - p16 patchy
  - Driven by *PTEN* mutations (Cowden syndrome)
- Posthormone therapy (progestins)
  - ↓ gland-to-stroma ratio
  - ↓ cellularity
  - ↓ mitotic figures
  - Bland
  - See Table 4.2
- Common histologic variants—must be seen in MAJORITY of tumor
  - Villoglandular
  - Ciliated
  - Squamous
    - Glycogenated squamous
    - Only endometrioid can have squamous differentiation (not clear cell or serous)

TABLE 4.2 ■ **Metaplasia vs. Endometrial Carcinoma**

Metaplasia	Endometrial CA (or EIC)
p53 heterogeneous	p53 strong and diffuse
ER+	ER− or weak

CA, Carcinoma; *EIC,* endometrial intraepithelial carcinoma; *ER,* estrogen receptor.

- Microcystic, elongated, and fragmented invasion (MELF)
  - Higher risk for lymphovascular invasion that is frequently missed
  - Small cysts filled with neutrophils
  - Fibromyxoid stromal reaction
- Endometrial intraepithelial neoplasia (EIN)
  - Controversial; not everyone uses it
  - Between complex hyperplasia and FIGO 1 endometrioid
- Corded and hyalinized variant of endometrial carcinoma (CHEC)
  - Favorable prognosis (do not confuse with carcinosarcoma)
  - Biphasic
    - Typical/villoglandular endometrial carcinoma
    - Distinct cords of epithelioid or spindle stromal cells (not malignant) in hyaline stroma
      - Rarely forms osteoid
  - Low stage even though they look like sarcomas
  - Two-thirds are grade 1; one-third are grade 2
  - Nuclear beta-catenin and loss of e-cadherin
- Undifferentiated/dedifferentiated endometrial carcinoma
  - Sheet-like, rhabdoid, in postmenopausal women
  - CK18+ EMA+ keratin-
  - Loss of MLH1 and PMS2 in 50%
  - Undifferentiated—no "classic component"
  - Dedifferentiated—adjacent FIGO 1 to 2 endometrial carcinoma
- Histologic changes
  - Secretory change (subnuclear vacuoles)
  - Clear cell change
    - Pitfall: confusing clear cell change for clear cell carcinoma
    - Clear cell carcinoma is high-grade and has hobnailing
  - Papillary change
    - Not just in serous/clear cell!

Other Rare Lesions

- Papillary proliferations of the endometrium
- Small cell neuroendocrine
- Large cell neuroendocrine

Uterine Mesenchymal Tumors

- Leiomyoma
  - Most common by far
  - Thick-walled vessels, cleft between normal tissue
  - Desmin+, SMA+, caldesmon+

- Can be treated with embolization or leupron (GnRH agonist) or progestins → may cause ischemia and necrosis
- Variants
  - Leiomyoma with bizarre nuclei
    - New name for simplastic/atypical leiomyoma
    - Reported cases of recurrence after myomectomy but BENIGN
    - Degenerative sort of atypia (like ancient schwannoma)
    - Can get intranuclear pseudoinclusions
    - Called smooth muscle tumor of uncertain malignant potent (STUMP)
  - Cellular leiomyoma
    - Can be CD10+
    - Very blue!
  - Fumarate hydratase deficient
    - Eosinophilic nucleoli, eosinophilic cytoplasmic globules, perinuclear halos
    - Renal cell carcinoma syndrome with cutaneous leiomyomas
    - Low Ki-67
- Common changes in leiomyomas: calcifications, hyaline change, ischemia, hydropic
  - Apoplectic change—young women on hormones—streaky hemorrhage in the center, increased mitoses in periphery
  - Locations: submucosal, mural, subserosal
- Smooth muscle tumor of uncertain malignant potentional (STUMP)
  - Smooth muscle tumor of unknown malignant potential
  - No necrosis (vs. leiomyosarcoma, which has tumor necrosis)
- Leiomyosarcoma
  - One of following = benign, 2 or more = malignant
    - Marked pleomorphism/atypia
    - Mitosis (≥10/10 hpf)
    - Necrosis
      - Only tumor/coagulative = karyorrhexis, debris, abrupt transition, alive blood vessels, ghost cells
      - NOT ischemic/hyaline necrosis—gradual zone of transition, dead blood vessels, lays down collagen
    - Infiltration
  - Malignant criteria do not apply to myxoid/epithelioid smooth muscle tumors
    - Need less
    - For example, ≥ 2/10 hpf (< would be STUMP)
  - Can have heterologous differentiation
  - Perinuclear clearing, lots of lymphovascular invasion (LVI)
  - Recur distantly (as opposed to stromal sarcomas, which recur locally)
- Endometrial stroma tumor
  - CD10+
  - Small vessels in spirals
  - NOT infiltrative (can have mitoses/necrosis)
- Endometrial stromal sarcoma (ESS)
  - Low-grade ESS
    - Infiltrative
    - Anastomosing tongues of small round blue cells into myometrium
    - Hyaline globules
    - Spiral arteries
    - Translocation of *JAZF1*

- High-grade ESS
  - Difficult to recognize
  - *YWHAE* family translocations
- Recur locally (as opposed to leiomyosarcomas, which recur distantly)
- Adenofibroma
  - Benign glands and benign stroma (looks like phyllodes)
- Adenosarcoma
  - Benign glands and malignant stroma
- Malignant mixed Mullerian tumor = carcinosarcoma
  - Older women, poor prognosis (usually deeply invasive)
  - HG epithelial component (endometrioid or serous) and HG mesenchymal component
  - Heterologous elements—rhabdomyosarcoma, chondrosarcoma, osteosarcoma
- PEComa
  - Epithelioid, looks like leiomyoma
  - Positive for smooth muscle tumor markers and melanoma markers

Ovaries and Fallopian Tubes

OVARIAN NEOPLASMS

Surface Epithelial

- General
  - Each should be categorized as serous, mucinous, or clear cell
    - Cystadenoma
    - Cystadenofibroma
    - Adenofibroma
      - Fibrous stroma with benign epithelial glands throughout
    - Carcinoma
  - Lymphovascular invasion and prototypical "invasion" are not really reported
  - Type 1—lower grade
    - Endometrioid, clear cell, mucinous, low-grade serous, transitional cell (Brenner)
    - Endometriosis related, HNF1beta+, *ARID1A* mutations
      - Retrograde menstruation; tubal ligation can decrease risk for type 1 carcinoma
  - Type 2—*TP53* mutations, higher grade
    - High-grade serous carcinoma, undifferentiated carcinoma, carcinosarcoma
  - Gross examination
    - Surface of mass (Is there a tumor on surface? Use ink sparingly for possible involvement.)
    - Weigh intact (if received intact), then open, drain if necessary, and weigh again
    - Is the tube present?
    - If frozen comes back as high-grade serous, do not need 1 section/cm → only if borderline or benign
  - Associations
    - Tubal implants → serous
    - Endometriosis → clear cell (papillary or tubulocystic pattern), mucinous, endometrioid
    - Walthard rests → Brenner
  - Biopsy of ovarian mass can upstage to T1c as a result of disrupted surface → patient should go straight to bilateral salpingo-oophorectomy (BSO)
  - Mucinous and serous ovarian carcinomas raise CA125, not clear cell
    - Intended to be used as one-time test after treatment to detect residual disease when considering "second-look procedure" (>35 U/mL)

- Benign/nonneoplastic lesions
  - Inclusion cysts
    - Common on ovaries
    - Simple cyst lined by cuboidal, columnar, or ciliated epithelium
    - Can have budding
    - If large, best referred to as *serous cystadenomas*
  - Follicular cysts
    - Cystic change of ovarian follicle
    - Lined by luteinized granulosa cells
    - Clinicians use FIGO instead of AJCC; they are very similar though
    - Surface of liver/spleen is stage III, parenchymal invasion stage IV
    - Node staging—isolated tumor cells = N0(i+) ≤0.2 mm
  - Pitfall—sarcoma-like mural nodules
    - Benign
    - Markedly pleomorphic osteoclast-like giant cells
    - Well-circumscribed, keratin–
- Mucinous
  - Most indolent of all surface carcinomas
  - Mucinous tumors (benign and malignant) love to "hang out" with Brenner tumors
  - Intestinal type (historical term, now just regular mucinous)
    - 85%, goblet cells, septated (honeycomb)
    - Can even get Paneth cells
  - Benign
    - Cystadenoma, cystadenofibroma
    - Thin-walled cysts, single cell layer, no atypia, basal nuclei
    - Intestinal differentiation is okay
    - Can get functional luteinized stroma → virilization, abnormal uterine bleeding
  - Mucinous borderlines
    - Like benign but have *cellular atypia* (>10% atypia) and glandular complexity
      - Do not have much papillae or gross clues to identify
      - Focal proliferation can still qualify as benign (<10%)
    - Low recurrence rate (1%)
    - Papillary tufts with pseudostratified nuclei
    - Necrosis may be present (resulting from extravasated mucin)
      - Okay—does not mean it is malignant
    - Do not have implants
    - …with intraepithelial carcinoma
      - *More atypia* than regular borderlines, no stromal invasion
      - Cribriform pattern
      - Papillae are very thin—minimal stroma
      - Survival 95%
    - …with microinvasion
      - No destructive invasion, moderate atypia
      - <5 mm in linear dimension (can be multiple)
      - Still pretty good outcomes
    - …with microinvasive carcinoma
      - Marked cytologic atypia
  - Invasive mucinous carcinoma
    - Confluent cribriform formation is suspicious for invasion
    - Expansile vs. destructive (traditional) invasion of mucinous carcinoma

- FIGO grading
  - Grade 1: <5% nonsquamous solid tumor growth
  - Grade 2: 5% to 50% nonsquamous solid tumor growth
  - Grade 3: >50% nonsquamous solid tumor growth
- Expansile may have a more favorable prognosis
  - Very large invading glands, no small glands/single cells, no desmoplasia
- Just too big/too much with decreased stroma
  - Suggests primary (over met)
- Anaplastic foci paradoxically portend a more favorable prognosis
- Mutations
  - *KRAS* (benign, borderline, carcinoma)
  - *CDKN2a*
  - Less commonly, *TP53*
- Prognosis is related to stage
  - Low grade—pretty good prognosis
- May be metastatic from gastrointestinal tract
  - If nuclear features are atypical throughout architecturally simple areas, think metastasis from appendix (low-grade appendiceal mucinous neoplasm—LAMN)
    - Tall mucin, think appendix
  - SATB2 negative in ovarian primary, positive in gastrointestinal metastases
    - PAX8, ER, and PR can be helpful if positive but can be lost in ovarian mucinous primary (negative staining does not rule out ovarian primary)
  - Clue—bilaterality
    - Mucinous ovarian carcinoma is very rarely bilateral
- Seromucinous
  - Probably endometriosis-related
  - Old term is *endocervical* type
  - Morphology
    - Serous (tubal type) and mucinous lining in same cystadenoma or cystadenofibroma
    - Low power—serous tumor (bulbous complex papillae)
    - Eosinophilic cytoplasm, may have implants or intraepithelial carcinoma, papillary architecture
    - Mucin-containing cells (no goblet cells) admixed with polygonal eosinophilic cells
    - May have squamoid proliferations
  - Mutations
    - *ARID1A*
      - Because of association with endometriosis
      - As does endometrioid type
    - *PTEN*
  - WT1−, ER+, PAX8+
  - Seromucinous borderline tumor is a distinctive entity but controversial
    - Papillary architecture lined by stratified mucinous cells and hobnail-shaped cells containing abundant eosinophilic cytoplasm
    - Stromal inflammatory infiltrate
    - Minimal cytologic atypia
  - Seromucinous carcinoma is a rare and controversial entity
- Serous
  - All should be WT1 positive, ER+ (low-grade > high-grade)
  - Tend to have psammoma bodies in low-grade lesions (variable in high-grade)
  - Completely *benign* serous lesions have cilia
    - Focal atypia okay if <10% ("with focal atypia")

- Serous cystadenofibroma, cystadenoma, adenofibroma, papillary adenofibroma, surface papillary adenofibroma
- Adenofibroma
  - May result in knobby papillae that can look like excrescences grossly but are firm
  - Composed of benign tubal-like glands and/or cysts (like endosalpingiosis) causing visible mass and broad fibrous stromal component
- Benign serous cystadenoma
  - Cyst with blunted cuboidal lining, rare cilia, and watery secretions
- Borderline serous
  - Hierarchical branching, can be very obvious
  - Can have microinvasion
    - If each is <5mm in largest dimension and nondestructive
    - Small island, cleft around it, no desmoplasia
    - Does not alter the tumor behavior but clues you in to look for implants
  - Common in 30s
  - Micropapillary variant (medusa head)
    - Can also be called
      - *Serous borderline tumor with micropapillary features*
      - *Noninvasive low-grade carcinoma*
    - Poorer prognosis than nonmicropapillary borderline serous
    - Papillae must be 5× as long as they are wide, must be >5 mm, must be >10% of tumor
    - Papillae may merge to have cribriform patterns
  - Borderline serous tumor with microinvasion
    - Isolated rounded eosinophilic cells or cell clusters within the stroma
      - Look like the epithelial cells lining the surface of the papillae
    - Surrounded by retraction spaces and a stroma rich in fibroblasts
    - *Cannot exceed **5 mm** in the largest linear dimension*
  - Solid nests or cribriform glands → low-grade serous carcinoma
  - See Table 4.3.
  - *Low-grade serous carcinoma **does not** progress to high-grade serous carcinoma*
- High-grade serous

TABLE 4.3 ■ **Low-Grade vs. High-Grade Serous Carcinoma**

	Low-Grade Serous Carcinoma	**High-Grade Serous Carcinoma**
Mutations	*BRAF* and *KRAS*	*TP 53*
Precursor lesion	Borderline serous arising in cortical inclusion cysts	STIC from tubes
p53	Strong and diffuse *or* null (p16 strong and diffuse)	Wild-type
Architecture	Extensive simple papillae and glands Many psammoma bodies	Slit-like spaces and papillae to solid nests Variable psammoma bodies
Stroma	Fibrous	Fibrous, edematous, myxoid, or edematous
Cytology	Uniform round nucleoli with evenly distributed chromatin +/− nucleoli	Ugly, cherry macronucleoli

STIC, Serous tubal intraepithelial carcinoma.

- ↑ mitotic activity, ↑ apoptotic debris, pleomorphic, hyperchromatic, psammoma bodies
- Papillary, micropapillary, solid, nests with slit-like spaces
- Diffuse+ or p53−, Napsin−, WT-1+, CA125+
- 65% bilateral, may arise from serous tubal intraepithelial carcinoma
- High-grade serous vs. FIGO 3 endometrioid
  - Serous has slit-like spaces, very ugly, common periadnexal/omental involvement, lots of LVI
  - Endometrioid has rounded glands, can get ugly too
- Solid, pseudoendometrioid, and transitional-like (SET) patterns are more common in *BRCA*-mutated cases
- Psammocarcinoma
  - Low-grade serous carcinoma with so many psammoma bodies that you can barely see any epithelium
  - Nests with <15 cells in largest dimension
  - 75% of tumor has psammoma bodies
- Implants
  - Only occur in serous or seromucinous borderline tumors
    - Carcinomas have metastases
  - Can be epithelial noninvasive or desmoplastic noninvasive
    - Do not need to differentiate—just call them *implants*
  - If invasive → no longer borderline, now carcinoma
    - Destroys underlying tissue, micropapillary invasion
  - Must distinguish from benign mimics (endosalpingiosis)
- STIC—serous tubal intraepithelial carcinoma
  - Precursor for high-grade serous adenocarcinoma
  - High-grade nuclei, heaped up on each other
  - Use SEE-FIM grossing protocol to avoid missing them
    - Sectioning and extensively examining the fimbriated end of the fallopian tube
  - ~10% of BRCA 1/2 patients undergoing prophylactic bilateral salpingo-oophorectomy (BSO) will have STIC
  - p53 strong and diffuse, Ki67 high
  - See "Algorithm for STIC" paper
- Clear cell carcinoma
  - "Mesonephroid"
  - Associated with endometriosis and hypercalcemia
  - Benign clear cell tumors are RARE
  - Frozen sections to not have typical "clear cell" morphology
    - Clearing is an artifact of fixation, so frozen sections will not be clear but *will still show hobnailing*
    - Resembles mucinous
  - Morphology
    - Clear cells in papillary, glandular, nested, trabeculae patterns
      - Mixed patterns
    - Tend to fall out of centers of nests → *hobnail!*
      - See Fig. 4.2
    - Hyalinized fibrovascular cores
    - Hyaline globules
    - Can have prominent fibrous component, can be cystic
      - Versus fibroma or thecoma
        - CCC has admixed tumor cells
        - Ex. borderline clear cell adenofibroma

Fig. 4.2 Hobnail appearance of clear cell carcinoma caused by high-grade cells falling out of lumens.

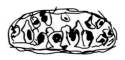

- Immunophenotype
  - Positive: CK, Leu-MI, PAS-D, VHL, HNF1β, napsin, racemase
  - Negative: AFP, WT1, ER/PR, GPC3
  - p53 wild-type
- Mixed tumors of endometrioid, and clear cell is not uncommon
  - But watch out for clear cell change in endometrioid
    - Need all features of clear cell carcinoma to call it a mixed tumor
  - Mixed endometrioid and serous are rare
  - Need to do MMR panels on endometrioid portion
- Chemo-resistant! Surgery and chemo
- Endometrioid
  - Benign
    - Adenofibroma or cystadenoma
  - Borderline
    - Looks like endometrial atypical hyperplasia
    - Microinvasion is uncommon
  - Endometriosis-associated in 42% (younger patients)
  - Typically stage 1 grade 1
  - Adenocarcinoma with squamous differentiation helps diagnose endometrioid
  - Sertoliform variant (no inhibin+)
  - Not *TP53* mutated, ER/PR+
  - Can be mistaken for metastatic colorectal adenocarcinoma
    - Colorectal: CK7+/−, CK20+, CDX2+
    - Endometrioid: CK7+, CK20−, CDX2−
- Brenner
  - Benign or malignant
  - Very hard to cut when fixed
- Small cell carcinoma of ovary, hypercalcemic type
  - Young patients—early 20s
  - Two-thirds of patients have hypercalcemia
    - Disappears after surgical resection
    - Poorer prognosis than normocalcemic
  - Morphology
    - Diffuse sheets of small, closely packed round cells with scant cytoplasm
    - Follicle-like structures with eosinophilic fluid
    - Small hyperchromatic nuclei with irregular chromatin clumps
    - Small but identifiable nucleoli
    - Cytoplasmic hyaline globules
    - Frequent mitotic figures and tumor necrosis with perivascular sparing
    - Rhabdoid
  - No Azzopardi effect
  - Large cell variant
    - Must be at least 50%
    - Abundant eosinophilic cytoplasm and large nuclei with prominent nucleoli

- Positive: CAM 5.2, vimentin (50%), variable chromogranin, laminin, PTH-related protein and EMA (30%)
  - *SMARC B1/INI1* loss
- Small cell carcinoma of ovary, pulmonary type
  - Older patients—late 50s/early 60s
  - Morphology
    - Sheets and nests of size round-to-spindle cells with hyperchromatic nuclei
    - Fine regular chromatin (not clumped)
    - Inconspicuous nucleoli and minimal cytoplasm
    - Crush artifact, Azzopardi effect
  - Occasionally associated with endometrioid carcinoma
  - May have squamous, mucinous, and Brenner differentiation
  - Immunophenotype
    - Positive for keratin, EMA, NSE; occasional chromogranin
    - Negative for vimentin
- Odds and ends
  - Ovarian tumors with follicles/follicle-like spaces
    - Clear cell carcinoma
    - Endometrioid carcinoma
    - Struma ovarii
    - Sertoli-Leydig
  - PARP inhibitors
    - Assist in base-excision repair
      - Inhibition stops single strand repair → single base mutations add up → double strand breaks occur
      - Best if used in homologous recombination deficient tumors that cannot fix double strand breaks
        - Like those with *BRCA* mutations!
- Goblet cell carcinoid of the ovary
  - Signet ring, goblet cell, some salt and pepper
  - Causes ascites (may get cytologic specimens)
  - Mucicarmine+
  - Chromogranin and synaptophysin is positive in some cells

Germ Cell Tumors (GCTs)

- General
- AFP is high in yolk sac tumor
- HCG in choriocarcinoma
- Both in embryonal
- Neither in teratoma
  - Teratoma
- Mature
  - Epidermoid cyst—keratinizing squamous epithelium without appendages
  - Dermoid cyst—keratinizing squamous epithelium with appendages and Rokitansky's tubercle
  - Struma ovarii—monodermal teratoma of only thyroid tissue
    - Strumal carcinoid = struma ovarii + trabecular carcinoid
    - Malignant struma = thyroid carcinoma (usually papillary thyroid carcinoma)
  - Fetiform teratoma—"homunculus"
  - Secondary carcinoid (insular > trabecular >> goblet cell)

- Secondary squamous cell carcinoma
- Teratoma + embryonal carcinoma = teratocarcinoma
- Immature
  - May come from (or progress through) embryonal carcinoma
  - Solid, usually do not metastasize to lymph nodes, need chemotherapy
  - Graded on amount of immature neuroepithelium (resemble tubules)
    - High-grade (can see primitive neuroepithelium easily) gets chemotherapy
    - Low-grade (have to hunt for it) may get chemotherapy
- Dysgerminoma
  - Seminoma counterpart
  - KIT, PLAP, OCT3/4, LDH
  - Most common immature GCT
  - May have syncytiotrophoblast component (with hCG secretion)
    - Do not worry about choriocarcinoma unless cytotrophoblasts are present
  - More common in those with dysgenic ovaries (i.e., Turner syndrome)
- Yolk sac tumor
  - (aka endodermal sinus)
  - Increased AFP, multiple patterns, PAS+ droplets, Schiller-Duval (SD) bodies
  - Patterns
    - Reticular (most common, lacy, "microcystic")
    - Macrocystic
    - Myxomatous
    - Papillary
    - Solid
    - Endodermal sinus (perivascular with SD bodies)
    - Alveolar-glandular
    - Polyvesicular
    - Hepatoid
    - Glandular (intestinal/primitive endodermal)
  - AFP+, CD30–, OCT3/4–
- Embryonal
  - CD30+
  - Highly pleomorphic
  - Polyembryoma—super rare variant composed only of embryoid bodies
- Choriocarcinoma
  - Solid sheets of large primitive cells
  - Admixed papillary areas with slit-like spaces
  - Numerous syncytiotrophoblasts (hCG+)
  - Positive for CD30, PLAP, NSE, and CK

Sex Cord–Stromal

- General
  - Normal component → malignant
    - Stroma → theca and Leydig
    - Sex cord → granulosa and Sertoli
    - Oocyte → germ cell tumors
  - Theca cells—stimulated by leutinizing hormone (LH), secrete androgens
    - Interna → thecoma
    - Externa → fibroma
    - Both → fibrothecoma

- Granulosa cells—stimulated by follicle-stimulating hormone (FSH), convert androgens to estrogen
  - Granulosa cell tumor
    - Pseudorosettes around gland-like spaces (rare)
    - Call-Exner bodies: hyaline globules
    - Cleaved coffee bean cells
    - Causes ER secretion → endometrial hyperplasia/carcinoma
      - Also thecomas and fibrothecomas
    - Inhibin+, CD99+
- All are positive for inhibin, calretinin, SF1
  - EMA−, may be cytokeratin+
  - Normal stroma is weak inhibin+, luteinized stroma is strongly positive
- Estrogenic tumors
  - Thecoma
  - Fibrothecoma
  - Granulosa cell tumor
  - Steroid cell tumor
- Fibroma
  - Most common sex cord/stromal tumor
  - Not hormonally active
  - Gorlin syndrome (nevoid basal cell carcinoma syndrome)
    - *PTCH1* mutation on 9q22.3
  - Meig syndrome (very large with ascites and pleural effusions)
  - Morphology
    - Bland wavy spindled cells without atypia, collagen bundles, storiform/whorls
    - Okay to be hypercellular and mitotically active—need to have a very high threshold for fibrosarcoma
      - Fibrosarcomas happen in Maffucci syndrome (enchondromas, hemangiomas, lymphangiomas)
    - Can have minor granulosa component
    - Can calcify
  - Benign but can recur (especially with rupture)
  - DDx includes granulosa cell tumor
    - Use reticulin! GCT → surrounds groups, fibroma → surrounds each cell
- Thecoma
  - Rare, benign
  - Estrogenic
  - Morphology
    - Polygonal cells with round nuclei, ill-defined cell borders, pink to pale gray cytoplasm, small nucleoli
    - Collagenized stroma that pushes follicles to the side
  - Reticulin stains similar to fibroma
  - Inhibin more strongly stains luteinized cells
  - *Bilateral luteinized thecomas with sclerosing peritonitis in younger patients*
    - Brisk mitoses, spindled, edema, trapped follicles
- Fibrothecoma
  - Both theca layers
  - Granulosa cell tumor
  - Meig and Gorlin syndromes
  - Can be estrogenic

- Adult granulosa cell tumor
  - Relatively common malignant stromal-sex cord tumor
  - Estrogenic, often symptomatic (bleeding)
    - Can cause atypical endometrial hyperplasia
  - Low-grade, rupture increases risk for recurrence
    - 20% to 30% recur—can be late (>5 but <20 years)
  - Can rarely be entirely cystic (difficult diagnosis)
  - Can be hemorrhagic
  - Small, round blue cells with nuclear grooves (coffee beans)
    - Delicate cords, solid, trabecular, watered silk
    - +/− Call-Exner bodies (microfollicles with eosinophilic secretions)
    - *Can look like anything*
      - *Pitfall—do not call carcinoma on frozen section!*
  - *FOXL2* mutations in almost all
  - May be CK+ (EMA− and CK7−)
  - Increased serum inhibin
  - Juvenile granulosa cell tumor
    - Maffucci syndrome
    - Precocious puberty
    - Low-stage, but can recur (<3 years)
    - No *FOXL2* mutation
    - Solid, hemorrhage, follicular (with eosinophilic secretions), ample cleared-out cytoplasm, *more atypia than adult*, less grooves than adult
- Benign Leydig or Hilus cells
  - Can surround rete ovarii, associated with hilar vessels and pseudoperineural invasion
  - More prominent in postmenopausal ovaries
  - Morphology
    - Reinke crystals—eosinophilic rod-shaped
    - Pink polygonal cells
    - Can have prominent clear cells (finely vacuolated) with anastomosing capillary network
  - Seen hyperplastic in stromal hyperplasia and hyperthecosis
  - + strong inhibin
  - + Melan-A and HMB-45
- Leydig cell tumor or Hilus cell tumor
  - Rare, androgen-producing
    - Hirsutism, androgyny
    - Very rarely, estrogenic presentation
  - Small mass, uniform polygonal cells in sheets and nests, rich capillary network
  - Occasional bizarre nuclei
  - Nuclear-rich and -poor zones (looks pseudopalisading)
    - Acellular eosinophilic regions
  - Fibrinoid necrosis of vessels
  - Reinke crystals
  - Can have associated nodular hilar cell hyperplasia and/or stromal hyperthecosis
  - Positive for inhibin, calretinin, Melan-A, SF1, and CD99
- Sertoli cell tumor
  - Grossly yellow, usually unilateral
  - Clinical
    - Usually estrogenic

- Uncommonly androgenic
- Very rarely both
- Most have a great prognosis
- Can be "malignant"
- Associated with Peutz-Jeghers syndrome
  - Tubular morphology
  - Heterologous elements, especially in intermediate and poorly differentiated
    - Most common is mucinous epithelium
  - Immunophenotype
    - Positive: CD99, calretinin, inhibin, CD19, AE1/AE3
  - Folliculoma lipidique = lipid-rich variant (oil red O positive)
- Sertoli-Leydig tumor (SLT)
  - Maybe from theca interna and granulosa layers
  - Unilateral, low stage
  - Leydig portion is tubular, Sertoli portion is solid between the tubules
  - Well-, mod-, poorly differentiated based on solid Sertoli component
    - More tubules—well differentiated
    - More solid—poor differentiated
  - Heterologous elements
    - Can be *very* prominent
  - Molecular classification
    - *DICER1* mutation
      - Young, high-grade, heterologous elements and/or retiform
      - Germline
        - Cystic nephroma
        - Nodular thyroid hyperplasia
        - Pleuropulmonary blastomas
      - 60% of sporadic SLTs have *DICER1* mutations
    - *FOXL2* mutation
      - Postmenopausal, high-grade, no heterologous elements or retiform
    - Wild-type
      - Intermediate age, low-grade
- Sex cord tumor with annular tubules (SCTAT)
  - Peutz-Jeghers (plus adenoma malignum)
  - Two cell layers separated by fibrillar cytoplasm
  - Basal lamina material accumulation in space
  - Sort of Call-Exner bodies
  - No benign vs. malignant—will recur
- Luteoma
  - Estrogenic (rarely androgenic)
  - Sixth to seventh decade of life
  - Organoid, sheets, nests
  - Round cells with prominent nucleoli
  - Associated with stromal hyperthecosis
- Luteoma of pregnancy
  - Androgenic → see painting of Magdalena Ventura with her husband and son
  - Abundant granular pink cytoplasm with round nucleus and single small nucleolus
  - Multinodular
    - Can be bilateral

- Steroid cell tumor, not otherwise specified (NOS)
  - Usually hormonally active
    - Androgenic > estrogenic > Cushing
    - Can be associated with endometrial hyperplasia
  - Poor prognostic features:
    - >7 cm
    - Necrosis
    - Hemorrhage
    - Nuclear atypia
    - >2 mitotic figures/10 hpf
  - Organoid, sheets, nests, polygonal cells with well-defined cell borders
  - Lipid-rich or -poor (depending on cytoplasm—granular or vacuolated, respectively)
- Sclerosing stromal tumor
  - Pseudolobular appearance
    - Hyper- and hypocellular areas
    - Edema, cystic
  - Bland, fibroblast-like spindled cells (can have polygonal/signet ring)
  - Hemangiopericytoma-like staghorn vessels
  - Low-power diagnosis
  - Positive for inhibin and calretinin
  - Can be luteinized in pregnancy
- Microcystic stromal tumor
  - Solid and cystic
  - Not hormonally active
  - *CTNNB1* mutations are common
  - CD10+ *FOXL2*+ SF1+ WT1+ nuclear beta-catenin+
    - calretinin−, inhibin−
  - Intracytoplasmic vacuoles
  - Eosinophilic secretions
  - Other
- Gonadoblastoma
  - Typically has germ cell tumor component (dysgerminoma) and a sex-cord stromal component (granulosa cell tumor with Call-Exner bodies)
    - 50% have coexisting dysgerminoma
    - Calcification and hyalinized stroma are common
    - Typically in gonadal dysgenesis (patients may be XXY). They do not metastasize but may undergo malignant transformation into a dysgerminoma → oophorectomy
- Metastases
  - Metastatic gastric adenocarcinoma is notorious for infiltrating in small glands with round, hyperchromatic nuclei
- Odds and ends
  - Ovarian tumors with papillary architecture
    - Serous
    - Clear cell
    - Yolk sac
    - Rarely endometrioid
  - Serous ovarian
    - High-or low-grade, WT-1+
    - Gets neoadjuvant

- VS serous endometrioid
  - Only high-grade, WT-1–
  - No neoadjuvant chemo
- Nests of urothelium in…
  - Tubes = Walthard rests
    - Paratubal cyst with chunky eosinophilic secretions and urothelial lining—cystic Walthard rest
  - Ovaries = Brenner rest

FALLOPIAN TUBE AND PERITONEUM

- Peritoneal leiomyomatosis
  - Disseminated leiomyomas, typically s/p morcellation of uterine leiomyoma
  - "Metastasizes" within vessels
- After removing immature teratoma, can get peritoneal gliomatosis
- *Front → Back, it's really f***ing obvious*
  - Round ligament, fallopian tube, ovary
- SCOUT—secretory cell outgrowths on fallopian tubes
  - Type I
  - Type II
  - Nuclear beta-catenin+ in epithelial and stromal cells
  - Associated with ovarian cancer but not directly linked
- Psammoma bodies suggest serous (but nonspecific)
- Endometriosis
  - Hemosiderin, capillaries, denser stroma, glands
  - CD10+ stroma
- Endosalpingiosis
  - Proliferation of benign plans and cysts lined by ciliated tube-like epithelium
  - Microscopic incidental finding

CHAPTER 5

Placenta and Products of Conception

Products of Conception and Normal Anatomy/Physiology

- 1 to 8 weeks—embryo, 8+ weeks—fetus
- Trimesters
    - 1st = 1 to 13 weeks
    - 2nd = 14 to 26 weeks
    - 3rd = 27 to 42 weeks
- "Term birth" = 38 weeks or later
- Possible components
    - Endometrium
    - Decidua
    - Chorionic villi
    - Fetal tissue
        - Myocytes are heavily glycogenized (pale)
        - Liver is full of extramedullary hematopoiesis
    - Fetal membranes
    - Blood clot
    - Implantation site
        - See Fig. 5.1
- Normal anatomy
    - See Fig. 5.2

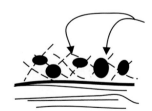

Fig. 5.1 Implantation site morphology. *CK*, cytokeratin.

Intermediate extravillous trophoblasts (CK+)

Nitabuch's fibrinoid

Decidua

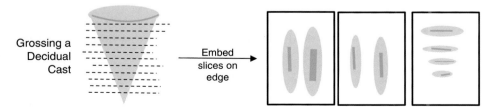

Grossing a Decidual Cast

Embed slices on edge

Fig. 5.2 Grossing a decidual cast.

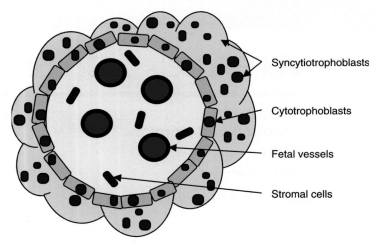

Fig. 5.3 Morphology of chorionic villi.

- Intermediate trophoblasts (X-cells, extravillous trophoblasts) invade decidua into the media of spiral arteries, keratin+
- Chorionic villi
  - Villi are part of the chorionic layer
  - See Fig. 5.3
  - Mature villi—<50% of stroma is dilated vessels (compared with >50% in terminal villi)
    - Immature villi are more bulbous with reticular stroma and Hofbauer cells
  - Intermediate trophoblasts = keratin (+) vimentin (−)
    - Decidua = keratin (−) vimentin (+)
    - Useful in accreta cases
    - Loss of decidua between chorion and myometrium
- Multiple gestations
  - Weigh placentas together even if submitted separately (but after trimming)
  - "Twin placenta, [two discs/fused disc], [mono]chorionic-[di]amniotic, term"
  - See Table 5.1
- Sexing a fetus
  - Gender identity is formed at ~12 weeks (crown-rump length of 6 cm and foot length of 1 cm)
  - Both have phallus, females have split labial swellings
  - Ovaries are sausage-shaped compared with egg-shaped testes
  - See Fig. 5.4
- Normal physiology pearls
  - Fetal hematopoiesis
    - Yolk sac to liver to bone marrow
    - Nucleated red blood cells (RBCs) start in villous capillaries at around 8 to 9 weeks, gone by around 16 weeks
- Our job is to
  - 1. Prove the pregnancy was intrauterine OR alert clinical team that ectopic pregnancy may be possible
    - Histologic proof
      - Chorionic villi

TABLE 5.1 ■ **Types of Intermediate Trophoblasts**

Type	Location	Morphology
Villous	At anchoring villi of trophoblastic column	Polyhedral, uniform nuclei, prominent cell borders
Implantation site	Implantation site	Pleomorphic irregular nuclei, hyperchromatic, large, +/– multinucleation Abundant eosinophilic to amphophilic cytoplasm Infiltrative growth into mother's vessels
Chorionic-type	At chorionic laeve of fetal membranes	Round nuclei, +/– multinucleation, cohesive growth

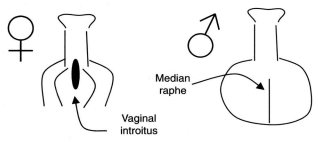

Fig. 5.4 Sexing a fetus over 12 weeks gestation.

- ▨ Embryonic/fetal tissue
- ▨ Implantation site
- ▪ Imaging ("fetal sac present")
- ▪ 2. Evaluate for molar pregnancy (see "Molar Pregnancy" section later)
- ▪ 3. Evaluate for fetal or placental defects, infections, or other causes of spontaneous abortion (SAB)
  - ▨ 50% of SAB are caused by chromosomal abnormalities
  - ▨ Growth disorganized
  - ▨ Specific developmental defect
  - ▨ Macerated, damaged, and so on
  - ▨ Inflammation (see "Placental Infections/Inflammation" section later)
- ▪ Pitfalls and red herrings
  - ▪ Arias-Stella reaction—well-formed glands with ballooning, cleared-out cytoplasm, and very pleomorphic nuclei but NO MITOSES
    - ▨ Normal pregnancy reaction
    - ▨ Endometrial glands with hobnailed and cleared cytoplasm, nuclear atypia
  - ▪ Villi in ectopic pregnancies look a little more compact with "juicier" syncytiotrophoblasts
  - ▪ Perivillous fibrinoid (not "fibrin")
    - ▨ Usually incidental, not usually important in small numbers
    - ▨ Do not mistake for infarcts
    - ▨ Looks gray and rubbery grossly
    - ▨ Massive perivillous fibrinoid = >⅓ involved
      - ▨ Can predict recurrent pregnancy loss
      - ▨ Caused by decreased placental function

- Villus with what looks like cytotrophoblast cap = anchoring column in early pregnancy
  - Do not mistake for trophoblastic hyperplasia
- Villi with degenerative changes = myxoid stroma, hypocellular, no blood vessels (endothelial apoptosis → extravasated RBCs)

Molar Pregnancies

- *TP 57*
  - Paternally imprinted tumor suppressor gene on chromosome 11 (only maternal allele is expressed)
    - See Table 5.2
  - Syncytiotrophoblasts are always negative
  - Extravillous trophoblasts are always positive
- Determine ploidy with cytogenetics, flow cytometry, short tandem repeats (STR, through CODIS), or FISH
  - Partial moles are diandric
- Complete hydatidiform mole
  - Diploid (46XX usually)
    - Empty ovum fertilized by sperm, then duplication of chromosomes
    - Rarely dispermy (46XX or 46XY)
    - No maternal genetic material
  - Higher risk for trophoblastic sequelae than partial moles
    - More aggressive, more likely to transform
  - Really high hCG
    - Can present with larger-than-dates uterus, preeclampsia, hyperemesis, hyperthyroidism, respiratory distress
  - Morphology
    - Diffusely hydropic villi, all villi involved
    - Diffuse (concentric) trophoblastic hyperplasia
    - Central cistern caused by necrosis
    - Marked atypia of implantation site
    - Amnion, yolk sac, and nucleated RBCs are absent
  - Early complete mole morphology
    - Can be difficult!
    - Irregular bulbous villi (claw-like or cauliflower-like)
    - Hypercellular blue stroma with network of stromal vessels
    - Prominent stromal karyorrhexis/apoptosis

TABLE 5.2 ■ *p57* Staining Patterns

Type	Cytotrophoblasts	Villous Stromal Cells
Normal conceptus	Positive	Positive
Complete mole	Negative	Negative
Partial mole	Positive	Positive
Mosaicism in mole	Some negative villi	Some negative villi
Mesenchymal dysplasia	Positive	Negative

- Circumferential syncytiotrophoblast hyperplasia
  - Can be rare or hard to find
- Exaggerated implantation site with frankly atypical trophoblasts
  - Also called *exaggerated placental site*
- Can get "complete mole with coexisting fetus" (CMCEF)
  - Relatively normal fetus with twin mole
  - Results from separate fertilization events ("fraternal")
- Biparental complete mole
  - Way of getting rid of mutated maternal gene (then spermatic DNA duplication) but not getting rid of *all* of mother's genome
  - Tend to have recurrent moles, less common live births
  - Several recurrent gene mutations
  - Use STR to differentiate from uniparental moles
- Partial hydatidiform mole
  - Triploid
    - Dispermic fertilization of normal ovum
    - 69XXX or 69XXY (>>>69XYY)
  - Low risk for trophoblastic sequelae
  - hCG < 100, 00 mIU/mL
  - Present as missed abortion
  - Morphology
    - Two distinct villous populations
      - Hydropic villi
      - Normal or sclerotic villi
    - Can have cisterns but not as abundant or prominent as complete moles
    - Can have fetal tissue or nucleated RBCs
      - May have polydactyly, cleft lip, and so on.
      - Do not need p57 stain to prove it is a partial mole
    - Focal trophoblastic hyperplasia (tufts) with scalloped or shaggy edges, plane-of-section artifactual "inclusions," lacy mounds
  - DDx = hydropic abortus (incomplete abortion with degenerative changes)—have continuum between normal villi and hydropic villi (not two distinct populations)
  - Retained p57 expression
  - Determine ploidy with cytogenetics, flow cytometry, STR (through CODIS), or FISH
    - Partial moles are diandric
    - Nonmolar triploid pregnancies are digynic
- Mosaicism
  - p57 is lost in some hydropic villi but retained in others
- Placental mesenchymal dysplasia
  - One-third of cases are seen in Beckwith-Wiedemann syndrome
  - Placentomegaly, enlarged and cystic villi but without syncytiotrophoblast hyperplasia
  - Thick-walled villous vessels with dilation and/or thrombi
  - p57 lost in villous stromal cells but retained in cytotrophoblasts
- Invasive moles—invade myometrium
  - Staged
  - Metastasize most commonly to the lungs
  - Increased risk for trophoblastic carcinoma
- Moles can metastasize
  - Monitor with quantitative hCG after dilation and curettage (D&C) or dilation and evacuation (D&E)

- Can repeat D&C or go straight to methotrexate if hCG level is increasing or not dropping appropriately
- Do not overlook a molar twin in a term gestation

Placental Infections/Inflammation

- Normally, there should be no plasma cells in the decidua and no inflammation in the villi
- In very macerated tissue, submit some tissue to assess for spirochetes
- Chorioamnionitis
  - Neutrophils and bacteria in fetal lungs and GI tract
  - When amnion gets reactive (proliferative, more juicy than plain cuboidal), look for chorioamnionitis!
  - Patterns are described by maternal and fetal response, both are staged and graded
    - Maternal response
      - Stages
        - 1—Acute subchorionitis or chorionitis
          - Neutrophils in subchorionic fibrin or with membrane trophoblasts
        - 2—Acute chorioamnionitis
          - Patchy diffuse neutrophils in fibrous chorion and/or amnion
        - 3—Necrotizing chorioamnionitis
          - Neutrophils undergoing karyorrhexis, amniocyte necrosis, amnion membrane thickening/hypereosinophilia
      - Grade
        - 1 to 2—(No special terminology)—not as severe as grade 3
        - 3—Severe acute chorioamnionitis OR subchorionic microabscesses
          - More than three large neutrophil collections between chorion and decidua OR continuous band of neutrophils
    - Fetal response
      - Stage
        - 1—Chorionic vasculitis or umbilical phlebitis
        - 2—Umbilical vasculitis (one or both arteries +/– vein)
        - 3—Necrotizing "funisitis" (inflammation of umbilical cord) or concentric umbilical perivasculitis
      - Grade
        - 1 to 2—(No special terminology)—not as severe as grade 3
        - 3—Severe fetal inflammatory response
          - Abundant intramural neutrophils in chorionic or umbilical vessels with destruction of muscular layer
      - Isolated umbilical phlebitis
        - Do not grade/stage
        - Could be secondary to prophylactic antibiotics given to mother for Group B streptococcus (GBS)
- Patchy villous edema in the setting of chorioamnionitis = poor prognosis
- Pigmented macrophages in membranes—"Pigment consistent with meconium"
  - If there is a lot, do an iron stain to check for hemosiderin (which should be darker and chunkier). Could indicate chronic hemosiderosis, which has pulmonary implications for the baby
  - Amnion undergoes coagulative necrosis
- Villitis
  - Plasma cells—CMV
  - Only lymphocytes—chronic villitis of unknown etiology

- Tends to be along maternal plate
- Graded and staged
- HSV, CMV, Treponema, toxoplasma stains
  - Check serum first for Treponema
- Tend to occur with chronic deciduitis
- Parvovirus
  - Erythroblasts with glassy intranuclear inclusions
  - With deep blue cytoplasm
- Candida—half-moon abscesses on outside of umbilical cord
- Listeria—rampant intervillositis (mother's blood space filled with neutrophils)

Gestational Trophoblastic Disease

- See Fig. 5.5
- Choriocarcinoma
  - Morphology
    - Biphasic
      - Mononuclear trophoblasts (intermediate and cytotrophoblasts) and syncytiotrophoblasts
      - Highly atypical
    - Do not get villi!
    - Prominent vasculature

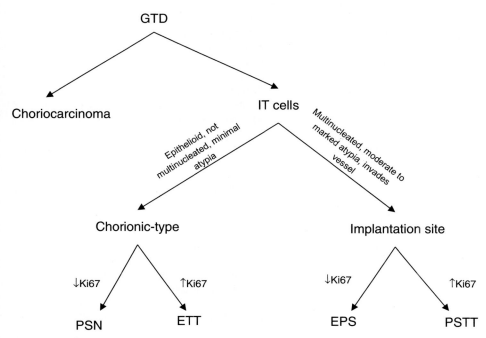

Fig. 5.5 Algorithm for categorizing gestational trophoblastic disease (GTD). *EPS*, exaggerated placental site; *ETT*, epithelioid trophoblastic tumor; *IT*, intermediate trophoblasts; *PSN*, placental site nodule; *PSTT*, placental site trophoblastic tumor.

- Antecedent pregnancy is most commonly a mole (50%) > miscarriage > normal pregnancy > ectopic
  - Usually several months but can be up to 14 years later
    - Variants or subtypes
  - Intraplacental choriocarcinomas are rare
    - Can metastasize to mother or baby
  - Nongestational choriocarcinomas are rare (germ cell tumor)
  - Somatic tumors (carcinomas with trophoblastic differentiation) are rare
- Present with vaginal bleeding
- Tends to metastasize to liver, lung, and brain
- hCG level is typically extremely high
- May be found admixed with epithelioid trophoblastic tumor or placental site trophoblastic tumor
- Lesions of extravillous trophoblasts
  - Implantation site-type intermediate trophoblasts (ITs)—express human placental lactogen (hPL)
    - Exaggerated placental site (EPS)
      - Nonneoplastic ("benign")
      - Intermediate trophoblasts proliferate around decidual vessels with fibrinoid material
        - Only mononuclear cells
      - Villi should be present unless there has already been a curettage
      - Ki67 ~0%
    - Placental site trophoblastic tumor (PSTT)
      - Malignant counterpart to EPS
      - 12 to 18 months after pregnancy (range 2 weeks to 17 years)
        - Most commonly after normal pregnancy (not molar)
      - Elevated serum beta-hCG (low levels <1000)
      - Do not respond to chemotherapy
      - Morphology
        - Almost all mononuclear cells with marked pleomorphism
          - Rare multinucleated cells but not enough for choriocarcinoma
        - Fibrinoid necrosis of decidual arteries (like deciduopathy)
        - Vascular invasion
        - No/rare calcifications
        - No villi
      - IHC
        - Positive for hPL (diffuse), MUC4, Mel-CAM, GATA3 (usually), inhibin (patchy), hCG (patchy)
        - Negative for PLAP and p63
        - Ki67 >10%
  - Chorionic-type ITs—express placental alkaline phosphatase (PLAP)
    - Placental site nodule (PSN)
      - Benign counterpart to epithelioid trophoblastic tumor
      - Interval after pregnancy 2 to 108 months, usually incidental
      - Morphology
        - Pink hyaline, paucicellular material with mostly mononuclear cells
        - Cord pattern
        - No villi
        - Invade vessels
      - IHC

- Positive for EMA, PLAP, inhibin A, p63, cytokeratin
- Negative for hCG, hPL
- Low Ki67 (3% to 10%)
- "Atypical PSN" has higher Ki67, more cellular, clinical significance unknown
- Epithelioid trophoblastic tumor (ETT)
  - Malignant
  - Resembles carcinoma
  - hCG mildly elevated (<2500)
  - Interval = 1 to 25 years (mean 6 years) after normal pregnancy
  - Can metastasize
  - Classically involves cervix, biopsied and misdiagnosed as squamous cell carcinoma
  - Morphology
    - Mononuclear cells (relatively uniform)
    - Hyaline-like material (similar to PSN)
    - Necrosis
    - Calcifications are common
  - *Does not invade vessels like PSTT; tumor cells are smaller than PSTT*
  - IHC
    - Positive for PLAP, focal hPL, p63, GATA3, inhibin
    - Ki67 ~10%

Other Placental Pathology

- More syncytial knots (multinucleated cap of syncytiotrophoblasts, no fibrovascular core) as placenta matures
- Intravillous hemorrhage
  - Cord accident
  - Abruption
  - Mechanical
- Chorangiosis = increased vessels in villi, seen in diabetics and pregnancies at high elevation
  - Rare, not just ectatic vessels (which is a normal change later in pregnancy)
  - 10 fields with 10 villi with 10 capillaries
  - *Chorangioma*—a single tumor (vs. diffuse increased vessels in chorangiosis)
- Diabetes effects on the placenta—chorangiosis, immature villi (especially distal villi) (rarely hypermature), large for gestational age
- Preeclampsia effects on the placenta
  - Decidual vasculopathy—fibrinoid necrosis of decidual vessels, luminal foamy macrophages and fibrin, destruction of arterial wall
  - Hypertrophic vasculopathy—retained muscular wall of maternal floor vessels
  - Increased perivillous fibrin, syncytial knots, and villous maturity
- Cord hypercoiling suggests fetal distress
- Amnion nodosum
  - Anucleate squamous cells and hair from fetus adhered to amnion
  - Secondary to oligohydramnios
- Dysmorphic villi = edematous villi
  - Nonspecific but can be seen in chromosomal abnormalities, vasculopathy, and so on
- Endothelial cushions—myxoid hump with fibrin
  - *Must* have sclerotic downstream villi
- Infarct (see Fig. 5.6)
  - Red infarct—massive congestion of villi, matted together, cannot tell villi apart

- Cell death (coagulative necrosis)
- Involution
- How to estimate percentage of placental disc involved by infarcts
  - Break into quadrants
  - Estimate how much of each quadrant is involved
  - Add all together and divide by 4
  - See Fig. 5.7
- Twin gestations
  - Fibrotic avascular villi indicate fetal thrombotic vasculopathy
  - Associated with poor outcomes
  - Circumvallate vs. circummarginate—see Fig. 5.8
  - Retroplacental hemorrhage = pathologic correlate of placental abruption
  - Clinical—vaginal bleeding and abdominal pain
  - Symptoms are not well-correlated with outcome (can bleed a lot and be fine)
  - Patchy retromembranous hemorrhage—fibrin, emulsified blood, hemosiderin-laden macrophages
    - Relevant if there is a lot of it
- Retromembranous = under decidua

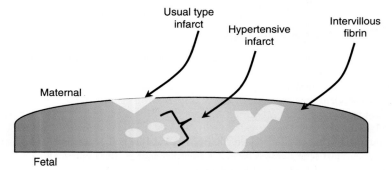

Fig. 5.6   Types of placental infarcts/lesions.

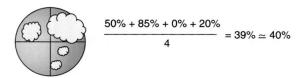

Fig. 5.7   Estimating percentage of placental involvement by infarcts/lesions.

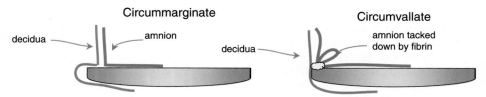

Fig. 5.8   How to differentiate between circummarginate and circumvallate membrane insertion.

- Intramembranous = between decidua and chorion or subamniotic
- Trisomy 21 placentas
  - Sometimes normal
  - Sometimes edematous and/or with dysmorphic villi (oddly shaped)
- Can get placental fibrosarcoma when the fetus gets congenital FS (secondary to field defect)
  - Placental tumors are rare; most common is chorangioma
- Villous stromal sclerosis secondary to stem villous thrombosis
- Nonmolar hydropic degenerative villi—round contours, thin trophoblastic rim, myxoid stroma

CHAPTER 6

Pediatric Pathology

Normal Anatomy and Physiology

- Hematopoiesis
  - Second trimester (after 6 to 7 weeks)—liver
    - Myelopoiesis in portal triads, erythropoiesis in lobules
    - Hematopoietic cells compose 50% of liver
    - After 32 weeks—little hematopoiesis in the portal triads
    - By 36 weeks—only small scattered lobular islands
- Transition to adult circulation
  - Pulmonary vascular resistance decreases
  - Pulmonary blood flow increases
  - Left atrial pressure increases
  - Foramen ovale closes
  - Ductus venosus closes
  - Liver blood flow increases
  - Proximal umbilical arteries stay patent as superior vesicle arteries
  - Prostaglandins drop
  - Ductus arteriosus closes

Metabolic Disorders

- Hurlers
  - Colloidal iron is positive in acid mucopolysaccharides
    - Stain also useful for necrobiotic xanthogranuloma
  - Will be in connective tissues (cannot see on H&E)
    - May see bluish edema/pools in rare cases
- Ornithine transcarbamylase deficiency → need liver transplants
  - Explanted livers are histologically normal

Genetic Collagen Disorders

See Table 6.1.

Gastrointestinal

- Immunohistochemistry pearls in the gastrointestinal tract
  - CD10+ in small intestine (and microvillous inclusion disease)
  - CEA+ in large intestine
  - SMA stains alpha-actin
  - MSA is supposed to stain alpha- and gamma-actin but really only stains gamma-actin
  - CD4– T-helper cells and macrophages
  - CD68– PGM1 more specific in KP1
  - Lysozyme—specific for enzyme

TABLE 6.1 ■ Genetic Collagen Disorders

Collagen I	Hard and soft tissues	Osteogenesis imperfecta
Collagen II	Cartilage, intervertebral disks, vitreous	Achondrogenesis type II, spondyloe Aptara
Collagen III	Hollow organs, soft tissues	Vascular Ehlers-Danlos syndrome
Collagen IV	Basement membrane (only nonfibrillar)	Alport syndrome
Collagen V	Soft tissue, blood vessels	Classical Ehlers-Danlos syndrome
Collagen IX and XI	Cartilage, vitreous	Stickler syndrome

- Esophagus
  - Eosinophilic esophagitis
    - Diagnostic criteria
      - Superficial pooling and microabscesses for eosinophilic esophagitis OR
      - Lots of eosinophils are present and the mid-esophagus is more involved than distal OR
      - Symptom relief with eliminating trigger
    - Eosinophils can be found in allergic and reflux esophagitis
  - Compact superficial squamous cells (almost parakeratotic) = reparative change
  - Candida esophagitis
    - Superficial neutrophils and microabscesses
    - Parakeratotic scale with hyphae that may flake off into specimen jar
      - Do not invade deeply
    - Best method of diagnosis = brushing (not biopsy)
      - DDx includes herpes ulcer (zebra stripes of neutrophils)
- Stomach
  - May have neutrophils in superficial lamina propria normally
  - Chronic PPI use—increased enterochromaffin-like (round with halos, cytoplasmic granules) cells and parietal cell pseudohypertrophy
  - Ferrous sulfate pills—crystalline → gray/black amorphous
  - Incidental appendectomy (88302) versus appendectomy for acute appendicitis charges (88304)
  - *Helicobacter heilmannii*—stains positive with *Helicobacter pylori* IHC, spirochete!
    - Reservoir in animals
    - Tend to have marked acute inflammation
- Duodenum
  - Children usually have ↑↑↑ tissue transglutaminase (TTG) IgA (but not in IgA-deficient patients)
    - Celiac
      - Villous atrophy, crypt hyperplasia, intraepithelial lymphocytes (>20 lymphocytes per 100 enterocyte nuclei)
      - Often a background of acute duodenitis (increased acute/chronic inflammation in the lamina propria)
      - Most commonly found in the duodenal bulb (sometimes not biopsied, can miss it)
      - If TTG IgA is minimally elevated (~20), may see some villous blunting (probably not rip-roaring celiac)

- Villous atrophy + crypt hypoplasia in duodenum +/− acute duodenitis → nutritional deficiency
- Microvillous inclusion disease (MVID)
  - Villous blunting
  - Vacuoles with microvilli in them that cannot fuse with apical cytoplasm to create brush border
  - Mainly small bowel, can include colon
  - PAS+ vesicles, CD10+
  - Congenital (young children), present as neonates
  - Loose stool → malnutrition → failure to thrive → death
  - Can also have progressive familial intrahepatic cholestasis
- Autoimmune enteritis—antibody against Paneth, parietal, or goblet cells
- Brunner glands all have a round profile and tiny dark nuclei against basal plate
  - Versus antral crypts, which are branching with larger, paler nuclei up off basal plate
- Inflammatory bowel disease
  - Clinical
    - Children may have self-limited colitis without real chronicity
    - Do not need to distinguish between Crohn's disease (CD) and ulcerative colitis (UC); that is a clinical call
  - Morphology
    - Cryptitis, crypt distortion, basal plasmacytosis
    - Paneth cells are okay to be in the right colon
    - Widening of lamina propria, diminished surface mucus production
    - Up to 10% of CD can have Schaumann-like crystals
    - Order CMV immunostains if there are prominent lymphocytes and plasma cells
  - Differences in pediatric patients versus adults
    - Children with ulcerative colitis will often get rectal sparing
    - Children with CD can get pancolitis and no involvement of terminal ileum
  - Pitfall
    - Granulomas in the ileum can be caused by *Campylobacter jejuni*, mycobacteria, mucous granulomas, sarcoid
- Hirschsprung's disease (HD)
  - Must assess for ganglia
    - Ganglions = ganglion cells and enteraglia in a rosette with central neuropil
      - Adult ganglion features
        - Low N:C ratio with eccentric nucleus
        - Peripheral Nissl substance
        - Prominent nucleolus and pale chromatin
        - Loose rosette or cluster
      - Pediatric ganglion features
        - High N:C ratio with central nucleus
        - Minimal Nissl substance
        - Dispersed "salt and pepper" chromatin without nucleolus
        - Distinct rosette pattern
    - Only present below the muscularis mucosae (none in the lamina propria)
    - Ganglia outside outer longitudinal muscle layer do not "count" for Hirschsprung test
      - They must be between muscular layers (Auerbach/intermuscular plexus) or in submucosa (Meissner/submucosal plexus).
    - Will get a circumferential "donut" margin → need to identify ganglia in at least 7 of 8 sectors to ensure good function after anastomosis

- Physiologic aganglionic zone
  - Up to 2 cm past the dentate line
  - May have a calretinin+ network
  - Ganglia gets more sparse distally
    - More likely to see single scattered ganglia
- Dysmotility without HD = "intestinal neuronal dysplasia"
  - Wait for children to mature, do ACE (anterograde continent enema, uses tip of appendix as stoma for saline flushes), use colon manometry
  - Rarely take colon out if secondary infection or inflammation occurs
- Staining in HD
  - Acetylcholine esterase stain (enzymatic stain)
    - Need fresh tissue
    - Total colonic HD may have normal staining pattern
  - Calretinin
    - Any bona fide calretinin plexus fibers present is not compatible with HD
    - Does not stain intermuscular fibers; does not stain submucosal fibers that hug glands
  - PTEN is the universal ganglion stain
  - Trichrome
    - Muscle = red
    - Collagen = dark blue
    - Neuropil = light blue to pink
  - CD56 ("NCAM")—stains neuromuscular junctions, enteraglia, and neuropil
  - S100 is positive in ganglion cells
  - NSE is positive in ganglion cells, inner circular fibers, and neural processes
- General intestine
  - Adenovirus can cause intussusception via mesenteric adenitis
    - Treatment is appendectomy and surgical reduction
    - Cowdry nuclear inclusions and smudged nuclei
  - Short gut or malabsorption leads to increased luminal fatty acids that binds Ca^{++}, freeing up oxalate to be reabsorbed (primarily in the colon)
    - Increased oxalate kidney stones
  - Melanosis coli
    - Negative for Prussian blue (not iron)
    - Positive for melanin (but light brown, not normal dark diffuse black) and Fontana-Masson
  - Stages of necrotizing enterocolitis
    - Stage 1 is coagulative necrosis—everything is pale pink
    - Stage 2 is acute inflammation
    - Stage 3 is sloughing of mucosa and granulation tissue
    - Stage 4 is resolution of granulation tissue and reepithelialization with stricture formation (if they live)
  - Tufting enteropathy
    - Teardrop tufts
    - Failure to thrive
    - Electron microscopy: intracellular junctions
    - EpCAM loss
- Liver
  - Normal anatomy, physiology, and phenotype
    - Liver parenchyma is derived from the foregut (endoderm), and the connective tissue elements (stroma and capsule) derive from the transverse septum (the mesodermal plate that separates the thoracic from abdominal cavities).

- Regenerative hepatocytes at limiting plate can pick up CK7
  - Normally bile ducts and capsule are the only positive tissues in liver
- CD31 stains hepatic sinusoids, and CD34 does not
- Ceroid-laden macrophages in liver (PAS-D+)
- Biliary atresia
  - Morphology
    - Widening of portal areas with portal fibrosis and bile duct proliferation
    - Bile plugs in ducts, canalicular bile stasis, intrahepatic bile
    - +/− portal-portal bridging fibrosis
  - Kasai procedure
    - One-third go to transplant right away
    - One-third do okay for a while and then go to transplant
    - One-third do well for a long time
  - "Changes consistent with extrahepatic biliary obstruction (see microscopic description)"
- Hepatoblastoma
  - Mixed epithelial and mesenchymal = epithelial hepatoblastoma + fibroblasts, osteoid, skeletal muscle, or chondroid
  - "Hepatoblastoma with teratoid features" = mixed epithelial and mesenchymal hepatoblastoma features + stratified squamous epithelium, mucinous epithelium, neuroglial tissues, and/or melanin-containing cells, among others
  - See Fig. 6.1
  - Prognosis associated with epithelial components
    - Pure fetal histology—favorable prognosis
    - Small cell/undifferentiated—poor prognosis
    - Embryonal—between the two
  - Can get islands of extramedullary hematopoiesis
  - Increased in those with FAP and Beckwith-Wiedemann
  - Use AFP to monitor for recurrence
- Pancreas
  - Pancreatoblastoma
    - Children 2 to 3 years of age
    - Solid and lobulated
    - Epithelial (solid, acinar, "squamoid corpuscles") and stromal
    - Positive for nuclear beta-catenin, trypsin, and lipase
    - Surgical resection for primary and metastases
      - Long-term survival is pretty high

Soft Tissue Neoplasms

- Immunohistochemistry
  - CD99
    - Ewing sarcoma
      - 60% are NKX2.2+
      - Depending on translocation, can use FLI1 IHC
    - Synovial sarcoma
      - CD56, bcl2, CD99
      - Do genetics
      - May have dim INI1 (heterozygous loss)
    - Benign lymphocytes
  - Myogenin for rhabdomyosarcoma

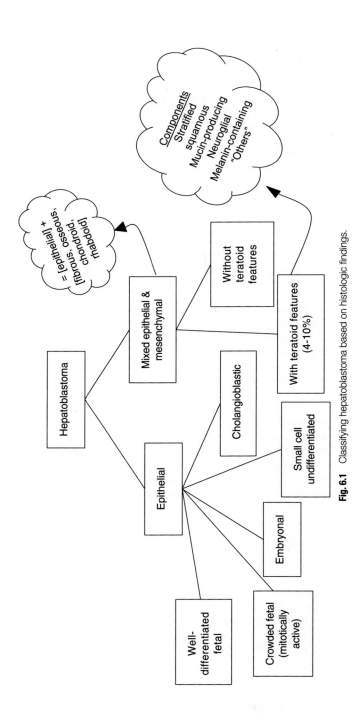

Fig. 6.1 Classifying hepatoblastoma based on histologic findings.

- myoD1+ for embryonal rhabdomyosarcoma
- Reticulin
  - Wraps around smooth muscle tumors but not fibroblastic tumors
- Osteosarcoma
  - Large, pleomorphic, distinct cell borders and a large single nucleolus
  - Telangiectatic osteosarcoma
    - Radiology looks benign (like aneurysmal bone cyst)
    - Frankly malignant histology with blood lakes
    - There is a high-grade variant
- Fibrous dysplasia—medullary lesion (not keratin+)
  - Osteofibrous dysplasia (OFD)—anterior cortical lesion
  - OFD-like adamantinoma—can have epithelium, starts in the anterior cortex but can become medullary, one trisomy is not found in OFD
    - Spindle cells are keratin+
- *NTRK* neoplasms
  - Infantile fibrosarcoma, spindle cell sarcoma, secretory breast carcinoma, mammary analog secretory carcinoma (salivary gland), congenital mesoblastic nephroma
    - Provisional—*NTRK*-related sarcoma
  - CD30+
  - Superficial CD34+
  - *NTRK3-ETV6* translocation
- To count/quantify treatment effect, need to see ***necrosis or viable tumor***—not just fibrosis
  - Reactive changes—be careful!
- *USP6* rearrangements in aneurysmal bone cysts (ABC) → "blue bone fragments"
  - Nonossifying fibroma can get ABC-like changes
    - Collagenous/fibrous background
  - Rule out telangiectatic osteosarcoma
  - Can get solid ABCs; may have a little atypia, bone formation, mitoses
  - DDx also includes giant cell tumor of bone
    - Sea of monotonous ladybug cells and giant cells
- Inclusion body fibromatosis
  - Aka infantile digital fibrosarcoma
  - Benign, recur locally
  - Most <1 year of age, hands and feet
  - Bland fibroblastic proliferation with eosinophilic paranuclear inclusions
- Fibrous hamartoma of infancy
  - Older than 1 year of age, males > females, trunk
  - Components
    - Adipose
    - Fibrous tissue
    - Primitive mesenchymal cells
  - Benign, may recur locally

Genitourinary

GENITAL PATHOLOGY

- Gonadal dysgenesis
  - Most common causes = XO or XY chimera
  - Get gonadoblastomas more frequently
    - Dysgerminoma/seminoma + abnormal granulosa cells or Sertoli/Leydig cells

- Can get separate dysgenetic testis and ovary OR intermingled tissue
  - Vas deferens has three separate muscle layers; epididymis has two (both lined by columnar cells with stereo-cilia
  - Balanitis xerotica obliterans—peak in children and middle aged

PEDIATRIC RENAL NEOPLASMS

- Wilms tumor (WT, "nephroblastoma")
  - Children 3 to 5 years of age, most unilateral and unicentric *but* those treated for unilateral WT are at increased risk for a subsequent second WT (presumably because the patient has increased nephrogenic rests)
  - Bilateral in 5% (higher in those with autosomal dominant-inherited familial nephroblastoma disease)
  - WAGR
    - Deletion on 11p13 (*WT1* gene)
    - Wilms tumor, aniridia, genitourinary malformation, retardation
  - Classic triphasic morphology has
    - Blastemal—small round blue cells with neuroendocrine nuclear features
    - Epithelial—tubules, rosette-like structures, glomeruloids
    - Stromal—stellate cells in a myxoid background, spindle cells, smooth muscle, striated muscle, fat, cartilage, osteoid, neuroglia
  - Can have any component by itself
  - Immunohistochemistry
    - *WT1* is positive in primitive epithelial and blastemal components
      - Negative in stromal and well-differentiated epithelium
    - Epithelial component is keratin+
    - Blastemal component is strong and diffuse CD56+
    - 75% of anaplastic WT has nuclear p53
  - Needle core with blastema only
    - DDx includes neuroblastoma, synovial sarcoma, PNET, clear cell sarcoma of the kidney, renal rhabdoid tumor, renal lymphoma·
  - Prognosis
    - Poor prognosis
      - Anaplasia
        - Nuclear pleomorphism—one 3× as big as others
        - Atypical mitotic figures
        - Hyperchromatic
        - Can be focal or diffuse
      - Loss of heterozygosity of 1p and 16q
      - TrkB neurotrophin receptor expression
      - *MYCN* amplification
        - Those <1 year of age can have metastases to liver, skin, and bone, and still have a 3-year overall survival of 93%, but if *MYCN* is amplified, 3-year overall survival drops to 10%
    - Favorable prognosis
      - Hyperdiploid
      - Expression of TrkA neurotrophin receptor
- Cystic renal lesions
  - Cystic renal dysplasia
    - If severe and bilateral → Potter's sequence, incompatible with life

- Potter's sequence findings are all caused by oligohydramnios because fetal urine is the primary component
  - Pulmonary hypoplasia, flattened facies, clubbed feet
- Cystic nephroma (CN)
  - Cystic well-circumscribed lesion with septa that have no solid nodules and only mature elements
- Cystic partially differentiated nephroblastoma (CPDN)
  - Septa also contain embryonal elements but do not form nodules (conform to the shape of the septa)
  - Side note—the plural of septum is *septa*, not *septae*
- Cystic Wilms tumor (CWT)
  - Classic components of WT forming nodules that distort septal contours
- CN and CPDN treated by excision only, CWT is treated like WT (chemo)
- Clear cell sarcoma of the kidney
  - 3% of malignant pediatric renal tumors
  - Average age at diagnosis is 3 years old
  - No diagnostic IHC, numerous morphologies
    - Vimentin, bcl2+
    - Cytokeratin, *WT1*, CD99−
  - Classical pattern = nests (or cords) of ovoid cells separated by fibrovascular septa
    - May be ovoid, epithelioid, or spindled with bland nuclei without prominent nucleoli
    - Septa have "chicken wire" type vascular
    - Infiltrative on high power (though may look circumscribed on low power)
    - May also have varying amounts of any pattern—myxoid, sclerosing, cellular, epithelioid, palisaded, spindled, storiform, anaplastic
    - May be deceptively bland
- Renal rhabdoid tumor
  - Rare high grade malignancy
  - Average age at diagnosis is 1 year old (essentially never in children older than 5 years)
  - Loss of nuclear INI1, located on chromosome 22
  - Not encapsulated, extensive vascular invasion, nuclear pleomorphism
    - Open vesicular chromatin, prominent nucleoli, scattered hyaline eosinophilic cytoplasmic inclusions → paranuclear, keratin+
    - Rhabdoid morphology can be present in varying proportions
- Congenital mesoblastic nephroma
  - Low-grade spindle neoplasm in renal medulla
    - Typically cured with nephrectomy
  - 90% present in first year of life
  - Most common renal neoplasm in those younger than 3 months of age
    - >95% event-free survival but 3 months or older have poorer prognosis
  - Solid pale cream tumor with slight whorling and infiltration of adjacent kidney
    - May have marked areas of hemorrhage and cystic change
  - Associated with polyhydramnios
  - Morphology
    - Classical subtype: 25% to 50%
      - Bland spindle cells in variably collagenous stroma
      - Interlacing fascicles
    - Cellular subtype: 40% to 60%
      - Morphologically indistinguishable from infantile fibrosarcoma

- Solid sheets of ovoid tumor cells with relative ↓ cytoplasm, ↑ cellularity, ↑ mitoses, focal necrosis
- Associated with *ETV6-NTRK3* (t12;15)(p13;q25)
  - Same as congenital/infantile fibrosarcoma
- More likely to recur compared with classic or mixed
  - Though most important risk factor for local recurrence is complete excision at primary surgery
- Mixed subtype: <10%
  - Some areas classical, some areas cellular
- Infiltrative growth
- Metanephric adenoma (MA)
  - Most cases in adults but has been reported in childhood
  - Small uniform embryonic-appearing cells with no atypia that form branching tubular structures
    - Variable adenomatous to collagenous stroma may be present
    - +/− psammoma bodies
  - Epithelial areas are keratin and vimentin+; WT may be positive
  - Metanephric adenofibroma is like MA plus spindle cell component
    - Fibroblast-like cells in collagenous stroma (hyaline and myxoid change focally is okay)
    - Stromal component may be CD34
    - +/− heterologous differentiation

Neuro and Musculoskeletal

- Neonatal encephalopathy (NE) = hypotonia, apnea, coma, and seizure
  - 13% develop cerebral palsy (CP); 24% of CP patients have history of NE
- SMA (spinal muscular atrophy) involves SMN (superior motor nucleus)
- Pterygium = web between forearm and arm, keeps flexed
- Arthrogryposis multiplex congenita = flexion contractures
  - End phenotype of multiple conditions including oligohydramnios, neurologic disease, muscular disease, SMA, and so on
- Osteogenesis imperfecta, type 2
  - Poorly ossified, soft cranium
  - Small thorax for gestational age
  - Crumpled/collapsed/fractured long bones > ribs > others
- Best differentiated to worst differentiated
  - Ganglioneuroma
  - Ganglioneuroblastoma, intermixed
  - Ganglioneuroblastoma, nodular
  - Neuroblastoma, differentiating
    - Neuropil
    - >5% ganglion differentiation
    - Gains on 17q are associated with poor prognosis
  - Neuroblastoma, poorly differentiated
    - Neuropil
    - <5% ganglion differentiation
  - Neuroblastoma, undifferentiated
    - No neuropil
- Hereditary neuroblastoma
  - Germline activating *ALK* point mutations

- Germinal matrix hemorrhages
  - Grade 1—confined to germinal matrix
  - Grade 2—extend into ventricles
  - Grade 3—fill and expand ventricles
  - Grade 4—extend into parenchyma

Odds and Ends

- Zeus is for immunofluorescence, glutaraldehyde is for electron microscopy
- Limbal dermoid—"open-face" dermoid
  - Plaque-like lesion on area where cornea and sclera meet
  - DDx includes cystic nevus—small glands with nevus (conjunctival-entrapped normal glands)
- Thymic changes in trisomy 21
  - Paucity of Hassall's corpuscles (become large and calcified)
  - Taken out incidentally during endocardial cushion defect surgery
- Cystic fibrosis—inspissated mucus in dilated glands/ducts

CHAPTER 7

Gastrointestinal and Pancreatic Pathology

Syndromes

- Hamartomatous polyps
  - Juvenile polyposis syndrome—*SMAD4* and *BMPR1A*
    - Retention polyps in rectum
      - Inspissated mucin in dilated crypts
  - Peutz-Jeghers syndrome—*STK11*
    - Throughout gastrointestinal (GI) tract
      - Most common in small bowel
    - Atypical formations of smooth muscle and reactive/hyperplastic mucosa
      - Looks like Christmas tree at low power
      - Mucosa is arranged normal for the abnormal orientation of the smooth muscle
    - Freckles on oral mucosa
    - Adenoma malignum and sex cord tumor with annular tubules (SCTAT)
  - Cronkhite-Canada syndrome—unknown
  - Cowden syndrome—*PTEN*
- Lynch syndrome—hereditary nonpolyposis colorectal cancer (HNPCC) syndrome
  - Use modified Amsterdam criteria to assess risk
  - More carcinomas than adenomas
  - Sessile architecture
  - Mismatch repair (MMR) genes mutated → microsatellite instable cancers
    - Also 15% of sporadic carcinomas
    - MSH2 and MSH6, MLH1 and PMS2 heterodimers
      - MLH1 is a methylator
    - CIPM—CpG island methylator phenotype
    - Preexisting serrated adenoma is not required
  - Need annual screening!
  - 80% of all colorectal carcinoma (CRC) is microsatellite stable (MSS), and 20% are microsatellite instable (MSI)
- Familial adenomatosis polyposis
  - More adenomas than carcinomas
  - *APC* gene mutation (tumor suppressor)
  - Classic adenoma-carcinoma sequence (tubular adenoma → high-grade dysplasia → carcinoma with acquisition of *KRAS* mutation)
- Von Hippel-Lindau (VHL) syndrome—pancreatic microcystic serous cystadenoma and clear cell pancreatic neuroendocrine tumors

Esophagus

- Parakeratosis in esophagus can be caused by *candida*

- Glycogenic acanthosis—hyperplastic with clear cells
- Gastroesophageal reflux disease (GERD)
  - Increased intraepithelial eosinophils
  - Elongation of vascular papillae (>⅔ thickness of epithelium)
  - Basal cell hyperplasia (>15%)
  - +/− Ulcer, intraepithelial lymphs, balloon cells
- Eosinophilic esophagitis (EE)
  - Technically, the American Gastroenterological Association defines as a minimum of 15 eosinophils per high-power field (eos/hpf)
  - <8 eos/hpf → favor reflux
  - >24 eos/hpf → favor EE
  - May be responsive to PPIs *or* steroids
- Sloughing esophagitis (esophagitis dissecans superficialis)
  - Necrosis and sloughing of superficial squamous mucosa
  - Elderly and chronically ill
  - May be caused by direct contact with multiple medications (like a diffuse form of pill esophagitis), skin conditions, or trauma
  - "Two-tone esophagus"
- Granular cell tumor in lamina propria
  - Overlying mucosa showing pseudoepitheliomatous hyperplasia
- Complete intestinal metaplasia—goblet cells + ciliated absorptive cells
  - Lower cancer risk than incomplete metaplasia (goblet cells + foveolar epithelium)
- Three *M*s of herpes—molding, margination (Cowdry type A inclusions), multinucleation
- Barrett's esophagus
  - Barrett's-dysplasia-adenocarcinoma sequence involves: MSI, *MYC* amplification, *p53* mutations, *KRAS* mutations
    - Less commonly—*EGFR, CTNNB1, HER2, MCC, DCC*
  - True intestinal metaplasia is Alcian blue + (at pH 2.5)
    - Acid mucin to counteract basic pancreatic secretions
    - Sialomucin
  - Incomplete intestinal metaplasia
    - Sialomucin + neutral mucin
  - Inadvertent sampling of cardia will be PAS+
    - Neutral mucin to counteract stomach acid
  - MUC subtyping
    - Positive for MUC2
    - Negative for MUC1, MUC5AC, and MUC6
  - Frequent biopsies to assess for dysplasia (low-grade or high-grade)
- Gastric foveolar-type dysplasia
  - More eosinophilic, glandular crowding
  - Graded by nuclear size
    - Low-grade—2 to 3× the size of a lymphocyte
    - High-grade—3 to 4× lymphocyte size
  - Seen in up to 20% Barrett esophagus-associated dysplasia, may be mixed in with traditional intestinal dysplasia

Stomach

INTRODUCTION

- Challenges with gastric biopsy
  - Lack of clinical information on submitted requisition

- Incorrect clinical information provided
- Small biopsies
- Multiple biopsies or fragments submitted in same container
- Poor correlation between endoscopic findings and histologic features
- Is the biopsy done for screening (no symptoms), diagnosis (symptoms), or surveillance (Barrett's, *H. pylori*, dysplasia, metaplasia, celiac, inflammatory bowel disease, cancer resection)?
- Normal
  - Fundic/oxyntic glands found in fundus and body
  - Mucinous glands in pylorus/antrum and cardia

INFLAMMATORY

- Proton pump inhibitor (PPI) effect
  - Cystic/dilated fundic (mixed cell-types) glands (like foveolar hyperplastic polyps)
  - With apical snouts
- Reactive gastropathy
  - Caused by reflux, alcohol, NSAIDs
  - Foveolar hyperplasia, tortuous/corkscrew glands, smooth muscle fibers aberrantly in lamina propria
  - Inflammation is mild to absent
  - Loss of mucin
- Erosive gastropathy
  - Like reactive gastropathy but with eroded superficial epithelium and fibrin deposition
  - Acute inflammation okay near erosion
- Chronic gastritis
  - Lymphoplasmacytic diffuse infiltrate in lamina propria, increased lymphoid follicles (with germinal centers)
  - Lymphoid aggregates higher than base = abnormal
  - Old rule—"two plasma cells touching each other" = chronic gastritis
  - "Active" = neutrophils in lamina propria, epithelium, or lumens
    - *H. pylori*, partially treated *H. pylori*, medication-induced
  - Grade severity—mild, moderate, severe
- Gastric antral vascular ectasia (GAVE)—"watermelon stomach"
  - Named for endoscopic appearance, need the appropriate endoscopic impression to diagnose it on biopsy
  - Morphology
    - Proliferation of foveolar epithelium with congested vessels
    - Superficial granulation tissue and fibrin thrombi (caused by erosion)
    - Looks like hyperplastic polyp with congested/dilated capillaries
  - Long-standing—smooth muscle bundles extending upward, dissecting glands
- Autoimmune metaplastic atrophic gastritis (AMAG)
  - Body and fundic biopsies
    - Look like antrum (just mucous glands, no oxyntic) (pseudopyloric metaplasia) + lamina propria lymphoplasmacytic inflammation
    - Other—intestinal metaplasia, endocrine cell hyperplasia
    - Gastrin−
  - Antral biopsies
    - Only mild inflammation
    - Gastrin+
      - Gastrin+ G cells should be sparse and interspersed in normal antrum. In AMAG, there are six or more in a row.

- - Autoantibodies against parietal cells → low hydrochloric acid but high gastrin
  - Increased risk for carcinoma
- Gastric calcinosis
  - Occurs in renal failure
  - Calcifications in lamina propria
- Gastritis cystica profunda
  - Prolapse/misplacement of glands in muscularis mucosae with no desmoplasia
  - Typically status post-partial gastrectomy → *flat* endoscopically
    - If *nodular* endoscopically → gastritis cystica polyposa
- Pancreatic heterotopia
  - Stomach = most common site
  - Lobular with central duct
  - Ductal, acinar, and/or islet portions
    - Type 1 = three components
    - Type 2 = two components
    - Type 3 = one component
- Gastric antral vascular ectasia
  - Thrombi (CD61+) in dilated superficial vessels
  - Differential diagnosis (DDx)—portal gastropathy
- Inflammatory fibrous polyp of GI tract
  - Stomach and small intestine
  - Whorling/onion skinning spindle cells around vessels, CD34+
- Menetrier disease
  - Adults (in children—usually self-limited)
  - Protein-losing enteropathy
    - Weight loss, diarrhea, peripheral edema
  - Diffuse hyperplasia of rugal folds, oxyntic gland loss
- Granulomas in stomach → Crohn's vs. sarcoidosis
- Whipple disease
  - Lamina propria expansion of foamy macrophages, bulbous villi, dilated lymphatics
  - PAS+, *T. whippelii* immunohistochemistry (IHC)+
  - DDx—xanthoma (most common site = stomach, CD68+)

NEOPLASTIC

Mesenchymal Proliferations

- Smooth muscle proliferation in gastrointestinal (GI) tract
  - Gastrointestinal stromal tumor (GIST) vs. leiomyoma vs. schwannoma
  - IHC panel = desmin, S100, CD117
    - Others—DOG1, SMA, caldesmon
- GIST
  - Interstitial cells of Cajal
  - Activating *c-Kit* mutation
  - 25% malignant
  - Associated with NF1
  - Imatinib or sunitinib or dasatinib
  - Skeinoid fibers (small bowel only, large)
  - Express *c-Kit* (CD117), DOG1, S100, CD34

- Negative for SMA and desmin
- Carney triad (in young women)
  - Epithelioid GIST
  - Pulmonary chondroma
  - Extraadrenal paraganglioma
- *KIT* mutated
  - Exon 9 or 11, imatinib sensitive
  - Spindled/mixed
  - CD117/DOG1+
- *PDGFR* mutated
  - D842V, imatinib resistant
  - Epithelioid cells
  - DOG1+
- Succinate dehydrogenase (SDH) deficient
  - Lobules or nodules separated by fibromuscular tissue (plexiform)
  - Epithelioid cells
  - Pediatric
  - Genetics/syndromes
    - Carney triad
      - Young women
      - Gastric GIST, pulmonary chondroma, and extraadrenal paraganglioma
      - Unknown genetic mechanism
    - Carney-Stratakis syndrome
      - Germline *SDH* mutations
      - GIST and paragangliomas
      - Autosomal dominant inheritance
    - Other mutations that are important in GISTs—*KIT* and *PDGFR*
  - Immunohistochemistry
    - Loss of mitochondrial SDHB
    - CD117 (*KIT*)
    - DOG1+
  - Although most other GISTs rarely recur at anastomotic sites, SDH-deficient often recur locally in stomach (years or decade after primary resection)
- *RAS-P* mutated
  - Spindled
  - SDHB+
- Quadruple wild-type
  - SDHB+
- Spindled morphology—short intersecting fascicles, uniform cells, no cell borders, no nucleoli
- Epithelioid morphology—nested epithelioid cells, vesicular chromatin with nucleoli, prominent cell borders
  - Bland epithelioid cells infiltrating around normal glands
  - Amphophilic cytoplasm
  - CD117 is not as positive in epithelioid GIST, as in other patterns
- Leiomyoma
  - Esophagus in younger men, distal, present with dysphagia
  - Colorectal polyps, small
  - SMA and desmin strong positivity
    - Negative for S100, CD34, and CD117
  - Usually PINK on low-power (low to mod cellularity)

- Cytology—no single cells, big fragments
- (Myo)fibroblastic tumors
  - Plexiform fibromyxoma
    - Stomach, antrum
    - Bleeding and gastric outlet obstruction
    - Benign
    - Multinodular (DDx = SDH-deficient GIST), bland spindled cells in myxoid/collagenous background, prominent arborizing capillaries
    - 80% SMA+
    - Vascular invasion may happen (significance not known)
  - Inflammatory fibroid polyp
    - *PDGFRA* mutations, older females
    - Gastric antrum, polypoid submucosal lesions +/− mucosal involvement (with ulceration)
    - Concentric "onion" rings around vessels with tons of eosinophils
  - Inflammatory myofibroblastic tumor
    - Children and young adults, omentum and mesentery
    - Systemic inflammatory symptoms
    - Recur frequently, may metastasize
    - Vague fascicles of bland spindle cells with prominent nucleoli and lymphoplasmacytic infiltrate
    - SMA+, focal AE1/AE3 and CAM5.2+ in one-third (pitfall!)
    - 35% to 60% have *ALK* mutations
  - Desmoid fibromatosis
    - If in children or young adults, consider FAP/Gardner syndrome, mesentary
    - ≥10 cm with infiltrative margins, recur
    - Long fascicles, collagenous/myxoid stroma, dilated thin-walled vessels and extravasated RBCs
    - SMA+, nuclear beta-catenin+
  - Fibromatosis
    - Sweeping fascicles
    - β-catenin positive (nuclear)
    - Gaping vessels
    - Invasive through fat
- Nerve sheath/neural tumors
  - Schwannoma—most common
    - Myenteric plexus—most common in stomach
    - Characteristics—* = important GI-only feature
      - Discontinuous lymphoid cuff with follicles*
      - No capsule*
      - "Fish hook" nuclei, wavy
      - No Antoni B areas*
      - No association with NF*
      - Strong, diffuse S100+
      - Focal atypia
      - Wavy collagenous fibrils
    - Cytology—syncytial, bent nuclei with pointed ends, lymphocytes in background

Epithelial Proliferations

- Gastroesophageal junction (GEJ)—obtain frozen sections on esophageal margin

- Open stomach along greater curvature
- Masses that cross GEJ will be staged as esophageal/GEJ *unless* the epicenter of the mass is >2 cm into stomach
- Staged by DOI
- Gastric polyps
  - Asymptomatic usually, almost always incidental
  - Hyperplastic polyp (HP) <5 mm (but can be larger)
    - Ectatic glands lined by all hyperplastic/elongated foveolar epithelium
      - Looks like antrum
    - Splaying of muscularis mucosae with bundles extending into lamina propria
    - May have mitotic activity
    - Background of active gastritis
  - Polypoid gastritis → smaller HP associated with *H. pylori*
  - Polypoid foveolar hyperplasia → long cells, no cysts, some nuclear atypia, large and round nuclei, loss of mucin, history of NSAID use
    - No active gastritis
    - Looks papillary, can get serrations
    - *Polypoid gastropathy* or *gastropathy* can also be used
  - Fundic gland polyp → flattened fundic mucosa with cystic dilation, lined by both parietal (hydrochloric acid, intrinsic factor) and chief (pepsinogen)
    - Sporadic (β-catenin mutation, low dysplasia risk) or syndromic (*APC* gene FAP, usually multiple, *high dysplasia risk*)
    - Most common polyp
  - (Tubular) adenoma → dysplasia, solitary, intestinal type (with goblet cells) >> gastric type
    - Sessile or pedunculated
    - Up to 2 cm
  - Gastritis cystica polyposa → HP with cystic glands in muscularis, associated atrophic gastritis
  - Juvenile polyp → hamartomatous, similar to HP with smooth muscle cells in stroma
  - Peutz-Jeghers polyp → hamartomatous, arborizing muscle
  - Menetrier's disease → diffuse hyperplasia
  - Others → pancreatic heterotopia, pancreatic acinar metaplasia, Brunner's gland nodule, neuroendocrine tumor (associated with atrophic gastritis and intestinal metaplasia), polypoid carcinoma, xanthoma, amyloidosis, granuloma, calcium deposition
  - *Rare* nonepithelial polyps (boards-fodder) → glomus tumor, granular cell tumor, inflammatory fibroid polyp, GIST, inflammatory myofibroblastic tumor, lymphoid hyperplasia, lymphoma
- Dysplasia
  - Mucin depletion, glandular crowding, nuclear elongation, and pseudostratification
  - Low- and high-grade do *not* have surface maturation
  - High-grade has cribriforming and loss of polarity
    - Should be seen by *at least* two pathologists

Small Intestine

- Celiac disease
  - Hypersensitivity to α-gliadin+
  - Tests—antitissue transglutaminase or anti-endomysial serologies
  - Villous blunting, crypt hyperplasia, intraepithelial lymphocytes (>6 lymphocytes/20 tip enterocytes), dense lamina propria lymphoplasmacytic infiltrate, enterocyte damage (flattening and vacuoles)

- ■ Use modified Marsh criteria for severity
- ● Peptic duodenitis—foveolar epithelium in duodenum
  - ■ Small mucin cap on what look like normal absorptive intestinal cells
  - ■ Indicates increased acidity in duodenum
  - ■ *Always* report
- ● Heterotopia of body-type glands (fundic glands) in duodenum
- ● Ileum with gastric mucosa → Meckel with gastric heterotopia
- ● Peutz-Jeghers polyps in duodenum
  - ■ Smooth muscles = arborizing, Christmas tree
  - ■ Foveolar and intestinal epithelium
  - ■ Hamartomatous polyp
- ● Tufting enteropathy
  - ■ Congenital enteropathy → intractable diarrhea
  - ■ Arabic ancestry
  - ■ Bowel transplantation or lifelong parenteral nutrition
  - ■ Complicated by cirrhosis

Colon and Rectum

INFLAMMATORY

Inflammatory Bowel Disease

- ■ Crohn's disease (CD) and ulcerative colitis (UC)
- ■ Dyspepsia, diarrhea, bloating, indigestion, pain, bleeding, weight loss
- ■ Colonoscopy will have gross findings
- ■ Active inflammation (cryptitis, abscess) and chronic injury (crypt architectural distortion)
- ■ Mimics
  - ■ Infectious—no chronic injury, neutrophilia, acute, young
  - ■ Ischemic—splenic flexure, transverse colon, history of other ischemic events
  - ■ NSAID—history, colonoscopy findings
- ● Features of both
  - ■ Active inflammation
    - Cryptitis
    - Crypt abscesses
    - ↓ Mucin
  - ■ Chronicity
    - Crypt architectural distortion
      - Rule out rectal prolapse (trichrome highlights muscle)
    - Paneth metaplasia distal to hepatic flexure
    - Pyloric gland (pseudopyloric) metaplasia
      - Can also be seen in chronic cholecystitis
      - More frequently in CD
    - Crypt intraluminal budding
      - Looks like telescoping
      - Also graft-versus-host disease (GVHD)
  - ■ Basal lymphoplasmacytic infiltrate
- ● Features of Crohn's disease
  - ■ Transmural lymphoid aggregates
  - ■ Noncaseating granulomas

- Most common in young adults
- Children may not have granulomas, tend to present with perirectal fistula/abscess
  - Granulomas in the upper GI tract are highly diagnostic
- **UC can have granulomas from gland rupture**
- Mucosal edema
- Free neutrophils
- Glandular destruction
- Aphthous ulcers
- Serpiginous ulcers
- Transmural fibrosis
- Features that favor CD over UC
  - Lymphoid aggregates without germinal centers
  - ↑ Inflammation without crypt distortion
  - Submucosal lymphatic dilation
- Not resected, recurs
- Features of ulcerative colitis
  - Only inflammation is in large bowel
  - Must involve rectum
  - No skip areas (gross or micro)
  - No fissures
  - No granulomas
    - **May get foreign body giant cell response in damaged crypts**
  - Mucosal atrophy
  - Features that favor UC over CD
    - Muscularis mucosae thickened to >15 cells thick
  - Resected to limit cancer risk (no recurrence)
- Surveillance—llook for active inflammation and dysplasia
  - Dysplasia in IBD—flat dysplasia or dysplasia-associated lesion/mass (DALM)

Other Inflammatory

- Radiation colitis like IBD but with mucosal telangiectasias and ↑ atypical fibroblasts and *with the history*
- Ischemic colitis—surface enterocyte injury, crypt mucin loss, hyalinized lamina propria, closely packed glands (collapsed)
- Microscopic colitis
  - Chronic watery diarrhea, no architectural distortion, minimal endoscopic findings, no gross abnormalities
  - Collagenous colitis
    - Females > males
    - Irregular collagen table under surface epithelium with entrapped eosinophils and capillaries
  - Lymphocytic colitis
    - Lymphoplasmacytic inflammation in lamina propria, superficial injury with loss of surface mucin
    - Uniform involvement of epithelium by intraepithelial lymphocytes (IELs)
    - Versus normal colon
      - Normal colon has IELs over lymphoid aggregates
      - More in right colon than left (<5 lymphocytes/100 epithelial cells)
  - May be side effect of PPIs, selective serotonin reuptake inhibitors (SSRIs), NSAIDs

- Treated with budesonide
- >2 apoptotic cells in 1 crypt → GVHD vs. mycophenolate
- Active nonspecific colitis DDx—bowel prep effect, infectious, drug, mechanical injury

NEOPLASMS

Mesenchymal Neoplasms

- Mucosal perineurioma
  - Colon polyps in adult, recto-sigmoid
  - Benign
  - Lamina propria spindle cell proliferation displacing crypts, serrated overlying epithelium (which may harbor *BRAF* mutation)
    - Possible that perineurioma component is reactive
  - EMA+, S100–
- Mucosal Schwann cell hamartoma (MSCH)
  - Benign, left colon, no syndromic association, incidental polyp
  - Displaces crypts, bland
  - S100+ EMA–
- Ganglioneuroma
  - Schwann cell component + ganglion component in lamina propria
  - Cowden syndrome (polyposis in lamina propria), MEN IIB (polyposis throughout wall), and NF1 (polyposis throughout wall)
  - Like MSCH with ganglion cells in clusters

Epithelial Neoplasms

- "Advanced adenoma"
  - >1 cm
  - Villous architecture
    - >25% villous—tubulovillous adenoma
  - High-grade dysplasia
- Serrated neoplasia of the colon
  - For difficult-to-name lesions with mixed features (and/or dysplasia), essentially they just need a complete excision
- Hyperplastic polyps (HPs)
  - *BRAF/KRAS*—can be wild-type for both or mutant for one (never mutant for both)
  - Left (distal colon)
  - No mucin in bottom proliferative zones
  - Usually <5 mm (definitely <10 mm)
  - Microvesicular HPs
    - Mucin poor
    - *BRAF*
    - Small vacuoles of mucin, flocculant, serrated, 70% to 80% of HPs
    - Controversial whether they are precursors or related to sessile serrated adenomas (SSAs)
    - CIMP high (hypermethylation) and *BRAF* mutations
    - Usually <5 mm, mostly in left colon (but right-sided do occur)
    - Impaired superficial senescence, so lower cells "pile up"
  - Goblet cell-rich HPs
    - Can cluster in the rectum
    - *KRAS*

- Sessile serrated adenoma
  - Recognized by gland architecture! 99% are flat
  - Most common on right side
  - Hypermethylation and *BRAF* happen early in pathogenesis
  - Dysmaturation—basal cells resemble gastric foveolar epithelium
  - Irregular proliferative zone so cells migrate up *and* down, glands grow sideways at base (near muscularis mucosae) → boots and boats
    - Deep crypt branching
    - Crypt dilation
    - Generally accepted that *one crypt* is enough
      - Rex 2012 review and Bettington 2014 paper (critical appraisal)
  - Can percolate into submucosa without being "true invasion"
  - Tendency to have submucosal lipomas below
    - More protuberant than normal SSAs
    - Also perineuriomas and fibroblastic polyps associated
  - **Use morphology to differentiate between HPs and SSAs; use location and size as "tie-breaker"**
    - SSAs tend to be larger and more common in proximal/right colon, but exceptions do exist!
    - A polyp >10 mm in right colon—virtually always SSA
  - Endoscopically tend to have "fecal cap"—feces sticks to surface
  - SSA with cytologic dysplasia
    - Current guidelines are 3-year follow-up. Probably need 1 year follow-up initially
    - Acquires *MLH1* silencing via methylation
      - Stain loss in dysplastic portion, intact in background SSA
      - *BRAF* immunostain positive in all
        - Normal TAs are not positive for *BRAF* → this is how we tell it is not a mixed SSA/TA
    - Subgroups—minimal deviation, serrated, adenomatous, NOS
  - Serrated polyposis syndrome
    - Multiple serrated polyps (HP and SSAs)
    - See WHO for criteria
    - 1-year follow-up recommended
  - Serrated epithelial change (SEC)
    - In random sampling from IBD patient
    - May just be "furry surface"
    - "Field effect"—background mucosa is hypermethylated
- Traditional serrated adenomas (TSA)
  - *APC* mutation, *KRAS* mutation, microsatellite stable, CIMP low
  - Intense serrations from ectopic crypts
  - Mostly left-sided
  - Can develop conventional dysplasia
  - Pinecone at low power (filiform)
- Adenocarcinoma
  - Grading
    - Low grade: >50% gland formation (or medullary subtype)
    - High grade: <50% gland formation (or signet ring or clear cell subtypes)
  - Microsatellite tumors are more likely to have mixed phenotypes
    - Peritumoral Crohn's-like reaction also
      - Lymphoid aggregates = favorable prognosis
  - Classically has central/luminal necrosis with desmoplastic stromal response

TABLE 7.1 ■ **Colon Adenocarcinoma Staging (AJCC)**

Stage	Depth-Extent	Treatment
0	Mucosa; CIS	Polypectomy +/− surgery
1	Submucosa or muscularis propria	Surgery
2	Serosal involvement or direct invasion of local organs	Surgery +/− chemotherapy
3	+LNs	Surgery +/− chemotherapy
4	+Distant metastases	Chemotherapy +/− surgery

AJCC, American Joint Committee on Cancer; *CIS*, carcinoma in situ; *LNs*, lymph nodes.

- Incomplete glands are also helpful clues to CRC
  - Staging—see Table 7.1

Molecular Pathways

- Microsatellite instability can be caused by either Lynch syndrome or CIMP hypermethylation
  - CpG island methylator (CIMP)
    - Right-sided lesions
    - Methylation of cytosine turns off genes
    - Type A genes normally methylated with age and development
    - Type C genes are methylated in cancer
    - Screening new carcinomas
      - Cancer? Get MMR IHC panel
      - Loss of MLH1 alone or MLH1/PMS2? Get hypermethylation testing or *BRAF* testing
      - See Fig. 7.1
    - Lynch is *not* hypermethylated
  - CIMP hypermethylated are more responsive to PDL1 therapy (have more intratumoral lymphocytes) but not as responsive to traditional chemotherapy (5-FU)
    - Favorable prognosis
    - Develop interval cancers (develops between short-interval colonoscopies)
- *KRAS* mutations
  - TSAs
    - Left colon
    - Villous and pink; ectopic crypts and enteric metaplasia
    - 50% to 70% have *KRAS* mutations, 20% to 40% have *BRAF*
  - Goblet cell-rich HPs
    - Can cluster in the rectum
- *BRAF* mutations
  - Microvesicular HPs (mucin poor)
  - SSAs
    - Usually right-sided
    - No cytologic atypia, only architectural
    - Can be CIMP+
  - All sporadic CRC
    - Quickly develops ("interval" cancer)
- Adenoma-carcinoma sequence
  - Based on *APC* gene (tumor suppressor) mutated cancers
    - *KRAS* associated

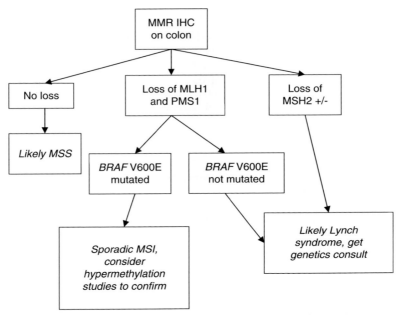

Fig. 7.1 How to interpret immunohistochemical (IHC) stain results for mismatch repair (MMR) genes in colorectal carcinoma. *MSI*, Microsatellite instability; *MSS,* microsatellite stability.

Appendix

GENERAL

- Clinical settings
  - Acute appendicitis
  - Appendiceal mass/swelling
  - As part of staging procedure
  - As part of any other procedure (incidental appendectomy)
- Mesoappendix—unique because it is not attached to posterior abdominal wall, instead to terminal ileum
  - True surgical margin?

NEUROENDOCRINE TUMORS

- Well-differentiated neuroendocrine (NE) tumor (carcinoid)
  - Grades 1 to 3 based on mitotic activity
  - Staged by size (starts in submucosa so not staged like epithelial neoplasms)
    - T1≤2 cm, T2 = 2 to 4 cm, T3 = 4 cm or more, T4 = peritoneum or adjacent structures
  - Cords, trabeculae, nests with CLEFTS
  - Stimulate stromal fibrosis
  - Ample eosinophilic cytoplasm, monomorphic small, round nuclei
- Goblet cell carcinoid
  - May be combined with conventional adenocarcinoma
- Poorly differentiated neuroendocrine carcinoma (NEC)

EPITHELIAL TUMORS

- Adenoma—adenomatous proliferation with intact muscularis mucosae
- Low-grade appendiceal mucinous neoplasm (LAMN)
  - Adenomatous epithelium with destruction of muscularis mucosa *or* nondestructive involvement of wall/peritoneum
- High-grade appendiceal mucinous neoplasm (HAMN)
  - Like LAMN with high-grade cytologic features
  - Very rare, not *usually* used
- Invasive adenocarcinoma
  - Destructive invasion and desmoplasia
  - Looks like colorectal
  - If >50% mucinous → mucinous adenocarcinoma
- Signet ring adenocarcinoma
  - Goblet cell carcinoid
  - Goblet cell carcinoid—adenocarcinoma
  - Large cell NEC
  - Small cell NEC
- Staging
  - Tis—not past muscularis mucosae
  - Tis—sitting on mucosa
  - T1—submucosa
  - T2—into muscularis propria
  - T3—through muscularis
  - T4a—serosa
  - T4b—adjacent structures
  - M1a—acellular mucin only on peritoneum
  - M1b—mucin with floating tumor cells on peritoneum
  - M1c—any other site than peritoneum

NONNEOPLASTIC

- Endometriosis is common
  - Long-standing—atrophic epithelium with minimal stroma
  - Can also get endosalpingiosis
- Gangrenous appendicitis (frankly necrotic)
- Acute appendicitis requires inflammation in the muscular layer
- Diagnose "serositis" if there is acute inflammation of the serosa
  - "Peritonitis" is a clinical diagnosis of acute abdomen
- Fibrous obliteration of the tip with atrophy of mucosa and lymphoid tissue
- Pinworms

Anus

NORMAL ANATOMY

- Anal verge—mucocutaneous junction (nonkeratinizing to keratinizing)
- Dentate line—transitional epithelium (columnar to squamous, resembles urothelium)
- Anal glands empty into anal sinuses (between anal papillae/columns)
  - CK7+, CK20+

COMMON BENIGN LESIONS

- Hemorrhoids
- Fibroepithelial polyp—hypertrophied anal papillae, "anal tags"
  - Can have bizarre stromal cells
- Inflammatory cloacogenic polyp
  - Mucosal prolapse disease at anorectal junction
  - Serrated/villous surface composed of multiple types of epithelium
  - Angulated crypts
  - Reactive changes—ischemia, atypia, ulceration
  - Irregular muscularis mucosae that extends into lamina propria
  - Acellular mucin

MALIGNANT OR PREMALIGNANT

- Condyloma acuminatum
  - Hyper-, para-, dyskeratosis
  - Superficial viral change—koilocytes
  - Exophytic verruciform
  - Dilated vessels and chronic inflammation
- Anal squamous intraepithelial neoplasia (AIN)
  - Low-grade—AIN1—koilocytic change
  - High-grade—AIN2 or 3—dysplasia >⅓ of mucosa
    - Can extend into anal gland
    - p16+ (block-like nuclear and cytoplasmic)
- Perianal squamous cell carcinoma in situ (Bowen disease)
  - Large plaques, Bowenoid papulosis = small widespread papules
  - Like high-grade dysplasia or squamous cell carcinoma in situ in perianal skin
  - Recurrences are common
  - Rare progression
- Squamous cell carcinoma
  - Treated with chemoradiation, not surgery
  - HPV16
  - Types
    - Keratinizing
    - Nonkeratinizing
      - Large
      - Basaloid
    - Verrucous carcinoma (giant condyloma acuminatum of Buschke-Lowenstein)
      - HPV6 and 11, >10 cm frequently, exo- and endophytic growth with broad-pushing border
- Paget disease of the anus
  - p16−, mucin+
  - Primary—intraepithelial apocrine neoplasm—GCDFP, CK7+
  - Secondary—extension of underlying colorectal adenocarcinoma—CK7−/+, CK20+, CDX2+
- Primary adenocarcinoma
  - Anorectal sinuses secondary to Crohn's, associated with fistulas
    - Abundant mucin, CK20+, CDX2+

- Anal glands—well-differentiated, irregularly shaped glands
  - CK7+, CK20–
- Poorer prognosis than squamous cell carcinoma
- Anal melanoma
  - Melanocytes present in transitional epithelium
  - Bleeding polypoid mass near dentate line (like hemorrhoids)
  - Most common primary melanoma of GI tract

Pancreas

NONNEOPLASTIC (INFLAMMATORY, CONGENITAL, ACQUIRED)

- Chronic pancreatitis
  - Lobular arrangement of cell clusters surrounding duct structure; may be only islet cells remaining (no or atrophic acinar cells with loose acinar stroma)
    - Dense interlobular fibrosis, loose intralobular fibrosis
    - Not an established "precursor" to ductal adenocarcinoma—likely adenocarcinoma causes chronic pancreatitis
    - Glands in fat, around nerves, or encroaching on vessels → more likely carcinoma
      - Nuclear variation of ≥4:1 → more likely carcinoma
      - Pitfall—islet cells can rim nerves! Can do CD56, chromogranin, synaptophysin. No nuclear variation. Neuroendocrine nuclear features
- Hereditary pancreatitis
  - Mutations in *PRSS1* (cationic trypsinogen) and *SPINK1* (serine protease inhibitor, Kazal type 1)
- Autoimmune pancreatitis
  - Type 1—IgG_4
    - ≥50 IgG_4 + cells/1 hpf
    - Storiform fibrosis
    - Obliterative venulitis
    - Obliterative vasculitis → autoimmune pancreatitis type 1
      - IgG_4
      - Hypergammaglobulinemia, mass-like lesion/stricture, fibrosis, lymphoplasmacytic infiltrate
      - 50 IgG_4/hpf
  - Type 2
    - Periductal lymphoplasmacytic infiltrate
    - Microabscesses (granulocytic epithelial lesions—GELs) near vessels
  - Unclassifiable
    - Features of both
- Congenital nesidioblastosis
  - Congenital hyperinsulinism
  - Islets close to ducts, forming ductuloinsular complexes
  - Beta cell hypertrophy with nuclear anisocytosis *required!*
    - Cells should be 3 to 4× other cells within the same islet
    - Compose ~ 70% of islets
  - Diffuse type (no nodules on ultrasound) vs. focal type (nodular on ultrasound)
    - No nodules → biopsy sent for frozen section.
    - If positive for beta cell hypertrophy on each → near-total pancreatectomy

- AR mutation of the sulfonylurea gene or *ABCC8* mutation
  - Homozygous or compound mutations → diffuse
  - Heterozygous mutation → focal
- DDx—neuroendocrine tumor—just tons of islets composed of one cell type
- Banff criteria for pancreas acute cell-mediated rejection
  - Grade I—active septal inflammation, venulitis, ductitis, perineural inflammation *or* focal acinar inflammation (<2 foci/lobule)
  - Grade II—multifocal acinar inflammation with spotty acinar cell injury *or* drop-out *or* minimal intimal arteritis
  - Grade III—diffuse acinar inflammation with focal *or* diffuse necrosis *or* moderate-to-severe intimal arteritis *or* transmural necrotizing arteritis
  - Neutrophils, eosinophils, apoptosis

NEOPLASTIC

- If there is a mass in the pancreas, biopsy is performed by endoscopic ultrasound-guided fine-needle aspiration
- Whipple resections
  - Usually distal duodenum becomes dusky from surgeon tying off vessels
  - Margins = proximal stomach, distal duodenum, vascular groove (may have SMV), pancreatic neck, bile duct, uncinate (dissected off SMA)
  - Cannot really tell posttreatment tumor bed vs. tumor
  - Staging based on *size* for exocrine tumor
    - Neuroendocrine tumors staged differently
    - Ampullary/duodenal masses are staged by depth of invasion *not* size
  - Frozen sections—bile duct and pancreatic neck margins

Cystic and Ductal Lesions

See Tables 7.2 and 7.3.
- Pseudocysts
  - Really high amylases
  - History of pancreatitis
  - Amorphous material with inflammatory cells, no epithelium
- Lymphoepithelial cyst
  - Uni- or multilocular
  - Middle-aged to older men

TABLE 7.2 ■ **Pancreas Cyst Differential Diagnosis**

Malignant	Benign
IPMN (↑ CEA)	Retention cyst
MCN (↑ CEA)	Lymphoepithelial cyst
Cystic solid neoplasms (e.g., cystic PanNET)	Acinar cystic transformation
Solid pseudopapillary neoplasm	Pseudocyst
	Serous cystadenoma

IPMN, Intraductal papillary mucinous neoplasm; *MCN*, mucinous cystic neoplasm; *PanNET*, pancreatic neuroendocrine tumor.

TABLE 7.3 ■ **Pancreatic Cysts**

	IPMN	**MCN**	**SCA**	**SPN**	**Pseudocyst**
Gender	M>F	M<<F	M<F	M<<F	F>M
Location	Head	Only tail	Head	Tail	Anywhere
Viscosity	↑	↑	↓	↓	↓
CEA	↑↑	↑↑	0	~↑	~↑
Amylase	↑	↓	↓	↓	↑
Cytology	Mucinous	Mucinous	Scant, bland, PAS+	Papillary and vascular	Pigmented histiocytes
Molecular	*KRAS, GNAS*	*KRAS*	*VHL*	*CTNNB1*	None

F, Female; *IPMN*, intraductal papillary mucinous neoplasm; *M*, male; *MCN*, mucinous cystic neoplasm; *SCA*, serous cystadenoma; *SPN*, solid pseudopapillary neoplasm.

- *Not* associated with HIV or autoimmune conditions (like lymphoepithelial lesions in other anatomic locations)
- Morphology
  - Cyst wall is stratified squamous epithelium with variable keratinization
  - Surrounded by lymphoid aggregates with germinal centers
- Serous
  - Serous cystadenoma
    - Clinical
      - Elderly female
      - Looks spongy on ultrasound and grossly
      - Associated with VHL
      - Do *not* get resected, no risk for recurrence, malignant transformation is rare
      - May become very large
    - Arise from centroacinar ductal cells
    - Microcystic is more common than macrocystic or solid
    - Clear bland cuboidal cells with sharp, distinct cell walls
    - Central scar
    - PAS+, diastase-sensitive
- Mucinous
  - Have really high CEA
  - Look for intracellular mucin on cytology
    - Positive for Alcian blue and mucicarmine
  - Intraductal papillary mucinous neoplasm (IPMN)
    - Main duct, >1 cm, grossly visible
      - Main duct type is more likely to be harboring high-grade dysplasia
      - Branched duct type has less risk
    - Papillary architecture with epithelium of types
      - Gastric—foveolar
      - Intestinal—long slender villi
      - Pancreaticobiliary—complex, cuboidal, cribriform, and micropapillary
    - Can have low-grade (cytologic) or high-grade (architectural) dysplasia, can progress to invasive adenocarcinoma
      - Pancreatic intraepithelial neoplasia (PanIN)

- Main duct is more likely to transform than side duct (40% to 50% vs. 10% to 20%)
- Can get concomitant carcinoma in 4% (caused by field effect)
- Associated with *colloid carcinoma* (must be 80% or more mucinous)
- Rule out *intraductal oncocytic papillary neoplasm* (IOPN, have *PRKACA* and *PRKACB* mutations)
  - These mutations are also associated with IOPN of the bile duct and fibrolamellar hepatocellular carcinoma
- Intraductal papillary neoplasm of the bile duct (IPNB)
  - Precursor lesion similar to IPMN
  - Elderly men
  - Types
    - Gastric
      - Most common, low-grade dysplasia
    - Pancreaticobiliary*
      - CK7+, CDX2–
      - High-grade dysplasia
    - Intestinal*
      - Looks like villous adenomas, intermediate- to high-grade dysplasia
    - Oncocytic
      - High-grade dysplasia
    - *Higher risk for becoming adenocarcinoma
- Mucinous cystic neoplasm (MCN)
  - Only ever solitary, usually multilocular
  - Strong female predominance (not frequently seen in males), middle-aged
  - Can have low- or high-grade dysplasia
  - Risk for malignancy = 6% to 36%
    - 10% have associated invasive carcinoma
      - Must submit *entire* specimen
    - Larger lesions → higher risk of malignancy (especially if >10 cm)
  - *Ovarian stroma* (ER/PR+, inhibin +) with epithelium of same types as IPMN (pancreaticobiliary, gastric, intestinal) and oncocytic
  - *KRAS* and *RNF43* mutations (not *GNAS* or *BRAF*)

Solid Tumors

- Solid pseudopapillary neoplasm (SPPN)
  - Tail or body, adults, slight female predominance
  - Solid and cystic on imaging
  - Low amylase and CEA
  - Cytology
    - Very cellular
      - DDx of very cellular pancreas smear—SPPN, PanNET, acinic cell carcinoma (has acini)
    - Naked nuclei, small/low-grade cells with nuclear grooves (coffee bean)
      - Neuroendocrine-like nuclear features, bland
    - Tadpole-like cells (cercariform cells)
    - Hyaline globules on Diff Quik (α_1-antitrypsin)
  - Histology
    - Solid tumor with cell death away from vessels (pseudofibrovascular cores) → pseudopapillary
    - Cholesterol clefts

- Myxoid stroma, "cylindroid" stromal hyalinization
- Central scar
  - Nuclear beta-catenin+, LEF1+, CD117+, CD10+, PR+
    - Pitfall—synaptophysin can be positive! Chromogranin should be negative
    - Nuclear beta-catenin is *also positive in cribriform morular neoplasms of the thyroid, fibromatosis, and aggressive* chronic lymphocytic leukemia/small lymphocytic lymphoma
  - Beta-catenin mutations
- Acinar cell carcinoma
  - Tend to be very big (10 cm) and well-circumscribed
  - Nests with vague rosetting (forming acini)
  - No stroma (soft consistency)
  - Fine chromatin, round basal nuclei, single small nucleoli
  - PAS-D+, chymotrypsin+, trypsin+
  - May have focal neuroendocrine differentiation/features
  - Can become cystic
- Islet cell (pancreatic neuroendocrine tumors—PanNET)
  - May be functional
    - Insulinoma
    - VIPoma
    - Glucagonoma
      - Can cause necrolytic migratory erythema
  - Morphology
    - Prominent hyalinized stroma (use for differentiating from acinar cell carcinoma)
    - Predominantly dyscohesive cells and occasional rosettes/clusters
    - Plasmacytoid low-grade cells with amphophilic cytoplasm, one nucleolus
  - Chromogranin/synaptophysin+
  - Use Ki67 or mitotic rate to grade
    - See Table 7.4
    - Note—all are well-differentiated tumors
  - For poorly differentiated neuroendocrine tumors, use carcinoma protocol
  - Can become cystic
  - MEN1, NF1, and tuberous sclerosis patients
    - Clear cell PanNETs—VHL
- Pancreatoblastoma
  - Rare, early childhood (~4 years) with second peak in mid-30s
  - 7 to 18 cm—large! Well-demarcated
  - Sheets of round cells with moderate cytoplasm and *scattered squamoid corpuscles* (pathognomonic) +/− nuclear pseudoinclusions
    - May have differentiation into (most common to least common)—acinar, ductal, endocrine

TABLE 7.4 ■ Grading Well-Differentiated Pancreatic Neuroendocrine Tumors

Grade	Mitoses/10 hpf	Ki67 Index
Low	<2	<3%
Intermediate	2–20	3%–20%
High	>20	>20%

hpf, High-power field.

- Nuclear beta-catenin and overexpression of cyclin D1, especially in squamoid corpuscles
- May have elevated AFP
- Rarely associated with Beckwith-Wiedemann or familial adenomatous polyposis
- 5-year survival <25%
- Adenocarcinoma
  - Most common—ductal adenocarcinoma
    - At time of diagnosis—70% are unresectable—may not see
  - Adenosquamous (>30% squamous), colloid (>80% mucinous), hepatoid, medullary, signet-ring, undifferentiated +/− osteoclast-like cells
  - Patterns—no prognostic implication!!
    - Foamy gland variant (usually say "suspicious for adenocarcinoma, foamy gland variant")
      - Foamy or microvacuolated cytoplasm with prominent cell borders, apical cytoplasm condensation (eosinophilic, resembles brush border)
      - *Bland nuclear features*
    - Solid nested pattern
      - Focal neuroendocrine features but with nucleoli
      - Organoid, squamoid look
    - Micropapillary pattern
  - Extrapancreatic extension no longer included in staging
  - IPMN with invasive mucinous adenocarcinoma
    - Background of chronic pancreatitis
    - Need to give the size of the IPMN and the size of the invasive component
      - Invasive component size is prognostic
      - Need to also give subtype because they have different therapies
      - Need to say main duct versus branched duct
    - IPMN-related adenocarcinomas have *KRAS* and *GNAS* mutations
      - Non-IPMN pancreatic ductal adenocarcinomas have activating mutations in *KRAS* and *p53*
  - Features supporting a diagnosis of pancreatic ductal adenocarcinoma
    - Haphazard growth pattern
    - Glands next to muscular vessels
    - Perineural invasion or lymphovascular invasion
    - Nuclear variation >4:1
    - Necrotic glandular debris
    - Incomplete lumina
    - Glands touching fat
    - Abnormal mitotic figures
    - *SMAD4* loss or *p53*+

Gallbladder and Biliary Tree

NONNEOPLASTIC

- Anatomy
  - In 5% of people, pancreatic and common bile duct remain separate
  - Rokitansky-Aschoff sinuses can be normal if superficial
    - If deep, likely represents chronic cholecystitis and/or cholelithiasis
  - Luschka ducts
    - Bland cuboidal/columnar cells surrounded by fibromuscular ring
    - At hepatic surface of gallbladder

- Peribiliary tubulovesicular glands
  - Peribiliary in neck of gallbladder
  - Lobular architecture
- Acute cholecystitis
  - Calculous—most common
  - Acalculous—severely ill patients, likely secondary to ischemia
  - Can become gangrenous
- Cholesterolosis
  - Strawberry gallbladder
  - Can form polyp (nonneoplastic)
- Subacute cholecystitis—eosinophils and lymphocytes
- Chronic cholecystitis
  - Associated with stones in 90%
  - Morphology
    - Thickened/fibrotic wall with mucosal herniation
    - Lymphoplasmacytic inflammation in lamina propria
    - Rokitansky-Aschoff sinuses
      - Cystically dilated = adenomyoma (single) or adenomyosis (diffuse)
      - CK7+
    - Can get metaplasia
      - Pyloric metaplasia—small round glands, pale
        - Pitfall—peribiliary glands
          - Similar to nests of pyloric metaplasia but not as pale and without lamina propria inflammation (both entities are benign)
      - Intestinal metaplasia—less common than pyloric
      - Associated with higher risk for dysplasia and malignancy
  - Subtypes
    - Chronic follicular
    - Eosinophilic
    - Chronic active
    - Xanthogranulomatous (associated with stones, clinically looks like cancer, rupture of Rokitansky-Aschoff sinuses)
- Complete porcelain gallbladder is not associated with an increased risk for carcinoma
  - Entire wall is think and sclerotic without muscle or epithelium
  - Incomplete porcelain and hyalinizing gallbladder *is* associated with high risk for carcinoma

NEOPLASTIC

Preinvasive

- Mass-forming
  - Intracholecystic papillary (or tubular) neoplasms (ICPN)
    - Less than 1 cm—polypoid metaplasia
    - More than 1 cm—"adenomas"
      - Biliary phenotype = cuboidal cells with large cherry red nucleoli
        - May be eosinophilic, clear, or with a perinuclear halos
  - Mucinous cystic neoplasm with ovarian-type stroma
- Flat dysplasias = "intraepithelial neoplasia"

- Most cancers arise from these
- Papillary, micropapillary, tubular, clinging, FLAT
- Can involve Rokitansky-Aschoff sinuses (mimicking invasion)
- Grading dysplasia
  - Low-grade
    - Columnar cells with minor changes
    - Submit four more blocks from gallbladder
    - Clinically insignificant
  - High-grade
    - Significant/severe changes with abrupt transition
    - Looks like a "wildfire"
      - Extensive, important, easily recognized
    - Submit the entire gallbladder!
      - Must look for T2 invasion
        - Most clinically significant "step" in staging
        - Poor prognosis
        - T2a—peritoneal side of gallbladder
        - T2b—hepatic side of gallbladder
  - Dysplasias have abrupt transitions, reactive changes have gradual changes
    - Reactive morphology—no nucleomegaly or architectural atypia, surface maturation preserved

Carcinoma

- 50% found incidentally on routine cholecystectomy for stones
  - Present late
  - 30% to 70% are missed grossly
- Most are adenocarcinoma
  - Biliary type most common
    - Other types—foveolar, intestinal (classical; looks like colorectal adenocarcinoma, goblet cell variant), clear cell, signet cell, hepatoid, mucinous
  - Well-formed, widely spaced glands
  - Haphazard densely fibrotic stroma
  - *Very* atypical cytology

EXTRAHEPATIC BILE DUCTS

- Muscle layer and peribiliary mucous ducts/glands are better formed closer to the common biliary duct
- Flat dysplasia (biliary intraepithelial neoplasia—BIN I, II, III) or mass-forming (same as gallbladder)
- Stage based on depth of invasion
  - <5 mm—T1
  - 5 to 12 mm—T2
  - >12 mm—T3
- Papillary intraductal neoplasm with low-grade dysplasia and invasive adenocarcinoma
  - Edematous stalks
- Well-differentiated cholangiocarcinoma arising in end-stage primary sclerosing cholangitis/cirrhosis
  - Onion-skinning fibrosis, obliterated bile ducts with bile ductule proliferation

- Usually large and medium bile ducts
- Large bile plug with bile stasis and biliary duct reaction

Gastrointestinal Hematolymphoid Neoplasms

NONNEOPLASTIC

- Conspicuous benign lymphoid aggregates
  - Normal (terminal ileum, appendix, rectal tonsil, idiopathic)
  - Diversion (colectomy)
  - Complicating IBD, *H. pylori*, celiac sprue, giardia (reactive)
  - Immunodeficiencies or hypogammaglobulinemia
  - *"Reactive lymphoid aggregates. Negative for neoplasm."*
- Confirming benignity
  - CD20 and CD3 behaving well
  - No CD20/CD43 coexpression
  - No *BCL2* in reactive germinal centers
- Gut intraepithelial T-lymphocytes are a mix of γ/δ and α/β

MALIGNANT

- Gut is common site for primary extranodal lymphoma
  - Stomach > small bowel > large bowel > esophagus
- Risk factors for GI lymphoma
  - Helicobacter-associated gastritis—extranodal marginal zone lymphoma (EMZL, "MALToma" or MALT lymphoma)
  - Celiac—enteropathy-associated T-cell lymphoma
  - Immunosuppression/HIV—all (60 to 200×)
  - Inflammatory bowel disease/thiopurine—EBV-associated lymphomas
  - Transplant—posttransplant lymphoproliferative disorders
- See Table 7.5
- Gastric mucosa-associated lymphoid tissue (MALT) lymphomas
  - Extranodal marginal zone lymphoma (EMZL)
  - Essentially three types
    - Type 1—Responsive to *H. pylori* eradication, gene fusion negative—60%
    - Type 2—Not responsive to eradication, gene fusion negative—20%
    - Type 3—Not responsive to eradication, positive for gene fusion—20%

TABLE 7.5 ■ **Small B-cell Lymphoma Immunophenotypes (CD20+/CD3−)**

Lymphoma	CD5	CD43	Cyclin D1	BCL2	CD10	CD23
Extranodal MZL (MALT)	neg	neg/pos	neg	neg	neg	neg/pos
Mantle cell	pos	pos	pos	neg	neg/pos	neg
Follicular	neg	neg	neg	pos	pos/neg	neg/pos
CLL/SLL	pos	pos	neg	neg	neg	pos

CLL/SLL, Chronic lymphocytic leukemia/small lymphocytic lymphoma; *MALT*, mucosa-associated lymphoid tissue; *MZL*, marginal zone lymphoma; *neg*, negative; *pos*, positive.

- t(11;18)(q21;q21)—*API2-MALT1*
  - Normally disappears in 80% in <12 months, very low rate of relapse
  - Be aware that persistence of a clone by ancillary testing ≠ lymphoma
  - Diffuse large B-cell lymphoma of the stomach is usually *H. pylori*/MALT-related
    - Treated with antibiotics and chemotherapy
- Intestinal MALT lymphoma
  - Large mass, indolent disease course
  - B-cell receptor gene rearrangements and κ:λ ratios help diagnosis
- Immunoproliferative small intestinal disease (IPSID)
  - Young adults, proximal small bowel, low socioeconomic status
  - Mediterranean, Middle Eastern, Asian, African descent
  - Like EMZL but with prominent CD20+ plasma cell population
- Mantle cell lymphoma
  - Intermediate-grade neoplasm
  - Causes most cases of lymphomatous polyposis
  - Cyclin D1 (BCL1), SOX10
  - Treated with chemotherapy
  - Looks bland
- Follicular lymphoma—prominent follicles in duodenum, very indolent
  - Middle aged to elderly
  - BCL2+ follicles with +/– BCL2 gene rearrangement
  - Usually no therapy
- Chronic lymphocytic leukemia/small lymphocytic lymphoma of the gut
  - CD20+, CD43+, CD23+, CD5+, cyclin D1–, BCL2–
- High-grade lymphomas
  - May want to rule out carcinoma, GIST, melanoma, and so on.
  - Usually B-cell lymphomas
  - Diffuse large B-cell lymphoma (DLBCL)
    - Must use Hans algorithm to classify
      - Germinal center subtype (more favorable prognosis) vs. nongerminal center
    - *MYC, BCL2, BCL6* FISH
  - Burkitt lymphoma
    - Children/teens
    - HIV-associated in some
    - Starry sky
    - Intermediate-sized cells, monomorphic
  - Plasmablastic lymphoma
    - HIV, EBV, large cells +/– plasmacytoid
  - High-grade B-cell lymphoma
    - NOS—morphology between Burkitt and DLBCL
    - With rearrangements of *MYC* and *BCL2* and/or *BCL6*
- Enteropathy associated T-cell lymphoma (EATL)
  - 10% to 25% of primary GI lymphomas
  - >50 years of age, poor prognosis
  - Jejunum > ileum > duodenum
  - Type 1—Northern European, 80% to 90%
    - Associated with celiac sprue that does not respond to gluten-free diet and HLA types
  - Type 2—Southeastern Asian
    - Not associated with sprue or HLA
  - Sprue that *did* respond to gluten-restricted diet, then symptoms return →

- Noncompliance
- Refractory celiac sprue
  - Still see intraepithelial lymphs
    - Type 1 refractory sprue → CD3+, CD8+, polyclonal (no *TCR* gene rearrangements) Try treating with steroids
    - Type 2 refractory sprue → CD3+, CD8–, higher risk for EATL, diffuse in GI tract, ↑ small intestine ulcers

Spleen

- Sclerosing angiomatoid nodular transformation (SANT)
  - Nonneoplastic
  - Micronodular plump endothelial cells and spindle cells
  - CD31+, CD34+/–, CD8+/–
  - "Spoke and wheel" on imaging
- Littoral cell angioma
  - Large nodules of anastomosing sinus-like vascular channels
  - Tall endothelial cells
  - CD31+, Factor VIII+, CD34–
- Hemangioma
- Angiosarcoma
- Hematolymphoid neoplasms
- Metastases

CHAPTER 8

Liver Pathology

Medical Liver

BASIC LIVER PATHOLOGY

- Blood flows from portal triad to central vein
- Zones
  - 1—periportal
  - 2—midzonal
  - 3—centrilobular (curvilinear)
- Bile duct should be about the size of the arteriole
  - Primary biliary cholangitis → bile duct larger than arteriole in triad
- Pigments
  - Lipofuscin really normal, especially centrilobular
    - More in Dubin–Johnson
    - Positive with PAS–D stain
    - Accumulate in Kupffer cells after acute hepatitis
  - Bile is only identifiable in spaces (canaliculi)
    - Cholangiolar cholestasis usually implies systemic infection (e.g., sepsis)
  - Iron—not normal outside neonatal period, location matters
    - Prussian blue highlights in Kupffer cells
- Stains
  - PAS stain for α_1 antitrypsin
  - Trichrome is good for fibrosis, identifying bile ducts, vascular stain, nodular regenerative hyperplasia
    - Iron stain also in "standard stain" subset
  - Reticulin
    - Reticulin—black
    - Mature collagen—brown
    - Used to demonstrate thickening of hepatic plates in hepatocellular carcinoma
    - Reticulin can be lost in areas of steatosis
  - CD34 stains capillary endothelium but not normal sinusoids
    - CD34+ sinusoids could mean adenoma, carcinoma (usually stains everything), or focal nodular hyperplasia (usually patchy)
    - *Not* positive in regenerative nodules
    - Most useful in chronic liver disease with loss of reticulin/widened portal plates
      - Hepatocellular carcinoma (stains positive) versus regenerative nodule (stains negative)
  - Liver fatty acid–binding protein (LFABP)
    - Positive in normal liver and negative in HNF-1α–mutated adenoma
    - Rarely used
  - Victoria blue or orcein stains
    - Copper–binding protein
    - Increased in periportal hepatocytes in chronic cholestasis of any etiology

- Most commonly unrecognized abnormalities
  - Loss or absence of bile ducts
  - Proliferation of bile ducts
  - Subtle sinusoidal infiltrates
  - Mallory's hyaline in nonalcoholic steatohepatitis (NASH)
  - Abnormal or compressed central veins
  - Nodular regeneration
  - Abnormal or missing portal veins
- Cirrhosis = advanced fibrosis with regenerative nodules that is diffuse
- Nodular regenerative hyperplasia → drugs or ischemia
  - Thick and thin hepatic plates
- Regeneration
  - Slightly thickened plates, mitoses, hepatocyte rosettes forming gland–like spaces
  - No normal structures
  - Can form very circumscribed, round nodules that appear to be expanding

LABORATORY VALUES

- Autoantibodies
  - Antismooth muscle → autoimmune hepatitis (low titers can be seen in steatohepatitis)
  - Antimitochondrial → primary biliary cirrhosis
- Transaminases = aspartate aminotransferase (AST) and alanine aminotransferase (ALT)
  - Acute hepatocellular disease—10 to 20× normal
  - Chronic hepatitis C infection—2 to 4×
  - Acute biliary tract—5 to 10×
  - Chronic biliary tract—2 to 3×
  - AST > ALT → more likely alcoholic liver disease or muscle origin
    - "toAST" to your liver!
  - Causes of increased transaminases and normal bx
    - Inadequate biopsy (at least 2.5 cm) or inadequate portal tracts (11 or more)
    - Focal lesion in liver
    - Transient hepatitis no longer present
    - Transaminases from other sources
    - Macrotransaminasemia
      - Like macroprolactinemia, this represents the target molecule bound to an antibody that is cleared from the kidney inefficiently
      - Increased measured serum levels, but not increased function
      - AST only, does not happen with ALT
    - No chronic liver disease!
- Alkaline phosphatase
  - Can separate by isoenzymes but usually not needed
  - Causes of increased alkaline phosphatase and normal biopsy
    - Inadequate biopsy
    - Focal lesion (including granulomatous disease)
    - Transient elevation caused by a passed stone
    - Sources other than liver
      - Also found in placenta and bone
        - Pregnancy
        - Broken bones, prolonged bed rest, pediatric patient during bone growth
      - Nodular regenerative hyperplasia

- Granulomas
- Tumors
- Advanced chronic liver disease
- Reevaluate biopsy for subtle bile ductular proliferation or nodular regenerative hyperplasia or loss of ducts
- Bilirubin
  - Most common cause—drugs
  - Second most common—heart failure (caused by hemolysis and congestive hepatopathy)
- ↑ Immunoglobulins
  - IgG
    - <1.5×—nonspecific, cirrhosis, inflammation
      - "Polyclonal hypergammaglobulinemia"
        - End–stage liver disease of any cause
        - Pathogenesis
          - Too few Kupffer cells left to remove excess immunoglobulins
    - *And* decreased antigen sequestering in the liver → increased antigen stimulation
    - >1.5×—autoimmune hepatitis, hepatitis E, drug-induced hepatitis
  - IgM— primary biliary cholangitis (PBC)
  - IgA—alcohol
- Patterns
  - GGT is increased in biliary and hepatocellular disease, and creatine kinase increases in muscle disease
  - Direct bilirubinemia, normal alkaline phosphatase and ALT/AST → drug reaction or sepsis
  - Alkaline phosphatase >2× normal, ALT <2× normal → biliary disease
  - Liver disease → increased conjugated (direct) bilirubin
  - Indirect bilirubinemia—Gilbert's or hemolysis
  - Direct bilirubinemia with normal alkaline phosphatase and transaminases → medication reaction or sepsis
    - Congenital/neonatal cholestatic syndromes (jaundice during pregnancy)

HEPATITIC DISORDERS

- Neutrophils in lobules (microabscesses) differential diagnosis
  - Cytomegalovirus (CMV)
    - Only in immunosuppressed patients or neonates
  - Surgical hepatitis (from surgical manipulation)
  - Alcoholic steatohepatitis
  - Sepsis or bacteremia
  - Mini–microabscess disease
- Nonalcoholic steatohepatitis (NASH)
  - Steatosis + ballooning degeneration (cells get larger, cytoplasm gets thin and granular)
    - Sometimes referred to as "rarified" cytoplasm
  - Can also get Mallory hyaline
  - Usually macrovesicular; microvesicular indicates higher disease activity and predicts faster progression
  - Delicate pericellular fibrosis
  - Differential diagnosis: acute alcoholic hepatitis (coarse Mallory hyaline and *neutrophils*)
  - NASH staging
    - I—pericellular fibrosis only

- II—start septal fibrotic bands
- III—distorting fibrous bands
- IV—advanced chronic liver disease, no spared areas
- Alcoholic steatohepatitis and sequelae
  - Acute foamy degeneration
    - Binge–drinking → diffuse microvesicular steatosis
  - Classic alcohol–associated liver disease
    - Micronodular (<3 mm), uniform
      - May become macronodular with time
    - Narrow fibrous bands
    - No gross nodules
    - Mallory hyaline with associated neutrophils
      - Stays for 6 to 12 months after cessation
  - If a patient with chronic alcohol liver disease stops drinking, they lose steatosis in ~1 week and Mallory hyaline in ~6 months
- Autoimmune hepatitis
  - Females, adolescents and 40s to 50s, high transaminases
  - Antismooth muscle
  - Morphology
    - Plasma cells, eosinophils, and lymphocytes in portal tracts
    - Plasma cells in sinusoids
    - Significant plasma cells in the parenchyma are abnormal
    - Emperipolesis
    - Diffuse ballooning degeneration and piecemeal necrosis (interface hepatitis) leading to fibrosis
      - Not delicate pericellular fibrosis (this favors NASH)
    - Can get confluent necrosis
  - Treat with steroids → azathioprine
  - Can be drug–mediated
    - Nitrofurantoin
    - Minocycline
    - Black cohosh
    - Herbalife
    - Valerian root
    - Diclofenac
    - Alpha–dopamine
    - Hydralazine
    - Statins
    - Anti–TNF–alpha drugs
    - Biologics (pembrolizumab)
  - Differential diagnosis (DDx): viral hepatitis superimposed on chronic liver disease, hepatitis E
  - Overlap syndrome
    - Autoimmune hepatitis *plus* PBC or primary sclerosing cholangitis (PSC)
    - Should have very high transaminases
- Viral hepatitis
  - Patterns
    - Whenever you have lymphoid aggregates, consider hepatitis C (HCV) (even superimposed on other diseases)
    - ↑ Hepatic mitoses without apoptoses—EBV and CMV

- Confluent necrosis (small groups of cells)—HSV or acetaminophen toxicity, autoimmune hepatitis
- Hepatitis C (HCV)
    - Only see chronic infection
    - Genotype 1 is most common
        - Not a lot of lobular infiltrate, patchy portal inflammation, mostly lymphocytes (lymphoid aggregates are pathognomonic)
    - Genotype 2—more eosinophils and plasma cells
    - Genotype 3—fatty change
    - Fibrosing cholestatic form of HCV—pericellular fibrosis, cholestasis, acidophil bodies
        - Acidophil, Councilman, apoptotic, or hyaline bodies all refer to dying hepatocytes with condensed hypereosinophilic cytoplasm and hyperchromatic nuclei
- Hepatitis B
    - Patchy portal triad lymph infiltrate with mild sinusoidal infiltrate
    - Ground–glass cells
        - Cells filled with cytoplasmic hepatitis B surface antigen pushing nuclei off to side
        - Classic finding but actually not seen very often
    - Rule out phenobarbital (central nucleus), disulfiram, glycogen storage disease type 4
- Hepatitis E
    - Can look histologically like autoimmune hepatitis
- HHV-6
    - Small clusters of lobular lymphocytes with acidophil bodies
- CMV
    - CMV inclusion disease of the newborn or status post–liver transplant
    - Neutrophil microabscesses in lobules
- Adenovirus
    - Nuclear inclusions—large, eosinophilic, indistinct borders
    - *No* multinucleation (unlike HSV and VZV hepatitis)
- Herpetic hepatitis (HSV and VZV)
    - Little inflammation with confluent necrosis
- Other hepatitic disorders
    - "Fulminant" microvesicular steatosis
        - Acute steatosis of pregnancy
        - Reye syndrome (kid with viral infection given aspirin)
        - Tetracycline toxicity
    - Interface hepatitis = piecemeal necrosis—destruction of limiting plate with little inflammation
        - Prominent in autoimmune hepatitis (antismooth muscle)
        - Rule out drugs (including nitrofurantoin)
    - Hypertrophied stellate cells in very high vitamin A and medication reaction
    - Kwashiorkor
        - Protein deficiency
        - Massive fatty change

CHOLESTATIC DISORDERS

- Congenital
    - Impaired biliary conjugation
        - Gilbert disease
            - Autosomal recessive

- Unconjugated bilirubinemia
- Missense mutation of *B-UGT* or *UGTA1* genes
- Lipofuscin in zone 3
- Indolent
- Crigler-Najjar syndrome
  - Autosomal recessive
  - Complete absence of *B-UGT* gene product (nonsense mutation)
  - Type 1 (most severe) and type 2
- Impaired biliary excretion
  - Dubin–Johnson
    - Autosomal recessive
    - Conjugated bilirubinemia
    - Mutation of *MPR/cMOAT* gene
    - Coarse pigment in zone 3 → black liver
    - Indolent
  - Rotor
    - Autosomal recessive
    - Conjugated bilirubinemia
    - Mutations of *SLCO1B1* or *SLCO1B3* genes
    - No pigment
    - Indolent
- Intrahepatic cholestasis
  - Primary biliary cholangitis (PBC)
    - Formerly primary biliary *cirrhosis*
    - Small, intrahepatic ductules
    - Antimitochondrial antibodies (*not* 100%)
    - Morphology
      - Some portal tracts have loss of bile ducts, some with ductular proliferation
      - Portal tract fibrosis, granulomas
      - Eosinophilic–rich inflammatory infiltrate
  - Primary sclerosing cholangitis (PSC)
    - Large (extrahepatic biliary tree) ductules, males, imaging important
    - Diffuse ductular proliferation
    - Atypical ANCA+ (*not* pANCA or cANCA)
  - Drugs and toxins
    - Big bile plugs
    - Erythromycin—bile stasis without inflammation
    - Augmentin—bile duct damage, inflammation, and bile stasis
  - Sepsis
    - ↑↑↑ Bilirubin (in excess of alkaline phosphatase and AST/ALT)
    - Enteric enzymes paralyze cilia that move bile along in canaliculi into bile duct
    - Look for cholestasis near central vein
  - Malignancy
  - Granulomatous liver disease
    - Infections
    - Chemistry
    - Drugs
    - Miscellaneous
  - Intrahepatic cholestasis of pregnancy
  - Hepatitis (viral and alcoholic)

- Genetic disorders
- Total parenteral nutrition–associated cholestasis
- Post–liver transplant cholestasis
- Acute vanishing bile duct syndrome (VBDS)
  - GVHD or failing allograft
  - Classic Hodgkin lymphoma
  - Sarcoidosis
  - CMV infection
  - HIV infection
  - Medication effect
- Extrahepatic cholestasis
- Obstruction
  - Stone, malignancy, cholangitis
  - Portal tract edema → fibrosis → cirrhosis
- Cholangitis lenta—causes jaundice after sepsis
  - Marker of poor prognosis
  - Bile within dilated bile ducts
  - Bile duct proliferation ("ductular reaction")
  - Ballooning degeneration, fibrosis, *not* a lot of inflammation
- Bile ductular proliferation

VASCULAR DISORDERS

- Ectatic vessels
  - Aberrant shunt vessels
  - Dilated and pressing out into parenchyma without surrounding collagen
  - Now called *herniated veins*
  - Polyarteritis nodosa—necrotizing arteritis
  - Budd–Chiari syndrome
  - Thrombosis of the vena cava or hepatic vein
- Veno-occlusive disease (VOD)
  - Also known as *sinusoidal obstructive syndrome*
  - Associated with alkylating agents and bone marrow transplants
  - Central versus obstruction
  - Decreased endothelial impermeability → space of Disse filling with red blood cells and endothelium sloughs off → occludes outflow of blood → thrombosis
- Congestive hepatopathy
  - Congestion from right-sided heart failure
  - Centrilobular
- *Congestive hepatopathy and Budd–Chiari affect the whole liver, and VOD is patchy*
- Hepatoportal sclerosis (idiopathic portal hypertension)
  - Aberrant shunt vessels (portal veins directly abutting hepatic plates without collagen)
  - Also has hepatosplenomegaly and thrombocytopenia

TRANSPLANT PATHOLOGY

- Liver transplant acute cellular rejection
  - Portal inflammation
  - Bile ducts inflammation and damage
  - Central vein endothelialitis

- See rejection activity index (RAI) grading from Banff 1997 conference
- Mild
  - Inflammation in a minority of portal triads
  - No extension into lobules
  - No confluent necrosis
- Moderate
  - Inflammation in most or all portal triads
  - Rare (if any) necrosis
- Severe
  - Robust inflammation with lobular extension
  - Areas of confluent necrosis near central vein

CONGENITAL

- Cystic fibrosis
  - Massive steatosis
  - Focal biliary fibrosis with proteinaceous debris in all ducts
- Hemochromatosis and Wilson's can present with lots of fatty change and glycogenated nuclei
  - Can diagnose Wilson's disease by 24-hour urine copper or quantitative copper level on liver biopsy
  - Staining for liver copper is not helpful
    - Copper is accumulated in any end–stage liver disease (not just Wilson disease)
  - Wilson causes hemolysis and liver failure (mixed bilirubinemia)

OTHER DISORDERS

- Zonal necrosis
  - Zone 1 (periportal)
    - HELLP syndrome (hemolysis, elevated liver enzymes, low platelet count)
    - Direct toxic/medicine injury (phosphorus), ferrous sulfate
  - Zone 2 (midzonal)
    - Hemorrhagic fevers (Ebola, yellow fever, dengue fever)
    - Heat stroke
  - Zone 3
    - Shock, ischemia/hypoxia
    - Toxicity from chloroform, halothane, mushroom (Amanita species), carbon tetrachloride
    - Acetaminophen
  - Nonzonal
    - Viral hepatitis (especially herpes)
- Hormonal change
  - Peliosis (vascular lakes, random, no endothelial lining)
    - Also in spleen
    - Risk for rupture and hemorrhage
  - Bland cholestasis
- Glycogenic hepatopathy
  - Poorly controlled diabetes or glycogen storage disease
  - Prominent cell borders (plant–like)

- Combined variable immunodeficiency can present with nodular regenerative hyperplasia or granulomatous hepatitis
  - Amiodarone toxicity
- Lots of Mallory hyaline, not much fatty change, cholestasis
  - (Band–like) atrophy—drugs, chronic ischemia, outflow obstruction/congestion
  - Unpaired arterioles in portal tract differential: PBC or hepatic adenoma
- Does not count in areas of fibrosis
  - Inflammatory pseudotumors in liver—mixed inflammation causing tumor
- Probably represent healing abscesses

Neoplastic Liver

BENIGN

Bile Duct Tumors

- von Meyenburg complex = biliary hamartoma
  - Dilated bile ducts of different sizes
  - Associated with autosomal recessive polycystic kidney disease (ARPKD)
    - Also can get congenital hepatic fibrosis (both ductal plate proliferation)
  - Bile duct adenoma
  - Bile ducts that are not dilated, are all the same size

Focal Nodular Hyperplasia (FNH)

- Usually incidental, solitary, small association with oral contraceptive pills (OCPs)
- Classic radiographic appearance, so usually not biopsied (early homogenous enhancement with visible central scar)
- No risk for rupture
- Morphology
  - Multinodular lesion with central fibrosis and an abnormal (dystrophic) hyalinized feeding artery
  - No capsule
  - Bile ductular reaction (bile ductule proliferation) and inflammation at nodule septa
  - Normal hepatocytes (cell plates <2 cells wide)
- Glutamine synthetase—geographic, map–like around central vein
- Can have fatty change!

Hepatocellular Adenoma (HA)

- The majority have no portal tracts or central vein, lobular interface with normal liver
- HNF-1α mutated = type 1
  - Nearly all have macrovesicular steatosis (fatty liver) and no atypia
  - LFABP loss is abnormal and diagnostic
  - Important!
  - Associated with OCPs
  - Rarely transform
  - Not β-catenin mutated, not positive for glutamine synthetase
    - When differential includes hepatocellular carcinoma (HCC)
      - Positive glutamine synthetase can rule in HCC
      - Negative glutamine synthetase cannot rule out HNF-1α adenoma
- β-catenin mutated = type 2

- "Noninflammatory"
- Atypia is present
- One-third have cytologic abnormalities (small cell change and pseudoglands)
- One-fourth have macrovesicular steatosis
- β-catenin stain (+) nuclear
  - Normal is membrane
  - Rule out inflammatory by morphology
- Glutamine synthetase is uniform, diffuse, and strong
  - Normally (+) just around central vein
  - "Geographic" pattern in focal nodular hyperplasia
  - Global (+) → "atypical HA"
  - Can get odd staining patterns in Osler–Webber–Rendu syndrome = hereditary telangiectasia
  - β-catenin is also mutated in colorectal carcinoma and HCC
  - Occur in approximately 40% of men
  - Associated with anabolic/androgenic steroids and glycogen storage diseases
  - Atypical HAs are more likely to progress to HCC
- Inflammatory (telangiectatic) = type 3
  - Males, androgenic steroids, pseudoglandular
  - Women, obesity, diabetes, increased CRP
  - 10% are β-catenin mutated
  - 60% have gain-of-function mutation in interleukin-6 ST (IL6ST)
  - Most likely to rupture, associated with obesity
  - Serum amyloid A+ (diffuse), patchy glutamine synthetase
  - CD34+ sinusoidal epithelium (normally negative in sinusoids and positive in capillary endothelium)
  - Features—a little central fibrosis, (focal or diffuse) inflammation, +/− bile ductule proliferation, sinusoidal dilation, blood pooling, and ectatic thick-walled vessels (congestion)
- No known mutation ("null") = type 4
  - Normal LFABP staining (+)
- See Table 8.1

TABLE 8.1 ■ Comparison of Focal Nodular Hyperplasia and Hepatocellular Adenoma

Focal Nodular Hyperplasia	Hepatocellular Adenoma
Solitary	Usually multiple
Bile ductule proliferation	No bile ductule proliferation
No drug association (small OCP association)	Androgenic steroids (β-catenin), OCPs (HNF-1α and inflammatory)
No BMI association	High BMI association (chronic inflammation)
No malignancy association	Malignancy history (chronic inflammation)
Glutamine synthetase is geographic	Should be resected before pregnancy to avoid rupture

OCP, Oral contraceptive pill; BMI, body mass index.

MALIGNANT

Hepatocellular Carcinoma (HCC)

- Association with chronic hepatitis (mostly HCV)
- Atypia does not really help because reactive/regenerative can have a lot of atypia
  - Widened hepatic plates!
- Almost always has nuclear pseudoinclusions—benign does not!
- Can have rosette–like patterns
  - Fetal components
- Stains for benign (focal nodular hyperplasia versus adenoma versus normal) versus well-differentiated HCC
  - Reticulin—widened hepatic plates
  - CD34—marks sinusoids in neoplasms
    - HCC is diffuse and uniform staining
    - Adenoma and FNH positive too
  - Glypican 3—oncofetal protein
    - Strong and diffuse staining in HCC
    - May be negative in well–differentiated
  - Arginase+, Hep Par+
- HCC can be combined with cholangiocarcinoma
  - HCC—CK18, arginase
  - Cholangiocarcinoma—CK19, CD7
- Steatohepatitic HCC
  - Macrovesicular steatosis, balloon cells, +/– Mallory bodies, inflammation and pericellular fibrosis
  - Well-differentiated are hard to distinguish from HNF-1α–inactivated HA
  - Reticulin stain shows thickened hepatic plates, LFABP not lost

Cholangiocarcinoma

OTHER MALIGNANCIES

- Low–grade lymphomas infiltrate portal triads and high–grades form masses
- Angiosarcoma can be mass–forming *or* sinusoidal
- Kaposi sarcoma
  - HHV8+
- Ocular melanoma classically metastasizes to the liver
  - Classic vignette: Patient with one yellow eye
    - They have had their involved orbit removed, and it metastasizes to the liver and causes jaundice
    - Their eye prosthetic obviously does not become icteric
  - Metastatic melanoma will probably lose HMB45, may lose Melan-A, will probably keep S100

CHAPTER 9

Genitourinary Pathology

Prostate Pathology

ANATOMY

- Transition zone—hyperplasia
  - Peripheral zone—carcinoma
- "Median lobe" of prostate is transitional zone benign prostatic hyperplasia that protrudes into the floor of the bladder

PROSTATE ADENOCARCINOMA AND PRECURSOR LESIONS

Precursor Lesions

- ASAP—atypical small acinar proliferation
  - <5% of tumor glands, grade 4 or less
  - p63/racemase is helpful—no basal cells (p63 negative) and neoplastic epithelial cells (racemase positive)
- High-grade prostatic intraepithelial neoplasia (HGPIN)
  - Pleomorphic, stratified with upper nuclei larger than lower, nucleomegaly, and nucleoli *but* normal architecture
  - Not much increase in prediction of carcinoma (CA) compared with benign biopsies
  - Seminal vesicle bases look similar
  - Differential diagnosis (DDx): intraductal carcinoma—high-grade carcinoma spreading in ducts, necrosis, infiltrating carcinoma elsewhere
  - 30% of HGPIN patients progress to cancer

Adenocarcinoma

- Classic acinar adenocarcinoma
  - Cancer cells are monomorphic, and nuclei are same size with nucleoli
  - *Always adenocarcinoma → 1-glomeruloid formation, 2-mucinous fibroplasia, and 3-perineural invasion*
  - Prostate dual stain—racemase (AMCAR) + basal cell marker (SPACE)(p63, CK5/6, etc.)
  - Highest inherited component of any major cancer
    - One relative—2×, two relatives—5×, three relatives—15×
- Adenocarcinoma variants
  - Ductal variant of adenocarcinoma
    - Very rare
    - Looks like endometrial carcinoma
    - Large cribriforming or papillary nests
    - Looks like a tubular adenoma with long papillary fronds
    - Can have comedo necrosis (upgrades from 4 to 5)
    - HGPIN is smaller
    - 4 + 4 by definition

- Intraductal carcinoma
  - "Cancerization" of ducts by HG cancer, looks like carcinoma elsewhere in the specimen
    - Tends to be associated with HG invasive carcinoma
  - Morphology
    - Dark, small "eyeliner" of basal cells with malignant proliferation inside
    - Solid, dense cribriform, micropapillary*, and loose cribriform*
      - * + marked atypia or comedonecrosis
    - Disorganized (less organized than ductal variant), ↑ pleomorphism
  - Usually loss of *PTEN*
- Mucinous carcinoma
  - Neoplastic cells floating in pools of mucin, ≥25% of tumor (if <25%, "with mucinous features")
  - Classic acinar pattern is usually present elsewhere
  - Rule colorectal carcinoma
  - Grade by "subtracting" mucin and pretending it is stroma
- Staining of metastases—NKX3.1 > PSA-P
- Criteria for active surveillance of prostate cancer
- No higher composite Gleason than 6
- PSA ≤ 0.15
- ≤2 involved cores
- ≤50% involvement
  - May be replaced by unilateral disease
- May still get routine biopsies
- May not be applicable to African-American men, as they tend to have anterior tumors
- Predictive testing for prostate adenocarcinoma is available

Cancer Mimics

- Clear cell cribriform hyperplasia
- Basal cell hyperplasia—atrophic prostates, PSA or p63 can help, keeps glandular structure
- Atrophy
  - Simple atrophy—larger glands with small dark cells
  - Simple atrophy with cyst formation—small and large (cystic) glands
  - Postatrophic hyperplasia—simplified glands, small acini in lobular formation, central dilated duct
  - Partial atrophy—can have cleared cytoplasm and nucleoli (in leftover basal cells), irregular thickness of gland epithelium and "broken" basal layer
  - Proliferative (inflammatory) atrophy—mixed inflammatory infiltrate with simple atrophy or postatrophic hyperplasia
    - WATCH OUT FOR ATROPHIC CANCER
- Nephrogenic adenoma
  - Arises from urethra, edematous stroma with inflammation, papillary or glandular architecture, dilated vessels
  - Racemase+, PAX8+
- Cowper glands in lateral prostate
  - Tightly grouped glands around central duct, foamy to clear cytoplasm, hyperchromatic nuclei pushed to base
  - Rule out foamy gland carcinoma
- Treatment effect
  - Inflammation, edema, sclerosis, atrophy, squamous metaplasia, atypia
  - Racemase is helpful, look for lack of normal architecture

- Urothelial carcinoma
  - Umbrella cells not found in high-grade
  - Especially PUNLMP—papillary urothelial neoplasm of low malignant potential

Gleason Grading

- Major and minor features
- Small glands without lumen = 4, if they open up = 3
- Grade 4 architecture
  - Ductal
  - Glomeruloid
  - Cribriform
  - Regular (poorly formed glands)
  - Hypernephroid (clear cell nests, like clear cell renal cell carcinoma)
  - Collagenous micronodules—only found in carcinoma, considered modified Gleason 4
  - Signet ring—on trabeculae = 4
- Grade 5
  - Cribriform + comedo necrosis = 5
  - Single cells or sheets = 5
- International Society of Urologic Pathologists (ISUP) grade group
  - Grade 1: ≤ 3 + 3
  - Grade 2: 3 + 4
  - Grade 3: 4 + 3
  - Grade 4: 4 + 4
  - Grade 5: ≥ 4 + 5

OTHER NEOPLASMS

- Small cell carcinoma
  - Like small cell carcinoma in other anatomic locations
  - No response with androgen deprivation therapy, treat with platinum–based chemo
- Stromal malignancies
  - Leiomyosarcoma
  - Rhabdomyosarcoma
  - Stromal sarcoma (phyllodes tumor type)

PROSTATE ODDS AND ENDS

- Granulomatous
  - Secondary to tuberculosis, fungus, prior biopsy, post-BCG therapy
  - AFB may be positive in post-BCG
- "Benign prostatic stromal hyperplasia"
  - Histologic correlate of benign prostatic hypertrophy

Testis Pathology

NONNEOPLASTIC

- Stroma
  - Inflammation (acute, chronic, granulomas)
  - Tumor

- Leydig numbers
  - Each seminiferous tubule should have a small cluster
  - Old Leydig cells get lipofuscin
- Tubules
  - Three tubules/hpf
  - Atrophy—thickened basement membrane
  - Cell type
    - Only Sertoli cells? → Sertoli cell-only syndrome
  - Look for maturational arrest
- Maturation pattern
  - Spermatogonia (no nucleolus)
    - If spermatogonia acquires a nucleolus, it is likely germ cell neoplasia in situ (GCNis)
  - Primary spermatocyte (very granular chromatin)
  - Secondary spermatocyte
  - Immature spermatid (look like lymphocytes)
  - Mature spermatid (very small and elongated)
    - On average, each tubule should have ~20
  - Spermatozoa (acrosomal vesicle and flagella)
- Most common diagnoses
  - Obstruction
  - Mixed hypospermatogenesis
  - Sertoli cell-only syndrome
- Granulomatous orchitis—may be submitted as "mass"
  - Pain, BCG treatment, epididymitis
  - Differential diagnosis (DDx)
    - Bugs! Do fungal, mycobacterial, and treponemal stains
      - Syphilitic infection—more plasma cells
      - Urinary tract infections
    - Trauma (sperm granulomas form secondary to mature sperm in surrounding tissue)
    - Intravesical BCG therapy for urothelial carcinoma
    - *Seminoma!! Always look for GCNis in residual seminiferous tubules*
- Fibrous pseudotumor (nodular periorchitis) with entrapped mesothelium
  - Inflammatory, benign
  - Tunica and paratesticular soft tissue, painless mass
  - Associated with hydrocele or trauma
  - Multinodular (rarely diffuse and encasing testis)
  - Collagenous with calcifications and focal inflammatory cells
- Splenogonadal fusion
  - Spleen remnant in scrotum
  - Can swell with mumps
- Müllerian duct remnant
  - Anastomosing cords with single layer of ciliated cells
  - No stratification/tufting/atypia
  - Negative for calretinin
  - DDx: adenomatoid tumor (calretinin+) and Wolffian duct remnant (hamartoma, cyst lined by ciliated cuboidal-to-columnar cells)

NEOPLASTIC

Germ Cell Neoplasms

- Most common prepubertal testicular tumors
  - 60% yolk sac tumor, 40% teratoma

- Alpha fetoprotein (AFP)
  - Half–life = 4 to 5 days
  - Elevated in yolk sac tumor and *some* teratomas *(not seminoma or embryonal)*
- From worst to best
  - Choriocarcinoma, embryonal, yolk sac tumor, seminoma, teratoma
  - All germ cells are PLAP+
    - OCT3/4—nuclear transcription factor
      - Positive in seminoma and embryonal
    - CD30—only positive in embryonal
    - CD117—in seminoma
  - All germ cell tumors have isochromosome 12p *except* prepubertal teratomas
- Cryptorchidism is associated with 3 to 5× risk for cancer and 3% to 14% lifetime risk for germ cell tumor
- Nonseminomatous germ cell tumors—2% to 5% chance of having contralateral tumor
  - 20× risk for general population
  - Also 5% to 6% risk for contralateral GCNis (see later)
- Seminoma
  - 10% bilateral
  - Serum LDH mildly elevated
  - Morphology
    - Sheets of fried egg–appearing cells, prominent eosinophilic nucleoli
    - Dense lymphocytes (cytotoxic T cells), focal reticular areas
    - Cleared out cytoplasm in seminoma is only present in well-fixed specimens
      - May rarely contain red blood cells
      - T1a and T1b cutoff—3 cm (pure seminoma only)
    - Can have syncytiotrophoblasts → can have increased serum hCG
      - Outcome is the same as pure seminoma
    - Rare cases have sarcomatoid degeneration
  - Positive for PLAP, p53, OCT3/4, CD117, and EMA
  - Staging
    - Pagetoid spread in the rete testis does not change outcome
    - Hilar invasion is now pT2 instead of pT1 (higher risk for recurrence)
  - In situ → intratubular germ cell neoplasia (GCNis)
    - If combined with other component, it is enough to call *mixed germ cell tumor*
    - Check lymphocytic infiltration for small foci of invasion
    - Pagetoid spread of large atypical cells within tubules
    - Treat with orchiectomy and chemo (same as seminoma)
  - Spermatocytic seminoma
    - Three cell types: very small (lymphocyte–like), intermediate (classic seminoma cells), and very large (with macronucleoli; "spireme" chromatin)
      - Do not stain for normal seminoma stains
    - Not associated with cryptorchidism, 50 to –55 years of age
    - Not associated with extratesticular sites, GCNis, or other germ cell tumors
    - OCT3/4–
    - Can have bilateral synchronous or metachronous tumors
    - Now called *spermatocytic tumor*—less aggressive
      - Very rarely associated with sarcomatoid differentiation
      - Does not metastasize as seminoma, only sarcoma left
      - Treated with orchiectomy alone
    - Counterpart not seen in ovary
  - Anaplastic seminoma no longer exists

- When it occurs outside of testis → germinoma
  - Sacrum, mediastinum, sella, pineal gland
- Yolk sac tumor
  - Schiller–Duval bodies
  - Most common germ cell tumor in prepuberty
  - Many patterns
  - See "Gynecologic Pathology" chapter
- Embryonal carcinoma
  - Dirty necrosis, vague nuclear border, overlapping cells, pleomorphic nuclei
  - Prominent lymphovascular invasion
  - Immunohistochemistry (IHC) typically not used
    - Positive for CD30, OCT3/4, cytokeratin
    - Negative for EMA
    - Variable for PLAP
- Choriocarcinoma
  - Hemorrhage
  - Cytotrophoblasts
    - Large pleomorphic cells
  - Clustered syncytiotrophoblasts (only ones that stain positively for hCG)
    - Dark pink to purple cytoplasm
- Teratomas
  - Mature teratomas can get sarcomatoid degeneration
    - Chondrosarcoma, rhabdomyosarcoma, leiomyosarcoma >> osteosarcoma, angiosarcoma
    - Surgery is best treatment
      - Chemotherapy not used because it causes "unmasking" of sarcomatous components—metastases are pure sarcoma
  - Ovarian teratomas tend to develop carcinomas; testes → sarcomas
  - Grading mature teratomas is not important in testes
  - "Epidermoid cyst" alone (without hypercellular stroma) → testicular–saving excision
    - If *with* hypercellular stroma → mature teratoma
  - PREPUBERTAL—diploid and benign
  - POSTPUBERTAL—aneuploid and malignant
    - *Therefore teratomas in adults are never called "benign"*
- Mixed germ cell tumors (MGCTs)
  - Must note all components
  - >40% embryonal and lymphovascular invasion → stage II
    - Goes to retroperitoneal lymph nodes

Sex Cord–Stromal

- Leydig cell hyperplasia
  - If diffuse or involving the entire testis → McCune–Albright
    - Fibrous dysplasia → bone pain, cafe-au-lait spots, endocrine abnormality
    - Check for *GNAS* mutations
- Leydig cell tumor
  - Oncocytic (looks like oncocytomas of other organs) cells outside of tubules
  - Can get bilateral
  - Positive for α-inhibin, Melan-A, calretinin, synaptophysin
    - Intermediate filaments are positive for vimentin
    - *May* be positive for S100
  - Associated with cryptorchidism and Klinefelter

- Produce androgens → precocious pseudopuberty and gynecomastia
- Occasionally have characteristic Reinke crystalloids
- 10% have malignant behavior (atypia, large, necrosis, mitoses, infiltrative border, lympho-vascular invasion) and do not produce androgens
- DDx: TTAGS (see next entity), Leydig cell hyperplasia, adrenogenital syndrome (21-hydroxylase deficiency)
- Testicular tumors of adrenogenital syndrome (TTAGS)
  - Babies
  - 21-hydroxylase deficiency
  - Bilateral tumor of rests
  - Look like pleomorphic Leydig cells separated by thick fibrous bands
- Sertoli cell tumor
  - Grossly small yellow-tan nodules
  - Solid to hollow, poorly formed small tubules
    - Cores, ribbons, trabeculae
  - Hyalinized stroma
  - +inhibin, +vimentin, +/–keratin (if positive, focal)
  - Uniform nuclei (mild nuclear pleomorphism is okay), cleared-out cytoplasm
  - Variants
    - Sclerosing
      - Do not confuse with Müllerian duct remnants
    - Large cell calcifying
      - Benign, young, syndromes
        - Carney complex—mucocutaneous pigmentation, atrial myxoma, endocrine tumors, bilateral large cell calcifying Sertoli cell tumor
      - Old, malignant, spontaneous
      - Large eosinophilic Leydig–like cells forming cords and tubules with or without calcifications
    - Lipid rich
    - With heterologous elements
  - DDx: primary carcinoid
  - Can also occur as metastases or in teratomas
- Sertoli–Leydig cell tumors
  - *DICER1* mutations
  - See "Gynecologic Pathology" chapter 4
- Granulosa cell tumor
  - Multiple growth patterns
    - Pseudoglandular/dyscohesive cells in center = microfollicles
    - Solid is the most common pattern in the testis
  - Uniform nuclei
    - Nuclear grooves are classic but may be rare to absent
  - Rare
  - Gynecomastia
  - Calretinin+, inhibin–

Other Neoplasms

- Papillary cystadenomas of *epididymis* is associated with Von Hippel Lindau syndrome (especially bilateral)
  - Account for one-third of all primary epididymal tumors
- Melanoma is the most common tumor to metastasize to testis

- Renal, prostatic, and colorectal cancer tend to go to testes too
- Can be mass–forming
- Usually amelanotic
- Rarely can have melanospermia
- Lymphoma
  - Interstitial pattern (between tubules)
  - Small lymphocytic lymphoma, diffuse large B cell lymphoma
- Adenomatoid tumor
  - Most common benign lesion in spermatic cord
    - Most common malignant is liposarcoma (from peritoneal adipose tissue tracking down inguinal canal)
  - Unencapsulated lesion composed of cuboidal to flat cells forming cords and channels with dilated lumina (sort of like vessels)
  - No atypia
  - Calretinin+, WT1+
- Dedifferentiated liposarcoma (MDM2+), extending through inguinal canal
  - Can have heterologous elements including malignant cartilage

Adrenal Pathology

- Inner—medulla—epinephrine and norepinephrine
- Outer—cortex (out → in)
  - Glomerulosa—aldosterone—thin—neural crest derived
  - Fasciculata—corticosteroids—largest—mesoderm derived
  - Reticularis—sex steroids
- Hypercortisolism
  - Adrenocorticotropic hormone (ACTH)-independent (primary)
    - Neoplastic
      - Adrenocortical adenoma (ACA)
      - Adrenocortical carcinoma (ACC)
    - Nonneoplastic
      - Macronodular cortical hyperplasia
      - Primary pigmented nodular adrenocortical disease
        - *PPKAR1A* mutation, associated with Carney complex
  - ACTH-dependent (secondary)
    - Pituitary adenoma
    - Tumor outside of pituitary–adrenal axis secreting ACTH

LESIONS

- Heterotopias: extra-adrenal, secondary to neural crest migration; aortic bifurcation (tumor of Zuckerkandl) or celiac axis
- Cysts
  - No lining, uniloculated = pseudocysts
  - Typically incidental
  - Worry about Wunderlich syndrome
    - Retroperitoneal hemorrhage and abdominal pain caused by rapid expansion
    - Echinococcal cysts—deep eosinophilic lining, usually associated with liver cysts
    - Can get pseudoangiomatous hyperplasia from inflammation and hemorrhage
    - Rule out angiosarcoma (small pseudovascular spaces, invasive, can be epithelioid)
- Waterhouse–Friderichsen syndrome

- Fulminant adrenal gland failure from adrenal hemorrhage
- Typically caused by *Neisseria meningitidis*
- Life–threatening
- Myelolipoma
  - Bone marrow elements in hamartomatous growth
  - No vascular or smooth muscle components (angiomyolipoma)
  - Lipid–rich on imaging
- Incidentalomas
  - <4 cm = follow
  - 4 to 6 cm = indeterminant
    - Follow for rate of growth
    - If decreased lipid content, resect
  - >6 cm or functional or invasive/necrotic = resect
- Ganglioneuroma—neural tissue (wavy spindled cells) with large pink ganglion cells
  - Benign
  - Adipocytic metaplasia can be present
- Calcifying fibrous tissue
  - Densely fibrotic tissue with psammomatous calcifications (scattered, small), well-circumscribed, macrophages
  - Positive for vimentin, F13a, CD34
  - Negative for SMA, desmin, S100, Alk-1, CD31
- Adrenal cortical adenoma
  - Nodule of cortical tissue, benign, less cords than normal architecture
  - Can get lipomatous/myelolipomatous metaplasia
  - Pigmented (black) adenoma (neuromelanin)
  - Functional
    - Aldosterone–secreting → Conn syndrome
    - Paradoxical cortical hyperplasia
    - Cortisol–secreting → Cushing syndrome
    - Cortical atrophy
  - Nonfunctional
- Adrenocortical carcinoma
  - Higher percentage are functional (secrete cortisol or sex hormones) than ACAs, but ACAs are much more common
  - Metastasizes to liver frequently, poor survival
  - Brown on gross examination (instead of yellow, like adenomas)
  - Pleomorphism, usually nonfunctional, hyalinized, flocculent eosinophilic cytoplasm, prominent cell borders, very *round* nuclei
  - Positive for synaptophysin, inhibin, steroid factor 1 (SF1)
  - Difficult to differentiate from ACA
    - Modified Weiss criteria (currently in use)
      - 5 mitotic figures per 50 hpf (+2)
      - Clear cells ≤25% of tumor (+2)
      - Abnormal mitoses (+1)
      - Necrosis (+1)
      - Capsular invasion (+1)
      - *If total ≥3 = malignant*
    - Helsinki score adds Ki67 but not proven to be better than Weiss
  - Massive DNA loss with whole genome doubling
- Pheochromocytoma—tumor cells in small ball–like structures, slit–like vascular spaces
  - Use PASS score for determining benign vs. malignant (aggressive)

- *SDHB* and *SDHD* mutations can predict malignancy
- Hypertension (epinephrine) or diarrhea (VIP)
- 30% to 40% are hereditary
  - MEN IIA/IIB, VHL, NF1, Sturge–Weber
- Can get hybrid tumor—looks like adrenal cortical adenoma, acts like pheochromocytoma
- Extrarenal sites: organ of Zuckerkandl (between inferior mesenteric artery and bifurcation of the abdominal aorta), carotid bifurcation
  - *"Paraganglioma"* —not "pheochromocytoma" when outside kidney

Bladder Pathology

BLADDER ANATOMY AND HISTOLOGY

- Bladder is different from other luminal organs because there is fat between muscle fascicles and into the lamina propria
  - Makes staging a bit more difficult
- Staging is most important determinant of prognosis and management
- Normal urothelium is three to six layers thick with overlying multinucleated umbrella cells
  - High-molecular-weight keratin–, full-thickness +
  - CD44– full-thickness+
  - p53– wild-type staining
  - CK20 and p63– umbrella cells
- Lamina propria—has muscularis mucosae and is irregular in thickness
  - Invasion through lamina propria = T1
    - But must include in reports how deep in the lamina propria it is invading (above or below muscularis mucosae)
  - Invasion through muscularis propria = T2
- Muscularis propria extends to epithelium in the trigone (where the ureters insert) and at bladder neck (where prostate merges with bladder muscle)

NONNEOPLASTIC

- Proliferative papillary cystitis
  - Reactive entity
  - Signet-ring–like cells ("mucinous metaplasia"), lymphocytes, plasma cells, neutrophils
  - Bulbous (edematous) papillae is usually not seen in neoplasms
- Cystitis cystica
  - Cystitis glandularis
  - Cystitis cystica et glandularis
  - Granulomatous cystitis
  - Status post-BCG treatment or transurethral resection of bladder tumor (TURBT)
  - Caseation vs. no caseation (respectively)
- Ectopic prostate glands
  - Prostatic urethra > bladder trigone > others
    - Bladder diverticulum
  - Lots of degenerating neutrophils
  - Reactive squamous cells
  - High residual post-void volume
    - Ileal loop neobladder cytology
  - Degenerative change, mucus, neutrophils, debris

- Can get papillary fragments
- BK/polyomavirus
  - Densely basophilic smudged nucleus
    - "Decoy cells" concerning for high-grade urothelial carcinoma (HGUC)
  - Significant in transplant patients because it may cause loss of graft
    - Insignificant in immunocompetent patients

UROTHELIAL NEOPLASIA CONCEPTS

- Neoplasms: flat vs. papillary, benign vs. malignant
- Low-grade has a 2% risk of invasion
  - Can usually default to diagnosing as high-grade urothelial carcinoma if invading
- High-grade pathway
  - *p53* and *RB* mutations
  - Usually flat
  - All flats are high-grade!
- High risk for invasion and multifocality
- Not treated with TURBT
- Precursor lesion is urothelial carcinoma in situ (CIS)
- Low-grade pathway
  - *FGFR* mutation
  - Papillary
  - May turn high-grade
  - Less likely to be multifocal
- Stains
  - Reactive urothelium
    - CD44 block+, CK20+ (in umbrella cells only), *p53* is heterogeneous (wild-type), GATA3–
  - Neoplastic urothelium (at least CIS)
    - CD44 basal+/–, CK20 block+, p53 block+, GATA3+
      - GATA3+ in normal breast and T cells too
- Umbrella cells are usually present in benign and absent in cancer, but cannot use alone to determine malignancy

UROTHELIAL NEOPLASMS

- Papilloma
  - Benign, extremely papillary, delicate fronds, normal thickness of urothelium
  - No atypia, no to rare mitosis
- Inverted papilloma
  - Endophytic growth, bland polytypic cells, umbrella cells may be vacuolated
- Papillary urothelial neoplasia of low malignant potential (PUNLMP)
  - PUNLMP can be used in younger patients to whom you do not want to give the label *cancer*
  - Like papilloma but with increased urothelial thickness, NO ATYPIA
  - Should be used *very* sparingly
- Low-grade papillary urothelial carcinoma
  - Always noninvasive (Ta)
    - If invasive, there must be some area of high-grade cytology
  - Small nuclei, thickened layer, some focal nucleomegaly, organized/polarized, monotonous
  - Rare-to-occasional mitotic figures

- Any atypia at all → low-grade!
- Can have rare focal whorling (disorganization, loss of polarity)
- *Nuclear grooves = pathognomonic for low-grade*
- High-grade urothelial carcinoma
  - Can be papillary or flat, can be noninvasive or invasive
    - Noninvasive flat high-grade = Tis
    - Papillary came from low-grade papillary urothelial carcinoma
  - Increased mitotic figures, apoptotic bodies, atypical mitoses, rarely necrosis
  - Demonstrates paradoxical maturation in invasive groups
  - Big distinction between T1 and T2—invasion into muscularis propria
    - Guides treatment and follow-up
  - Micropapillary variant
    - No fibrovascular core, clefting/retraction artifact (multiple nests in lacunae)
    - Needs immediate surgery, no neoadjuvant chemotherapy
  - Plasmacytoid variant
    - Single plasmacytoid cells with some cytoplasmic clearing, dyscohesive
    - Similar in behavior to diffuse gastric (signet ring) adenocarcinoma and lobular breast carcinoma
  - Nested variant
    - Deceptively bland and can confuse with Brunn nests—PITFALL!
    - High-grade nuclei and extension into muscle help DDx
  - Sarcomatoid variant
    - Lymphocytic infiltrate, extremely pleomorphic in areas
    - Need surgery first, and then adjuvant chemotherapy
    - DDx: includes inflammatory myofibroblastic tumor, leiomyosarcoma, benign myofibroblastic proliferation
    - C-kit−, CK5/6+, p63+

Staging for Bladder (Urothelial) Carcinoma

Ta—noninvasive papillary
Tis—flat CIS
T1—invades lamina propria
T2—invades muscularis propria
   A—superficial (inner half)
   B—deep (outer half)
T3—invades perivesical soft tissue
   A—microscopically
   B—mass–forming macroscopically
T4—directly invades adjacent tissues
   A—prostate, seminal vesicles, uterus, vagina
   B—pelvic wall, abdominal wall

PARIS SYSTEM FOR URINE CYTOLOGY

- Low sensitivity but good specificity
- Paris 2013, goal to detect high-grade urothelial carcinoma (HGUC)
1 Negative
   a. Can include "cannot exclude low-grade urothelial carcinoma" comment
2 Atypical urothelial cells (↓ quality and quantity)
   a. Nuclear-to-cytoplasmic (N:C) ratio >0.5 plus one of the following:

      i. Hyperchromasia
      ii. Clumped chromatin
      iii. Irregular nuclear membrane
   b. Should account for <10% of all diagnoses
   c. Cornish hat—pinched–off, pointy cells
3 Suspicious for HGUC ($\downarrow$ quantity)
   a. N:C > 0.7 plus hyperchromasia +/− clumped chromatin or irregular nuclear membrane in <10 cells
4 HGUC (need at least 10 cells)

- No minimum number of cells for adequacy, but there are criteria for "suboptimal" (including obscuring elements)
- Do not need to mention clusters of cells
  - In previous iterations, clusters were noted as possible low-grade urothelial neoplasms (LGUNs)
  - LGUNs include papilloma, papillary urothelial neoplasm of low malignant potential, and low-grade papillary urothelial carcinoma
  - Now we know these can be caused by stones, instrumentation, infection, and so on
- Melamed–Wolinska bodies = red or green cytoplasmic bodies seen in degenerating urothelial cells
  - Helpful to avoid the pitfall of dark/scary nuclei in degenerated cells

UROVYSION

- Used as an adjunct to cytology
- Polysomy is the most common abnormality
- Probes:
  - 9p21 (gold)—locus–specific
    - p16 location
    - Need $\geq$12 cells with homozygous deletion
  - Centromere enumeration probes (need 3+ copies)
    - 3 (red)
    - 7 (green)
    - 17 (aqua)
- We like to see odd numbers for polysomy
  - Even number of signals could represent a multinucleated cell (such as umbrella cells)
- Need abnormalities in at least 2 of 3 CEP probes and at least 4 cells out of 25
- Use DAPI alone or with probes to stain nucleus
- Not always covered by health insurance

OTHER NEOPLASMS

- Can get a neoplasm that resembles low-grade appendiceal mucinous neoplasm as primary in urachal remnant (dome of urinary bladder)
- Nephrogenic adenoma
  - Benign reactive pattern
  - Dilated vessels, loose edematous stroma, usually seen on transurethral resection of prostate (TURP)
  - Racemase+! PSA−, PAX8+
    - PITFALL! Do not mistake for prostate cancer
- Prostate adenocarcinoma with direct extension

- Collision tumor
  - Urothelial carcinoma + prostatic adenocarcinoma
- Inflammatory myofibroblastic tumor
  - Sarcomatous–look with inflammation
  - Pankeratins+, ALK+
  - PITFALL! Do not confuse with sarcomatous carcinoma!
- Small cell carcinoma
  - Salt-and-pepper chromatin without prominent nuclei
  - May compose small part of a tumor with more traditional urothelial carcinoma morphology
  - Use platinum–based therapy
- Paraganglioma (positive for neuroendocrine markers)

Penile Pathology

GENERAL

- Glands have mucosa and spongiosum
- Shaft is skin with spongiosum around urethra, paired cavernosa surrounded by tunica albuginea, and Buck/dartos fascia around all except skin
- Dartos muscle underlies penile skin
- "Bulbar urethra" is distal to prostatic and membranous urethra, just proximal to penile
- Penile squamous cell carcinoma is typically secondary to balanitis xerotica obliterans (BXO)/lichen sclerosis

STAGING FOR PENILE SQUAMOUS CELL CARCINOMA

Tis—CIS
Ta—noninvasive localized
T1—all have no lymphovascular invasion (LVI), no perineural invasion (PNI), low-grade
    Glans: invades lamina propria (not through dartos fascia)
    Foreskin: invades dermis, lamina propria, or dartos fascia
    Shaft: invades connective tissue between epidermis and corpora, regardless of location
    1a—no LVI/PNI *and* not high-grade
    1b—either no LVI/PNI *or* not high-grade
T2—invades corpus spongiosum (either glans or ventral shaft) with or without urethral invasion (through dartos fascia)
T3—invades corpora cavernosa (including tunica albuginea) with or without urethral invasion
T4—invades adjacent structures (scrotum, prostate, pubic bone)

Kidney Pathology

For medical renal, see renal section

Nonneoplastic

- Oxalate crystals—acquired kidney disease
- Renal cystic diseases
  - Genetic

- Autosomal dominant polycystic kidney disease (ADPKD)
- Autosomal recessive polycystic kidney disease (ARPKD)
- Juvenile nephronophthisis
- Medullary cystic disease
- Rare autosomal recessive disease (VHL and tuberous sclerosis)
- Nongenetic
  - Multicystic dysplastic kidney
  - Benign multilocular cyst
  - Simple cyst (hypertension–related)
  - Medullary sponge kidney
  - Sporadic glomerulocystic kidney disease
  - Acquired renal cystic disease
  - Calyceal diverticula
- Klippel–Trenaunay
  - Venous and lymphatic malformations
  - Kidney hemangiomas → gross hematuria
    - Can be bilateral or multifocal

RENAL CELL CARCINOMA AND RELATED NEOPLASMS

General Concepts

- Cytologic grading based on International Society of Urological pathology system
  - See Table 9.1.
  - PMID: 24025520
  - No nuclear grading on kidney biopsies
    - May be heterogeneous
  - Sarcomatoid change (ugly–looking spindly cells typically with lots of necrosis) and rhabdoid change (eccentric high-grade nuclei with abundant eosinophilic cytoplasm and occasional pink globules)
    - Automatically upgrades nuclear grade to 4
- Encapsulation → almost always seen in classic papillary renal cell carcinoma (RCC) and clear cell papillary RCC, also frequently in chromophobe
- Metastasizes to lung, liver, bone, lymph node > adrenal, brain, other kidney, heart, spleen, skin
- Ugly renal tumors
  - Medullary (looks like yolk sac/embryonal)
  - Collecting duct

TABLE 9.1 ■ The International Society of Urological Pathology Grading System for Renal Cell Carcinoma

Grade 1	Nucleoli are inconspicuous or invisible with 40x objective
Grade 2	Nucleoli conspicuous with 40x objective but inconspicuous with 10x objective
Grade 3	Nucleoli eosinophilic and distinct with 10x objective
Grade 4	Extreme nuclear pleomorphism, tumor giant cells, sarcomatoid and/or rhabdoid dedifferentiation

- Translocation–associated
- Molecular in renal tumors
  - Hereditary papillary RCC—7q31.1-q34—*MET* oncogene
  - Nephroblastoma—11p13—*WT1*
  - Beckwith–Wiedemann (nephromegaly, cysts, other)—11p13—*p57/kip2*
  - Clear cell RCC associated with VHL syndrome—3p25—*VHL*
- Staining patterns
  - See Table 9.2.

Clear Cell Renal Cell Carcinoma

- Gross: yellow, predominantly solid (but may have cysts)
- Trabeculated, clear/lacy cytoplasm, pronounced cell borders, uniform round nucleoli
  - "Optically clear" cytoplasm resulting from glycogen (PAS+)
  - Only gets eosinophilic granular cytoplasm when high-grade
- Look for nested vascular pattern
- Like chromophobe except no raisinoid nuclei
- Rule out xanthogranulomatous pyelonephritis
- CD117–, CK7–, CA9+, rarely AMACR (racemase)+
- Hemangioblastoma should be in the differential diagnosis of CCRCC
- **Papillary variant of CCRCC differs**
  - Never high-grade! Never metastasizes
  - Piano–key nuclei (apically oriented)
  - IHC
    - CA9+, CK7+ diffuse, CK90+
    - AMACR–, CD10–

Papillary Renal Cell Carcinoma

- Usually circumscribed with pseudocapsule
- Focal clear cell–like areas may be present
- CK7+, racemase+, EMA+, CD10+, CA9–
- Fibrovascular cores may contain foamy macrophages, psammoma bodies, hemosiderin
- Has an oncocytic variant
- *Hereditary papillary RCC syndrome*
  - Multiple bilateral RCCs
  - *c-MET*–activating mutations
- Type 1

TABLE 9.2 ■ Staining Patterns of Common Kidney Tumors

Tumor	CD10	CA-IX	CD117	CK7	Racemase	Other
Clear cell RCC	+	+ (box)	–	–		EMA+
Papillary RCC	+	–	–	+	+	
Chromophobe (classic) RCC	–	–	+	+		
Chromophobe eosinophilic variant RCC			+	focal		
Clear cell papillary RCC	–	+ (cup)	–	+	–	
Oncocytoma	–		+	–		

- Small cuboidal cells in a single layer, scant pale cytoplasm, low-grade nuclei
- Tubules and glomeruloid structures are possible
- +7, +17, *MET* mutations, Birt–Hogg–Dubé syndrome
- Type 2
  - Pseudostratified layers of cells, abundant eosinophilic cytoplasm, high nuclear grade
  - Multiple genetic aberrations

Chromophobe Renal Cell Carcinoma

- Grossly well-circumscribed, tan to light brown, occasional central scar
- Pale polygonal cells, binucleate with perinuclear halo in optically foamy (or flocculent) cytoplasm with many lysosomes, wrinkled nuclear membranes (raisinoid)
  - Microvesicles/lysosomes also seen in intercalated cells of collecting duct
- Three types of cells
  - Type 1—small with solid, slightly granular eosinophilic cytoplasm
  - Type 2—perinuclear halo in a background of pale, flocculent (not clear) cytoplasm
  - Type 3—large, polygonal cells with hard cell border, abundant reticular cytoplasm
- Sheets, cords, trabeculae in hyalinized stroma
- CD117+, EMA+, CK7+, colloidal Fe+, CA9–
- Moderate pleomorphism, ISUP nuclear grading not clinically relevant
- Intranuclear pseudo–inclusions
- DDx: oncocytoma (CK7–)
- Birt–Hogg–Dubé
- Chromophobe, eosinophilic variant
  - Archipelago, nests of eosinophilic cells without distinct cell borders, round nuclei, conspicuous nucleoli
  - Subtle nuclear atypia (not like oncocytoma)
  - Mostly oncocytoma–like but with characteristic foci

Oncocytoma

- Mitochondria = granules
- Can have atypia (oncoblasts)
- Nests with delicate vessels (+/– tubules)
- Can be bilateral or multifocal in 5% to 10%
  - Connection with Birt–Hogg–Dubé syndrome
    - Can have hybrid tumors
      - Features between chromophobe and oncocytoma ("checkerboard pattern")
      - Fibrofolliculoma (skin)
      - Pulmonary blebs → spontaneous pneumothorax
- CAIX+, CK7–
  - On biopsy "oncocytic neoplasm, cannot rule out chromophobe"
- 10% have concurrent RCC (ipsilateral or contralateral)

Translocation–Associated Renal Cell Carcinomas

- Often negative for epithelial markers (keratins and EMA)
- Occur most frequently in childhood; present at high stage
- *TFE3* gene mutations—Xp11.2, t(X;17), and t(X;1)
  - Also *TFEB* mutations t(6;11)
  - Mixed nested and papillary architecture
  - Cells with abundant clear cytoplasm and prominent cell borders, high nuclear grade, large red nucleoli

- Psammoma bodies
- IHC for TFE3 (nuclear) and TFEB proteins, retained PAX8+
  - CK7 and pankeratins are patchy and weakly positive (if any expression at all)
    - HMB45+ and Melan-A+
- Poor prognosis
- *Note: t(X;17)(p11.2;q25) is also seen in alveolar soft part sarcoma*
- t(6;11)
  - Biphasic population of cells
    - Large clear cells with bulbous cytoplasm
    - Small cells that form clusters around dense hyalinized cores
  - HMB45+, cathepsin K+
  - TFEB fusion protein by FISH (difficult by IHC)
  - Solid/cystic/nested architecture
  - Favorable prognosis
- SDHB−
  - Other SDHB− tumors: pheochromocytomas/paragangliomas and GISTs
  - Circumscribed, microcystic with pale proteinaceous fluid, eosinophilic cytoplasm, nests/solid
  - SDHB−, CK7−, CD117−, PAX8+
  - Favorable prognosis
- Hereditary leiomyomatosis and renal cell carcinoma syndrome (HLRCC)
  - Also known as *Reed syndrome*
  - Autosomal dominant, ↓ fumarate hydratase
  - Resembles papillary RCC type 2 with large red nucleoli
  - PAX8+, CD10+, CK7−
  - Poor prognosis

Acquired Cystic Disease–Associated Renal Cell Carcinoma

- Usually on dialysis
- Not an aggressive neoplasm
- Many micro- and macrocysts
- Oxalate crystals
- Eosinophilic cytoplasm

Multiloculated Renal Neoplasm of Low Malignant Potential (MRN-LMP)

- Old name = *multilocular cystic CCRCC*
- One layer of cells lining a multiloculated cyst
- Can have small clusters of cells in stroma
- DDx: CCRCC with cystic changes—nodular nest of clear cells in stroma

OTHER NEOPLASMS

- Angiomyolipoma
  - Dystrophic hyalinized vessels with smooth muscle cells streaming off, increased adipo- cytes scattered throughout
  - Okay to have nuclear atypia
  - SMA+, HMB-45+, Melan-A+
  - PEComa cells—perivascular epithelioid cells
- Myelolipoma
  - Bone marrow elements and adipocytes forming a mass

- Frozen–section diagnosis can be difficult
- Can occur in adrenal glands
- Cystic nephroma
  - More frequent in females, adults
  - Consistent gross appearance—all multilocular without solid areas, smooth cyst lining
  - Cyst lining—single layer epithelial cells and stromal cells
  - Fluid is weakly proteinaceous
  - Collagenous hypocellular stroma to pseudo-ovarian stroma
    - Can have areas that look like corpora albicantia (they are actually perivascular sclerosis)
    - Inhibin+ in some cells, ER/PR+ in some, SMA+, desmin and caldesmon variables
  - DDx: multilocular cystic neoplasm of uncertain malignant potential
    - Clear cells embedded in septa (cytologically identical to CCRCC cells)
  - Cured by resection, no recurrent genetic changes
- MESTs—mixed epithelial and stromal tumors
  - Cystic neoplasm with ovarian–like stroma
  - 7:1 female-to-male incidence
    - Exposure to hormones (including in utero DES exposure)
  - Gross
    - Can occur in pelves, medullae, cortices
    - May grossly appear completely solid
    - Mural nodules can be numerous
  - Incredibly variable features with many combinations
    - 20% have ≥7 types of epithelial elements; 50% have ≥3.
      - Small glands/tubules, sheets, elaborately branched channels, multicystic, complicated glands, stratified (urothelial–like), ciliated, fat papillae (spatulate papillae), micropapillary
      - All in septum
    - 50% have ≥3 stromal components
      - Spindled stromal cells—nondescript cellular, smooth muscle, *loose pseudo-ovarian stroma*, collagenous
    - Additional components
      - Mucin
      - Fat
      - Sclerotic vessels
      - Densely vascular
      - Corpora albicantia–like structures
  - Immunophenotype
    - SMA+, actin+ (usually), desmin+ (usually), ER/PR+ (in some), HMB45–, inhibin–, Melan-A–
  - May grow with estrogen therapy (either hormone replacement therapy or oral contraceptives)
  - Malignancies (carcinomas and sarcomas) rarely arise in MESTs
  - Cured by resection, no recurrent genetic changes
  - Unknown whether a completely different entity than cystic nephroma, or if they are two entities on a spectrum
    - Sort of related neoplasms
      - Partially differentiated nephroblastoma
      - *DICER1* mutations and pleuropulmonary blastoma
      - Impact on cystic nephromas later in life is unknown
- Medullary fibroma

- Fibrous nodule in renal medulla
- May have myxoid stroma
- Metanephric adenoma
  - Occur in all age groups
  - Up to 12% have polycythemia as a paraneoplastic syndrome
  - Primitive–appearing
  - Benign "counterpart" to Wilms tumor, thought to arise from nephrogenic rests
  - Cytologically bland
  - Psammoma bodies can be frequent
  - *BRAF V600E* mutations

CHAPTER 10

Renal Pathology

Introduction to Medical Renal Pathology

- Classified with four parameters: histologic, pathogenetic, clinical presentations, syndromes
- Stains
  - H&E
    - Least useful
    - Crystals and tubular pathology only; eosinophils
  - PAS
    - Basement membranes, Bowman's capsule, mesangial matrix, apical brush borders = pink–purple
  - PAMS silver stain
    - Extracellular matrix = black
    - Highlights capillary loops
    - Use silver stain to look for mesangial thickening
      - Silver (+) deposits >1.5 nuclei
      - Can also look at PAS stain. Also gives you hyperproliferation if >3 nuclei/branch
  - Trichrome
    - Blue = collagen and mesangium, highlights scars and deposits
    - Red = cytoplasm
    - Brown = nucleus
    - Use trichrome stain to look for podocyte detachment (pseudodeposits)
- Light microscopy (LM) and immunofluorescence (IF) more important than electron microscopy (EM)
  - LM specimen goes into formalin (you can *maybe* do EM on)
  - IF specimen goes into Zeus fixative (only usable for IF; must do in *all* transplant evaluations)
  - EM specimen goes into glutaraldehyde (you can *maybe* do LM on)
- Hypercellularity—What type of cells?
  - Mesangial (>3/glomerulus)
  - Endocapillary
  - Extracapillary/urinary space = CRESCENT
    - If neutrophils → infection
    - If anything else, deal with later (on permanent sections)
    - Can also be HIV-associated
  - Nonspecific patterns
    - Insudates/hyalinosis—entrapped protein (IgM and C3, red on trichrome)
    - Crescents—from glomerular basement membrane (GBM) defects/injury
      - WBCs, fibrin, reactive epithelium
      - anti-GBM antibodies, vasculitis, and so on
      - Phases
        - Cellular—acute and reversible

- Fibrocellular
  - Fibrous—chronic and irreversible
- Double contours of GBM in capillary loop
  - Large proteinuria
- Immunofluorescence
  - IgG, IgM, IgA, light chain, C3, C1q, (C4d for transplant), fibrin, albumin
  - Linear direct immunofluorescence (DIF)—anti-GBM
  - Granular DIF—deposits = membranous
  - Mesangial DIF—IgA
- Electron microscopy
  - Deposit location
    - Subendothelial (inside GBM)
    - Mesangial
    - Subepithelial (outside GBM)
  - Usually electron–dense (dark)
- Wedge biopsy—it can be NORMAL for subcapsular sclerosis in kidney and liver
- Normal % = (age/2) –10
- Proximal tubule—reabsorbs glucose, amino acids, proteins, lots of water and salt
- Basal nuclei, brush border
- More abundant eosinophilic cytoplasm
- Fanconi anemia has defects here
- Distal tubule—thiazides act here, nuclei are *apical*
- Collecting ducts—distinct cell membranes, cuboidal, central nuclei, larger lumen
  - Principal cells—antidiuretic hormone
  - Intercalated cells—bicarbonate
  - Medullary—clearer cytoplasm
- Parietal epithelial cells are progenitor cells for proximal tubule
  - Become columnar, ciliated, basal nuclei
  - If inflamed for a long time → reactive metaplasia
- Tubular casts
  - White blood cells
    - Granular tubular structure with lymphocytes
    - Tubulointerstitial disease (like interstitial nephritis and pyelonephritis) and transplant rejection
  - Red blood cells
    - Glomerulonephritis
  - Tubular epithelium
    - Abundant granular cytoplasm
    - Acute tubular necrosis (ATN), viral infection, drug toxicity
  - Granular cast
    - Brown amorphous granules
    - ATN and chronic renal failure
  - Hyaline cast
    - Normal, seen especially after periods of relative dehydration (such as first urination of the morning or after long exercise)
    - Composed of Tamm–Horsfall protein
  - Waxy cast
    - Chronic renal failure
  - Fatty cast

- Oval, formed in distal nephron
- Nephrotic syndrome

DONOR KIDNEY EVALUATION PEARLS

- A small wedge biopsy of a kidney (typically from a deceased donor) that will be transplanted into a patient with renal failure
  - Performed to check for underlying kidney disease and severe hypertensive changes that will limit kidney performance
  - Biopsy is also performed on all gross lesions (besides rare small simple cysts)
  - Not done at every institution
- Err on the side of *under* calling
- Do not call *rare/mild acute tubular injury*
- Arteriosclerosis—vessel with elastic lamina
- Hyalinosis—vessels without elastic lamina
  - Homogenous pink protein deposits
- Some amount of sclerotic glomeruli is normal (see earlier)
  - Globally sclerosed glomeruli/total glomeruli
  - Count at least two levels
- Always call for help when unsure

Glomerular Disease

GENERAL CONCEPTS

- Subendothelial deposits stimulate inflammation and endothelial proliferation
  - Subepithelial deposits do not
- Systemic and genetic causes for nephrotic syndrome
  - Diabetes mellitus (DM), systemic lupus erythematosus (SLE), amyloidosis
  - Finnish–type congenital nephropathy (nephrin mutation)
- Nephrotic syndrome
  - Prone to infections (loss of complement and immunoglobulin), thromboemboli (loss of antithrombin III)
  - >3 g per day
  - In nondiabetic patients, membranous nephropathy (MN), focal segmental glomerulosclerosis (FSGS), and minimal change disease (MCD) are three leading causes of nephrotic syndrome
  - Underlying pathology
    - FSGS
    - MN
    - MCD
    - Amyloidosis
    - Diabetic glomerulonephropathy
    - Membranoproliferative glomerulonephritis (MPGN)
- Nephritic syndrome
  - Hematuria and small proteinuria
  - Underlying pathology
    - Acute postinfectious (poststreptococcal) glomerulonephritis
    - Rapidly progressive glomerulonephritis

- IgA glomerulopathy (Berger disease)
- Alport syndrome
- MPGN (can be either nephritic or nephrotic)

Minimal Change Disease (MCD)

- Nil disease or lipoid nephrosis
- Most common cause of nephrotic syndrome in children, usually steroid–responsive
- Primary = idiopathic
  - Associated with immunization or allergies
  - Also secondary to NSAIDs, Hodgkin lymphoma, bee stings
- Selective albuminuria
- Genetic mutation in podocin
- Appear normal by light microscopy, podocyte effacement on EM (may have microvilli formation)

FOCAL SEGMENTAL GLOMERULOSCLEROSIS

- Most common nephrotic syndrome in African–American adults
- Vacuolated cytoplasm of podocytes on EM with effacement
- Usually idiopathic but can be from genetic mutations of podocyte proteins, viral infections, and drugs
  - ApoL1, podocin, *TRPC6* mutations
  - Parvovirus, HIV
  - Heroin, pamidronate, anabolic steroids
  - Obesity, vesicoureteral reflux
- First glomeruli affected are juxtamedullary glomeruli
- Trichrome dark, PAS pink deposits
- Can recur in transplanted kidneys
- Plasmapheresis for circulating "permeability factor"
- Collapsing variant
  - Tip lesions (foamy of macrophages at the start of proximal tubule), hilar fibrosis
  - Associated with HIV infection
  - Basement membrane collapses in on itself and obstructs capillaries
  - Hyperplastic epithelium

MEMBRANOUS GLOMERULOPATHY/NEPHROPATHY

- Most common cause of nephrotic syndrome in non-African–American adults
- Morphology
  - GBM thickening with spike formation on silver stain
  - "Lumpy bumpy" subepithelial electron–dense immune deposits—polyclonal IgG, C3, kappa, lambda
    - Granular on IF for IgG, kappa, and lambda
  - Effacement of foot processes
  - Thickened capillary walls without inflammation
- 75% are idiopathic (primary) = antibodies against basement membrane (anti-PLA2R in 80%)
  - Serum level correlates with disease level
- Secondary forms seen with

- Autoimmune or collagen vascular disease (SLE, rheumatoid arthritis, sarcoidosis)
- Drugs (gold, penicillamine, NSAIDs)
- Infection (syphilis, hepatitis B, hepatitis C)
- Malignancy (carcinomas of prostate, lung, or gastrointestinal)
- One-third spontaneously remit, one-third stay with chronic course, and one-third progress to renal failure

MEMBRANOPROLIFERATIVE GLOMERULONEPHRITIS

- GBM duplication, mesangial cell interposition (mesangial cells grow inside GBM and splits into "train tracks") and *subendothelial* electron–dense deposits
  - Lobular accentuation
- Seen in mixed (type 2) cryoglobulinemia (thumbprint on EM, microtubules), usually associated with hepatitis C infection
- Nephrotic range proteinuria, microhematuria, C3 and C4 low
- Type 1
  - Associated with immune complex depositions
  - Can only differentiate on IF or EM
  - Type 1 has smoother IF than type 2
- Type 2—"dense deposit disease"
  - Intensely electron–dense glomerular C3 deposits (more granular than type 1)
  - Dysregulation of alternative pathway resulting from autoantibodies that stabilizes C3 convertase (C3 nephritic factor)
- May recur in transplant

AMYLOIDOSIS

- Group of diseases characterized by extracellular, amorphous, eosinophilic protein deposits
  - Apple–green birefringence with Congo red
    - Congo red should be read on thick sections (10 μm)
  - Nonbranching fibrillar substructure—10 nm (8 to 12)
  - Antiparallel beta–pleated sheet structure
  - Expand the mesangial matrix and thicken GBM
- May involve many organs or one organ
  - Renal involvement is common in AL and AA amyloidosis
    - Can differentiate using stains for SAA, kappa, lambda
    - Vessels of all calibers are involved by progressive amyloid accumulation in the medial and intimal layers → rigidity
- AL amyloidosis
  - "Primary amyloidosis"
  - Monoclonal light chain (most commonly lambda), secondary to plasma cell dyscrasia
  - Most common
  - *Globular* deposits
- Light chain deposition disease (LCDD)
  - *Linear* deposits composed of kappa or lambda light chains
    - Most commonly kappa light chains
  - Granular–powdery light chain deposits in all basement membranes including glom, tubules, and vessels
  - Congo red negative
- Myeloma cast nephropathy

- Casts composed of kappa chain
- Manifests as acute renal failure
- Distinct tubular casts and widespread tubular injury
- AA amyloidosis
  - "Secondary amyloidosis"
  - Derived from SAA—an acute phase reactant from the liver
  - Develops with chronic inflammatory disorders
    - Autoimmune: rheumatoid arthritis, psoriasis, ankylosing spondylitis, Crohn's disease, familial Mediterranean fever
    - Infections: tuberculosis, chronic osteomyelitis, bronchiectasis, intravenous drug abuse

DIABETIC GLOMERULONEPHROPATHY/DIFFUSE DIABETIC GLOMERULOSCLEROSIS

- Develops in approximately 50% of patients with diabetes mellitus (DM, types 1 and 2)
- Typically develops concurrently with diabetic retinopathy
- Clinically first sign is microalbuminuria
  - Not picked up by dipstick
- Can get chronic pyelonephritis and papillary necrosis
- Afferent and efferent arteriosclerosis is DM until proven otherwise
- Morphology
  - First change—capillary and arteriolar basement membrane thickening
    - Caused by excessive synthesis of collagenous proteins and glycoproteins
  - Second change—mesangial thickening
    - Associated with microaneurysms, insudates
  - Kimmelstiel–Wilson nodules—use PAS to highlight
    - Nodular mesangial sclerosis
  - Armanni–Ebstein lesions (subnuclear vacuoles in proximal tubule)
  - Capsular drop—fibrin deposits hanging on capsule in urinary space
    - Light pink on silver stain
    - Red on trichrome stain

IgA nephropathy

- Results from autoantibody to underglycosylated IgA_1 molecules with subsequent glomerular deposition of IgA-containing immune complexes
- Mesangial hypercellularity and inflammation

POSTSTREPTOCOCCAL GLOMERULONEPHRITIS

- Streptococcus pyogenes
- IF: granular mesangial C3 deposits

RAPIDLY PROGRESSIVE GLOMERULONEPHRITIS (RPGN)

- Crescents
- Types
  - Immune complex deposition
  - Goodpasture syndrome
    - Linear IF resulting from antibodies against the basement membrane

- ▪ Treat with plasma exchange and steroids
- ▪ Usually favorable prognosis without relapses
- ■ Pauci–immune

Lupus Nephritis

- ■ A subset of RPGN cases
- ■ Anti-dsDNA antibodies
- ■ Morphology
  - ▪ Crescents
  - ▪ Increased cellularity in urinary space
  - ▪ Linear IgG on IF
  - ▪ Granular subepithelial deposits on EM (under foot processes)
  - ▪ Need treatment as soon as possible or will progress to chronic kidney failure quickly
- ■ Classification
  - ▪ Class I—minimal mesangial
    - ▪ Normal light microscopy
    - ▪ Immune deposits in mesangium
      - ▪ "Full house" (like in poker) = IgA, IgM, IgG, C1q, C3, +/– light chains
        - ▪ Three immunoglobulins and two complement proteins
  - ▪ Class II—mesangial proliferative
    - ▪ Mesangial hypercellularity and/or mesangial matrix expansion
    - ▪ Capillary growth—increased endothelial cells and wall leukocytes
    - ▪ IF—mesangial (rare subepithelial or subendothelial) deposits
  - ▪ Class III—focal endocapillary proliferation
    - ▪ Active or inactive, segmental or global, endo- or extracapillary glomerulonephritis involving <50% of glomeruli typically with focal subendothelial deposits +/– mesangial alterations, neutrophils
    - ▪ A—active
    - ▪ A/C—active and chronic
    - ▪ C—chronic
  - ▪ Class IV—segmental or global endocapillary proliferation
    - ▪ LNIV-S for segmental and LNIV-G for global
    - ▪ Same as class III but >50% of glomeruli
    - ▪ Most common on presentation biopsy because they are more symptomatic
  - ▪ Class V—membranous lupus nephritis
    - ▪ Normocellular glomeruli with diffuse thickening of capillary walls (with or without mesangial deposits)
      - ▪ Subepithelial spikes
    - ▪ If endocapillary proliferation is present, classify as *LNIII and LNV* or *LNIV* and *LNV* (depending on extent)
  - ▪ Class VI—advanced sclerosing lupus nephritis
    - ▪ >90% of glomeruli are globally sclerotic without residual activity
- ■ Do not necessarily progress linearly through the classes

Crescentic Types of Glomerulonephropathy (Not Necessarily Rapidly Progressive)

- ■ Linear deposits
  - ▪ Goodpasture syndrome
- ■ Granular deposits
  - ▪ Lupus nephritis

- MPGN
- Poststreptococcal glomerulonephritis
- IgA nephropathy
- Pauci–immune
  - Granulomatosis with polyangiitis (Wegener's granulomatosis)
    - *Pauci–immune necrotizing crescentic glomerulonephritis* when seen on biopsy
  - Microscopic polyangiitis
  - Eosinophilic granulomatosis with polyangiitis (Churg–Strauss syndrome)

FIBRILLARY GLOMERULONEPHRITIS

- Congo red negative glomerular deposits that are positive for IgG, C3, kappa, lambda
  - Larger than amyloid fibrils (30 nm)
- Autoantibodies against DNAJB9 (chaperone protein)
- Associated with chronic inflammatory states (such as hepatitis C and lupus)

THROMBOTIC MICROANGIOPATHY

- Mucoid intimal edema
- Most common cause in children is Shiga toxin–producing *E. coli* (STEC)
  - *E. coli* O157:H7
  - Clinical syndrome is hemolytic uremic syndrome
- Can also be caused by disseminated intravascular coagulopathy (DIC), thrombotic thrombocytopenic purpura (TTP), hemolysis with elevated liver enzymes and low platelets (HELLP) syndrome or preeclampsia in pregnancy, malignant hypertension, scleroderma, lupus anticoagulant

Tubulointerstitial and Vascular Disease

ACUTE TUBULAR NECROSIS OR ACUTE TUBULAR INJURY (ATN/ATI)

- A cause of acute kidney injury
- Normal glomerulus with diffuse dilation of proximal tubules and attenuated cytoplasm
- Tubular simplification, loss of brush border, sloughing of necrotic epithelial cells
- Ischemia
  - Cardiogenic shock
  - Heart failure
  - Trauma with severe blood loss
- Toxins
  - Cisplatin
  - Heavy metals (including arsenic)
  - Organic solvents
  - Radiation
  - Contrast dye
  - Hemoglobin/myoglobin
  - Aminoglycoside antibiotics
- On autopsy or explanted kidney, must distinguish from autolysis
  - See Table 10.1

TABLE 10.1 ■ Features of Acute Tubular Injury vs. Autolysis

Acute Tubular Injury/Necrosis	Autolysis
Proximal tubules mostly affected	All nuclei pyknotic
Flattened epithelium (normally tall with brush border)	Retraction and loss of continuity
Mitotic figures	
Loss of brush border	

BILE CAST NEPHROPATHY

- Setting of marked hyperbilirubinemia
- ATN/cd7 ATI with brownish–green casts

MALIGNANT HYPERTENSIVE NEPHROSCLEROSIS

- May arise de novo or in a patient with preexisting hypertension
- Severe blood pressure elevation (>200/>130) with acute renal failure, blurry vision, and headache
- Fibrinoid necrosis of the intrarenal arterioles and mucoid intimal edema of interlobular arteries
- Over time, progressive ischemia leads to glomerulosclerosis, tubular atrophy, interstitial fibrosis

CHRONIC PYELONEPHRITIS

- Pathologic features
  - Grossly shrunken
  - Broad *U*-shaped cortical scars
  - Blunting of papillae → calyceal deformity (especially at upper and lower poles)
  - Thyroid-type tubular atrophy
  - Relatively spared glomerulus
- Insidious onset of renal insufficiency and low–grade proteinuria
- Usually caused by bacterial organisms
- Seen in chronic urinary obstruction and vesicoureteral reflux
- May have negative cultures
- Tubular dysfunction → nocturia and polyuria because the kidney cannot concentrate urine

FIBROMUSCULAR DYSPLASIA

- Beading of the distal portion of the renal artery with "sausage–string" deformity
  - Compared with more common atherosclerotic stenosis (70%), which occurs in proximal segment in older adults
- Young women with hypertension → can cure with surgery or angioplasty

PAPILLARY NECROSIS

- Necrotic black tips of renal papillae

- Seen in four clinical settings (HIGHLY TESTABLE)
    - Sickle cell anemia—occlusion of the vasa recta renis of the pyramids → hypertonicity, acidosis, and ischemia
    - Analgesic (NSAIDs and aspirin) abuse—chronic interstitial nephritis and papillary necrosis caused by direct toxic effects of phenacetin metabolites on tubular cells + drug–induced inhibition of prostaglandins → vasoconstriction
    - Diabetic glomerulosclerosis—combination of severe small vessel disease and repeated infections
    - Obstructive pyelonephritis—infection and increased pressure on renal papillae secondary to outflow obstruction

XANTHOMATOUS PYELONEPHRITIS

- Inflammatory mass that can mimic renal cell carcinoma
- Unilateral, females more frequently effected, in the setting of chronic renal infections in an obstructed kidney and diabetes
    - Bacterial infections (most commonly *E. coli*)
- Yellow color grossly caused by foamy macrophages, single or multiple masses

Congenital Syndromes and Lesions

AUTOSOMAL DOMINANT POLYCYSTIC KIDNEY DISEASE (ADPKD)

- AD inheritance
    - One inherited mutation, then second acquired "hit"
- One of the most common human heritable diseases (1 in 500 to 1000)
    - Accounts for ~10% of all end-stage renal disease (ESRD) in the United States
- Mutations in polycystin-1 (*PKD1;* chromosome 16) or polycystin-2 (*PKD2*; chromosome 4)
- Bilateral cysts → massively enlarged kidneys
- Clinical presentation
    - Onset 20 s to 40 s (rarely in childhood)
    - Renal insufficiency, hypertension, hematuria, renal colic
    - Slowly progressive
    - End–stage disease after 40 years of age
- Associated with liver cysts and berry aneurysms

AUTOSOMAL RECESSIVE POLYCYSTIC KIDNEY DISEASE (ARPKD)

- Far less common than ADPKD, 1 in 20,000
- Most result in stillbirth or death in early neonatal period
- Oligohydramnios in third trimester → pulmonary hypoplasia and Potter facies
- Enlarged but externally smooth kidneys
    - Bilateral diffuse cortical and medullary cysts that are elongated, perpendicular to surface
- Liver disease is always present
    - Bile ductule proliferation and cyst formation
    - Those who survive neonatal period develop congenital hepatic fibrosis

RENAL DYSPLASIA

- Abnormal development of the kidney secondary to aberrant differentiation of the metanephric blastema

- Associated with teratogenic syndromes or anomalies elsewhere in the genitourinary tract (e.g., posterior urethral valves, urethral atresia)
- May be unilateral or bilateral
  - Unilateral may be clinically silent or a palpable flank mass in neonate
  - Severe and bilateral is incompatible with life
- Oligohydramnios, pulmonary hypoplasia, and Potter facies
- May be cystic or noncystic
- Microscopy recapitulates renal development with aberrant differentiation
  - Most commonly
    - Primitive dysplastic medullary tubules lined by cuboidal/columnar epithelium
      - Resembles ureteric bud derivatives
    - Encircled by immature, loose spindle cells ("mesenchymal cuff")
  - Heterotopic elements may be present

ALPORT SYNDROME

- Mutation in collagen IV α_5 chain (X-linked)
- "Basket weave" lamellation of glomerular basement membranes

TRANSPLANT PATHOLOGY

- Acute cellular rejection—lymphocytic interstitial infiltrates, tubulitis, endarteritis
- Acute antibody–mediated rejection—interstitial capillaritis, glomerulitis
  - C4d staining and donor–specific antibodies of peritubular capillaries
- Cyclosporine/tacrolimus (calcineurin inhibitors) toxicity →
  - *Isometric vacuolization of proximal tubules*
    - All vacuoles are the same size
    - Most frequently proximal tubules, can also affect distal
  - Acute, potentially reversible
- BK polyomavirus infection
  - Basophilic intranuclear inclusions in tubular epithelium
  - SV40+
- Transplant rejection—C4d mediated (linear IF staining of capillaries for C4d)
  - T-cell mediated—endarteritis
- Entities that recur in transplanted kidneys—FSGS, MPGN

Odds and Ends

- NSAIDs are associated with MCD, acute interstitial nephritis, and ATN
- HIV—collapsing glomerulopathy (variant of FSGS)
  - Tubuloreticular inclusions
- Glomerulonephritis with *C3 only* deposits = dysregulation of complement alternative pathway
- Hypertensive kidney disease—medullary rays and outer stripe of outer medulla
  - Thick ascending limb
  - Straight proximal tubule
  - Idiopathic longstanding hypertension (not malignant hypertension)
- Antibody mediated—endarteritis, interstitial capillaritis, and C4d staining of peritubular capillaries

CHAPTER 11

Forensic Pathology

Introduction to Forensic Pathology

- In general, deaths to report include sudden, unexpected, and/or caused entirely or in part by anything other than natural causes
  - Has not seen doctor in >10 years
  - Drug use
    - Exception—death after prolonged hospitalization with no preserved admission samples for drug testing
  - Sudden death
  - No history of underlying disease
  - In emergency department
  - In operating room
  - Within 24 hours of arrival in health care facility
  - No physician present (outside of licensed health care/hospice facility)
- Manners of death
  - Natural (disease entity is responsible)
    - Only manner that can be selected by noncoroner/nonmedical examiner certifier
  - Accident (include drug toxicities, traffic accidents, falls)
  - Suicide
  - Homicide
  - Undetermined (conflicting or insufficient data)
- Proximate (underlying) cause = underlying condition that started the terminal chain
  - Last line of death certificate cause-of-death hierarchy
- Intermediate cause = link between proximate and immediate
- Immediate cause = last event in terminal sequence (first line of death certificate cause-of-death hierarchy)

Toxicology and Chemistry

GENERAL TESTING

- Tubes
  - Gray—preservative stops serum cholinesterase from breaking down cocaine
    - Drug confirmation/quantitation
  - Purple—EDTA
    - Genetic studies
  - Red—no preservative
    - Immunoassays, serologies, TSH, chemistries

ALCOHOL AND DRUGS

- Alcohol is produced postmortem
- If vitreous is negative for alcohol but blood is positive, it is most likely postmortem production (decomposition)

- Postmortem alcohol production generally <0.2
- Blood alcohol content (g/dL)
  - 0.30 to 0.40—obtunded, stupor, impaired
  - 0.40+—coma, death possible
- Test for drug overdose in peripheral blood (central can get leakage from organs—falsely elevated from perimortem ingestion)
  - Use femoral/subclavian
- Delayed death after drug use → check subdural hemorrhage blood, intracranial hemorrhage, admission blood tubes
  - If unavailable and you want to check for opiates → check bile!
  - Subdural and intracranial hemorrhages are very slowly resorbed. They are typically a "picture" of blood content at time of bleed
- Methamphetamine is ONLY seen in illicit use
- 6-MAM (6-monoacetylmorphine) is a breakdown product of heroin (specific)
- Levamisole is a cutting agent (antihelminth agent)
  - Enhances cocaine's effect
  - Can cause agranulocytosis
- Cocaine active metabolites: norcocaine, cocaethylene, benzoylecgonine (BE)
  - Enough to say "acute cocaine toxicity"
  - Benzoylecgonine cannot prove cocaine use alone
  - Can only say "recent use"
  - BE is not an active metabolite
- Embalming fluid can contain methanol, isopropanol, formaldehyde, and so on
  - Vitreous is well protected
- Normal vitreous concentrations
  - Sodium: 130 to 155 mEq/L
  - Chloride: 105 to 135 mEq/L
  - Potassium: <15 mEq/L
  - Urea nitrogen: <40 mg/dL
  - Creatinine: <1.0 mg/dL
  - Glucose: <200 mg/dL
- Vitreous chemical patterns
  - Reference ranges
    - Sodium (Na): 130 to 155 mEq/L
    - Chloride (Cl): 105 to 135 mEq/L
    - Potassium (K): <15 mEq/L
    - Urea: <40 mg/dL
    - Glucose: <200 mg/dL
  - High Na, high Cl, normal or high urea and creatinine
    - Dehydration
  - Low Na, low Cl, normal K/urea/glucose/creatinine
    - Low salt
  - Low Na, low Cl, high K, normal urea/glucose/creatinine
    - Decomposition
  - High/normal Na, very high glucose, variable everything else
    - Diabetes
      - Important to have beta–hydroxybutyrate on vitreous panel in addition to acetone—some diabetic ketoacidosis and alcoholic ketoacidosis can be negative for acetone

- Armanni–Ebstein lesions—subnuclear vacuoles in renal tubules
  - Seen in ketoacidosis (diabetic, alcoholic, starvation)
- Very high urea and creatinine, variable everything else
  - Uremia

ASSOCIATIONS

- Pink brain with necrosis of the globus pallidus—*carbon monoxide poisoning*
  - Differential diagnosis (DDx): hypothermia and cyanide
- Pistachio green brain—*hydrogen sulfide*
  - DDx: methylene blue treatment
- Mee's lines in nails—*heavy metal poisoning* (arsenic, lead, thallium)
- Armanni-Ebstein lesions (subnuclear vacuoles in renal tubule cells)—*ketoacidosis*
- Polarizable crystals in renal tubules (calcium oxalate)—*ethylene glycol*
  - Toxicity phases
    - Central nervous system
    - Cardiorespiratory
    - Renal

HIGH–YIELD POINTS

- Peripheral blood is the most accurate specimen for postmortem toxicology analysis
  - Understand postmortem redistribution (elevations of drug concentrations in central blood after diffusion from solid organs or gastric contents)
- Positive drug screen results should be confirmed by a second method of analysis
- Heroin's main metabolite = 6-monoacetyl morphine
- Cocaine's main metabolites = benzoylecgonine (BE) and ecgonine methyl ester
  - Must be collected in gray–top tube (sodium fluoride)
- The ethanol concentration of a subdural hematoma may more accurately reflect the concentration at the time of injury than will peripheral blood
- Hospital admission specimens will more accurately reflect drug levels at the time of an incident than will postmortem specimens
- Ethanol is produced in the body postmortem
- Recognize postmortem vitreous humor electrolyte patterns for dehydration, uremia, hyponatremia, decomposition, and hyperglycemia

Sharp and Blunt Force Injuries

- Cutting/incised: longer than deep
- Stabbing: deeper than wide
- Ambiguous? "Sharp force injury"
- Comminuted fracture—broken bone in more than two pieces
- LeFort facial fractures—skull fractures in a variety of patterns
- Commotio cordis
  - Sudden death from cardiac arrest after blow to chest *without* structural damage
  - Probably caused by ventricular arrhythmia
- As little pericardial fluid as 150 mL can be lethal
- Clots

- Postmortem—large "layers" of currant jelly and chicken fat (or just soft maroon)
  - Soft, shiny, smooth, easily falls apart
- True clot—coiled upon itself, relatively uniform maroon, gritty/granular/fibrinous surface
  - Firm, retains vessel shape after removal
- Explosion injuries
  - Primary—direct impact of blast—tympanic membrane rupture, pulmonary barotrauma
  - Secondary—flying debris and bomb fragments
  - Tertiary—person being thrown by blast wind
  - Quaternary—exacerbation of preexisting conditions (angina, COPD, asthma)

Asphyxia

- Greek for "breathlessness"
- Oxygen deprivation
- Interference with mechanics of breathing, reduced or absent environmental oxygen, cellular poisons
- Anoxia
  - Complete deprivation of oxygen
  - *Complications of anoxic encephalopathy*
  - Unconscious in seconds, death in 4 to 5 minutes
- Petechial hemorrhages
  - Not specific
  - Caused by acute rise in venous pressure
  - Scalp, eyelids, conjunctivae, sclera, pleura, pericardium, epiglottis
  - Can coalesce into Tardieu spots
- Suffocation
  - Failure of oxygen to reach blood
  - Entrapment/environmental hazards
    - High altitude, natural gas leaks, trapped in small airtight spaces
  - Smothering
    - Mechanical obstruction of external airways
    - Cause of death cannot be determined if the bag is removed
    - Overlay
    - 90 seconds
  - Choking
    - Obstruction within air passages
    - Swallowed object, obstructive airway swelling
  - Mechanical asphyxia
    - Pressure on neck/chest/abdomen preventing inspiration/expiration
  - Positional asphyxia
    - Trapped in restricted space or position by own body
    - Prone restraint—overweight, on stomach, +/− knee on back, hogtie restraint position
    - Riot crush
  - Suffocating gases
    - Carbon dioxide, methane, nitrogen, helium
  - Mechanical asphyxia + smothering
    - Outside pressure plus external obstruction
    - Overlaying
- Strangulation
  - External compression of neck resulting in closure of the vasculature and/or trachea
  - Hanging
    - Pressure needed to compress

- 4 ppsi (pounds per square inch)—compress jugular veins
- 11—carotids
- 33—trachea
- 66—vertebral arteries
  - Dissect neck last
  - Sexual asphyxia
- Ligature strangulation
  - Furrow is horizontal (hanging has upward cant)
- Manual strangulation
  - Excessive force often used
- Chemical
  - Hydrogen cyanide
    - Can happen in fires
  - Hydrogen sulfide
    - Sewers
    - Can stain internal structures green
  - Fires and carbon monoxide toxicity
    - Cherry red (also hypothermia)
    - Soot in airways
  - Recreational inhalants

Child Abuse Deaths

- Mostly children younger than 1 year of age
- Differences in infant autopsies
  - Skeletal survey—close–up views of every bone
  - Many cultures
  - Strip pleura off ribs
  - Unroof orbits, and look at optic nerves
    - Save and bisect to look for retinal hemorrhages
  - Reverse Y incision
- Neural injuries/findings
  - Mostly in "shaken baby syndrome"
  - Shearing contusions at gray–white junction, corpus callosum, brainstem
    - Microscopically looks like a lake of blood
    - *Diffuse axonal injury* is usually cause of death
  - Axonal spheroids—18 to 24 hours to develop
    - Can used immunostain for bAPP for earlier changes
  - Subdural hemorrhage (95%)
- Fractures
  - Cannot give specific age, just broad categories (acute or healing)
  - Subperiosteal new bone formation
    - Thin gray line on radiographs
  - Classic metaphyseal fracture/lesion = bucket handle fracture
    - Most specific finding for inflicted trauma
    - Other, most specific to least specific
      - Posterior rib fractures (caused by abusive squeezing)
      - Scapula
      - Sternum
      - Multiple or different ages
      - Others

- Inflicted abdominal injury
  - Crushing solid organs against vertebral column
  - Compressing and rupturing hollow organs
  - Mesenteric laceration
  - Toddlers and older kids
  - 40% have no external injuries
  - Second only to head injury for cause of death in abuse
- Inflicted chest trauma
  - Cardiac lacerations
  - Rare
- Homicidal infant suffocation/smothering
  - 70 to 90 seconds
  - Fewer than 50% have any signs

Odds and Ends

- Sleep–related deaths and airway obstruction
  - Plastic bags causing smothering
    - Findings are minimal
    - Diagnosis made with scene investigation and history
  - Strangulation and hanging
    - Clothing, cribs, cords, furniture
    - Cribs are most common
  - Hennepin County (Minnesota) sees 15 to 20 deaths per year caused by unsafe sleep environments
    - More than one-half were in adult beds (alone or cosleeping)
  - Reenactment is important
  - Rarely still call it *sudden unexplained infant death/undetermined*, then list stressors or contributing causes
    - More frequently, *accident*
- Pulmonary barotrauma
  - Ascending too rapidly
  - Alveoli diffusely rupture
    - Pneumomediastinum
    - Pneumothorax
    - Subcutaneous emphysema
    - Arterial air embolism
- "The bends"
  - Decompression sickness
  - Dissolved nitrogen coming out of solution, forms bubbles in blood, pumped to body
  - Rashes, joint pain, altered mental status, paralysis, death
- Time to third–degree burns for adults
  - 120° F: 5 minutes
  - 130° F: 30 seconds
  - 140° F: 6 seconds
  - 150° F: 2 seconds
- Shotgun wounds
  - 0 to 2 feet away—smooth margins
  - 2 to 4 feet away—scalloped margins
  - 4 to 10 feet away—some satellite wounds
  - 10+ feet away—great variation, many satellites

CHAPTER 12

Lung and Cardiac Pathology

Nonneoplastic Lung

MAIN CONSIDERATIONS

- Pattern of fibrosis
- Severity
- Spatial and temporal heterogeneity

ENTITIES

- Asthma–related changes
  - Goblet cell hyperplasia
  - Thickened basement membrane
  - Eosinophilic inflammation (especially in untreated)
  - Charcot–Leyden crystals
    - Eosinophilic, short, linear
    - Made from lysophospholipase from eosinophil granules
    - Curschmann's spirals
    - Gray to black loose spirals
    - Casts of small bronchioles, made of mucous and dead epithelial cells
- Chronic bronchitis
  - Increased mixed inflammation
  - Reid index (RI) = gland/wall
    - 0.5 is chronic bronchitis, <0.4 is normal
- Usual interstitial pneumonitis (UIP)
  - Clinical term = *interstitial pulmonary fibrosis*
  - Temporal and spatial heterogeneity
  - Dense active fibroblastic foci
    - Subpleural lower lobes
    - Center is relatively spared
  - Diffuse interstitial thickening, accentuation of subpleural scar, honeycomb change, +/– chronic inflammatory infiltrate
    - Honeycomb change alone is not diagnostic of UIP—it is the common end stage of many lung pathologies
  - Progressive fibrosis of lung parenchyma, unknown etiology
  - Chronic dyspnea, dry cough, fatigue, digital clubbing
  - Respiratory and heart failure (cor pulmonale) in 3 to 5 years
  - Can be confused with pleuroparenchymal fibroelastosis but has a faster progression
- Nonspecific interstitial pneumonitis (NSIP)
  - Like UIP minus subpleural scar accentuation and honeycomb change
    - Thickening of alveolar septae
    - Lots of lymphocytes in septae
  - Cellular stage responds well to steroids, can be idiopathic

- Fibrotic stage (irreversible)
  - Collagen deposition and less cellular
- Can be idiopathic or as part of systemic process
  - Connective tissue/autoimmune, drug reaction, chronic hypersensitivity pneumonitis, graft-versus-host disease (GVHD), hematopoietic malignancy
- Airway-centered interstitial fibrosis (ACIF)
  - Like UIP but central with involvement of alveolar walls, and respiratory epithelium extending into adjacent alveoli ("peribronchiolar metaplasia")
- Desquamative interstitial fibrosis (DIP)
  - Pigmented macrophages filling alveoli, spatially heterogeneous, +/– ↑ interstitial fibrosis, +/– intra-alveolar eosinophils
  - Less filled alveoli → "respiratory bronchiolitis-associated interstitial lung disease"—less severe version of DIP (continuum)
  - Respiratory bronchiolitis—smoking association, pigmented macrophages (fine granules)
- Hypersensitivity pneumonia (HSP)
  - Airway-centered fibrosis, organizing pneumonia, focal, peribronchial chronic inflammation, granuloma, upper–lobe predominant
    - Poorly formed, small, necrotizing granulomas in interstitium +/– multinuclear giant cells
      - Compared with sarcoid—larger, nonnecrotizing, tight granulomas
  - 45 to 60 years of age; exposure to allergen
- Cryptogenic organizing pneumonitis (COP)
  - Old term—*bronchiolitis obliterans–organizing pneumonia* (BOOP)
  - Nodular (haphazard) at low power, obliterative bronchiolar process with branching pattern and Masson bodies (intrabronchiolar fibrosis), inflamed and vascularized fibrosis
  - Differential diagnosis (DDx)
    - Aspiration with organizing pneumonia—dispersed nodules with ↑ lymphs around bronchioles +/– food particles
    - Langerhans cell histiocytosis—stellate nodules, not round
    - Sarcoidosis
      - Discrete small, nodular granulomas in linear arrangement or groups
      - Lymphangitic spread
      - Diagnosis of exclusion
    - Organizing pneumonia—fibroblastic plugs in airspaces
- Diffuse alveolar damage (DAD)
  - Histopathologic correlate of acute respiratory distress syndrome (ARDS)
  - Lung injury with fibrinous exudate and type 2 pneumocyte hyperplasia
  - Consolidated and basophilic at low power; hyaline membranes, fibroblasts filling alveoli, thrombosed small vessels
    - Stage 1—exudative—hyaline membranes
    - Stage 2—proliferative—fibroblasts and macrophages
    - When resolved—fibrosis of interstitium
- Lymphocytic interstitial pneumonitis (LIP)
  - Cellular NSIP + lymphoid aggregates near airways
  - DDx
    - Lymphoma—bronchus–associated lymphoid tissue (BALT) lymphoma (extranodal marginal zone lymphoma)
    - Connective tissue disease (e.g., rheumatoid arthritis, Sjogren's syndrome)
- Eosinophilic pneumonitis
  - Many eosinophils, pulmonary edema (alveolar proteinosis), alveolar macrophages; vasculitis

- DDx
  - Desquamative interstitial pneumonitis (DIP) has no eosinophils and many macrophages
  - Churg–Strauss (eosinophilic granulomatosis with polyangiitis) would have an eosinophilic infiltrate within the vessel wall, necrosis, and infarcts
    - Idiopathic
  - If no vasculitis is seen with the same picture → eosinophilic pneumonitis secondary to asthma/allergies
    - May have peripheral eosinophilia
    - Can be secondary to parasites (e.g., *Entamoeba histolytica, Ascaris*)
- Pulmonary alveolar proteinosis
  - PAS +/– D
  - Nocardia
  - Autoantibodies to GM-CSF
  - Surfactant protein B mutation (lethal)
- Granulomatosis with polyangiitis (GPA)
  - Formerly Wegener's granulomatosis
  - pANCA
  - Morphology
    - Bronchovascular distribution
    - Poorly defined
    - Geographic necrosis
    - Granulomas with multinucleated giant cells
    - Vasculitis with fibrinoid necrosis
    - Mixed inflammation (including eosinophils)
      - Eosinophils can be prominent in drug reactions, Hodgkin, collagen vascular disease, eosinophilic granulomatosis with polyangiitis
    - Differential diagnosis includes infection
- Eosinophilic granulomatosis with polyangiitis (EGPA)
  - Formerly Churg-Strauss syndrome
  - Very rare
  - cANCA
  - Two components
  - Eosinophilic pneumonitis
  - Eosinophilic vasculitis
  - Immune complex deposition
  - Associated with pulmonary hemorrhage and necrosis
- Bronchopulmonary dysplasia
  - Acute = necrotizing bronchiolitis obliterans
  - Chronic = submucosal fibrosis, mucous gland atrophy, medial hyperplasia of pulmonary arteries, squamous metaplasia
- Idiopathic pulmonary hemosiderosis
  - Associated with peripheral eosinophilia and iron–deficiency anemia
- Pleuroparenchymal fibroelastosis (PPFE)
  - Lots of deposited elastin in subpleural upper lobes, sharply demarcated
- Pulmonary malakoplakia
  - From *Rhodococcus equi* infection
    - Can rarely come from *E. coli*
  - Accumulation of histiocytes that form large areas of consolidation and even masses
  - Concentric bodies that contain calcium and iron (Michaelis–Gutmann bodies)
  - Usually in immunosuppressed patients (AIDS)

DIFFERENTIAL BY LOCATION

- Alveolar space, alveolar septum/interstitium, airways, vascular, pleura
- Alveolar space pathology
  - Pulmonary edema (cardiogenic)
  - Acute lung injury (ALI)
    - Acute onset of bilateral pulmonary infiltrates with hypoxemia
    - Clinical/imaging correlate = ARDS
    - Diffuse consolidation and heavy on autopsy
    - Etiologies/patterns
      - Pneumonia
        - Clinical diagnosis, categorized histologically by whether acute inflammation or organizing fibrosis predominates
        - Organizing pneumonia (OP)—Masson bodies (wavy fibroblast aggregates in alveoli)
        - Acute fibrinous pneumonia (AFP)—fibrin and inflammatory cells in alveolar (mostly neutrophils)
          - Note: fibrinous and fibrous are not the same! Fibrin is acellular/paucicellular, and fibrous tissue has fibroblasts
        - Acute fibrinous and organizing pneumonia (AFOP)—combination of previous two
      - Diffuse alveolar damage (DAD)
      - Noncardiogenic edema
  - Atelectasis
  - Emphysema
  - DIP
  - COP (formerly BOOP)
- Airway
  - Bronchitis
  - Asthma
  - Bronchiectasis
  - Obstruct bronchiolitis
  - Respiratory bronchiolitis interstitial lung disease
- Septum
  - Inflammatory
  - Fibrotic
  - Neoplasms
- Vascular
  - Embolus
  - Hypertension
    - Primary (idiopathic)
      - *BMPR2* in familial cases
      - 25% sporadic
    - Secondary
      - Chronic obstructive pulmonary disease (COPD)
      - Chronic interstitial pulmonary disease
      - Chronic heart failure
      - Recurrent pulmonary emboli (PE)
        - Especially small "showers" of PEs
      - Obstructive sleep apnea

- Drugs
  - Pulmonary veno–occlusive disease (PVOD)
  - Thickened arteriole walls and plexiform changes (revascularization) +/– intravascular thrombosis
- Inflammatory vasculitis
  - GPA (granulomatosis with polyangiitis/Wegener's granulomatosis)
  - EGPA (eosinophilic granulomatosis with polyangiitis/Churg–Strauss syndrome)
- Pleura
  - Inflammatory/infectious
  - PPFE
  - Malignancy

LOW–POWER DIFFERENTIAL

- ACUTE
  - Floridly fibrotic consolidation—DAD
  - Fluid and cellular consolidation—hemorrhage, edema, infection, eosinophilic pneumonia
- CHRONIC
  - Linear—interstitial (e.g., UIP)
  - Lobular filling—DIP or respiratory bronchiolitis–associated interstitial lung disease (RBILD)
  - Nodular dispersed—bronchiolar (BOOP, aspiration)
  - Nodular lymphangitic—sarcoid
    - Peripheral and central
  - Cystic
    - Microcystic
    - Langerhans cell histiocytosis usually in burned–out phase
    - Lymphangioleiomyomatosis
    - Emphysema, bronchiectasis, overinflation due to obstruction, cystic adenomatoid malformation

LUNG TRANSPLANT REJECTION

- Two components
  - Vessels away from airway with lymphocytic cuffing (graded 1 to 4)
  - Airway—need intact smooth muscle (low versus high)
- Chronic rejection
  - Fibrosis → ↓ lumen of airway (bronchiolitis obliterans)
  - Typically requires bronchial stenting
- The International Society for Heart and Lung Transplantation (ISHLT) grading system

Neoplastic Lung

- Can get salivary gland neoplasms from minor salivary glands in bronchial tree (see Chapter 13, Head and Neck Pathology)

BENIGN NEOPLASMS

- Pulmonary hamartoma
  - The fibromyxoid stroma is key (immature cartilaginous material)

- Usually seen in older men with smoking history
- "Popcorn" calcifications with soft tissue density on imaging
- Usually not sampled unless rapid growth
- Paraganglioma
  - Can be described as in the lung but is usually between lung lobe and central structures (like aorta)
  - Solid/vaguely nodular mass, glassy amphophilic cytoplasm, low N:C
  - S100 stains sustentacular spindled cells
  - Atypia/pleomorphism does not mean malignant
    - Invasion, necrosis, metastasis do
  - "Zellballen"—cell balls
  - Pheochromocytoma = paraganglioma in the adrenal gland
  - Positive for CD56, synaptophysin, chromogranin, SDHA (can be positive for melanoma markers)
    - SDHB+ weak in sustentacular cells
    - *SDH A/B* mutation can be germline (shown by loss of expression)
      - B mutated more frequently than A
- Lymphangioleiomyomatosis
  - Cystic lymphatic dilation lined by smooth muscle
  - ER/PR+
  - HMB45+, Melan-A+
    - Like PEComa
    - Is commonly associated with renal angiomyolipoma
  - Usually diagnosed radiographically, not surgically
  - Virtually all are women; lesions are proliferative during menstrual years
  - Mutations in tuberous sclerosis genes (*TSC1* and *TSC2*)
- Pulmonary meningothelioid nodule
  - Minute and diffusely distributed (<0.5 cm)
  - Swirled bland cells around vessels
  - Resembles meningioma
  - EMA+, vimentin+, CK–, S100–, CD34–
- Inflammatory myofibroblastic tumor
  - Peripherally located, in children
  - Grows into large airways and vessels
  - Associated with hypergammaglobulinemia, leukocytosis, thrombocytosis, weight loss, fever
  - Low mitotic rate (no necrosis)
    - Biologically a borderline lesion
    - Recurs in 25%, may undergo malignant transformation
  - Calcifications
  - Translocation of ALK receptor on 2p23
- Pulmonary sclerosing "hemangioma"
  - Actually pneumocytomas of epithelial origin
  - Positive for cytokeratins and TTF1
  - Negative for CD34 and CD31
  - Rarely multifocal
  - Patterns: papillary, solid, sclerotic, angiomatoid

MALIGNANT NEOPLASMS

- Neuroendocrine
  - General considerations

- Can have other component (e.g., adeno) in "combined tumor"
- Based on WHO → do not require neuroendocrine marker expression!
  - Small cell may lose all
- TTF-1 expression does not mean lung primary
- Tumorlet
  - Looks like carcinoid, but 1 to 5 mm in greatest dimension
    - If <1 mm = tumor nodule
  - Associated with airways
  - Multiple tumorlets → will have symptoms (shortness of breath, slowly progressive)
- Diffuse idiopathic pulmonary neuroendocrine hyperplasia (DIPNECH)
  - 5-year survival of 85% to 98%
  - No treatment
  - Can progress to carcinoids (rarely atypical carcinoids)
- Typical carcinoid
  - <2 mitoses, no necrosis
  - Loosely cohesive, rosette–like structures, plasmacytoid
  - Low–grade cells with neuroendocrine (salt and pepper) and ample granular cytoplasm
  - No or very rare mitoses
  - No necrosis
  - Immunohistochemistry
    - Positive for synaptophysin, chromogranin, CD56
    - Negative for TTF-1
    - Ki67 low
  - Classic presentation is an endobronchial mass
  - ~95% survival
- Atypical carcinoid
  - 2 to 10 mitoses or necrosis present
  - 60% survival
- Small cell carcinoma
  - High–grade neuroendocrine carcinoma
  - Molded chain (or clusters) of cells with salt-and-pepper chromatin and very high N:C ratios
    - Classically small–sized cells but not required
  - Pleural effusion only occurs in 3% of patients
    - Most common lung malignancy to cause effusion is adenocarcinoma
  - Usually central, can be peripheral
  - 15% to 20% of total primary lung malignancies
  - Standard is chemotherapy only (in the US)
    - Other countries may do resections
  - Paraneoplastic syndrome
- Large cell carcinoma
  - Size does not actually matter when differentiating large versus small
  - Large nucleoli, solid large nests with central necrosis
    - *Does not have salt-and-pepper chromatin*
    - *Can have prominent nucleoli*
- Non-small–cell lung carcinoma (NSCLC)
  - General
    - 70% to 75% of lung primaries
    - Adenosquamous, sarcomatoid, squamous, adenocarcinoma
    - On limited biopsies, a dual stain may be useful

  ▫ TTF-1 (for adenocarcinoma) and p40 (for squamous) is widely used
  ▫ Okay to say, "NSCLC, favor adenocarcinoma"
- Adenocarcinoma
  - Most common lung cancer caused by smoking reduction
  - One-third are central and two-thirds are peripheral
  - Very heterogeneous
  - Immunostains
    ▫ Positive for TTF1 (SPT24 < 8G7G3/1), Napsin A, CK7
  - Patterns (most favorable prognosis to poorest)
    ▫ Lepidic
      ▪ Means malignant cells involve the pre-existing alveolar structures without destroying them or causing desmoplasia
      ▪ Categorized by size
        ▫ ≤0.5 cm = atypical adenomatous hyperplasia
        ▫ 0.5 cm and ≤3 cm = adenocarcinoma in situ
        ▫ Formerly known as *bronchoalveolar carcinoma*
        ▫ ≤3 cm with ≤0.5 cm invasion = minimally invasive adenocarcinoma (invasive part not lipidic)
        ▫ 0.5 cm invasion or >3 cm or other growth patterns = invasive adenocarcinoma
    ▫ Acinar
    ▫ Papillary
    ▫ Micropapillary
    ▫ Cribriform
    ▫ Solid
  - Other variants
    ▫ Mucinous
      ▪ May look in situ/lepidic but with mucinous cells—still call *invasive*!
    ▫ Colloid
      ▪ Cells floating in pools of mucin
    ▫ Adenosquamous
      ▪ Squamous elements and vacuolated cells in a dyscohesive pattern
      ▪ Full squamous pattern is <1%
      ▪ Cannot make diagnosis on limited biopsy or FNA
    ▫ Signet ring
      ▪ Associated with *KRAS* or *EGFR1* mutations
      ▪ All mutations in lung cancers are mutually exclusive
      ▪ Panel
        ▪ CK7 and CEA (confirm adenocarcinoma, nonspecific)
        ▪ CK19 and CA19-9 (favor pancreaticobiliary met)
        ▪ TTF1 (must be nuclear)
        ▪ CK20 negativity is nonspecific and does not help
      ▪ CK20 may favor GI primary
  - Important factors in staging
    ▫ Size
    ▫ Single versus multiple
    ▫ Pleural invasion
    ▫ Lymph nodes (LN)
      ▪ LN staging trick: If the node station number is 1 digit = N2, if node station number is 2 digits = N1
    ▫ Metastases

- Must obtain molecular testing on all invasive primary lung adenocarcinomas to predict response to targeted treatment
  - Mutually exclusive aberrations
    - *EGFR*—exon 19 and 21, activating mutation, susceptible to erlotinib
    - *ALK*—3% to 13% of all lung adenocarcinomas have *EML4-ALK* translocations
      - Younger nonsmokers
      - Most commonly found in signet ring or acinar
    - *ROS*—1% to 2%
      - Sensitive to crizotinib
    - *KRAS*
  - PDL1 (see Chapter 1)
- Squamous cell carcinoma (SCC)
  - Stains for CK5/6, p40, p63, CK903/34 βE12
    - Basaloid SCC—p63/p40
    - Spindle cell or pleomorphic
      - Giant cell carcinoma of the lung (CK+, TTF−, Napsin A−)
- Malignant mesothelioma
  - Starts from parietal pleura (not visceral)
  - Localized
    - Very rare
    - Not related to asbestos
    - Favorable prognosis with just resection
    - Grossly papillary
  - Diffuse
    - May have dominant mass
    - Most favorable survival to poorest: epithelioid → biphasic → sarcomatoid
      - 20% to 30% are epithelioid and can be positive for adenocarcinoma markers
      - Sarcomatoid subtype: desmoplastic (looks like pleuritis)
    - Important to show invasion into adipose *or* skeletal muscles
      - Papillary fronds can be reactive
      - Tumor formation also helpful for malignant versus reactive
  - Immunostains
    - Expresses: calretinin, WT-1, cytokeratins
      - PITFALL: MOC31 and BerEP4 can be +
      - N240 in sarcomatoid
    - Negative for Napsin A/TTF-1, CEA, claudin-4
      - These will all be positive in adenocarcinoma
    - BAP1 *absence* is specific for mesothelioma (but presence does not rule out)
  - p16 deletion by FISH
  - DDx includes serous carcinoma (CEA would be positive)
- Other malignant neoplasms
  - Hemangioendothelioma
    - Well–demarcated areas of collagen deposits, epithelioid cells with intracytoplasmic lumens
    - CD34+, ERG+
    - Low–grade neoplasm but can metastasize
  - Solitary fibrous tumor
    - CD34+ (can be patchy or weak), STAT6+, TLE1−
    - Staghorn vessels, hypercellular, "patternless pattern," whorled around vessels
    - Can be malignant

- Increased mitoses (>5/10 hpf, most are >10/10 hpf) and necrosis
■ Monophasic synovial sarcoma
  - Plump spindle cells in fascicles; hyperchromatic and some pleomorphism
  - CD34+, TLE1+, STAT6–

Lung Odds and Ends

■ Can get subpleural nodule with dystrophic calcifications
  - Can have ossification, even with adipose tissue and marrow elements
■ Number–one tumor in the lung—metastasis
■ Number–one primary tumor in the lung—adenocarcinoma
  - Smoking is decreasing
  - Current cigarette filters only allow smaller particulates through, which penetrate deeply and cause peripheral adenocarcinomas
■ Clara cells
  - Columnar nonciliated bronchial cells
  - Secrete surfactant and protease inhibitors
■ Kulchitsky cells
  - Basally oriented cells with tons of neuroendocrine granules
  - Function unknown
■ Giant cells and granulomas in a bronchovascular distribution can be seen in
  - Intravenous drug abuse
  - Granulomatosis with polyangiitis
  - Methotrexate toxicity
  - Henoch–Schönlein purpura
  - *Not* seen in systemic lupus erythematosus
    - Acute phase → siderophages, pleuritis, capillaritis
    - Chronic → lymphoplasmacytic interstitial pneumonia with fibrosis (NSIP)
■ α_1-antitrypsin = protease inhibitor
■ Do not diagnose emphysema on histology (other than in autopsy)
■ Asbestos–related lung disease
  - Most common manifestation is pleural plaque formation
  - Can get bronchogenic carcinoma, pleural effusions, interstitial fibrosis, mesothelioma, laryngeal neoplasms

Cardiac

■ Aschoff bodies
  - Acute rheumatic carditis
  - Intramyocardial aggregates of large histiocytes (Anitschkow cells) with basophilic cytoplasm, vesicular nuclei with central bar of chromatin
■ Myocarditis associations
  - Giant cell—*horrible* prognosis
  - Neutrophilic with necrosis—bacterial
  - Eosinophilic—hypersensitivity to drug or parasite
  - Amastigotes in sarcoplasm—Chagas disease
  - Neutrophilic and granulomatous with *extensive* necrosis—fungal
■ Antibody–mediated cardiac rejection
  - Myocyte edema, ↑ macrophages in capillary walls, capillary C4d
    - Quilty lesion

- Dense endocardial lymphocytic aggregate, predominantly T cells
- Idiosyncratic reaction to immunosuppression post–transplant
  - PITFALL—*not* cell rejection!
- Cardiac amyloidosis
  - Vessel wall deposits → luminal obstruction → ischemia
- Anthracycline cardiotoxicity
  - Extensive sarcotubular dilation on EM
  - Hydroxychloroquine—curvilinear bodies
  - Fat vacuoles—fatty acid metabolism disorder
  - Fibrillary—amyloid
  - Lamellar myelin—Fabry disease
- Cyanotic congenital heart disease = think T
  - Tetralogy of Fallot
  - Tricuspid atresia
  - Transposition of the great arteries
  - Truncus arteriosus
  - Total anomalous pulmonary return
  - Coarctation of the aorta
  - Severe stenosis of aortic or pulmonic valve
- Neoplasms
  - Most common primary malignant cardiac tumor is angiosarcoma
  - Papillary fibroelastoma
    - Benign, second most common primary cardiac tumor
    - On surface of valves, usually aortic
    - Resemble Lambl excrescences grossly and microscopically
      - Look like sea anemone under water/saline
      - Fine avascular papillae lined by endothelium/endocardium
    - Histogenesis is unknown
    - Tumor MOBILITY (not size) predicts embolism and death
  - Cardiac myxomas
    - 90% sporadic
      - Females, approximately 50 years of age, left atrium near fossa ovalis
    - 7% as part of the Carney complex
      - Females, 25 years of age, right atrium, multiple tumors
      - Also freckles and nevi
    - Positive for CD34, CD31, calretinin, S100
    - May be confused for thrombus with myxoid changes
    - May have heterologous elements and/or extramedullary hematopoiesis

CHAPTER 13

Head and Neck Pathology

Salivary Gland

NORMAL AND NON-NEOPLASTIC

- Duct types
  - Striated ducts—luminal/ductal and basal cells, rigid
    - Low–molecular–weight keratin (LMWK) highlights luminal/ductal cells
      - CAM5.2, CK7
    - High-molecular-weight keratin (HMWK) highlights basal cells
      - p63, p40, CK5/6
  - Intercalated—smaller, less rigid, distal to striated
    - Myoepithelial cells—S100, SMA (also stains vessels), calponin, and all basal cell markers ("basal cell plus")
      - Polymorphous low–grade adenocarcinoma (PLGA), mammary-analog secretory carcinoma (MASC), epithelial–myoepithelial carcinoma
  - Excretory—most proximal, can undergo squamous metaplasia
- Acinar cells can be serous, mucous, or both
  - Major salivary glands
    - Parotid—serous
    - Submandibular—seromucous
      - Can be mistaken clinically/radiologically for lymph node
      - Can undergo squamous metaplasia (sialometaplasia)
    - Sublingual—mucoserous
    - Minor glands—vary based on location
  - Purple granules in serous acini = zymogen granules (use PAS-D)
  - Stain with DOG1 even if zymogen–poor
    - Canalicular pattern (apical membrane)
  - Can have sebaceous rests
  - Can have intraparenchymal lymph nodes
    - Can get tumor-associated lymphoid infiltrate (especially in satellite tumor nodules)—do not mistake these for involved lymph nodes
- Lymphoepithelial cysts
  - Watery cyst fluid
  - Lymphocytes, histiocytes, and squamous cells
  - Increased in HIV patients
    - Bilateral and multiple
  - Reactive condition secondary to duct obstruction or obliteration

NEOPLASTIC

- General considerations
  - Indolent but persistent
  - Must be able to distinguish benign, low-grade, and high-grade

- *It is usually okay to get the diagnosis a little wrong if they are in the same category*
- *Or say "low-/high-grade salivary gland tumor"*
- Fine needle aspiration (FNA) is more than just a screening tool
- Treatment = surgical resection with clear margins
  - Low-grade tumors have limited resection, and high-grade tumors may have nerves sacrificed
- Tumor and normal interface
  - Circumscribed (benign)
  - Encapsulated (benign)
  - Pushing border (low-grade)
  - Nodular expansion (low-grade)
  - Infiltrative (high-grade)
- Signs of malignancy
  - Perineural invasion
  - Angiolymphatic invasion
  - True tumoral necrosis (sudden transition to necrotic tissue)
- Painful?
  - Warthin tumor with infarction
  - Adenoid cystic carcinoma with nerve invasion
  - Acinic cell or adenoid cystic carcinoma on FNA
- Milan classification system for salivary gland neoplasms
  - Nondiagnostic
    - ≤10% should be nondiagnostic in your institution
    - Less than 60 lesional cells
    - Benign salivary gland in the setting of a mass is nondiagnostic
    - Cell-free mucin is nondiagnostic
  - Non-neoplastic
    - Acute/chronic/granulomatous sialadenitis
    - Reactive lymph node
  - Atypia of unknown significance (AUS)
    - Should be smallest category, rarely use!
    - Should compose <10% of cases
    - Rebiopsy or resection
  - Neoplasm: benign
    - Gets limited resection
    - Warthin tumor
    - Pleomorphic adenoma
    - Schwannoma
  - Neoplasm: SUMP (salivary gland neoplasm of unknown malignant potential)
    - Basaloid cells with irregular hyaline stroma
      - Pleomorphic adenoma (PA) or adenoid cystic carcinoma (AdCC)
    - Basaloid cells
      - Adenoma or carcinoma
    - Benign lesion with worrisome features
  - Neoplasm: suspicious
    - Suggestive of malignancy but lacks material to make diagnosis (because of quantity or quality)
  - Neoplasm: malignant
    - Radical dissection with facial nerve sacrifice
    - Myoepithelial carcinoma

- Mammary analog secretory carcinoma (MASC)
- Mucoepidermoid carcinoma
- Carcinoma ex PA
  - A carcinoma that has arisen from a PA
- Lymphoma
- Sarcoma
- Metastases
- Differential diagnoses
  - WHO risk levels
    - Low risk
      - Acinic cell carcinoma, low-grade mucoepidermoid carcinoma, epithelial–myoepithelial carcinoma, polymorphic low–grade adenocarcinoma, clear cell carcinoma, basal cell adenocarcinoma, low–grade salivary duct carcinoma, myoepithelial carcinoma, sialoblastoma
    - High risk
      - Sebaceous carcinoma, high–grade mucoepidermoid carcinoma, adenoid cystic carcinoma, mucinous adenocarcinoma, squamous cell carcinoma, small cell carcinoma, large cell carcinoma, lymphoepithelial carcinoma, carcinosarcoma
  - Basaloid neoplasms (high nuclear-to-cytoplasmic ratio)
    - Benign
      - Basal cell adenoma (peripheral palisading), cellular pleomorphic adenoma, sebaceous/nonsebaceous (lymphocytic) adenoma, myoepithelioma
    - Malignant
      - Adenoid cystic carcinoma, pleomorphic low–grade adenoma (PLGA), basal cell adenocarcinoma, metastatic basaloid squamous cell carcinoma, metastatic basal cell carcinoma, epithelial-myoepithelioma, carcinoma ex pleomorphic adenoma
    - Mimics
      - Metastatic or primary nonkeratinizing or basaloid squamous cell carcinoma
      - Small cell carcinoma—CK7+
      - Adamantinoma–like Ewing sarcoma—*EWSR1* translocation but positive for keratins
      - Rhabdomyosarcoma—myogenin
      - Synovial sarcoma
      - Metastatic melanoma
      - Merkel cell carcinoma—dot–like positivity for CK20, polyoma-virus+
  - Clear cell neoplasms
    - Hyalinizing clear cell carcinoma (*EWSR+*), epithelial–myoepithelial carcinoma (myoepithelial cells are clear), myoepithelioma, myoepithelial carcinoma, clear cell mucoepidermoid carcinoma (can become cystic)
    - Mimics—metastatic renal cell carcinoma, focal change of *any* tumor
  - Oncocytic neoplasms
    - Oncocytoma, oncocytic carcinoma, many duct–derived tumors
    - Growth patterns—trabecular, tubular, solid, cribriform, cystic (micro and macro)
  - Biphasic
    - Benign—pleomorphic adenoma, Warthin tumor
    - Malignant—epithelial–myoepithelial carcinoma, adenoid cystic carcinoma, basal cell adenoma, basal cell carcinoma
  - Monomorphic
    - Benign—canalicular adenoma, myoepithelioma
    - Malignant—PLGA, mucoepidermoid carcinoma, salivary duct carcinoma, squamous cell carcinoma

- Acinus–derived versus duct–derived
- Benign neoplasms
- Pleomorphic adenoma
  - Also known as *benign mixed tumor*
  - Most common salivary tumor, usually within the superficial parotid gland
  - "Pleomorphic" = 2 cell types+matrix
    - Not a marker of malignancy in this case
    - Morphology
      - Two cell populations
      - Honeycomb epithelial cells
      - Myoepithelial cells
        - Spindled or plasmacytoid
        - "Hyaline cells"
        - Glassy, embedded within matrix
      - "Metachromatic" matrix
        - Magenta on Diff Quik, fibrillary, cotton candy–like
        - Chondromyxoid
        - Classically tyrosine crystals (daisy–head)
    - If the patient has a long history of a small mass and new rapid growth, worry about carcinoma ex pleomorphic adenoma
    - Excellent prognosis with complete excision
- Warthin tumor
  - Second most common salivary tumor
  - Male with a smoking history
  - "Doughy" parotid mass
  - "Motor oil" on aspiration
  - Dirty/grungy cystic background
  - Monomorphic oncocytic cells (plasmacytoid with abundant cytoplasm in a sheet) with a background of polymorphic lymphocytes
  - May have squamous metaplasia or reactive atypia
  - Differential diagnosis (DDx): oncocytoma (less or no lymphocytes) and acinic cell CA (PAS-D+, 3D clusters, vacuoles/granules)
    - Can just call it "low–grade salivary gland neoplasm" if you cannot differentiate
      - *Increased risk for lymphoma*
      - Recurrences are common
- Oncocytoma
  - Looks like Warthin without lymphocytes
  - Plump, round cells with finely granular cytoplasm
- Malignant neoplasms
- Acinic cell carcinoma
  - Low–grade tumor
    - Can undergo high–grade transformation
  - Parotid gland only (serous–derived)
  - Cytology
    - Cellular aspirate with papillary structures
    - Dirty/blood background
    - Fibrovascular cores with polygonal bland serous epithelial cells with wispy cytoplasm
    - Small dark, plasmacytoid cells in clusters
    - Can be painful to do FNA like adenoid cystic

- Histology
  - Hyperchromatic cells in invasive nests/clusters/cords
  - Purple, *finely granular* cytoplasm
  - Variable nuclei with inconspicuous nucleoli
  - Rare lumens
  - PAS-D+ zymogen granules, DOG1+
  - Vascular pattern similar to renal cell carcinoma
  - DDx: sebaceous carcinoma (diastase sensitive), mucoepidermoid, normal salivary gland
- Carcinoma ex pleomorphic adenoma
  - Fibrotic (can be chondromyxoid) stroma, some lumen formation
  - Some nuclear atypia
  - Invasion through capsule with pushing border
  - Low grade
    - Minimally invasive with low–grade histology
  - High grade
    - Widely invasive with high–grade histology
  - Bimorphic
    - Basal cells—p63+
      - Luminal cells—CK7+
- Adenoid cystic carcinoma
  - High risk for local recurrence
  - Frequent perineural invasion
    - Painful to perform FNA!
  - Hyalinized stroma, infiltrative glands
    - "Gumballs and taffy" on cytology
    - 3D hyaline globules with oval myoepithelial cells stuck to it (not running through matrix)
  - Jigsaw of tubular, cribriform, solid glands
  - Bimorphic—luminal and abluminal
  - Grading
    - ONLY tubular, no cribriform = grade 1
    - Grade 2 = between 1 and 3
    - ≥30% solid = high-grade (grade 3)
  - Can get high–grade transformation, which has a higher risk for nodal metastases
  - CD117+
- Mucoepidermoid carcinoma
  - Background of mucin
  - Three types of cells
    - Mucinous goblet cells
      - Necessary for diagnosis!
    - Squamoid/epithelioid
      - Hyperchromatic nucleus, orange or dense cytoplasm
    - Intermediate cells
      - Small, bland, easily overlooked
  - Obvious malignant cytologic features
    - Irregular nuclear contours
    - Coarse/clumped chromatin
    - Prominent nucleoli
  - Common in parotid

- Cytoplasmic vacuole of mucin (mucicarmine+)
- Grades
    - Low grade: predominantly mucinous cells
    - High grade: predominantly squamous cells
- t(11;19)(q21;p13) *CRTC1-MAML2*
- See Table 13.1
■ Salivary duct carcinoma
- High grade
- Infiltrative, perineural invasion
- One cell type—pleomorphic plasmacytoid cells, looks like breast ductal carcinoma in situ
- Hyalinized/fibrotic stroma
- DDx includes high–grade mucoepidermoid
- p63–, ↑ Ki67, mucin–, AR+
- *HER2* amplification (17q21.1)
■ Polymorphous low-grade adenocarcinoma
- Low grade
    - If many mitotic figures are present, consider cribriform carcinoma (high grade)
- Only minor salivary glands (classically on palate)
- Morphology
    - Rugated/corrugated gross surface
    - Architecturally, can have MANY growth patterns, hence "polymorphous"
        - Classic swirling ("eye of the hurricane")
    - One cell type, polygonal to spindled
        - Cytologically monomorphic cells that look like papillary thyroid carcinoma
        - Indistinct cell borders
        - Vesicular chromatin
        - Rare mitoses
    - Slate gray myxoid stroma (can become hyalinized)
- Immunostains
    - Positive: *S100 strong* and p63+
        - Other S100+ salivary tumors—mammary analog secretory carcinoma and low–grade ductal adenocarcinoma
    - Negative: p40 *(paradoxical)*
- *PLAG1* rearrangement (8q12)
■ Mammary analog secreting carcinoma (MASC)
- Low grade
- t(12;15)(p13;q25) *ETV6–NTRK*
- Morphology
    - Usually microcystic/glandular
    - Brightly eosinophilic luminal secretions

TABLE 13.1 ■ **High–Grade Salivary Gland Carcinoma Immunophenotypes**

	AR	HER2	p63	CK5/6
Salivary duct carcinoma	+	+	–	–
HG mucoepidermoid carcinoma	–	–	+	+

AR, Androgen receptor; *HG*, high-grade.

- Finely vacuolated cytoplasm
- Immunophenotype
  - Positive for S100 and mammaglobin
  - Negative for p63 and DOG1
- Hyalinizing clear cell carcinoma
  - Rare
  - t(12;22)(q21;q12) *EWSR1-ATF1*
- Epithelial–myoepithelial carcinoma
  - Low grade
  - Multinodular
  - Inner dark ductal epithelial cells rimmed by myoepithelial cells
  - Three alternate names based on morphology
    - Glycogen–rich adenoma—clear cells predominate
    - Myoepithelioma—spindle cell and plasmacytoid cells
    - Myoepithelial carcinoma—no significant epithelial differentiation, markedly atypical cells
  - Can dedifferentiate
- Basal cell adenocarcinoma
  - Low–grade but infiltrative (perineural and vascular invasion is prominent)
  - Small dark palisading cells and larger epithelioid cells with eosinophilic/amphophilic cytoplasm
  - Malignant counterpart to basal cell adenoma
  - Associated with dermal cylindromas
- Adenocarcinoma, not otherwise specified (NOS)

Sinonasal

NORMAL AND NON–NEOPLASTIC

- Types of cells
  - Respiratory mucosa
    - Surface epithelial
      - Ciliated and nonciliated columnar cells—adenocarcinoma
      - Goblet cells—adenocarcinoma
    - Minor salivary glands—acinar, ductal, basal, myoepithelial
      - Myoepithelial cells stain with S100!
      - Can get any salivary gland neoplasm!!
        - Arise from seromucinous glands and surface epithelium of the nasal cavity and paranasal sinuses
  - Neuroepithelium (cribriform plate)
  - Squamous mucosa
  - Also melanocytes and hematolymphoid cells
    - Normal myoepithelial cells stain with p63, SMA, calponin, vimentin, S100
    - Eosinophils in nasal polyp? "Inflammatory/allergic–type polyp"

BENIGN NEOPLASMS

- Benign salivary gland neoplasms
  - Pleomorphic adenoma (most common salivary–type tumor)
  - Basal cell adenoma

- Pure epithelial
- Pure myoepithelial (also known as *myoepithelioma* or *cellular PA*)
- Other benign
  - Papillomas
    - Schneiderian papilloma
      - Benign but can be locally destructive
      - One–third to one–half are associated with human papillomavirus (HPV)
      - Lined with sinonasal mucosa
      - Can be exophytic, inverted, oncocytic
      - Keratinization may predict transformation to squamous cell carcinoma
    - Squamous papilloma
  - Respiratory epithelial adenomatoid hamartoma (REAH)
    - Uncommon polypoid mass with prominent glandular proliferations lined by ciliated respiratory epithelium originating from the surface epithelium
    - May be confused with adenocarcinoma or inverted polyp
  - Seromucinous hamartoma
    - Looks like prostate cancer

MALIGNANT NEOPLASMS

- Most common cancers
  - First—squamous cell carcinoma (SCC)
  - Second—adenoid cystic carcinoma (AdCC)
    - 10% to 18% of all sinonasal malignancies
  - Third—adenocarcinoma
- Malignant salivary gland neoplasms
  - Includes all those listed earlier
- Squamous malignancies
  - Carcinoma characteristics
    - Marked nuclear pleomorphism and hyperchromasia
    - Frequent mitotic figures beyond basal layer including the atypical forms
    - Tumor necrosis
    - Frank invasion with infiltrative irregular nests and desmoplastic stromal reaction
  - Can range from well–differentiated and keratinizing to poorly differentiated squamous cell carcinoma (SCC)
    - In general, similar to other mucosal SCC malignancies
  - Sinonasal undifferentiated carcinoma (SNUC)
    - No glands, no squamous differentiation
    - Sheets of high–grade cells with increased apoptosis and mitosis
    - ~Sixth decade, males > females
    - Rapid growth, destructive
    - Diagnosis of exclusion
    - No specific mutations (rule out midline NUT carcinoma, INI-1, Brg-1, IDH2)
- Nonsalivary gland malignant neoplasms
  - Adenocarcinoma
    - Intestinal
      - Low grade and high grade
      - Second most common type of adenocarcinoma after AdCC
      - Architectural types
        - Colonic

- Most common
  - CK20+, CDX2+, CK7–/+, villin+, MUC2+
- Papillary
  - Looks like normal small intestinal mucosa
  - Columnar cells, resorptive cells, Paneth cells, and so on.
  - *Must use immunohistochemistry (IHC) to prove "intestinal type" because papillary nonintestinal can happen*
- Solid
- Mucinous
- Mixed
- Looks like colonic tubular adenoma (but malignant), stains like intestinal epithelium
- Nonintestinal
  - One cell population
  - Low grade and high grade
  - Must use IHC to rule out intestinal type and salivary type adenocarcinomas
    - CDX2–, CK20–, CK7–
- Neuroendocrine (NE) carcinomas
  - Low grade
  - High grade
  - p16+, chromogranin/synaptophysin+, p63+, S100–, dot staining for cytokeratin AE1/AE3
  - Mutation–associated sinonasal carcinomas
    - Midline NUT carcinoma
      - Females > males, 20 s, very aggressive
      - Like SNUC with abrupt/sudden keratinization (without transition)
      - Positive for nuclear NUT; NUT is only expressed in testes in normal tissues
      - *NUTM1* rearrangement
- Therapeutic targets
  - INI-1 negative carcinoma
    - "Rhabdoid cells" to undifferentiated
    - Can happen in almost any organ
    - Other neoplasms with INI-1 loss—epithelioid sarcoma, renal medullary carcinoma, myoepithelial carcinoma of soft tissue, epithelioid malignant peripheral nerve sheath tumor, extraskeletal myxoid chondrosarcoma, gastrointestinal rhabdoid carcinoma
  - CK+, INI-1–
  - Brg-1– carcinoma
  - SNUC with *IDH2 R172* mutation
  - Viral–associated sinonasal carcinoma
    - Epstein-Barr virus (EBV)
      - Nasopharyngeal carcinoma
- Very blue on low power
- Lymphocytes and epithelial—"lymphoepithelial" by morphology
- "Nasopharyngeal" by location
- Immunophenotype
- Positive for pankeratin, CK5/6, p63, EBER in situ hybridization
- Focal positive for CAM5.2, S100, SMA
- Negative for p16 and CK7
- Favorable prognosis, do not grade because you would "overgrade"
- No such thing as *in situ*

- Multiphenotypic human papillomavirus (HPV)–related carcinoma
  - Surface atypia, two types of cells (epithelial and myoepithelial) with basement membrane, salivary gland/adenoid cystic look
  - c-Kit+
  - HPV–related (serotype 33), only in sinonasal tract
  - Cell of origin: excretory duct
  - Do not metastasize or kill patients
  - HPV—poorly differentiated (nonkeratinizing) SCC
- Alveolar rhabdomyosarcoma
  - Myogenin+, synaptophysin+, chromogranin+, keratin–/+
  - Younger patients
  - Nasal cavity is a classic site
  - Small round blue cell tumor
- Can get germ cell tumors or pituitary tumors that grow directly from sella into sinonasal
  - Merkel cell carcinoma
    - Associated with sun exposure and immunodeficiency (parvovirus)
    - Neuroendocrine morphology and immunophenotype *plus* dot–like CK20+
- Spindle cell neoplasms
  - If surface is intact, it means it is slow–growing
  - *Glomangiopericytoma*
    - New name for hemangiopericytoma in sinonasal tract
    - Benign, do not metastasize
    - Large vessels with monotonous cells that are derived from pericytes, scattered eosinophils
    - SMA+, CD34+ vessels, factor XIIIa, nuclear beta–catenin
  - Biphenotypic sinonasal sarcoma
    - Looks like glomangiopericytoma
      - Storiform spindle cells, very highly cellular with no/low mitoses
      - Tends to be highly infiltrative
    - Both neural and smooth muscle markers, nuclear beta–catenin
      - SMA+, S100+
    - t(2;4) pathognomonic *(PAX3-MAML3)*
  - Malignant peripheral nerve sheath tumor (MPNST)
    - Herringbone, high cellularity, mild-to-moderate pleomorphism
    - Occasional mitoses → high grade
  - Loss of histone methylator gene
    - Epithelial–myoepithelial carcinoma
    - Hemangiopericytoma–like vessels, highly cellular, vesicles, myxoid matrix
    - S100+, SMA–, calponin–, p63+, CK+
  - Sarcomatoid carcinoma (spindle cell squamous cell carcinoma)
  - Solitary fibrous tumor
    - Patternless pattern, staghorn vessel, hypo- and hypercellular zones, ropey collagen
    - STAT6+ (rearranged)
- Differential diagnosis for small round blue cell tumors (SRBCTs)
  - Sinonasal neuroendocrine carcinoma
    - Cytokeratin+
    - Positive for neuroendocrine markers synaptophysin, chromogranin, and CD56
    - S100: variable
    - Negative for other melanoma markers (Melan-A, HMB-45, tyrosinase)
  - Olfactory neuroblastoma (esthesioneuroblastoma)

- Uncommon malignant neuroectodermal neoplasm associated with cribriform plate
- Lobular/insular architecture, vascularized stroma, neuropil matrix
- Homer Wright pseudorosettes (no lumen in middle)
- Flexner–Wintersteiner rosettes (lumen; indicates higher grade)
- Hyman grading system (I to IV)
- DDx includes ectopic pituitary adenoma (keratin+)
- Kadish staging (A to C)
- Cytokeratin: usually negative (rare cases positive)
- Neuroendocrine marker: positive
- S100: sustentacular pattern of staining
- Negative for other melanoma markers (Melan-A, HMB-45, tyrosinase); positive for calretinin
  - Malignant melanoma
    - Cytokeratin: usually negative (rare cases positive)
    - S100+
    - Positive for other melanoma markers (Melan-A, HMB-45, tyrosinase)
  - Ewing family of tumors (Ewing sarcoma, peripheral neuroectodermal tumor)
    - Cytokeratin usually negative (rare cases positive)
    - Neuroendocrine markers: variably positive
    - S100 variable
    - Negative for other melanoma markers (Melan-A, HMB-45, tyrosinase)
    - CD99+
    - FLI1 may be positive
  - Paraganglioma
    - Cytokeratin–
    - Positive for neuroendocrine markers
    - S100: sustentacular pattern of staining
    - Negative for other melanoma markers (Melan-A, HMB-45, tyrosinase)
    - GATA-3+
    - SDHB: loss of expression in patients with *SDH* mutations
  - Pituitary adenoma
    - Cytokeratin+ (80%)
    - Positive for neuroendocrine markers
    - S100–
    - Positive for pituitary hormones; most commonly prolactin (60%)
- Helpful tips:
  - Strong cytokeratin and neuroendocrine (NE) markers—NE carcinoma
  - Strong cytokeratin and weak NE markers—SNUC
  - Weak cytokeratin and strong NE markers—neuroblastoma
  - Neuroblastoma—S100+, calretinin+

Oropharyngeal and Laryngeal Squamous Neoplasia

- Locations of malignancy in decreasing frequency
  - Glottis
  - Soft palate
  - Floor of mouth
  - Lip
  - Gingiva

- Buccal mucosa
- Hard palate
- Benign and premalignant
  - Heck's disease
    - HPV–associated (types 13 and 32) proliferation of oral mucosa
    - Most common in children
    - Cobblestone appearance
    - "Mitosoid" cells—nuclei look like mitotic figures
  - *Leukoplakia*—clinical term—white patch/plaque, well–defined
    - 1) thickening, 2) parakeratosis, 3) hyperkeratosis
    - Blue swollen granular layer
    - Vast majority do not have dysplasia
    - 10% become dysplastic, <5% become malignant
  - Erythroplakia—less well–defined red patch
    - 40% to 50% are already dysplastic at biopsy
- Dysplasia
  - Features
    - Abnormal architecture
    - Thickened basal layer
    - Hyperchromatic round nuclei with dispersed chromatin
  - Risk for malignant transformation into invasive squamous cell carcinoma (SCC)
    - Mild dysplasia—5%
    - Moderate dysplasia—10% to 15%
    - Severe dysplasia—25% to 30%
  - Risk factors
    - Alcohol
    - Smoking
    - Male (3:1 M:F)
      - Except proliferative verrucous leukoplakia
  - Some differentiate between severe dysplasia and carcinoma in situ (CIS); some do not
    - Severe dysplasia = dysplasia top to bottom but not thickened
    - CIS = dysplasia top to bottom *and* diffusely thickened
- Management for dysplasia/CIS
  - Mild dysplasia—biopsy every 6 months to 1 year
  - Moderate dysplasia— biopsy every 3 months
  - Severe dysplasia/CIS—local excision
- Carcinoma
  - Mitoses might not be prominent
  - Architecture is very important!
    - Verrucous or papillary
      - Does not need invasion to be called *cancer*, just severe dysplasia
      - Verrucous hyperplasia, atypical verrucous hyperplasia, verrucous carcinoma
    - Flat
    - Inverted
  - Patterns of invasion
    - Type 1—broad pushing border
    - Type 2—broad pushing "fingers" or separate large tumor islands causing stellate appearance
    - Type 3—invasive islands of tumor greater than 15 cells per island

- Type 4—invasive tumor islands smaller than 15 cells per island
  - Type 5—widely dispersed pattern
  - Tumor satellites of any size with 1 mm or greater of normal tissue between satellites
- Prognosis: poorest pattern of invasion, lymphovascular invasion, and perineural invasion are all important
- Staging
  - Microinvasion is <1 mm
  - Depth of invasion (DOI) is most important in staging
    - Size of tumor second most important
    - How to measure DOI
      - Draw a horizontal line at the basement membrane of the adjacent normal epithelium
      - Draw a vertical "plumb" line down to the deepest invasion
    - DIFFERENT from tumor thickness which usually measures from the top of ulcerated tumor to deepest invasion (undermeasures DOI)
    - If DOI is >3 mm → neck dissection
- Lymph nodes
  - Number of nodes
  - Size of metastases
  - Ipsilateral or contralateral
  - Presence or absence of extranodal extension
    - Major >2 mm or identified grossly
  - Isolated tumor cells = N0
- Oropharyngeal HPV+ squamous cell carcinoma has excellent outcomes, now staged differently (has no CIS, only T4 without A/B)
  - p16+ by IHC or HPV+ by ISH in situ hybridization or polymerase chain reaction
    - IHC is only positive if 2+ or 3+ in ≥ 75% of tumor and in cytoplasm + nucleus
  - p16– oropharynx and hypopharynx are staged the same
    - Size of tumor is most prognostic
  - Lymph nodes
    - HPV+: only number of nodes (clinical or pathologic staging)
    - HPV–: number, *size of metastasis*, ipsilateral or contralateral
    - Extranodal extension

Thyroid
GENERAL CONSIDERATIONS

- FNA is common for nodules
  - Need 60 cells (6 groups of 10 cells) for adequacy
- If hypercellular and no atypia, call *benign* but with comment to rebiopsy if indicated
- Can get any thyroid carcinoma in a thyroglossal duct cyst *except medullary thyroid carcinoma*
  - C cells do not migrate with thyroid in embryogenesis
- Thyroid molecular reports
  - Afirma—"benign" or "suspicious"
  - ThyroSeq—"no mutation identified" or "[specific mutation] identified"
- PAX8+ in thyroid (may be only positive thyroid stain in undifferentiated thyroid carcinoma)
  - Driven by *p53* mutation
  - Can mimic anything
- Imaging

- TIRADS malignancy criteria: taller than wide, irregular borders, hypoechoic, solid or cystic with solid component
- Only sample >1 cm unless radiologically suspicious for malignancy

NON-NEOPLASTIC

- Squamous metaplasia
  - Can occur with thymic rests, follicular adenomatous hyperplasia, lymphocytic thyroiditis, ultimobranchial body rests/solid nodules
  - Can also occur in some tumors
    - Diffusing sclerosing variant of papillary thyroid carcinoma
    - Primary squamous cell carcinoma
    - Thyroid carcinoma showing thymic–like differentiation (CASTLE)
    - Cribriform–morular papillary thyroid carcinoma
    - Mucoepidermoid carcinoma
    - Anaplastic thyroid carcinoma
- Amiodarone–induced hyperthyroidism
  - Shows distended disrupted follicles with foamy macrophages in colloid
- Thyroiditis
  - Acute—rare!!
  - Subacute
    - De Quervain thyroiditis (granulomatous or giant cell thyroiditis)
    - Can initially cause hyperthyroidism
    - Usually regenerates and patient ends up euthyroid
    - Most likely caused by viral infection
    - Bilateral thyroid involved
    - No increased risk for subsequent carcinoma
  - Lymphocytic (Hashimoto) thyroiditis
    - Lymphocytic inflammation forming reactive follicles
- Benign follicular nodule
  - Most common entity in thyroid cytology, benign; includes:
    - Nodular goiter
    - Hyperplastic (adenomatoid) nodule
    - Colloid nodule
    - Nodules in Graves' disease
    - Macrofollicular subset of follicular adenoma

NEOPLASTIC

- Follicular neoplasms
  - Little-to-no colloid (↑↑ cell:colloid ratio), microfollicles, 3D aggregates
  - *Can never make diagnosis of follicular carcinoma on cytology!!*
    - "Suspicious for follicular neoplasm"
  - 10% to 15% risk for malignancy, but require surgery (hemithyroidectomy)
  - Follicular neoplasms on frozen section
    - One lesion
    - "Follicular neoplasm"
      - Need to submit the entire capsule
    - Two or more lesions *or* no capsule

- "Follicular lesions"
  - Do not need to submit all of the capsules
- Follicular carcinoma
  - t(2;3) *PAX8-PPAR*
  - Metastasizes hematogenously
  - Usually invades capsule with a pushing border—mushroom–shaped
- Hurthle cell neoplasm
  - 75% of cells must be oncocytic to be a Hurthle cell neoplasm
  - Can allow nucleoli, nucleomegaly, and slight atypia, but should *not* have papillary nuclear features
- Medullary thyroid carcinoma
  - Very highly cellular, dispersed single cells
  - Plasmacytoid (>spindled or polygonal) with very fine reddish cytoplasmic granules
    - Neurosecretory granules, best seen on Diff–Quik (DQ, modified Romanowsky stain)
  - Intranuclear pseudoinclusions can be seen in 50% of medullary
    - Internal appearance similar to cytoplasm, one-third of nuclear size or larger, nuclear condensation around it
  - Salt-and-pepper chromatin on Pap
  - Amyloid can be seen in up to 80% (best seen on DQ)
  - Calcitonin levels are elevated in most cases
  - CEA levels are elevated in most cases
    - Postsurgical rise is associated with distant metastases
  - If serum calcitonin is high and morphology matches, do not need cell block for stains
    - But can use calcitonin and Congo red
      - Must dedicate passes for cell block (not usually done in thyroid)
    - A noncalcitonin secreting variant has been described
- Papillary neoplasms
  - Cytologic features
    - Powdery chromatin, no nucleoli
    - Intranuclear pseudoinclusions, nuclear grooves
      - Need *many* grooves to call *papillary thyroid carcinoma without pseudoinclusions* (because grooves can be seen in hyperplasia)
  - Papillary thyroid carcinoma (PTC)
    - *BRAF* mutations in 45%
    - *RET/PTC1* or *PTC3* rearrangements in 20%
    - Morphology
      - Papillary architecture (if follicular, see later)
        - Papillary architecture without typical nuclear features is *not* papillary thyroid carcinoma
      - Overlapping nuclei, elongation, grooves, pseudoinclusions (or chromatin margination), nuclear pleomorphism
        - Pseudoinclusions are not specific for PTC on frozen sections, as they can be formed artifactually
      - Hyalinizing fibrosis of the capsule or within the lesion
      - Can have completely intact capsule and is still called *PTC* if papillary architecture is present
      - CK19 is diffusely and strongly positive in 80%
  - The follicular variant of papillary carcinoma (FVPC)
    - Nonfatal tumors that are overdetected and overtreated (similar to prostate carcinoma)

- 98.1% 5-year survival
- More than double the diagnoses in 10 years
- Female > male because of "opportunistic ultrasonography" in obstetric clinics
- Litigation concerns, no minimum criteria for diagnosis of FVPC
- Noninvasive follicular thyroid neoplasm with papillary–like nuclear features (NIFTP)
  - Essentially an encapsulated and nonaggressive–appearing FVPC
  - Encapsulated or clear demarcation
  - 99% follicular pattern, <30% solid growth
  - No psammoma bodies
  - <3 mitoses per hpf, no lymphovascular invasion or capsule invasion
- Anaplastic/undifferentiated thyroid carcinoma
  - Classic presentation is very rapid growth (like several weeks) in an elderly patient
  - May be de-differentiated from another carcinoma
    - Example pathogenesis: normal → *BRAF* or *RAS* mutation → PTC → *p53* or beta–catenin mutation → anaplastic carcinoma
  - Women > men
  - Diagnosis of exclusion
  - May lose every marker
    - Usually TTF1– and thyroglobulin–
    - Sometimes pankeratin+, sometimes PAX8+
  - Staged as T4 by definition
  - Poor prognosis (5-year survival 0% to 14%), surgery only for palliative care
    - May do well with *BRAF* targeted therapy
- Other malignancies
  - Primary thyroid lymphoma
    - Usually diffuse large B-cell lymphoma
    - Most commonly secondary to Hashimoto's thyroiditis
    - Rapid growth
  - Carcinoma showing thymus–like differentiation (CASTLE)
    - Solid nests, broad invasive border
    - "Lymphoepithelial–like"
    - Positive for p63, CD5, and high–molecular–weight keratin
  - Hyalinizing–trabecular tumor of thyroid—Ki67 stains *membranously*

Parathyroid

- Normal parathyroid is composed of chief cells and clear cells
- Parathyroid hyperplasia
  - Should have both cell types present
- Hyperplastic parathyroiditis
  - Possible autoimmune etiology
  - Lymphoid aggregates and reactive follicles
- Parathyroid adenoma
  - Clonal expansion of one cell type
  - Does not invade locally
- Parathyroid carcinoma
  - Invasion of vessels and/or local structures
  - Broad fibrous bands
  - *Not* helpful: increased mitotic activity, presence/absence of capsule, pleomorphism

- *Parathyroidosis*
  - Parathyroidectomy for hyperplasia, adenoma, or carcinoma leads to seeding of surgical field
  - Nodules of parathyroid tissue

Mandibular/Maxillary Lesions

- Inflammatory cysts—radicular or periapical cyst
  - Mandible and maxilla at tooth root
  - Lots of inflammation
  - Hyaline balls
  - No keratinizing squamous mucosa
- Glandular odontogenic cyst
  - Vacuoles in squamoid epithelium
- Compound odontoma
  - Morphology
    - Enamel matrix (looks like fish scales)
    - Remnants of enamel organ
    - Tubular dentin
  - Imaging: "multiple tooth–like structures"
  - DDx: complex odontoma (which has hard and soft structure)
- Central giant cell granuloma
  - In jaw, looks like giant cell tumors elsewhere
  - DDx: cherubism—multiple tumors, eosinophilic cuffing of vessels
- Dentigerous cyst
  - Forms as a result of fluid accumulation between unerupted tooth follicle (that has ↓ enamel) and crown
  - Vaguely squamoid but no keratinization, no rete ridges ever, loss of polarization
  - Most common odontogenic cyst
- Keratocystic odontogenic tumor (KOT)
  - New name for odontogenic keratocyst (OKC)
  - 8 to 10 layers of squamous cells + corrugated parakeratosis +/− squamous debris
    - Can be inflamed
    - Can get rete ridges
  - Posterior mandible, 25 to 45 years of age
  - Can recur if incompletely excised
    - Treated by resection with marsupialization (suture edges of slit and underlying cyst wall together to ensure *open* pouch formation, allows for drainage)
  - Gorlin syndrome (nevoid basal cell carcinoma syndrome) get multiple of these
    - *PTCH1* mutation
  - WHO calls it *keratinizing cystic odontogenic tumor* (KCOT)
- Ameloblastoma
  - Previously called *adamantinoma*
  - May arise from dentigerous cyst
  - Benign but locally aggressive
  - Mean age = 30 years of age, no gender predilection
  - Histology
    - Nests with central loose reticular cells
    - Can have granular, basaloid, or squamous cells

- Palisaded hyperchromatic basal cells (like an OKC!)
- Reverse polarity with subnuclear vacuoles
  - Very useful and specific for ameloblastoma
- Similar to mucoepidermoid carcinoma, but little to no atypia
- Cytopathology—palisading, epithelioid group, spherical cytoplasmic bodies
- Histologic types
  - Plexiform
  - Acanthomatous/acantholytic—prominent squamous features
  - Follicular—most common
  - Granular
  - Desmoplastic
  - Basal cell type
- Cystic ameloblastoma
  - Basal layer palisading and vacuolated (nuclei at top, vacuole at bottom)
  - Edematous squamoid epithelium that may keratinize
  - Cystic is less aggressive than "malignant" but have local recurrence risk
    - Malignant—pleomorphism, increased mitotic activity
    - Metastasizes typically to lung

CHAPTER 14

Neuropathology

Normal Anatomy and Physiology

- Fibrillary processes → glial
  - Ependymal—cerebrospinal fluid (CSF) production
  - Astrocytes—blood–brain barrier
  - Microglia—macrophages (cigar–shaped)
  - Oligodendrocytes—myelination
- Lateral geniculate nucleus
  - See Fig. 14.1
  - Gets input from optic nerves
- Hippocampus
  - See Fig. 14.2
- Clark nucleus in anterior thoracic cord
- Stripe of Gennari—in calcarine sulcus
- Entorhinal cortex
  - Neocortex
  - Islands of neurons normally
  - Lost in Alzheimer's disease
- Vessels in the globus pallidus, dentate nucleus, and red nucleus become mineralized (iron and calcium), black crystals in media
  - Not significant, can happen any time after middle age
  - Can also get perivenous vacuoles/edema
- Pituitary microinfarcts are common with age

Nonneoplastic

PATHOLOGIC REACTIONS OF THE NERVOUS SYSTEM, COURTESY OF H. BRENT CLARK

1. *The clinical presentation of neurologic disease is dependent both on the pathologic nature and the location of the underlying disease process.*
2. *Neurons are the cells most vulnerable to injury in the central nervous system (CNS), and there are numerous manifestations of neuronal pathology, differing with the nature of the underlying process.*
3. *Axonal pathology can be intrinsic (e.g., in degenerative disease) or extrinsic (e.g., secondary to trauma, ischemia, or inflammation).*
4. *Astrocytes and microglial cells are the principal cells of the CNS that react to injury.*
5. *The peripheral nervous system is a more favorable environment for regeneration of axons and restoration of myelination, primarily because of Schwann cells. The peripheral nervous system is a less favorable environment for regeneration of axons and restoration of myelination, primarily because of glial cells.*
6. *Increased intracranial pressure and cerebral herniation are common and clinically important complications of many types of CNS pathology.*

Lateral geniculate nucleus

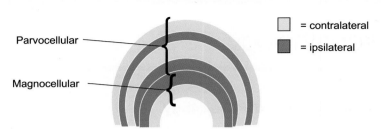

Parvocellular

Magnocellular

☐ = contralateral

■ = ipsilateral

Fig. 14.1   Anatomy of the lateral geniculate nucleus.

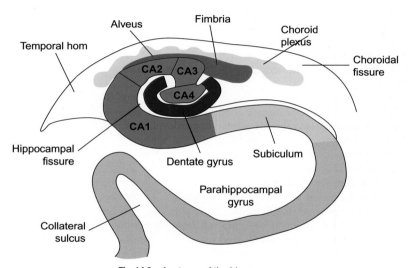

Fig. 14.2   Anatomy of the hippocampus.

- Perikaryon changes
  - Eosinophilic neuronal necrosis—seen after hypoxic ischemic injury
    - Pyknotic, hypereosinophilic DEAD neurons
    - Starts 3+ hours after injury (may be absent at autopsy)
    - Cerebral cortex in watershed areas, cerebellar Purkinje cells, and CA1 region of hippocampus
  - Neuronal somatic changes in neurodegenerative disease
    - Apoptosis—probably happens in several diseases, karyorrhectic debris
    - Simple atrophy—amyotrophic lateral sclerosis (ALS), degenerative ataxias, tiny soma
    - Pick bodies—tau protein, frontotemporal dementia
      - Can stain with immunohistochemistry (IHC) for ubiquitin or with silver stain (Bielschowsky)
    - Neurofibrillary tangles—phosphorylated tau protein, Alzheimer's
      - Can stain with IHC for ubiquitin or with silver stain (Bielschowsky)
    - Lewy bodies—eosinophilic, misfolded α-synuclein, in substantia nigra in Parkinson's
      - Can stain with IHC for ubiquitin

- Neuromelanin in neurons with dopamine (and all catecholamine) receptors
  - Pigment accumulates with age
  - Locus ceruleus, sympathetic ganglia, scattered in brainstem
- Anterograde transsynaptic degeneration
  - Presumably caused by loss of trophic signals (afferent signals that are supposed to stimulate the neuron in question) in very hardwired pathways (little collateral input)
  - Examples:
    - Lateral geniculate nucleus after optic chiasm/nerve lesion or enucleation
      - Ipsilateral—layers 2, 3, 5
    - Mammillary bodies after fornix lesion (from hippocampus)
      - Most common cause of damage—shearing
    - Gracile and cuneate nuclei after posterior column lesion
    - Inferior olives after lesion of central tegmental tract (from red nucleus and dentate nucleus)
      - "Hypertrophic olivary degeneration" before drop out
  - See Fig. 14.3
- Retrograde transsynaptic degeneration
  - Loss of target leads to loss of the neuron in question in very hardwired pathways (little collateral pathways)
  - Examples
    - Retinal ganglion cells after optic radiation lesion
    - Inferior olives after Purkinje cell loss (from alcoholic cerebellar degeneration)
      - Anterior-superior ⅓ of vermis (in midline) withered
  - See Fig. 14.4
- Central chromatolysis—somatic reaction to axon transection as it is trying to regenerate
  - ↓ Nissl substance—cholinesterase neurotransmitters (rough ER), do not need neurotransmitter production right now
    - Glassy pink cell body (smooth ER) with marginated pale nucleus
    - May recover
  - Seen after lower extremity amputation
- Axonal changes
  - Wallerian degeneration (WD)—axon distal to lesion (infarct or spinal cord lesion or distal to the cell body injury) eventually disappear (with loss of volume)

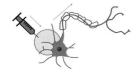

Fig. 14.3 Anterograde transsynaptic degeneration. **Anterograde**

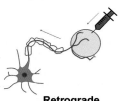

Fig. 14.4 Retrograde transsynaptic degeneration. **Retrograde**

- May be accompanied by chromatolysis of the cell body
- CAUSED BY EXTRINSIC CAUSES (like transection)
- Dying back toward cell body (proximal to lesion)
  - INTRINSIC to the neuron
  - Accompanied by simple atrophy of cell body
  - ALS, motor neuron disease, peripheral neuropathy
  - Greater propensity for regeneration in the peripheral nervous system (PNS)
  - Different than WD because it is caused by primary axonopathy
- Axonal spheroids = focal dilation of axon filled with accumulated organelles
  - Can happen after axonal injury
  - Take 1 to 2 days to form after trauma or ischemia
    - Example: Closed head injury with axonal shearing
  - Beta–amyloid precursor protein IHC can be positive in a few hours (autopsy)
  - Looks like long pink streaks in longitudinal plane and spheres in axials plane (beads on a string)
- Axonal torpedo = Purkinje cell axonal reaction = dilation of axon very close to cell body
  - Constipation of material in axon
- Dystrophic axon terminals = huge axon terminals (look vaguely like spheroid fungus)
  - Infantile neuraxonal dystrophy
- Corpora amylacea are brightly PAS+
  - Not pathogenic
  - Lots in spinal cord or subpial areas
  - Increase with age
- Astrocytes and their reactions
  - Major reactive cell in CNS
  - Nucleus is smaller than neuron but bigger than oligodendrocyte. Slightly vesicular, pale chromatin.
  - End feet (S100+) line small vessels to form blood–brain barrier
  - Reactive astrocytosis (gliosis)
    - Most sensitive marker for pathologic process in CNS (pretty fast to form too)
    - Hypertrophy (enlargement, filled up with GFAP or vimentin) and hyperplasia (proliferation of cells)
    - Gemistocytes
      - Plump GFAP+ reactive astrocytes, abundant glassy pink cytoplasm with eccentric round nucleus
      - Acute injury, gemistocytic astrocytoma, glioblastoma multiforme (GBM)
      - Seen in walls of infarcts 10 to 14 days after ischemic injury
      - Processes of these astrocytes form intracellular scars (rather than made of extracellular matrix like everywhere else in the body)
    - Isomorphic gliosis
      - Seen in demyelinating diseases like multiple sclerosis (MS)
      - Astrocytes fill in spaces where myelin was and conform to architecture (fill in missing volume)
      - Looks fascicular
  - Rosenthal fibers are a feature of chronic intense gliosis
    - Brightly eosinophilic amorphic globules (heat–shock protein called *alpha-B crystallin*)
  - Metabolic astrocytosis (Alzheimer's type 2 astrocytes)
    - Dilation of nucleus, marginated chromatin with inclusion–like appearance
    - Caudate and gray matter of cortex

- Hepatic encephalopathy
  - Glutamate recycling to glutamine by aminotransferases are damaged
  - Reversible and takes a few days to develop
    - Corpora amylacea are nonpathologic alterations (polyglucosan bodies)
  - Gray to blue, strong PAS+
- Oligodendrocytes (oligodendroglia)
  - Sunny–side–up fried egg appearance with small nucleus (looks like lymphocyte in a small lacuna), myelin–making cells
  - Single cell can supply myelin for up to 40 internodes (distance of axon between two nodes of Ranvier)
  - Second most vulnerable to ischemic damage (behind neurons)
  - Damage to oligodendrocytes causes primary demyelination (like MS) with preservation of axon
    - Luxol fast blue–PAS shows *loss* of blue–staining myelin in plaque, with *preserved* silver–staining (Bielschowsky) axons
  - Progressive multifocal leukoencephalopathy (PML)—oligodendrocytes selectively killed by measles virus
- Ependymal cells
  - Line ventricle, glial in origin, small cuboidal/low columnar cells
  - Negative for epithelial markers except EMA
  - Vulnerable to injury but we do not really need them
    - May try to regenerate but form "pitiful rosettes" that do not really line the ventricle (reactive ependymal hyperplasia)
- Microglia
  - Mesenchymal origin from bone marrow (not neuroepithelial)
  - Half–life of 30 days
    - Replaced by circulating cells of monocyte/macrophage lineage
  - Can give rise to macrophages (though most macrophages in large injuries are directly from circulating monocytes)
  - "Reticuloendothelial system of the CNS"
    - Primary source of CNS phagocytosis, antigen–presenting cells, recruit inflammatory cells via cytokine secretion
      - Tertiary syphilis and AIDS dementia are probably mostly caused by too much cytokine release
      - Number one responder to viral infections
  - Morphology
    - Bipolar with lateral dendrites
    - As they become activated, they elongate → microglial rod cells
    - Tendency to form nodular aggregates in viral diseases → microglial nodule (common)
      - Rickettsial (typhus, Rocky Mountain spotted fever) and poliovirus
  - CD45+, class II MHC+
  - Viral infections, syphilis, "leading wave" of microglia in infiltrative neoplasm
  - Foamy macrophage accumulation in resolving infarct
- Neuronal stem cells
  - Pluripotent stem cells may exist in the CNS (perhaps in bone marrow) that can turn into CNS-specific cells
  - Role in repair of injury is unclear
- Immune cell types seen
  - Macrophages seen in destructive/demyelinating processes (from blood monocytes or CNS microglia)

- Microglia = antigen–presenting cells of CNS, phagocytic, like monocytes or macrophages
  - Reactive—look rod–like, usually in viral infections, can cluster (microglial nodule)
- Neutrophils—acute infarcts, purulent infections
- Lymphocytes—viral/rickettsial infection, autoimmune (demyelinating, vasculitis, auto-immune encephalitis)
- Peripheral nerve reactions
  - See axonal injury from CNS
  - Similar to CNS, but far more efficient at functionally repairing damage to axons and myelin (regeneration and remyelination)
    - Schwann cell is the major reason for this difference
    - Basal lamina "case" is left behind, which leaves framework for regeneration
  - Regeneration much more rapid
  - CAN get complete recovery from demyelinating disease (Guillain-Barré)
    - Chronic form = CIDP (chronic inflammatory demyelinated polyneuropathy)
- Reactions of the brain as an organ
  - Increased intracranial pressure
    - Increased tissue—tumors
    - Increased blood—hemorrhage, venous congestion
    - Increased water—cerebral edema
      - Cytotoxic edema caused by failure of ATP-dependent ionic transport resulting in intracellular edema
        - Early ischemic injuries or after seizures
        - Can be reversible with thrombolytic therapies
        - Positive "diffusion–weighted MRI" (diffusion restriction)
      - Vasogenic edema is the most common, caused by increased vascular permeability (later infarcts and tumors) causing extracellular edema
        - Breakdown of blood–brain barrier
        - Positive T2-weighted MRI
  - Brain herniation
    - Subfalcine (falx cerebri)—cingulate
    - Transtentorial (tentorial incisura)—uncus
      - May be unilateral or "central"
        - Neither uncus is malformed but diencephalon is pushed down
      - Compression of CN3 (exits at midbrain)
      - Duret hemorrhages in midline rostral brainstem
      - Slit–like aqueduct
      - Compression of the contralateral cerebral peduncle (Kernohan notch) with hemorrhagic infarction
        - Paradoxical ipsilateral paralysis
      - Compression of posterior cerebral artery with infarction of the medial occipital lobe
    - Tonsillar (cerebellar tonsil)—foramen magnum
    - Extracranial
  - Hydrocephalus = dilation of ventricular system of brain
    - Noncommunicating; caused by obstruction within ventricular system
      - Tumor, aqueductal stenosis, Arnold Chiari malformation
        - Chiari type I
          - Most common, less severe, presents with headaches
          - Tonsillar displacement through foramen magnum
        - Chiari type 2
          - *Tonsils/vermis and medulla* protrude through foramen magnum and block flow of CSF → *meningomyelocele* and *hydrocephalus*

- Caused by small posterior fossa
- Fused tectum in the midbrain causing aqueductal stenosis
  - Most common spot is aqueduct (narrowest area)
- Communicating—caused by obstruction of CSF flow in the subarachnoid stenosis with decreased resorption into arachnoid granulations
  - After subarachnoid hemorrhage or granulomatous meningitis
  - Dandy–Walker
    - Enlarged fourth ventricle
    - Absence of cerebellar vermis
- Atrophic dilation (hydrocephalus ex vacuo)—ventricular enlargement secondary to loss of surrounding brain tissue
  - No hydrodynamic pathology

CNS VASCULAR DISEASE

- Assessment at autopsy
  - Perfuse cerebral vasculature through aortic arch
    - Most common site of stenosis = bifurcation of carotid (we cannot usually visualize on autopsy)
  - Palpate and examine external surface of brain and circle of Willis
    - Infarcts are soft, may be discolored (pale) depending on age
    - See what type of variability they have in anatomy of vasculature
- Middle cerebral artery (MCA) aneurysm → sylvian fissure
- Anterior cerebral artery (ACA) aneurysm → parenchymal, lateral ventricle, between hemispheres
  - Cannot find source on brain? Go back to body and check ophthalmic artery
- Risk factors for infarction: cardiac arrhythmia, hypertension (lacunar infarcts), vasculitis (systemic or CNS only), thrombotic thrombocytopenic purpura
  - Granulomatous angiitis = primary CNS vasculitis—lymphocytes and possible granulomas in small vessels, multinucleated giant cells in media
    - Only involves brain, no rheumatologic serum markers
    - Patchy (negative biopsies are common)
    - Scattered ischemic injuries
      - Distal, small injuries
    - Beading/narrowing on angiography
    - A mimic is intravascular lymphoma (but will have small infarcts throughout the body, not just the brain)
  - Systemic vasculitis—polyarteritis nodosa, lupus "vasculitis" (fibrinoid necrosis but no inflammation)
  - Infectious vasculitis—cryptococcus or tuberculosis
- Cerebral vessels have internal elastic lamina but *not* external elastic lamina
  - Saccular aneurysms lose internal elastic lamina and media
- Embolic strokes are hemorrhagic
  - Embolus breaks down and moves downstream quite early → reperfusion injury → ribbon–like hemorrhages of cortex (gyriform pattern)
- Venous infarction can be hemorrhagic, but hematoma–like and deeper in brain (white matter > gray)
  - Risks: hyperviscosity, hypercoagulation
- Contusions—located in base of frontal lobes (subfrontal) or occipital lobes (where brain hits skull), mostly cortical and superficial, covering multiple vascular distribution areas
  - Old = hemosiderin on crest of gyrus
- Watershed

- Between anterior cerebral artery and medial cerebral artery (ACA-MCA), superior cerebral artery and posterior inferior cerebellar artery (SCA-PICA)
  - Secondary to hypotension, may be incidental
- Infarcts timeline
  - Acutely get pallor and pericellular vacuoles (edema)
  - 1 to 2 days = red neurons and neutrophils with increased microglia (first endogenous, then systemic macrophages/microglia)
    - Neurons are first to die (then oligodendrocytes)
      - "Eosinophilic neuronal necrosis"
      - Pyknotic triangular nuclei
    - Infarcts grow for the first 2 to 3 days
      - Secondary to nitric oxide and other leukotrienes
  - 2 to 3 days = macrophage and monocyte dominant infiltrate, pyknotic/mummified
  - 3 to 4 days = vascular edema and hypertrophy
  - 7 to 10 days = lots of macrophages, astrocytosis (enlargement and proliferation—plump, glassy pink cytoplasm, many processes), gemistocytes
  - Chronic = cavitary surrounded by long–lasting gliosis
    - Spindled astrocytes
    - *Intra*cellular scar instead of extracellular fibrosing scar
- Ischemic strokes secondary to atherosclerosis—usually around circle of Willis
  - If stroke is more distal, likely embolic (gyriform pattern) or vasculitic (see earlier)
- Spinal cord
  - Anterior spinal artery and posterior vertebral arteries
  - T5 to T8 = watershed area → large collaterals enter inferiorly (artery of Adamkiewicz)
  - Gray is more susceptible than white
- Lacunar hypertensive strokes in the basal ganglia (two-thirds from thalamostriate and lenticulostriate arteries, also known as *penetrating arteries*) and basal pons (one-third from penetrating basal pons arteries off pontine basilar artery) > cerebellar white matter
  - Because of the abrupt step–down from large caliber to small caliber arteries/arterioles
  - *Lipohyalinosis* used for atherosclerosis of small vessels
  - Can lead to vascular dementia in a saltatory pattern (though often coexists with other dementias)
  - True lacune vs. artifact—has gliosis (reactive astrocytosis) at edges; ragged tissue inside with hemosiderin–laden macrophages
  - *Hypertensive hemorrhages*
    - Moderate amount of blood in midpons, inferior cerebellum, basal ganglia
- Anoxic brain injury
  - Chronically will have extremely thinned cortex and white matter in a shriveled brain (like half the weight of normal)
  - Almost no neurons present
  - *Purkinje cells and CA1 of the hippocampus* are very vulnerable
    - Neurons in layers 3 to 5 cortex
    - Selective vulnerability likely caused by glutamate toxicity
    - Can cause or worsen seizures
- Amyloid angiopathy—small and subcortical (gray–white junction)
  - Amyloid is not usually found near vessels in the white matter or deep gray
    - Occipital > frontal > temporal
  - Common >65 years of age
  - Caused by hemorrhage/leakage → accumulated amyloid and edema
    - Show up as white spots on T2—usually called *small vessel ischemic disease* erroneously by radiologists
  - Can have incomplete infarcts

- Scaffolding remains, neurons die off
- Arteriovenous malformation (AVM)
  - Subarachnoid layer and/or underlying brain
  - Spinal varices caused by dural AVM = Foix–Alajouanine
    - Leads to chronic cord infarct and progressive neurologic deterioration
  - Has intervening gliotic brain between very large, thick–walled vessels
    - Elastin stain to differentiate arteries and veins
  - Early: focal neuro deficits or seizures
  - Can get chronic ischemic changes locally caused by blood–stealing
  - Can get catastrophic bleeds
  - Difficult to treat
    - Can recruit new vessels after embolization
- Cavernous hemangioma
  - No intervening brain between tons of large vessels
  - Leaks can cause seizures or focal deficits
    - Hemosiderin–laden macrophages and gliosis
  - Venous, usually do not bleed catastrophically
- Arteriovenous fistula
  - Congenital or "acquired" (mechanism unknown)
  - One artery to one vein, frequently involves spinal arteries
  - Dilated venous system → slow venous infarct
  - Can prevent permanent damage by treating
- Capillary telangiectasia
  - Basal pons
  - Small dilated capillaries
  - Normal intervening brain tissue
- Mycotic aneurysm—small, superficial
- Vein of Galen aneurysm
  - High output heart failure
  - Developmental delay
  - Hydrocephaly
- Saccular (berry) aneurysm
  - Autosomal dominant polycystic kidney disease (ADPKD), aortic coarctation
  - Loss of elastic lamina and media (adventitia remains)
  - ~1 cm is the most common size to rupture
    - Sequelae = hemorrhage and infarcts
    - Risk highest for women in fifth decade
  - At branch points near circle of Willis
    - Ophthalmic artery and internal carotid cannot be seen on autopsy (left behind in body)
    - Most common at middle cerebral trifurcation
- Traumatic shearing—brainstem, corpus callosum, parasagittal white matter, not massive
- Hippocampal sclerosis
  - Can be secondary to epilepsy or hypoxic–ischemic damage
    - Hyperglutamate states, cannot run ATP-dependent glutamate transporters
      - CA1 is most susceptible, and CA2 is most resistant
  - Also can be primary degeneration of age, like Alzheimer's

MYELIN DISEASES

- Multiple sclerosis
  - Visual areas most commonly demyelinated in MS
    - Optic radiations (along lateral ventricles)

- Optic chiasm
- Cerebral cortical plaques
  - Hard to see
  - Gross not distinctive
  - IHC for myelin > LFB-PAS
- Weakness
  - Cerebral hemispheric involvement
    - Cortex
    - White matter
    - Internal capsule
  - Brainstem
  - Spinal cord
    - Gray matter
    - White matter
  - Or multiple hits!
- Acute lesions
  - Axonal spheroids
    - Stain with neurofilament
    - Form because of microtubule disruption
  - T-lymphocytic cuffing
    - CD4 first, then CD8
  - Macrophages
    - Main cell that causes damage
    - LFB-PAS will stain phagocytosed myelin
  - Reactive astrocytes
    - Plump, gemistocytic, homogenous eosinophilic cytoplasm with bland round to ovoid nucleus
    - Compensate for volume loss associated with myelin loss (which usually occupies 50% of volume)
  - **Tumefactive MS may be mistaken for tumor**
    - Frozen section is difficult, touch prep shows foamy macrophages
- Variants
  - Most common type = Charcot type (remitting–relapsing)
  - Marburg—acute, relentless progressive
  - Primary progressive—gradual without attacks or remissions
  - Secondary progressive—evolves from Charcot
  - Clinically silent
  - Schilder—diffuse hemispheric demyelination with MS-like pathology
    - Term is confusing because it is historically associated with multiple diseases
- MRI has helped by...
  - Identifying demyelinating lesions
  - Monitoring the activity of lesions
    - Contrast enhancement on T1
      - Old lesions are dark; new are bright
      - FLAIR sequence helps see all lesions, but does not distinguish old/new
- CSF water is dark, compared with T2 in which CSF is bright—lesions are at interface, so hard to see
      - More activity → more likely to undergo aggressive therapy early in course
        - Plasma exchange can help with even the very aggressive Marburg
  - Allows earlier diagnosis

- Helps differentiate MS from neuromyelitis optica (NMO)
  - Devic disease
  - Looks like MS that only affects spinal cord and optic nerve
    - Do not see oligoclonal bands
    - Later onset
  - Aquaporin-4 antibodies (astrocytic end feet)
    - Highly concentrated in spinal cord, optic nerve >> hypothalamus
  - Poorer prognosis than MS
    - Do not respond well to beta–interferon (sometimes do worse) and other MS drugs
    - PLEX is used (not sure if it helps)
- Central pontine myelinolysis
  - Acute demyelination of pons > striatum (caudate and putamen) > subcortical white matter
  - Rapid correction of severe hyponatremia (<120 mEq/L)
  - Triangle–shaped lesion that rarely extends into the tegmentum
    - Demyelinative lesions initially, then axonal loss and acute tissue destructive
    - Does not look like ischemia because neuronal bodies are relatively spared
  - Reversible forms may exist, but most are fatal
- Carbon monoxide (CO) toxicity (Grinker leukoencephalopathy)
  - Delayed (1 week) demyelination caused by injury to oligodendrocytes by CO
    - Probably killed at time of exposure but takes 7 to 14 days for the myelin to fall apart
  - Often fatal
  - Hypoxic ischemic damage to globus pallidus alone
    - Also manganese poisoning, which can also get injury to substantia nigra → Parkinsonism
- Other toxins that can cause demyelination
  - Organic solvents (toluene)
  - Chemotherapy (methotrexate + radiotherapy), diffuse
- Inflammatory demyelinating diseases
  - MS (multiple sclerosis)
    - Macrophages with PAS+ material
      - Blue on LFB
    - No oligodendrocytes in plaques, only astrocytes
    - Periventricular and subcortical plaques
    - Tumefactive MS → looks ring–enhancing on MRI
  - NMO
  - Acute demyelinating encephalomyelitis (ADEM)
    - Looks like Guillain-Barré in CNS
    - After vaccine (rabies, smallpox, pertussis) or viral infection
      - Vaccine is essentially experimental allergic encephalitis
    - Children have a more favorable prognosis than adults
    - Small perivascular plaques, may have remyelination with time
    - Patchy, brainstem and cortex
  - Acute hemorrhagic (necrotizing) leukoencephalitis (Weston–Hurst)
    - 70% mortality
    - During or immediately after viral infection (usually gastrointestinal)
      - Massive cerebral edema
    - Antibody–antigen complexes in CNS vasculature in white matter → injury → fibrinoid necrosis and edema
      - Surrounding demyelination and inflammatory cells
- Inborn errors of myelin metabolism

- Leukodystrophies—affect all white matter with thin ribbon of spared "U-fibers" under cortex
  - Metachromatic leukodystrophy
    - Acidified cresyl violet on frozen section stain golden brown
    - Strongly PAS+ macrophages
    - Arylsulfatase A defect
  - Krabbe
    - Multinucleated giant cells = globoid cells
    - Glassy on hematoxylin and eosin (H&E) stain
    - Beta–galactocerebrosidase defect
  - Adrenoleukodystrophy
    - X-linked
    - Perivascular lymphocytic cuff
    - Cerebral atrophy, adrenal atrophy, cytoplasmic inclusions
    - Very-long chain fatty acid defect (Lorenzo's oil)
  - Alexander disease
    - *Tons* of Rosenthal fibers
    - GFAP mutation

TRAUMA

- Focal contusions—olfactory deficits, subfrontal
  - Chronic issues—seizures
  - Resolve as holes (like infarcts) or divot in cortical ribbon with hemosiderin staining
- Intraparenchymal hemorrhage (IPH) secondary to shearing injury
  - Petechial to massive
  - Get *diffuse axonal injury* at lesser injuries than IPH → axonal spheroids
    - Diffuse axonal injury = traumatic axonal injury
    - Sudden acceleration or deceleration
    - Spheroids take time to develop (not present in instant death)
  - Side impact—corpus callosum, fornices (hippocampal connections to brain), long tracts in brainstem, superior cerebellar peduncles
  - Loss of consciousness from reticular activating system (RAS) injuries (rostral midbrain)
    - Punch to the jaw rotates brain up and sideways ("glass jaw")
  - Axonal spheroids need time to develop—will not be seen if injury happens immediately before death, only see petechiae

DEMENTIAS AND MOVEMENT DISORDERS

- Neurofibrillary tangles in cell body, flame–shaped, extend into primary process (dendrite)
  - Silver stain highlights plaques and tangles
    - Plaques occasionally have amyloid cores
  - Ghost tangles stay after neuron dies → lighter on silver stain
- Mesiotemporal involvement does not correlate well with clinical dementia, but frontal lobe involvement does
  - Other factors can affect (e.g., vascular dementia, Lewy body)
- Almost all patients with Alzheimer's disease (AD) will have amyloid angiopathy (replacement of media)—more frequent in apoE4
- Harano body—usually in dendrites, rod–like eosinophilic body
  - May be close to (and "stabbing") cell body

- Rarely seen outside of AD; most numerous in CA1/subiculum of hippocampus
- "Tombstones" = clusters of pigmented macrophages at site of dead neuron
  - Can also occur with advanced age
- Parkinson's (PD) and Lewy body dementia (LBD)—both have substantia nigra (SN) pallor and Lewy bodies
  - Dementia ≥1 year before Parkinsonism → Lewy body dementia
    - Relatively early compared with other dementias (60 s)
    - Clinical distinction, not pathologic
  - Triad: tremor, bradykinesia, and rigidity (plus dysautonomia and dementia)
    - Delusional, clearly formed visual hallucinations
  - Lewy bodies are large, round, only in cytoplasm, and positive for alpha–synuclein (also have ubiquitin and alpha–beta–crystallin)
    - PD has Lewy bodies in pigmented neurons in SN and locus coeruleus
    - LBD has them everywhere in cortex
      - Cortical Lewy bodies are very subtle
    - Marinesco bodies are a pitfall—nuclear and cytoplasmic, small
    - Can have overlap between Alzheimer's
      - Though usually milder and more fluctuating than Alzheimer's
  - Dorsal motor nucleus, raphe nucleus, locus nucleus, preganglionic sympathetics
  - Progression
1. Entorhinal cortex
2. Hippocampus
3. Neocortex
4. Cortex farther away
5. All cortex, even occipital lobe
   - Pattern of involvement by Lewy bodies not predictive of clinical dementia
   - 15% to 20% of AD patients have PD pathology and vice versa
     - Especially difficult to separate in end–stage disease
     - Both AD and PD get olfactory deficits early
   - Associated with REM disorder and restless legs syndrome
   - Substantia nigra usually involved midway through → movement disorder (Parkinsonism)
- Frontotemporal dementia (FTD)—subgroup = Pick (silver + round cytoplasmic inclusions, tau protein)
  - Balloon cells—larger neurons filled with phosphorylated neurofilament, silver+
  - Severe frontotemporal atrophy (<1 kg)
  - Familial—mutation in the *tau* gene on chromosome 17 = early onset FTD + Parkinsonism
  - TDP43 granules aberrantly in cytoplasm in sporadic, crystal (cat's eye) in nucleus of familial
    - Also implicated in familial ALS and PD
- Progressive supranuclear palsy—tau-opathy (neurofibrillary tangles and neuron dropout)
  - "Parkinson plus"
  - Tangles in brainstem and globus pallidus made of tau protein
    - Can also get glial inclusions
  - Vertical gaze center in midbrain → fall backward
    - Voluntary extraocular movements affected (first vertical gaze)
  - Substantia nigra pallor
  - 5-year median survival
  - Poor response to L-DOPA
  - Mickey mouse view on imaging of midbrain
    - Basal ganglia (globus pallidus and subthalamic nucleus)

- Midbrain (substantia nigra, red nucleus, periaqueductal gray nucleus, third nerve nucleus)
- Pons (locus coeruleus, raphe, basal pons, tegmentum)
- Inferior olives
- Dentate nucleus of cerebellum
- Corticobasilar degeneration—tau-opathy (neurofibrillary tangles and neuron dropout)
  - Caudate, cortical atrophy
  - Substantia nigra pallor and tangles in brainstem
- Multiple system atrophy (MSA) = striatonigral degeneration = Shy Drager syndrome
  - Part of olivocerebellar degenerative disorder group
  - Blue–gray putamen, substantia nigra pallor, ↓ basis pontis, ↓ olives, OK cerebellar peduncles (around fourth ventricle in pontine tegmentum/midbrain junction)
    - Demyelination
  - Looks like PD that is unresponsive to dopamine
  - Movement disorder and striking dysautonomia—orthostatic hypotension
- ALS (amyotrophic lateral sclerosis)
  - Denervation disease (not demyelinating)
  - Bilateral and symmetric degeneration of *lower and upper* motor neurons → muscular atrophy
    - Descending corticospinal tracts
  - The hypoglossal nuclei (CNXII) in floor of the fourth ventricle in medulla is almost always affected
    - Exits between medullary pyramid and inferior olive
  - Mutations in superoxide dismutase *(SOD1), TDP43, C9orf72*
  - Abnormal proteins like TDP-43
  - Survival depends on cervical (diaphragmatic) and bulbar (aspiration) involvement
- Subacute combined degeneration—B_{12} deficiency (pernicious anemia)
  - Posterior and lateral column demyelination
    - DDx: AIDS myelopathy and copper deficiency
  - Progressive paresthesias and numbness, weakness → bilateral spastic paralysis
    - Pressure/vibration/touch
    - Positive Babinski reflex (upgoing toes), positive Romberg test
- Spinal muscle atrophy
- X-linked spinal and bulbar muscular atrophy (Kennedy disease)
  - Androgen–receptor dysfunction
- Ataxias
  - Friedreich ataxia: trinucleotide repeat expansion disease
    - Intronic mitochondrial DNA
    - Childhood onset
    - Cardiomyopathy and diabetes
    - Posterior columns, spinocerebellar tracts of cords, corticospinal tracts (and posterior roots)
      - ↓ proprioception, ↓ coordination, ↓ strength
  - Ataxia–telangiectasia
  - ~4 dozen autosomal cerebellar ataxias
    - Similar disease course and inheritance pattern as Huntington
- Huntington
  - Loss of neurons and increased astrocytic gliosis
  - Can stain for Huntington protein
  - Intranuclear ubiquitin inclusion
- Granulovacuolar change—tubulin+
  - Associated with dementia, but not specific

- Most frequent in hippocampus
- Primary hippocampal degeneration of age
  - No tangles or plaques, but unilateral or bilateral neuron loss in hippocampal subiculum and CA1
  - Causes dementia (clinically like AD)

INFECTIONS

- Acute bacterial meningitis
  - Complications
    - Cranial neuropathy (most common is hearing loss)
    - Vasculitis → stroke
      - Occurs most frequently in granulomatous meningitis
    - Hydrocephalus from chronic leptomeningeal fibrosis
    - Altered mental status (caused by cytokine release, mitigate with steroids)
      - Most common pathogens: *Streptococcus pneumoniae, Neisseria, Escherichia coli* (neonates), group B streptococcus (neonates)
- Cerebritis (focal, caused by bacteria or fungus) and encephalitis (widespread, caused by viruses)
  - One of the rare causes of fibrosis in the brain
  - Typically a subacute bacterial infection
  - Can lead to abscess → happen at gray–white junction like metastases
    - Restricted water diffusion on imaging (compared with no restriction in metastases)
    - Usually caused by anaerobic organisms
- Granulomatous meningitis (usually at the base of the brain)
  - Nonnecrotizing—sarcoidosis (notorious to cause hydrocephalus)
  - Necrotizing
    - Tuberculosis
      - Only entity limited to base of brain involvement
      - Focal
    - Can be fulminant
    - Fungal
      - Blastomycosis
      - Coccidiomycosis
        - Large round yeast forms with refractile double wall
      - Cryptococcus
        - ≤ size of red cell (though size can vary), PAS+, refractile double wall
        - In immunocompetent—granulomatous with infarcts
        - In immunodeficient—bland with little inflammation
          - Can find organisms in perivascular spaces
- Hyphal fungi
  - Aspergillosis—essentially 100% mortality
    - Grossly create hemorrhagic infarcts
    - Micro: red dead neurons, edema, +/− gliosis
    - Equal diameter of trunks and branches, classically 45-degree branching (not necessarily true in histologic sections)
    - Imaging differential includes lymphoma
  - Mucor (zygomycetes)—no normal brain between foci of fungi
    - Type 2 diabetics, not septic
    - Ribbon–like, branches are smaller than trunk
    - Direct brain invasion from sinonasal area
  - Candida—pseudohyphae

- Not common in immunosuppressed anymore because of decreased use of corticosteroids
  - Less destructive than Aspergillus and Mucor
  - Miliary pattern with normal brain in between
  - Pinched branch points like balloon animals
- Bacteria
  - Listeria
    - Bacteria with lymphocytic inflammation
    - Children and adults
  - Whipple
    - *Tropheryma whippelii*
    - Foamy macrophages that stain brightly on PAS-LFB with chunky elongated dots, throughout brain
    - Looks similar to leishmaniasis
  - Neurosyphilis
    - *Treponema pallidum* (spirochete)
    - Increased microglia in gray > white, all pointing to surface
    - Plasmacytic perivascular inflammation
    - Damage and loss of neurons secondary to inflammation → irreversible
    - Similar to AIDS dementia complex (in which the microglia are infected by HIV)
    - Increased CSF protein
    - Tabes dorsalis—demyelination of posterior columns and dorsal root ganglia
      - ↓ proprioception (subsequent "ataxia") with positive Romberg sign (can stay standing with feet together if eyes are open but cannot with eyes closed)
- Viruses
  - In general, lymphocytes near blood vessels and around microglial nodules
  - Rabies
    - Negri body—eosinophilic cytoplasmic inclusion
  - Herpes simplex
    - Hemorrhagic, mononuclear inflammation
    - Do not usually see viral inclusions
    - Mesolimbic, temporal lobe, insula → memory loss and seizures
    - Diagnose with PCR of CSF
    - Herpes zoster—devastating, fatal in days in HIV patients
  - Coxsackie
    - Classic cause of "aseptic meningitis"
    - Common, may not seek health care
  - Measles (rubeola)
    - Subacute sclerosing panencephalitis
    - Gray and white matter involved
  - CMV
    - Necrotizing/cavitating lesion
    - Large cell, pink cytoplasm with nucleus pushed off to side—purple intranuclear inclusion with halo
    - No inflammation, smoldering infection
    - Can be secondary to CMV retinitis
    - More likely to be seen in HIV patients than posttransplant immunosuppressed patients
  - JC virus → progressive multifocal leukoencephalopathy (PML)
    - HIV/AIDS, opportunistic infection
      - Rare infections can occur in immunocompetent patients (will have inflammation)

- Oligodendrocytes become infected and die → demyelination → macrophages with large foamy cytoplasm with glassy inclusions
  - Astrocytes become infected and do not die but look very atypical (like diffuse large B cell lymphoma or GBM cells)
  - On imaging can look like demyelination patches, but *do not* enhance (because there is no inflammation)
  - MS treatment natalizumab can predispose to PML
- Arboviruses—West Nile, LaCrosse, St. Louis, Powassan
  - From mosquitoes and ticks
  - Most people do not get encephalitis, just meningitis (mild, do not present to health care)
    - Mild meningitis also caused by enteroviruses (Coxsackie)
  - North Americans get polio–like syndrome with West Nile virus
  - RNA viruses, no therapy, diagnosed with PCR
- HIV
  - Classic multinucleated cells, not seen frequently in reality
  - In microglia, cytokine release from microglia and macrophages causes damage
  - Reversible in early stages, irreversible neural and vessel damage → AIDS dementia complex/AIDS encephalopathy
    - White matter macrophages with 3 to 4 nuclei (not *quite* multinucleated giant cells), infected by HIV
    - Usually large viral load
    - Can see white matter lesions on imaging, not prognostically significant
  - CNS lymphoma can be driven by HIV and/or EBV
- Parasites
  - Cerebral malaria
    - *P. falciparum*
    - Rosetting of red blood cells
    - "Sequestered" to endothelium → plug → hemozoin pigment accumulation → hypoxia → ring hemorrhages with small collections of leukocytes
      - = "Durck granulomas"
  - Toxoplasmosis
    - One of the most common HIV-presenting infections
    - Causes profound anomalies in fetuses
    - Can be multifocal
    - Tachyzoites (1 to 3 μm, purple, look karyorrhectic) in a necrotic background
    - Large bradyzoites
    - Can stain with toxoplasma IHC
  - Rickettsial—typhus, Rocky Mountain spotted fever
    - Treatable but easy to miss rash
  - Cysticercosis—pork tapeworm
    - From contaminated water/food; get tapeworm from eating pork
    - Number-one cause of epilepsy in endemic countries
    - Look for scolex and tegument
- All viral and Rickettsial infections get microglial nodules and mononuclear infiltrate

Neoplastic

GLIAL TUMORS = GLIOMAS

- *Gliomas* include astrocytoma, ependymoma, glioblastoma (GBM), oligodendroglioma
- Do not jump sulci to neighboring gyri

- Neoplastic astrocytes have cleared cytoplasm with nucleoli, lots of cytoplasmic processes
- Calcifications in low–grade gliomas—ganglioglioma, oligodendroglioma, pilocytic astrocytomas
  - Diffuse astrocytomas almost never calcify
- First symptom is usually seizure
- All low–grade astrocytomas and oligodendrogliomas that progress to glioblastoma have *IDH* mutation
  - They have a more favorable prognosis than de novo GBMs
  - Increased mitotic counts in *IDH* mutants *are not* independent prognostic markers (R132H, arginine to histidine)
  - Median survival for *IDH*-wild type GBMs = 14 months
  - Virtually all astrocytomas have *ATRX* null deletion. Therefore, secondary GBMs have positive IDH1 staining (and R132H mutation) and loss of ATRX staining (null deletion). Furthermore, retained ATRX expression essentially rules out an *IDH1/2* mutation.
    - There can be some *IDH* mutations that do not express the target protein of the IHC stain, but still prognostically important. They will have loss of ATRX.
  - MGMT promoter hypermethylation has a better response to temozolomide (alkylating agent)
    - *IDH* mutated usually have hypermethylation
  - Morphologic clues of mutated *IDH*—younger patient (<55 years of age), gemistocytic, microcystic architecture, perivascular lymphocytes
- Contrast enhancement is caused by attenuated/weakened blood–brain barrier
  - Caused by VEGF-associated vascular proliferation (can ↓ with dexamethasone or bevacizumab)
    - Hyperplastic, thickened capillaries; may have capillaries or poorly formed vascular channels
  - Pilocytic astrocytoma
  - Diffuse astrocytoma
  - GBM—ring enhancing **(most common tumor to have contrast enhancement)**
  - Lymphoma—solid and homogenous
  - NOT low–grade oligodendroglioma (no vascular proliferation)
  - Extra–axial tumors
    - Meningiomas
    - Schwannomas
- Grading
  - Get 1 point for showing up + 1 point for each of the following
    - Nuclear pleomorphism
    - ↑ mitotic activity
    - Necrosis *or* microvascular proliferation (MVP, see above)
- Pilocytic astrocytoma
  - Grade 1 = glial tumor with the most favorable prognosis
  - Most common solid neoplasm in children
  - Excisable and indolent, circumscribed and cystic
  - Cerebellum > hypothalamus/third ventricle region > optic nerves > brainstem > cerebral hemispheres > spinal cord
  - Biphasic pattern: loose (microcytic) and compact fibrillary (piloid/pilar) background
    - Resembles Antoni A/B
  - Rosenthal fibers in compact areas
    - Heat shock protein alpha–B–crystallin

- Can also be seen in intense reactive gliosis ("chronic piloid gliosis," tends to happen near cysts)
- Eosinophilic granular bodies (EGBs, more frequent in loose areas with microcysts)
  - Can also be seen in pleomorphic xanthoastrocytoma
- Can have microvascular proliferation (and glomeruloid bodies) with associated contrast enhancement, nuclear atypia, and meningeal infiltration, but mitoses are rare to absent
- Treated with resection only
  - Malignant transformation is rare
- No *TP53* mutations; associated with NF1, may have *BRAF* mutations (−17q, non-V600E)
- Pleomorphic xanthoastrocytoma (PXA)
  - Not formally graded by usual criteria, is always grade 2
  - Rare, indolent, associated with seizures, second to third decade
  - Supratentorial (superficial cortex and leptomeninges), circumscribed and cystic, bizarre giant cells with one or more nuclei and xanthomatous cytoplasm (lipidized change)
    - Pleomorphic early → spindled late
  - Bizarre nuclei, EGBs, pericellular reticulin network, perivascular lymphocytes
  - GFAP+, S100+, CD34+ in a subset, PAS+ eosinophilic granular bodies
  - May have MVP and contrast enhancement (no mitoses, no necrosis)
  - 10-year recurrence-free survival of 60%
- Diffuse intrinsic pontine gliomas
  - Aggressive
  - Look like astrocytes but not IHC reactive, mitotic, mild-to-moderate pleomorphism, diffuse sheets
  - If histone 3.3 mutation (H3 K27M), *diffuse midline glioma*
    - New in WHO 2016, histologically looks okay (grade 2 to 3) but very poor outcome → always grade 4 (like a GBM)
    - Can be anywhere midline, not just pons
    - *IDH1* wild type
- Pilomyxoid astrocytoma—grade 2
  - Very young patients (<1 year of age) in the hypothalamus or optic chiasm
  - Indolent glial tumor, but more aggressive than pilocytic astrocytomas
  - Angiocentric, myxoid change
  - No Rosenthal fibers or eosinophilic granular bodies; no cystic component
    - Diffuse astrocytoma
  - Grade 2, very infiltrative
  - A cortical lesion with bright T2 and dark T2-FLAIR is called "T2-mismatch" and has 100% positive predictive value for an *IDH2*-mutated diffuse astrocytoma
  - Can get extensive microglial infiltration at leading edge (also in oligodendrogliomas)
    - May *aid* tumor
  - Mild atypia and enlargement of cells, very rare mitoses, never necrosis or vascular proliferation
  - Subtypes: fibrillary (GFAP+), gemistocytic (≥20% gemistocytes), protoplasmic (very small cells, looks like pilocytic astrocytoma but diffuse in mucoid or microcystic background)
  - *TP53* mutations in ~50% of cases
  - *IDH2* mutation—more favorable prognosis, can treat with temozolomide
- Anaplastic astrocytoma
  - Grade 3

- Looks like diffuse astrocytoma but with increased atypia, cellularity, and mitotic activity (Ki67 5% to 10%)
- Inactivation of CDKN2A/p16/ARF, CDK4, and RB
- Glioblastoma multiforme (GBM)
  - Grade 4
  - Most common primary brain tumor in adults (~50%)
  - De novo (primary) or from lower–grade astrocytoma (secondary)
  - Ring enhancing, classic "butterfly" pattern is spread across corpus callosum
  - High cellularity, marked nuclear atypia, mitoses (Ki67 15% to 20%), microvascular proliferation, necrosis (+/– pseudopalisading)
  - May have zones of better differentiation (fibrillary and gemistocytic astrocytes)
  - PITFALL—can be cytokeratin positive!
  - Variants
    - Small cell glioblastoma: small cells with poor GFAP expression and scant cytoplasm more typical of secondary (which usually have *EGFR* gene amplification)
    - Giant cell glioblastoma: rare, better circumscribed, abundant reticulin, *TP53* mutations
    - Gliosarcoma: biphasic mesenchymal and glial elements; reticulin+, GFAP– (in sarcomatous component); mimic meningioma on imaging (circumscribed, uniformly enhancing)
      - Superficial temporal lobes, perivascular distribution
      - Not treated differently than GBM
    - Other cell types (not true variants): glandular or epithelioid, oligodendrocyte–like, PAS+ granular, lipidized
  - Primary: inactivation of CDKN2A/p16/ARF, CDK4, and RB; loss of chromosome 10 (with PTEN), amplification/rearrangement of *EGFR*
  - Secondary: *IDH* mutation (most common is *IDH1*; IHC cytoplasmic+), *TP53* mutations
    - Retention of ATRX expression by IHC is highly correlated with *absence* of *IDH1* mutation. Thus, you do not need to do *IDH1* sequencing if you get a negative *IDH1* IHC as long as you have a positive ATRX.
    - 98% of *IDH*-mutant astrocytic tumors have *TP53* mutations
  - RECURRENT VS. RESIDUAL GBMs
    - Recurrent—highly cellular, microvascular proliferation, high mitotic activity
    - Residual treated—low cellularity, no mitoses/Ki67+, only telangiectatic/thin–walled vessels
  - Temozolomide
    - Used to treat GBMs with MGMT hypermethylation and lower–grade gliomas with *IDH* mutations
- Gliomatosis cerebri
  - Very diffuse, very infiltrative glioma involving more than two lobes, frequently bilateral and may extend to posterior fossa and spinal cord
  - Poor prognosis, even though histologic grading is low
  - Taken out of the World Health Organization (WHO) 2016 categorization
  - Neoplastic cells may resemble astrocytes or oligodendrocytes, variable GFAP
- Subependymal giant cell astrocytomas (SEGAs)
  - Benign intraventricular slow–growing tumors associated with tuberous sclerosis
    - TS patients also get hard white–tan cortical nodules (ill–defined, causing blurring of gray–white junction, = tubers) and ependymal hamartomas ("dripping candle wax")
  - Large cells resembling gemistocytes but having "ganglioid" cells with prominent nucleoli +/– spindled cells +/– atypia +/– occasional mitoses
  - May express either or both glial and neuronal markers

- *TSC1* gene on 9q and *TSC2* gene on 16p
- Usually left alone, often found incidentally
- Choroid glioma of the third ventricle
  - Nests and cords of strongly GFAP+ cells in mucinous stroma
  - Lymphoplasmacytic infiltrate, little to no mitotic activity
- Oligodendroglioma (grade 2)
  - Infiltrating (therefore incurable by surgery) but usually slowly progressive; can live >10 years; median survival 3 to 5 years
  - Peak incidence between 30 and 60 years of age
  - May be mucoid or cystic grossly
  - Fried egg or honeycomb appearance caused by swelling artifact causing clear halo around small nucleus; delicate branching capillaries (chicken–wire vasculature)
    - Remember frozen sections do not get swelling artifact that causes permanent sections to have "fried egg" morphology
  - Tumor cells aggregate around vessels, neurons, and pia
  - Occasional mitosis (Ki67 < 5%) and atypia okay
    - If significant mitotic activity, microvascular proliferation, or necrosis → *anaplastic oligodendroglioma* (grade 3)
      - GFAP+ minigemistocytes common
      - Survival is still not bad
      - Contrast enhancement, should be *very* ugly, 6 to 8 mitoses/10 hpf, MVP
  - May get microcalcifications or GFAP+ minigemistocytes
  - Curvilinear calcifications on imaging
  - 1p/19q codeletions in almost all
    - Considered defining characteristic now, regardless if histologic appearance, pathognomonic
    - When 1p/19q codeletion present, great response to chemotherapy (and survival >10 years)
      - Other alterations have poor prognosis (*PTEN* mutations, chromosome 10 loss, *EGFR* amplification, CDKN2A/p16/ARF deletion)
    - Usually *IDH1* or *IDH2* mutations, MGMT hypermethylated also present
    - Mutually exclusive with *TP53* and *ATRX* mutations
- Mixed gliomas
  - No longer exist in the WHO
- Filum terminale may be involved by m*yxopapillary ependymomas* (or *schwannomas*)
- Astroblastoma
  - Uncertain histogenesis
  - Perivascular pseudorosettes of GFAP+ tumor cells with processes that extend to thickened hyalinized wall
    - Shorter and thicker processes than ependymoma
    - Young adults > children
  - Not graded because of lack of data
- *Angioblastic glioma* is a descriptive term for gliomas with a lot of vessels

OTHERS TUMORS

- Neurocytic tumors
  - Central neurocytoma (grade 2)
    - Growing from putamen into the third or fourth ventricle
    - Looks like oligodendroglioma but positive synaptophysin
    - Well–behaved, occurs in young adults
  - Cerebellar liponeurocytoma (grade 2)

- Glioneuronal tumors
  - Gangliocytoma (grade 1)
    - Children and adults
    - Temporal lobe, associated with seizures, homogeneous and circumscribed
      - Variant in sellar or suprasellar location
    - Mature ganglion cells that may be binucleate or bizarre, fine pericellular reticulin network (especially superficially)
    - No mitoses or necrosis, no MVP
  - Ganglioglioma
    - Late in childhood, temporal lobe epilepsy, circumscribed and cystic, enhancing, grade 1
      - Discrete cyst with bright mural nodule on imaging
    - Neuronal = bizarre and binucleated with prominent nucleoli, synaptophysin+
    - Glial = GFAP+, S100+ (usually astrocytic though oligodendroglial differentiation can happen)
    - Behavior determined by anaplasia of *glial component* (document necrosis, mitoses, MVP)
    - Can have calcifications
    - Perivascular lymphocytes
  - Dysplastic gangliocytoma of the cerebellum (Lhermitte–Duclos disease)
    - Grossly visible expansion of folia in one hemisphere
    - Center of folia have Purkinje–like cells (large, bizarre ganglion cells) and small granular neurons; surface is covered by aberrant white matter bundles *inverted cerebellar cortex*
    - Best considered a hamartoma
    - Associated with Cowden syndrome (verrucous skin lesions, facial trichilemmomas, oral fibromas, hamartomatous gastrointestinal polyps, thyroid tumors, breast tumors; *PTEN* mutation)
  - Desmoplastic infantile ganglioglioma (grade 1)
    - Large, cerebral (superficial frontal and parietal), cystic, first year of life (up to 2 years of age)
    - Astrocytic and ganglion cell components—may be difficult to find ganglion component
    - Strong desmoplasia, sarcomatoid appearance but low mitoses, circumscribed
  - Dysembryoplastic neuroepithelial tumor (DNET) (grade 1)
    - Epilepsy, older, cortical, low–grade, associated with cortical dysplasia, indolent and cured with resection
      - May be an epileptic focus
    - Nodular, bland small round S100+ nuclei, myxoid material surrounding neurons and keeping glial cells away ("floating neurons")
    - Looks like oligodendroglioma cells in nodules
      - Heterotopic neurons (in white matter where there is usually none), pools of mucin (T2 bright)
      - Columns of synaptophysin positivity around tumor nodules
  - Papillary glioneuronal tumor (grade 1)
  - Rosette–forming glioneuronal tumor of the fourth ventricle (grade 1)
  - Paraganglioma
    - Extra–adrenal chromaffin tissue; essentially nonadrenal pheochromocytoma
    - Filum terminale > spinal/cranial nerve root with extension into cranium/spinal canal
      - Middle ear (sometimes into posterior fossa) = *glomus jugulare*
    - Zellballen of plump neuroendocrine cells with fine fibrovascular septa
    - IHC
      - Tumor cells chromogranin/synaptophysin+

- Sustentacular cells S100+
- +/− Focal ganglion differentiation
- Rarely produce catecholamines
- Prognosis related to anatomic extent and resectability
- Olfactory neuroblastoma (esthesioneuroblastoma)
  - Small round blue cell tumor
  - Late childhood through adulthood, presents with headache or nasal obstruction
  - Upper nasal cavity, through cribriform plate and into frontal lobes
  - Characteristic broad, nodular growth pattern
  - Homer–Wright pseudorosettes (neurofibrillary processes in middle) > Flexner–Wintersteiner rosettes (central lumina)
  - Low or high grade, depending on differentiation, mitotic activity, pleomorphism, and necrosis (Hyams grading system)
  - IHC
    - S100+ in sustentacular cells (highlights lobularity)
    - Calretinin+ in tumor cells
    - Some may be positive for epithelial markers (confused for small cell carcinoma)
- Ependymoma (grade 2)
  - Most common site in pediatrics = intraventricular (fourth > lateral)
    - Most common site in adults = spinal cord arising from central canal
    - CSF spread ("drop mets" to cauda equina)
  - Associated with NF2
  - Treated with surgery and adjuvant radiation; local recurrence is common
  - Strong contrast enhancement, well–circumscribed, +/− hydrocephalus
  - Polygonal cells with uniform nuclei and eosinophilic cytoplasm, minimal atypia
  - Perivascular pseudorosettes (with GFAP+ in cytoplasmic processes), true ependymal rosettes with ciliated lumens (tubules)
  - Occasional myxoid degeneration, focal hemorrhage, focal necrosis, rare bone/cartilage formation
  - Variants: cellular, tanycytic (look like schwannomas, fascicles), clear cell, myxopapillary, papillary
    - Myxopapillary ependymoma (MPE)
      - Occurs exclusively in the conus medullaris/cauda equina (arising from filum terminale)
      - Rare subcutaneous or presacral MPEs arise from ectopic ependymal remnants
      - Young adults, present with back pain or incidental, favorable prognosis
      - GFAP + cuboidal cells on fibrovascular cores with variable myxoid change
      - End feet are pushed back by mucinous material
        - Alcian blue+
        - PAS+
      - See Fig. 14.5.
    - Anaplastic ependymoma (grade 3)
      - Like grade 2 but with increased cellularity, atypia, mitoses, and (usually) microvascular proliferation and necrosis
        - Though necrosis alone does not indicate anaplastic change
        - Might not be prognostically relevant
- Subependymoma
  - Clinically silent unless large enough to block CSF flow
  - Well–demarcated, attached to ventricular wall and project into lumen (exophytic), most frequent in floor of fourth ventricle
  - Small nests of glial nuclei in hypocellular GFAP+ fibrillary matrix

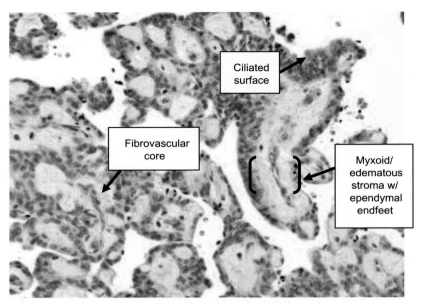

Fig. 14.5 Myxopapillary ependymoma histology.

- Rosettes with nothing in the center
- No mitoses, benign
- +/– microcysts, calcifications, focal hemorrhage, abnormal vessels
- Mixed ependymoma/subependymomas have been described
- Choroid plexus papilloma (CPP, grade 1)
  - Young, intraventricular (lateral > fourth > third)
  - Slightly more crowded and elongated papillae compared with normal
    - Cells are normally cuboidal, become columnar in papilloma
  - S100+, EMA+, CK+, transthyretin (focal GFAP) (glial and epithelial markers are expressed)
  - Low–grade → atypical CPP → *choroid plexus carcinoma*
    - Grade 3, atypia, frequent mitoses, more solid growth, loss of papillary architecture, brain invasion
    - *Infantile carcinoma* in lateral ventricles
    - Major differential consideration is metastatic carcinoma
- Pineal tumors
  - Germ cell tumors
    - Intracranial germ cell tumors
      - Most likely in pineal region or in suprasellar region
        - Pineal—under corpus callosum and in third ventricular
          - Can lead to Parinaud syndrome (dorsal midbrain)
            - Vertical gaze palsy
            - Convergence retraction nystagmus
            - Light–near dissociation
      - Include teratomas, embryonal carcinoma, yolk sac tumor, choriocarcinoma, mixed germ cell tumor, germinoma

- 90% in males (equal sex distribution in suprasellar region)
- Germinoma = most common (radiation cures)
  - Seminoma in testes, dysgerminoma in ovary
  - Lymphs, smudgy malignant cells
- Yolk sac, embryonal, choriocarcinoma, teratoma
- Gliomas
- Pineal parenchymal tumors
  - Neuroendocrine *and* retinal photoreceptor features, synaptophysin, NSE+
  - Pineocytoma (grade 1)
  - Pineal parenchymal tumor of intermediate differentiation (grade 2 or 3)
  - Pineoblastoma (grade 4)
    - See "embryonal tumors" later
  - Papillary tumor of pineal origin (grade 2 or 3)
- Craniopharyngioma
  - Suprasellar, from Rathke pouch (pituitary stalk)
  - Squamous epithelium with calcifications, cystic, keratinizing foci with pearls ("wet keratin")
  - Bimodal distribution—first decade and middle age
  - Adamantinomatous—most common, cystic, basaloid, nonlamellar growth pattern, beta-catenin mutations (nuclear expression)
  - Papillary—less cystic, less keratin, *BRAF* mutations
- Pituitary adenoma
  - Can be of basophilic (usually prolactin–secreting) or eosinophilic (usually GH-secreting) cells
    - Bland
  - Reticulin network is lost
  - 10 mm = macroadenoma
  - Imaging looks like decapitated snowman (one ball in the sella, a constriction, then another ball above the sella)
  - Normal pituitary
    - Anterior = adenohypophysis
      - From Rathke pouch
      - Basophils—"B-FLAT" mnemonic
        - Follicle–stimulating hormone, luteinizing hormone, adrenocorticotropic hormone, thyroid–stimulating hormone
      - Acidophils—growth hormone GH and prolactin
    - Posterior = neurohypophysis
      - From neuroectoderm
      - Antidiuretic hormone and oxytocin
    - Can have basophilic cell "invasion" into posterior pituitary normally
- Colloid cyst of the third ventricle
  - In foramen of Monro
  - Glandular and squamous, filled with colloid–like debris
  - Bright on CT
- Intraneural perineurioma (grade 1)
  - Adolescence/early adulthood
  - Peripheral nerves of extremities → localized tubular enlargement of nerve
  - Proliferations of perineurial cells in concentric layers (pseudo–onion bulbs) around nerve fibers
    - EMA+ S100−

- Soft tissue perineurioma is related but different
- Meningeal tumors
  - Can get meningeal tumors in ventricles (especially meningiomas) and primary meningeal melanoma because choroid plexus stroma is derived from neural crest cells (like melanocytes and arachnoid stroma)
  - Secretory meningioma—meningioma with CEA+, pseudoinclusions, psammoma bodies, lots of edema
  - Choroid meningioma—meningioma with pseudoinclusions and myxoid stroma
  - Meningiomas
    - Graded based on histologic appearance, associated with NF2
    - EMA+, keratin–, PR+ when low–grade
    - Postradiation meningiomas are usually grade 1
      - Grade 1
        - must have (1) mitotic index < 4/10 hpf, (2) have fewer than three atypical features, (3) not be grade 2 or 3 type, and (4) not show evidence of true brain invasion
        - Meningothelial
          - Epithelial–like cells with ill–defined cell borders (syncytial looking), pale nucleus with occasional intranuclear pseudoinclusions
          - Whorls *always*, psammoma bodies sometimes
        - Fibrous (fibroblastic)
          - Elongated fusiform cells arranged in fascicles
          - Well–developed collagen and reticulin network (pericellular)
          - Whorls and psammoma bodies may be present
          - S100+ (meningothelial is negative)
        - Transitional (mixed)
          - Intermediate features between meningothelial and fibroblastic
        - Psammomatous
          - Exceptionally numerous psammoma bodies, may be confluent
          - Frequent in spinal region
        - Angiomatous
          - Rich vascularization by small hyalinized vessels
        - Microcystic
          - Tumor cells have elongated processes that create multiple small cystic spaces +/– mucin
          - Pleomorphism and hyalinized vessels may be prominent
        - Secretory
          - Small eosinophilic PAS+ globular cytoplasmic inclusions
          - Cells are EMA+, CK+, CEA+
        - Lymphoplasmacyte–rich
        - Metaplastic
          - Includes those with xanthomatous change, myxomatous change, cartilage or bone, melanin pigment
      - Grade 2
        - Must belong to one of three categories: (1) atypical based on the criteria below, (2) chordoid or clear cell subtype, or (3) a meningioma that is histologically benign but shows *true brain invasion*
        - Atypical = increased mitotic activity (4 or more/10 hpf) and/or the presence of three or more of the following:
          - Increased cellularity

- Small cells with a high N:C ratio
- Prominent nucleoli at 10×
- Uninterrupted patternless or sheet–like growth
- Foci of spontaneous/geographic necrosis
- NOT A CRITERION: cytologic atypia (because it is usually degenerative in nature)
- Chordoid
  - Resembles chordoma with trabeculae of vacuolated cells in a myxoid matrix
  - May have conspicuous inflammatory infiltrate
  - High rate of recurrence
- Clear cell
  - Patternless proliferation of polygonal cells with clear PAS+ glycogen–rich cytoplasm
  - Lack other histologic features typical of meningioma
  - Spinal cord and posterior fossa of children and young adults
  - Biologically aggressive with frequent recurrences and occasional seeding of CSF
- Grade 3
  - Must be either anaplastic by the following histologic criteria or papillary/rhabdoid subtypes
  - Anaplastic = either having features that are clearly malignant and/or 20 or more mitotic figures/hpf
    - Can look sarcomatous, lose EMA
  - Papillary
  - Rhabdoid
    - *Normal INI* (compared with other rhabdoid tumors)
- Other meningeal tumors
  - Meningeal hemangiopericytoma (HPC)/solitary fibrous tumor (SFT)
    - Possibly fibroblastic meningioma is the lowest grade
  - Both have *NAB2-STAT6* fusion → one lesion!
    - Previously called separate lesions
  - Grade 1—SFT phenotype
    - Benign, surgery alone
    - Patternless pattern and hypocellular, perivascular hyaline collagen deposition
  - Grade 2 or 3—HPC phenotype
    - Malignant, adjuvant radiation
    - Hypercellular with little stroma, thin–walled branching blood vessels, more mitoses (grade 2 <5/10 hpf and grade 3 >5/10 hpf)
  - Hemangioblastoma (grade 1)
    - 7% of primary posterior fossa tumors, can occur at any age
      - Usually superficial and midline
    - If multiple, consider von Hippel–Lindau syndrome
      - Autosomal dominant loss-of-function mutation of tumor suppressor on chromosome 3p
      - Though most are sporadic
    - Cyst with mural nodule
    - Numerous ectatic capillaries/vascular channels of different sizes separated by trabeculae or sheets of clear neoplastic stromal cells with round or elongated nuclei and abundant lipid vacuoles (positive for vimentin and VEGF)
      - Foamy interstitial tumor cells

- May have extramedullary hematopoiesis
- Grossly looks like a raspberry
- Inhibin+
- Others
  - Lipoma and angiolipoma
  - Fibromatosis, intracranial fibrosarcoma, and fibrohistiocytic tumors
  - Leiomyosarcoma and rhabdomyosarcoma
  - Chondroma, osteoma, osteochondroma, chondrosarcoma, and osteosarcoma
  - Hemangioma, hemangioendothelioma, angiosarcoma, Kaposi sarcoma
  - Melanocytoma, malignant melanoma, neurocutaneous melanosis (diffuse melanosis and melanomatosis)
- Embryonal tumors
  - = CNS primitive neuroectodermal tumors (PNETs) (all grade 4)
  - Medulloblastoma
    - Poorly differentiated small cell tumor
      - Similar cells in the CSF of a premature neonate may represent normal germinal matrix cells
    - Clinical
      - Cerebellum only (usually in vermis), midline, usually first decade of life
      - Very responsive to treatment, but may have late recurrence
      - CSF spread—requires radiation to entire CNS
        - May hinder mental and skeletal development
    - VARIANTS (with survival rates)
      - Classical—80%
      - Nodular/desmoplastic—15%
        - Germinal center–like structures with synaptophysin + large cells
      - … with extensive nodularity—5%
      - Large cell/anaplastic—5%
      - … with myogenic differentiation
      - … with melanotic differentiation
    - Histology
      - Sheets of very malignant, small round blue cells
        - Similar to small cell carcinoma
      - NSE+, synaptophysin+
      - Homer–Wright pseudorosettes with central neurofilament
      - Confluent and single–cell necrosis, high mitotic count
      - NSE+, synaptophysin+
    - Genetics
      - Classic histology associated with isochromosome 17q
      - *MYC* amplification is associated with poor prognosis
      - Syndrome associations
        - Monosomy 6 and Turcot syndrome
          - Mutation in *APC* gene on 5q or MMR defect
            - Associated with nuclear beta–catenin → mutated → very favorable prognosis
        - Gorlin syndrome (basal cell nevus syndrome)
          - *PTCH* gene mutation on 9q
          - More likely to be large cell or anaplastic variants
        - Desmoplastic, large cell, or anaplastic variants may have sporadic *PTCH* mutations
        - Li–Fraumeni syndrome—*TP53* mutation
  - Pineoblastoma

- Looks like medulloblastoma, but genetically and biologically different
- Big and at tentorial notch—may be mistaken for medulloblastoma in the cerebellum invading downward
  - CNS/supratentorial PNET
    - Essentially medulloblastoma or pineoblastoma, but in cerebral hemispheres (not in pineal gland or cerebellum) and genetically distinct
    - Sort of like a PNET, not otherwise specified
  - Medulloepithelioma
    - Very rare, usually periventricular
    - Papillary, trabecular, or tubular growth pattern of small blue cells recapitulating embryonic neural tube
  - Ependymoblastoma
    - Rare, very aggressive
    - Characteristic "ependymoblastic rosettes" = multilayered rosettes with true lumina surrounded by ciliated neuroepithelial cells
  - Atypical teratoid/rhabdoid tumor (grade 4)
    - Young (infants), supratentorial ≥ infratentorial, CSF spread, poor prognosis, loss of *INI-1* staining (mutation of *SMARCB1* at 22q11.2)
    - Rhabdoid (eccentric eosinophilic cytoplasm, vimentin+) cells admixed with undifferentiated small blue cells (resembling medulloblastoma or PNET)
- Chordoma
  - Malignant midline tumor in clivus or coccyx (most frequently)
  - Arises from fetal notochord
  - Usually males, 50 to 60 years of age
  - Cords and lobules of "physaliferous" (bubbly or vacuolated) cells, fibrous septa, and extensive myxoid stroma
  - Cells may be quite large
  - CK+, EMA+, brachyury+
  - Number-one DDx = low–grade chondrosarcoma (EMA−)
- Metastases
  - MOST COMMON INTRACRANIAL NEOPLASM
  - Leptomeningeal carcinomatosis can be patchy, can extend down sulci and along vessels
    - Systemic lymphoma (meningitis–like)
    - Most common: lung > breast > melanoma, colon, and so on
      - Can get primary melanoma in meninges (neuroectodermal origin)
  - Most common to hemorrhage: melanoma, renal cell carcinoma, choriocarcinoma
  - RARE to metastasize to CNS: prostate, upper gastrointestinal, head and neck, thyroid, bladder, hepatocellular carcinoma, squamous cell carcinoma

PEDIATRIC TUMORS

See above for descriptions.

- Most are in posterior fossa
- Pilocytic astrocytoma and medulloblastoma most commonly found in children
- Brain tumors = most common solid neoplasm in children
- Glial tumors
  - Juvenile pilocytic astrocytoma (number-one most common)
  - Pleomorphic xanthoastrocytoma
  - Diffuse intrinsic pontine gliomas (midline gliomas)
  - Subependymal giant cell astrocytomas (SEGAs)
  - Diffuse midline glioma

- Neuronal + glial
  - Gangliocytoma
  - Ganglioglioma
  - Dysplastic gangliocytoma of the cerebellum (Lhermitte–Duclos disease)
  - Desmoplastic infantile ganglioglioma
- Dysembryoplastic neuroepithelial tumor (DNET)
- Ependymoma (third most common)
  - Myxopapillary ependymoma
  - Anaplastic ependymoma
- Choroid plexus papilloma
- Embryonal tumors
  - *Medulloblastoma* (second most common)
  - CNS primitive neuroectodermal tumors (PNETs)
    - CNS/supratentorial PNET
    - Medulloepithelioma
    - Ependymoblastoma
  - Atypical teratoid/rhabdoid tumor (grade 4)
- Pineal tumors/suprasellar
  - Germ cell tumors
  - Craniopharyngioma
- Extra–axial
  - *Meningiomas* = rare in pediatrics, neurofibromatosis (NF) 2 patients
  - Nerve sheath tumors
    - Schwannomas (NF2)
    - Neurofibromas (NF1)
    - To differentiate on imaging—If dumbbell–like growth through neural foramen, it is a NF. If nipple–like extension into the auditory canal, it is a schwannoma.

2016 WHO CHANGES

- Tries to incorporate more genetics
- Gliomatosis cerebri is out
- Solitary fibrous tumor and hemangiopericytoma are the same entity
- Recommend integrated diagnosis line
  - Histologic diagnosis
  - WHO grade
  - Molecular characteristics
    - Example: oligodendroglioma, grade 2, 1p/19q codeletion
      - Next line—MGMT methylated
- GBM subtyped by *IDH* status or CIMP (CpG island methylator phenotype)
  - *IDH* mutation—favorable prognosis (wild–type—poor prognosis)
    - *IDH1* >> *IDH2*
    - Mutation probably came from lower–grade tumor (while WT is probably an aggressive *de novo* GBM with *EGFR* mutations)
    - *IDH*-mutated tumors with rare mitoses (which would be grade 3) behave like grade 2
    - Younger patients
    - Longer survival (2 to 3 years)
    - Associated with 1p/19q codeletion
      - All codeleted are associated with *IDH* mutation
      - Nearly always associated with methylated MGMT

- CIMP (CpG island methylator phenotype)—activated (nonmethylated) MGMT can turn off alkylating chemotherapy agents (like temozolomide)
  - Methylated MGMT will respond better to chemo!
- *ATRX* mutation associated with *IDH* mutation that will likely be low–grade *astrocytic* tumor that may progress to GBM
- Diffuse midline glioma, *H3 K27M*-mutant
  - New entity
  - Histologically grade 2 to 3 but very poor outcome
  - Pons is the most common location

Odds and Ends

- Most common primary CNS tumors postradiation = anaplastic astrocytoma or glioblastoma
- Large rim–enhancing lesion—GBM, abscess, metastasis
- Nonenhancing lesion—astrocytoma (*ATRX* loss → anaplastic) and oligodendroglioma (calcifications, 1p19q codeletions)
- Schwannoma—fascicular pattern, S100+, EMA–
  - Can occur in the posterior roots of cranial nerves 5, 8, and 9
- Scotoma—a focal area of decreased or absent visual acuity surrounded by normal vision
  - One example is our blind spot (physiologic instead of pathologic)
- Abulia—the abnormal inability to make decisions
- Hurler—dilated perivascular spaces filled with mucopolysaccharide (removed in processing)
- Leigh syndrome—rare autosomal recessive disorder
  - Necrotizing encephalopathy
  - ↓ inferior olive (spongy), expanded anterior horn, bilateral and symmetric
  - Defective glycolysis/oxidative phosphorylation
- Amputation is the most common cause of a traumatic neuroma
  - Increased nerve fibers without perineurium
  - Morton neuroma is a traumatic neuroma of the second to third metatarsal
- *Etat crible* can mimic lacunae
- Imaging
  - Intra–axial vs. extra–axial
  - Enhancement = leaky blood–brain barrier
    - In intrinsic tumors, a bad sign!
  - T1—fluid is dark, looks like a black-and-white picture of the brain
  - T2—fluid is bright (inverted T1)
  - FLAIR—CSF is dark but tissue fluid (edema) is bright
  - DDx for enhancing vertebral lesion at T4—metastases, myeloma, myxopapillary ependymoma, +/− chordoma
- Lenticular opacities = cataracts
- Tumefactive perivascular spaces
  - Multicystic lesions, nonneoplastic, pia–lined
  - Can be alarming on imaging

CHAPTER 15

Soft Tissue and Bone Pathology

Nonneoplastic

Scar

- Dermal, moderately circumscribed spindle cell lesion
- Morphology
  - Fibroblastic, amphophilic cytoplasm with single nucleoli with fascicular growth pattern, more prominent collagen between cells
  - Extravasated red blood cells, anastomosing thin vessels
  - Dense scar–like collagen around mass
  - Large superficial nerves (or nerve–like structures)
- DDx
  - Superficial fibromatosis (would be larger lesion)
  - Dermatofibroma—polymorphic (fibroblasts, histiocytes, xanthoma cells, hemosiderin, chronic inflammation, touton giant cells)
  - Keloid (less cells and more glassy collagen)

PROLIFERATIVE MYOSITIS

- Has related entity
  - Proliferative fasciitis—histologically identical but in subcutis or fascial tissue
- Not really mass–forming, more infiltrative and nondestructive
- Some atrophy of muscle fibers near hypocellular fibrous areas with (myo)fibroblasts (some with rounded nuclei)
- Can see wavy cells, but cytoplasm is amphophilic
- Lots of ganglion cells! Some clustered, some mixed throughout
- Checkerboard pattern
- Beta catenin (nuclear + in fibromatosis—would also be mass–forming), S100 (+ in ganglioneuroma)

ACUTE OSTEOMYELITIS

- Neutrophils burrowing into lamellar bone
- Ragged edges and nonviable bone (empty lacunae)
- Need systemic antibiotics
- NOT granulation tissue–associated neutrophils under the ulcer

SEPTIC ARTHRITIS

- Neutrophil count per high–power field (hpf) is important
- >5 to 10 neutrophils per hpf increase likelihood of diagnosis
- "Synovial tissue with acute and chronic inflammation. Tissue neutrophil count up to 14/ hpf"

AVASCULAR NECROSIS

- Chronic steroids, alcohol, sickle cell anemia
- Wedge–shaped cartilage that separates from bone

PAGET'S DISEASE

- Mosaic bone matrix, increased bone remodeling with increased osteoclasts
- Woven bone with fibrosis rimmed by osteoblasts

Other Nonneoplastic

- Atrophic skeletal muscle can look atypical
- Cytoplasmic atrophy bunching nuclei together
- Osteoarthritis patients can get synovial fluid leaking into soft tissue or bone
  - Becomes cystic, looks like a ganglion cyst with degenerative changes
- Complex synovial/Baker's/popliteal cyst left for a long time organizes into a fibrous complex cyst in which cystic portion can be *very* minor
  - Can present as soft tissue mass → be careful!
  - Associated with degenerative joint disease
  - Hypovascular in myxoma–like area

Neoplastic

GENERAL APPROACH TO NEOPLASMS

1. Figure out cell of origin (rule out melanoma and sarcomatoid carcinoma)
   - Fibroblasts—tapered end of nucleus, amphophilic cytoplasm
   - Neural—tapered end but wavy
   - Smooth muscle—cigar nucleus, perinuclear vacuole (glycogen "snack"), eosinophilic cytoplasm
   - Myofibroblasts—corkscrew nuclei and cytoplasm, easier to see with condenser down
     - Positive for pankeratins but—for high–molecular–weight keratins (HMWK, like CK5/6)
2. Benign vs. malignant
3. Classify by what tissue it is differentiating toward
4. Stage, grade, evaluate margins, treatment effect
- Lesions that do not get graded
  - Malignant peripheral nerve sheath tumor
  - Embryonal/alveolar rhabdomyosarcoma
  - Extraskeletal myxoid chondrosarcoma
  - Alveolar soft part sarcoma
  - Clear cell sarcoma of soft tissue
  - Epithelioid sarcoma
- Do not grade after treatment

ADIPOCYTIC LESIONS

Lipoma

- Neck, shoulder, back (superficial trunk) tend to be benign (lipoma)
  - Almost never get liposarcomas in the trunk subcutaneous tissue
- Traumatized lipoma—fibrous septa, myxomatous change
- t(3;12)(q28;q14) *LPP-HMGA2*

Angiolipoma

- Angiolipomas on the extremities and upper back
- Mature fat cells with increased stroma between cells in *some* areas
- Dense ropey collagen, some areas of more myxoid stroma
- Lots of capillaries and extravasated red blood cells
    - Characteristically contain fibrin microthrombi and are usually painful!
- Never become malignant
- Will be S100+ in adipocytes and CD31/CD34+ in capillaries
    - HHV8– (if Kaposi is in differential)
- No characteristic karyotypic changes
- One of the FIVE PAINFUL SUBCUTANEOUS NODULES
    - Angiolipoma, angioleiomyoma, eccrine spiradenoma, schwannoma, glomus tumor

Spindle Cell/Pleomorphic Lipoma

- Fibrolipoma—not quite spindle cell lipoma
- Bland spindle cells with occasional hyperchromatic round cells
    - Some palisading and random fascicles ("school of fish")
- Variable amounts of admixed mature adipose tissue and ropey collagen
    - Radiologists will call if "fibrous stranding" is present → worry for malignancy, look for atypia
- No storiform, no atypia, no mitoses, no necrosis, no lipoblasts
- Some vascular proliferation
- Pleomorphic lipoma is all of this + "floret–like giant cells"
- CD34+ (liposarcoma is not)
    - One of the only useful uses of it, along with dermatofibrosarcoma protuberans (DFSP), solitary fibrous tumor (SFT), gastrointestinal stromal tumor (GIST)
- 90% males, 80% in subcutaneous posterior neck/shoulder/back
- Chromosome 16 losses

Atypical Lipomatous Tumor/Well–Differentiated Liposarcoma (Alt/Wdlps)

- If lipoma is 15 to 20 cm large, concerning for ALT/WDLPS
- Must submit one section per cm of mass and describe any grossly different areas
- Differentiating ALT from WDLPS
    - Histologically identical
    - ALT when in extremities—easily resected
    - WDLPS when in retroperitoneum—hard to resect
- Can also present in stomach as "giant fibrovascular polyp of the stomach" or in scrotum
    - Versus spindle cell/pleomorphic lipomas that are only in subcutaneous tissue
- Morphology
    - Increased stroma between cells
    - May have fibrous stranding
    - Very atypical hyperchromatic stromal cells with adipocytes
        - Atypical features of adipocytic lesions hyperchromasia, larger, anisocytosis, irregular nuclear borders
    - Lipoblasts—scalloped nuclear borders (very hard to identify in well–differentiated)
    - Can undergo myxoid changes
- Variants adipocytic, sclerosing, inflammatory, spindle cell
    - Can have prominent inflammatory and sclerotic components

- Sclerosing common in retroperitoneum and spermatic cord
- *MDM2/CDK4* not amplified in spindle cell type
- *MDM2/CDK4* amplification (12q13–15), S100+, p16
  - May have ring or giant marker chromosomes on karyotype
- Cannot metastasize without dedifferentiation

Dedifferentiated Liposarcoma

- Low–grade component *with* high–grade, nonlipomatous component
- Most common in retroperitoneum of adults
- Can have inflammatory infiltrate, which was previously called *inflammatory malignant fibrous histiocytoma* (MFH)
  - Antiquated term
- Can have heterologous components, meningothelioid swirls
- *MDM2/CDK4* amplification (positive nuclear staining), PPAR+
- Differential diagnosis (DDx) includes pleomorphic leiomyosarcoma
- 15% to 20% metastasis rate, most deaths caused by local destruction

Myxoid Liposarcoma

- Young patients, not a lot of atypia, pulmonary edema–like pattern
- Predominantly in limbs
- Tons of myxoid stroma (mucin pools), fewer discernible fat cells which are small → immature fat cells
  - Pulmonary edema–like pattern
- Vesicular chromatin, areas with less cellularity, uniform round cells, distinct nucleoli
  - Very little atypia
  - One or two fat vacuoles in each cell
- Delicate curvilinear vessels, arborizing, chicken–wire
- Patchy lymphocytic infiltrate
- When myxoid liposarcomas go bad, they form round cells *(round cell transformation—RCT)*
  - When cells start to touch each other, worry about RCT
    - Must be >5%
  - When WDLPSs go bad, they form spindle cells
- *DDIT3-FUS* translocation—t(12;16)
  - Not *CDK4/MDM2*
  - t(12;16)(q13;p11) or t(12;22)(q13;q12)

Pleomorphic Liposarcoma

- Tumor necrosis, lobulated solid mass
- Scattered huge cells (lipoblasts) with atypia, some vacuolated cytoplasm
- Atypical mitotic figures
- Largest cells that can be found in the human body were found in pleomorphic liposarcoma

Mixed Type

NEURAL

Perineurioma

- Rare benign nerve sheath tumor
- Small, superficial, circumscribed
- Bland elongated spindle cells with storiform/whorled pattern

- Immunohistochemistry
  - Positive for EMA, claudin-1, GLUT1
  - Negative for MUC4 and S100
  - CD34 is patchy

Schwannoma

- Verocay bodies, wavy nuclei, Antoni A and B areas, hyalinized vessels, circumscribed, encapsulated, chronic inflammation
- The second most common benign soft tissue tumor (after lipomas)
- Can have degenerative nuclei, myxoid degeneration, or ancient changes
  - Really atypical, no atypical mitoses, loss of Antoni A/B, fibrous background
- Huge spectrum in morphology
  - In neural lesions, always keep schwannoma in mind
- S100+ in all cells (unlike malignant peripheral nerve sheath tumor and neurofibroma)
  - Do not call it *malignant* unless some cells are negative
- Can be melanotic and malignant (HMB45+)
  - *PRKAR1a* loss, Carney complex (patients need to be checked for cardiac myxomas, which can throw clots)
  - Classic location is paraspinal
  - Psammomatous calcifications are almost always present (nonpsammomatous, not so much)
  - Normally look benign but are aggressive

Traumatic Neuroma

- Called *Morton's neuroma* on palmar foot
- Lobular on low power within adipose tissue
- Looks like a ball of nerves (with myxoid change around nerves—do not get that around smooth muscle), vaguely myxoid in areas, no high–grade feature
- S100+, GFAP+
- DDx: Palisading encapsulated neuroma (PEN)—females in dermis. More organized than this, looks like neurofibroma

Ganglioneuroma

- 10 to 30 years of age, retroperitoneum or posterior mediastinum
- Rare ganglion cells in a neural background, no necrosis or mitoses, thickened vessels
- Relatively hypercellular
- S100+

Neurofibroma (NF)

- Bland, spindled, eosinophilic cells
- "Shredded carrot" collagen with hypocellular nuclei sprinkled throughout
- (1) Inflammatory cells (lymphs), (2) fibroblasts, (3) neural cells (wavy nuclei), (4) perineural cells
- Loose stroma with more collagenized areas
- Positive for S100 and CD34
  - Schwann cells (schwannomas)—S100+
  - Perineural cells (perineuromas)—CD34+
    - Also EMA weakly positive
  - Neurofibromas—in between

- NF → atypical NF → malignant peripheral nerve sheath tumor (MPNST)
  - If slightly increased cellularity with some atypia but very rare mitoses—atypical neurofibroma
  - If nuclear atypia and mitoses are both present—MPNST
    - Condensed stroma around vessels
  - Do not get tricked by degenerative atypia—smudged chromatin, no mitoses, *not* high–grade
  - *Plexiform*
    - Worm–like sac, only seen in neurofibromatosis type 1 (NF1)—virtually diagnostic
  - *Diffuse*
    - Commonly seen in NF1 too, but also in normal patients
    - Infiltrative
  - NF1 patients get NFs with diffuse growth pattern and plexiform NFs, and increased risk for malignant transformation
    - Pseudo-Meissner corpuscles—almost always present in diffuse neuromas in NF1 patients—"organoid bodies"

Malignant Peripheral Nerve Sheath Tumor (MPNST)

- Can occur after radiation or sporadic or in NF1
- Clues to malignancy
  - Hypercellular
    - Atypical neurofibroma (no mitotic figures)—NF1 patients can have more hypercellular areas with atypia
    - Variable cellularity with some *very* hypercellular areas (marbled appearance on low power), frequent mitoses, wavy nuclei (so neural), sort of staghorn vessels with protrusions into vessels
    - Perivascular increase in cellularity
  - Fascicular growth pattern
  - Mitoses
  - Necrosis
  - Atypia +/−
    - Atypia is not a reliable feature
    - Degenerative neurofibroma or schwannoma nuclei can be very atypical
- S100 patchy + (in 30% to 40%), SOX10+ (in 30% to 40%), CD99+
  - S100 should *not* be diffuse and strong unless it is the epithelioid variant
- H3K27me3—trimethyl moiety of lysine 27 at histone H3 → made by PRC2 complex
  - Immunohistochemistry shows *complete* loss in…
    - 30% of low–grade MPNSTs
    - 60% of intermediate–grade MPNSTs
    - 85% of high–grade MPNSTs
  - Not lost in epithelioid variant
  - 7% of spindle cell melanomas (but should be S100 diffuse and strong), and 1% to 3% of dedifferentiated liposarcoma can show loss
- One of the most common to calcify
- May have glandular differentiation (positive for cytokeratin, EMA, and so on) or melanin in tumor cells
- Heterologous differentiation in 10%
  - Most common is rhabdomyoblastic—"malignant Triton tumor"

SMOOTH MUSCLE

Smooth Muscle Neoplasm by Site

- Gynecologic system—leiomyoma, stromal tumor of uncertain malignant potential (STUMP), leiomyosarcoma (acellular vs. mitotically active)—no grading
- Visceral—graded, leiomyoma vs. leiomyosarcoma
- Dermal—benign leiomyoma vs. "atypical smooth muscle tumor" vs. atypical fibroxanthoma

Leiomyoma and Variants

- Separated by location
  - Cutaneous
    - If diffuse/dermatomal, usually associated with fumarate hydratase mutation (1q42)
  - Subcutaneous and dermis
    - Fourth to sixth decade
    - Upper extremity—male, cavernous
    - Lower extremity—female, solid
    - May contain small nerve fibers or mature adipose tissue
- Fascicles of muscles
- Nuclei = blunt spindles (cigar) with perinuclear vacuoles (snacks)
- Cytoplasm = no borders, eosin, fibrillary
- Angioleiomyoma
  - Well–circumscribed, fascicular/nodular, smooth muscle cells, variably frequent vascular lumens (slit–like compressed vessels), occasional prominent vacuoles in endothelial cells
- Positive for SMA, desmin, and caldesmon
- Painful skin lesions = BLUE ANGEL
  - Blue rubber bleb nevus
  - Angiolipoma
  - Neuroma
  - Glomus tumor
  - Eccrine spiradenoma
  - (Angio)leiomyoma

Leiomyosarcoma

- Probably from a blood vessel wall (large veins have compact smooth muscle fibers like detrusor muscle)
  - Rounded because it fills and expands the vessel
- Morphology
  - Long fascicles/herringbone, hypercellular, well–circumscribed
  - Increased atypia, especially around edges
  - Eosinophilic vacuolated cytoplasms
  - Mitoses are present
  - Atrophic smooth muscle at periphery
- Bladder–like smooth muscle bundles, transitioning to sheets of cells with pleomorphism and increased mitoses
- Would not fulfill criteria for a leiomyosarcoma in GYN
  - Low threshold to call leiomyosarcoma outside of uterus
- If HIV+ or immunodeficient → EBV(+)
- SMA+

SKELETAL MUSCLE

Rhabdomyoma

- Most common in head and neck

Rhabdomyosarcoma

- Alveolar—children, small round blue cell tumor (SRBCT)
  - Dropout of cells resemble lung alveolus
  - Translocations with *FOXO1*
    - t(2;13) *PAX3-FOXO1*
      - More likely to involve the bone marrow
      - 8% overall survival with metastases
    - t(1;13) *PAX7-FOXO1*
      - Younger, localized on extremities
      - 75% 4-year survival with metastases
- Embryonal—toddlers, vagina, or bladder
  - Spindle cell (sarcoma botryoides) or SRBCT morphologies
    - Bunch of grapes
  - Primitive strap muscles
  - Cambium layer—condensation of spindle cells at edge

FIBROHISTIOCYTIC

Giant Cell Neoplasms

Giant Cell Tumor of Tendon Sheath

- 30- to 40-year-old female, digits, localized
- Lobular, well circumscribed, no villi
- Stromal cells, histiocytes, osteoclast–like giant cells (GCs), xanthoma cells (foamy histiocytes), siderophages
- Mature collagenous capsule
- Nodular (localized) vs. diffuse (infiltrative with cleft–like spaces)
  - Considerable overlap can occur
- In knee joint = "pigmented villonodular synovitis" (see later)
- Can *rarely* be malignant
  - Need lots of pleomorphism; do not rely on mitoses!

Pigmented Villonodular Synovitis (PVNS) ("Diffuse Giant Cell Tumor")

- <40-year-old female, usually younger than localized variant
- Villonodular masses involving most of synovium of large joints
- Invades, not well–circumscribed, few GCs, dyscohesion, pseudosynovial clefts
- Ladybug cells

Nonossifying Fibroma

- Storiform, osteoclast–like giant cells
- Lower extremity near metaphysis
- Younger than 20 years of age
- Asymptomatic lesions get no treatment; large/symptomatic lesions get curettage

Ossifying Fibroma

- Psammomatous calcifications

Elastofibroma

- Benign, poorly circumscribed scapular lesion in the elderly
- Slow–growing, from repetitive trauma
- Alternating bands of thick collagen and thick elastic fibers

Nodular Fasciitis

- Rapid growth after trauma
- Age range—children to ~40ish
- t(17;22), but considered a reactive process

Myositis Ossificans

- Very specific zonation
  - Central fibroblastic zone
  - Osteoblastic zone with woven bone (not calcified)
    - Plump epithelioid cells
  - Outer calcified zone

Myofibroma

- Usually sporadic
- Solitary (in dermis and subcutis of head and neck) or multicentric (superficial and deep)
- Biphasic
  - Peripheral—fascicular plump myofibroblasts
  - Central—hemangiopericytoma–like (staghorn vessels)
- May regress, may recur, rarely may metastasize and kill

Inflammatory Myofibroblastic Tumor

- ALK+ (gene fusion)
- Children and young adults
- Retroperitoneum, mesentery, lung, bladder
- Morphology
  - Loose fascicles
  - Chronic inflammatory infiltrate
  - Variable cellularity
  - Myxoid to sclerotic stroma

Fibromatosis (Desmoid Tumor, Desmoid Fibromatosis)

- Fibroproliferative process, benign but locally aggressive monoclonal proliferation
  - Does not metastasize
  - Can recur
  - Can dedifferentiate
- Three epidemiologic patterns
  - 1. Sporadic—on extremities or girdle, beta–catenin sporadically mutated
    - "Extra-abdominal" *or* "deep fibromatosis" *or*
    - "Superficial"
1. Synonymous with Dupuytren contracture/trigger finger of proximal interphalangeal (PIP) joints
2. Elderly men, alcoholism
3. Does not recur

- 2. Familial adenomatous polyposis patients
  - Intrabdominal
- 3. Young women, during or after pregnancy, on abdominal wall
  - **"Desmoid tumor"**
- Same density as skeletal muscle on imaging
- Median size = 6 cm, pseudocapsule
- Architecture
  - Fascicles, storiform, syncytial infiltrating fat and skeletal muscle
    - Long, sweeping, intersecting fascicles
  - More cellular than fibroma of tendon sheath
  - Can have myxoid or keloid–like collagenous stroma
    - "Classic" is bland collagenous stroma
  - +/− osteoid
- Vasculature
  - Slit–like, muscular, curvilinear/staghorn vessels between fascicles with extravasated red blood cells
  - +/− perivascular edema
- Cytology
  - Bland spindle cells—spindled nuclei with tapered ends and nucleoli
    - Usually wavy
    - Monomorphic
    - Smudge and hazy, "frosted glass" appearance
  - Sparse lymphocytes (inflammatory infiltrate)
  - Rare mitoses, no necrosis
- Trisomy 8 or 20, Gardner syndrome, inactivation of APC pathway, Wnt pathway alteration, activating mutation in beta–catenin
  - Nuclear beta–catenin+ (Wnt pathway, *APC* genetics)
  - Both beta–catenin and *APC* gene product are in the Wnt pathway
  - Germline *APC* mutation and sporadic *CTNNB1* (gene for beta–catenin) are histologically identical
- Also positive for SMA, MSA, desmin, ER
- DDx includes nodular fasciitis (smaller, superficial, circumscribed, loose fascicles)

Sclerosing Mesenteritis

- IgG$_4$-related, can treat with tamoxifen

Nodular Fasciitis

- Clinical
  - Short clinical course
    - Mitotically active with rapid growth → involution
  - Many patients endorse prior trauma in the same location, but this is *not* a reactive process
  - Tiny marble of firm tissue, rapidly growing
    - Must be <3 cm
  - Mostly superficial, associated with fascial plane that then grows "up" into subcutaneous tissue (sometimes grows "down" into muscle)
- Architecture
  - Short fascicles/storiform—"tissue culture growth"
  - Alternating areas of hypercellular and hypocellular
  - Older lesions are collagenous (can be striking—fibroma of tendon sheath is probably really late nodular fasciitis)

- Pseudopod–like extension into adjacent tissue
- Vasculature
  - Extravasated red blood cells, lots of delicate small vessels throughout
  - "Granulation tissue–like" vessels may be present
- Cytology
  - Myofibroblasts
    - Stellate
    - Rounded nuclei, multiple small nucleoli, pale chromatin
    - Amphophilic cytoplasm
    - Robust mitotic activity (especially if new)
    - Some atypia, no necrosis
  - Rarely can have osteoclast–like giant cells
- SMA (train track pattern), MSA, vimentin, calponin
- *MYH9-USP6* gene rearrangement (like aneurysmal bone cyst)

Ossifying Fasciitis
- Variant of nodular fasciitis plus foci of metaplastic bone
  - New woven bone
- Occurs after trauma
- Rapid growth, young, skeletal
- Extravasated red blood cells, chronic inflammation, high mitotic rate, do not care about margin
- Lacking zonation of myositis ossificans
- Lacks pleomorphism and hyperchromasia of extraskeletal osteosarcoma

Plexiform Fibrohistiocytic Tumor

- Children and young adults, on the shoulders and arms
- Clusters of histiocytes and osteoclast–like giant cells
- Surrounded and connected by spindle cells

Dermatofibroma—Also Known as Benign Fibrous Histiocytoma (BFH)

- Fibroblasts, Histiocytes, Hemosiderin, Touton Giant Cells
- Architecture
  - Lobular mass, no real pattern/vague storiform pattern
  - Cystic degeneration
    - Multinucleated Touton giant cells
    - Foamy macrophages
    - Cholesterol clefts debris
  - Collagen trapping
  - Admixed lymphocytes
- Vasculature
  - Reactive revved up endothelial cells in curvilinear vessels
  - Extravasated red blood cells
- Cytology
  - Plump spindle cells with finely vacuolated/foamy cytoplasm, prominent cell borders
  - Ovoid nucleus, single small nucleolus
- Factor XIIIa+, CD34 negative to weakly positive
  - Versus dermatofibrosarcoma protuberans (DFSP), which is diffusely CD34+

Cellular Fibrous Histiocytoma
- Borderline lesion between BFH and DFSP

Angiomatoid Fibrous Histiocytoma
- Rare soft tissue tumor of low–grade malignancy that usually occurs in children and young adults
- Solid arrays or nests of histiocyte–like cells, hemorrhagic cyst–like spaces, aggregates of chronic inflammatory cells, multifocal old and new hemorrhages
- t(12;22)(q13;q12) *ATF1-EWSR1* or t(12;16)(q13;p11) *ATF1-FUS*

Dermatofibrosarcoma Protuberans (DFSP)

- Dermal
- Intermediate–grade neoplasm
  - Recurs, locally aggressive
- May progress to…
  - Fibrosarcomatous DFSP
    - Herringbone patterns, high mitotic activity, rarely necrosis
    - Starts to lose CD34
  - Undifferentiated pleomorphic sarcoma (UPS)
    - See later
- Architecture
  - Storiform pattern, hypercellular, heterogeneous
  - Entrapped fat (honeycombing)
  - Collagenous stroma
- Cytology
  - Only one cell type
  - Hyperchromatic nuclei, not super high grade
  - Rare mitoses
  - Mast cells
  - CD34+ (diffuse and strong) CD99+, bcl2+
- t(17;22)(q21;q13) *COL1A1-PDGFRB*

Giant Cell Fibroblastoma
- Variant of DFSP that only occurs in pediatric patients
- Moderately cellular, infiltrative, bland fibroblasts, pleomorphic cells, multinucleated giant cells lining clefts
- Fibrous or myxoid stroma

Fibrosarcoma

- Herringbone, very high mitoses
- Mildly atypical fibroblasts
- May lose CD34 if from transformed DFSP; reticulin outlines each cell

Fibrous Dysplasia

- Somatic mutation during early embryogenesis
- Presents as a mass, pathologic fracture, or incidentally found
- Clinical
  - Seen in syndromes
    - McCune–Albright (polyostotic > monostotic)
      - Precocious puberty and café-au-lait spots

- Mazabraud syndrome
  - Muscular myxoma
- Monostotic (one bone)
  - Classically the mandible is involved
  - Craniofacial bones, ribs, and femur
- Polyostotic (multiple bones)
  - Femur > skull > tibia > humerus
  - Higher risk of transformation to sarcoma
  - Shepherd crook deformity
- Young adults/teens
- Intramedullary, well–defined, thinning of cortex
- Morphology
  - Hypocellular storiform fibrous tissue and bone trabeculae (irregular woven bone)
    - "Alphabet soup" with or without cementicles (dots on profile of trabeculae)
  - Inconspicuous osteoblastic rimming
  - Can get clusters of xanthomatous cells
- No IHC (spindle cells are negative for CK and EMA)
- If epicenter is in the anterior cortex of tibia or fibula = **osteofibrous dysplasia**
  - Trabeculae lined by osteoblasts
  - Spindle cells + CK and EMA (scattered)
  - Children → teens
  - Top DDx = well–differentiated adamantinoma

Chondromyxoid Fibroma

- Distinct radiographic findings
  - Sharp borders, lytic, parallel with bone
- Young patients, recurs
- Pseudolobules of cellular spindle cells in myxoid/chondroid stroma, separated by fibrous septa with giant cells
- DDx includes fibromyxoma (no specific architecture, older patients)

Intramuscular Myxoma

- Clinical
  - Intramuscular in older patients
- Architecture
  - Encapsulated
  - Uniformly hypocellular
  - Central areas are hypovascular
  - Abundant myxoid matrix with scattered small blood vessels
- Cytology
  - Spindle cells
  - Minimal atypia with variation in cell shape
- CD34+, SMA–, desmin–, S100–, EMA–
- Has mutation in codon 201 of *GNAS1* gene
- Common pitfall is calling it *malignant*

Low–Grade Fibromyxoid Sarcoma (LGFMS)

- Clinical
  - Young patients, thigh, more common in males
  - Known for late metastases (40%), locally aggressive

- Architecture
  - Has alternating myxoid and collagenous areas
    - Light and dark zones
    - Too compact and cellular for nodular fasciitis
  - Hypocellular
- Vessels
  - "Arcades" of thick, curvilinear vessels (not prominent)
  - No extravasated red blood cells
- Cytology
  - Looks bland but is malignant
  - Bland spindled cells with no atypia
  - Single nucleolus
- Frequently EMA+ and MUC4+
- Characteristic t(7;16)(q34;p11), *FUS-CREB3*
- DDx includes fibromatosis (beta–catenin), fibrosarcoma, perineuriomas (MUC4–, EMA+), nodular fasciitis (less cellular and compact than LGFMS)

High–Grade Myxofibrosarcoma

- Has been called *myxoid UPS* or *myxoid MFH* before
  - Synonymous with undifferentiated pleomorphic sarcoma (UPS) in elderly patients in subcutaneous tissue with myxoid change
- Clinical
  - Painless subcutaneous mass in thighs and hips of elderly
  - Can recur (usually with higher grade)
    - Rarely metastasize (5% to 25%)
- Architecture
  - Alternating hypocellular and hypercellular areas
  - Palisading necrosis in areas
  - Loose myxoid stroma
- Vessels
  - Curvilinear coarse blood vessels
  - Cytology
  - Cells spindled or pleomorphic
  - MAY have pseudolipoblasts or epithelioid cells
  - Graded (by FNCLCC) as low, intermediate, or high
    - Based on cellularity, atypia, necrosis, and mitoses
  - Prominent multinucleated cells
- No characteristic cytogenetic changes
  - Genomically complex
- Expresses vimentin, CD34, focal actin, MUC4
- DDx: fibromyxoid sarcoma, myxoid neurofibroma, nodular fasciitis, myxoid liposarcoma, myxoma

OSTEOBLASTIC

Osteosarcoma

- Most common bone tumor in teens
- Variants
  - Low–grade—medullary or juxtacortical parosteal

- Fibroblastic–like proliferation between woven or mature thick parallel trabeculae
- No osteoblast lining
- High–grade—surface
- Periosteal—cartilaginous surrounded by malignant osteoid
- Similar to parosteal
- Bland! Cytology does not help!
  - Looks almost normal
  - *MDM2+, CDK4+*
  - Trabecular arrangement, radiology, mets
  - Can have prominent chondroblastic differentiation

Osteoblastoma

- Neoblastic bone formation but *without* atypia or mitoses
- 10 to 40 years of age, males > females, spine > long bones > other
- Can get large but behaves indolently/benign
- Histologic overlap with osteoid osteoma
- Woven bone spicules with prominent *osteoblast rimming*

Differential Diagnosis For Multinucleated Giant Cells In Bone

- Aneurysmal bone cyst (ABC)
  - "Soap bubble" on imaging, metaphysis of long bones and vertebrae
  - Benign, second decade of life
  - Morphology
    - Blood–filled cyst
    - New bone formation in cyst wall
    - Smaller giant cells, aggregated near cyst wall with mononuclear cells, fibroblasts, and inflammatory cells
    - Can have solid growth pattern
  - t(16;17)(q22;p13) *USP6-CDH11*
- Giant cell tumor of bone
  - Skeletally mature patients, epiphysis
  - Expansile lytic lesion eroding cortex (soap bubble)
  - Multinucleated giant cells in sheet–like distribution, uniformly spread
    - Can get > 50 nuclei—very helpful in diagnosis!
    - CD68+
  - Two background cell populations—fibroblasts and mononuclear cells with nuclear features similar to those in the giant cells
  - Can have mitotic activity
  - Can have necrosis
  - Can metastasize but not called *malignant*
  - No new bone formation
  - In DDx
    - GC-rich osteosarcoma (have atypia)
    - Telangiectatic osteosarcoma (have atypia)
- Langerhans cell histiocytosis
- Osteoclast–rich osteosarcoma
- Telangiectatic osteosarcoma
- Chondroblastoma

CARTILAGINOUS

General

- Children, in long bones, no atypia = *enchondroma*
- Myxoid change, older, invade into bone, spindled cells, atypia = *malignant*
- Treatment
  - Enchondroma—curettage
  - Atypical chondrocytic neoplasm/atypical enchondroma/grade 1 chondrosarcoma—curettage or local excision only
  - Grade 2 chondrosarcoma and up—radical resection
- *Never* make chondrosarcoma diagnosis in patients older than 25 years of age without ruling out osteosarcoma with chondrocytic differentiation; they are treated differently
  - Chondrosarcoma—chemo then resection
  - Osteosarcoma—no adjuvant, resection
- Any mitotic figures → *at least* grade 2 chondrosarcoma
  - Grades 2 and 3 are pretty much treated the same
- *IDH1/IDH2* mutations are present in 56% of cartilaginous neoplasms

Ollier Disease

- Nonhereditary disease of appendicular enchondromas
- Most common on long bones of hand, unilateral, asymmetric
- Cortical surface
  - Versus *solitary enchondromas* that are typically intramedullary
- 15% to 30% risk of chondrosarcomatous transformation
  - Versus solitary enchondromas—0% risk
- Hypercellular, large atypical chondrocytes, myxoid stroma

Extraskeletal Myxoid Chondrosarcoma

- Low–grade (no high–grade atypia)
- Deep soft tissues
  - Trunk, paraspinal, retroperitoneum, THIGHS
  - Usually >10cm
- When they transform, go directly to dedifferentiated (undifferentiated pleomorphic sarcoma–like)
- Morphology
  - Hyper and hypocellular areas, lobular
  - Myxoid to cartilaginous matrix
  - Radially oriented cords/trabeculations/strands of bland, round, uniform epithelioid cells with reddish ("brick red colored") cytoplasm
    - Do not really look like chondrocytes—just atypical cells in a myxoid matrix
  - No prominent vascular network
- Focal weak S100 expression, S100+
- Local recurrence and late metastases
  - Survival—90% at 5 years, 60% at 15 years
- t(9;22) *EWSR1-NR4A3*

Chondrosarcoma

- Radiologic correlation is very important (erosion, soft tissue extension)
- Can be secondary to enchondroma

- Spindle cells and atypical lacunar–type cells
- Cellularity, atypia, myxoid change, mitotic figures
  - Most important diagnostic feature is destruction/invasion of trabecular bone
- Grading
  - Grade 1 is hard to differentiate from enchondroma
  - Grade 3 is sheet–like with lots of pleomorphism and mitose

Mesenchymal Chondrosarcoma
- Biphasic
  - Primitive round cells in sheets and fascicles
  - Variably mature hyaline cartilage
- Staghorn (hemangiopericytoma–like) vessels
- Head and neck of young adults
- del(8)(q13q21) *HEY1-NCOA2*

Chondroblastoma

- Clinical
  - Teens (skeletally immature)—end of long bones
  - Epiphyseal tumor
    - Greater trochanter is a secondary epiphysis ("apophysis")
    - Most common sites = distal tumor, proximal tibia
  - Benign behavior, 10% recur, rare benign lung implants
    - Treated with curettage
- Imaging
  - Sharply demarcated small lesion with a rim of sclerotic bone
- Architecture
  - Looks like oligodendroglioma with chicken wire calcifications ("pavement–like")
  - Can have chondroid matrix (but not required for diagnosis)
  - Can undergo aneurysmal degeneration
  - If decalcified, can do reticulin stain to pick up scaffolding
- Cytology
  - Polygonal histiocytoid cells with longitudinal cleft, uniform, small
  - +/– multinucleated giant cells in clusters
- S100+

VASCULAR

Masson Lesion (Reactive Papillary Endothelial Hyperplasia)

- Subepithelial, thrombus with spindled epithelioid cells—granulation tissue!
- Hemosiderin–laden macrophages
- Placenta–like villi—actually large anastomosing vascular channels, bland endothelium

Aggressive Angiomyxoma

- Deep soft tissue of vulva/perineum in reproductive–age female
- Need negative margins on resection—locally aggressive
- Morphology

- Poorly circumscribed, myxoid stroma, low cellularity
- Mast cells and extravasated red blood cells
- Numerous thick–walled medium–sized vessels with hyalinized walls
- Chromosome 12 translocations
- Immunohistochemistry
  - Positive for *HMGA2*, ER/PR, desmin, SMA
  - Negative for S100

Epithelioid Hemangioendothelioma

- Clinical
  - Lung, liver, bone, deep soft tissue
  - Truly a sarcoma, but lower–grade than angiosarcoma
  - Can met in 25% to 30%—intermediate malignancy
- Architecture
  - *Inside* a thick artery or vein
  - Central sclerosis, peripheral hypercellularity
  - "Myxohyaline" stroma (chondroid/myxoid)
  - Blister cells (intracytoplasmic lumina)
  - Cannot form vessels → cords and nests of cells
- Cytology
  - Bland and uniform cells
  - Intracellular vacuoles that look like lumens (signet ring–like)
- CAMTA1+, CD31/34+, CAM5.2+, ERG+ (and angiosarcoma, so are some prostate CA)
- t(1;3) *WWTR1-CAMTA1*
  - Nuclear *CAMTA1+*

Kaposiform Hemangioendothelioma

- Benign, locally aggressive
- Young children
- Superficial and deep extremities and retroperitoneum
- Kasabach–Merritt syndrome—fatal coagulopathy
- Morphology
  - Lobular nodules separated by fibrous septa
  - Vascular slits
  - Can have intracytoplasmic hyaline globules
  - Bland, low mitotic rate
- D240+, GLUT1–
  - GLUT+ in infantile hemangioma

HEMANGIOMAS

Intramuscular Hemangioma

- Also known as *venous malformation*
- Young women (hormone effect?)
- Spindled, staghorn vessels with thickened smooth muscle walls, increased capillary networks, lymphocytes
- Conspicuous small nucleoli in otherwise bland epithelioid cells
- DDx: epithelioid hemangioendothelioma, angiosarcoma, other hemangioendotheliomas

Cavernous Hemangioma

- Closely packed largely dilated vessels
- Flattened endothelium
- Fibrous septa

Spindle Cell Hemangioma

- Distal extremities
- Syndromes: Maffucci (enchondromas and hemangiomas), Klippel–Trenaunay, Milroy
- Cavernous spaces with thrombosis or phleboliths separated by bland spindle cell proliferations

Infantile Hemangioma

- Lobules of plump, mitotically active capillaries
- Delicate fibrous septa
- Thick basement membrane surrounded by pericytes
- Presents at birth, grows rapidly for 1 year, and then involutes
- GLUT1+

Angiohamartoma Of The Lymph Node Hilum

- Vessels with bland endothelium
- Sort of a vascular transformation
- Benign, most common in pelvic nodes
- Also sinus histiocytosis

Glomangioma

- Myxoid degeneration, staghorn vessels
- Lots of stroma
- Round punched out nucleoli with syncytial cytoplasm, condensing around vessels (vascular)
- Diffusely positive for SMA, areas of spindled smooth muscle cells positive for vimentin
- DDx
  - Not to be confused with hemangiopericytoma, which is the head and neck version of solitary fibrous tumor (STAT6+)
  - Glomus tumor has smaller vessels and more hypercellular
  - Glomangiomyoma has a more prominent spindle cell component

Glomus Tumor

- Clinical
  - Benign myoepithelial tumor
    - Modified smooth muscle cells forming masses around vascular channels
  - PAINFUL HEMORRHAGIC NODULE ON FINGER/TOE
  - Recur, rarely can be malignant. More common in NF1
- Architecture
  - Cords and "archipelagos"
  - Abundant myxoid matrix
  - Cells border slit–like vascular channels
- Cytology
  - Epithelioid bland cells

- Eosinophilic cytoplasm, centrally placed round nucleus with uniform chromatin (occasional intranuclear pseudoinclusions)
- Expresses SMA, MSA, vimentin
- Rare subtype glomangiomyoma
  - Looks like angioleiomyoma areas mixed with glomus areas
  - Subungual

Myoepithelioma

- Cords and trabeculae
- Reticular pattern
- Immunohistochemistry
  - Pankeratin+, EMA+
  - Can express S100, GFAP, SMA, calponin
  - Rarely has loss of INI1
- *EWSR1* or *PLAG1* rearrangements
- DDx includes ossifying fibromyxoid tumor, extraskeletal myxoid chondrosarcoma, and epithelioid schwannoma

PEComa

- Perivascular epithelioid cell tumor
- Synonymous with monotypic epithelioid angiomyolipoma (AML) in kidney, lymphangioleiomyomatosis in lung, uterine PEComa, cardiac rhabdomyoma, clear cell "sugar" tumor of pancreas
  - AMLs have PEComa cells growing in vessel wall
- Clinical
  - Middle-aged, females > males (71)
  - Tuberous sclerosis gene complex aberrations
    - *TSC1* and *TSC2* gene mutations
    - 20% have *TFE3* gene rearrangements
    - *TP53* mutations in malignant PEComas
- Architecture
  - Well circumscribed, at least partially encapsulated, epithelioid spindle cells in vague fascicles and nests
  - Thick hyalinized vessels and thin capillaries, areas of extravasated red blood cells
- Cytology
  - Granular eosinophilic to clear cytoplasm, well–defined cell borders
  - Vesicular chromatin with small conspicuous (red) nucleoli
  - Some nuclear atypia
  - Some multinucleated giant cells
- Myomelanocytic in origin
  - Positive for HMB45, Melan-A, SMA, desmin
  - Negative for S100

Well–Differentiated Angiosarcoma

- Too many cells and vascular channels in the superficial dermis
- Solar elastosis, anastomosing vascular channels
- Pleomorphism and hobnailing of endothelial cells
- Classic on scalp

- Think of Kaposi (patch stage) when you see promontory sign
  - Vascular channels wrapping around adnexal structures

Epithelioid Angiosarcoma

- Superficial dermis to subcutaneous fat, ill–defined and infiltrative (splitting collagen fibers), apoptosis
- *Amphophilic* cytoplasm, prominent cherry red nucleoli, epithelioid, syncytial (not discrete like melanoma), vascular spaces lined by epithelium
- AE1/AE3+, EMA+ (when epithelioid), ERG+, FLI1+
- Very aggressive

Pulmonary Artery Intimal Sarcoma

- MDM2/CDK4+, *MDM2* amplifications, chromosome 12 rearrangements

UNKNOWN ORIGIN

Undifferentiated Pleomorphic Sarcoma (UPS)

- Can be the result of many different mesenchymal tumors undergoing dedifferentiating
  - All roads to dedifferentiation end here
- High–grade tumor with variable cellularity, many multinucleated giant cells, myxoid background, necrosis.
  - UPS with some myxoid change can be called *high–grade myxofibrosarcoma*
- Giant cells, myxoid stroma, fibrous
- Poor prognosis
- IHC may be aberrant focally

Solitary Fibrous Tumor (SFT)

- Previously called *hemangiopericytoma*
- Syndromes
  - Pierre–Marie–Bamberger
    - 10% to 20%, benign and malignant SFTs
    - Digital clubbing and pulmonary osteoarthropathy
  - Doege–Potter
    - Refractory hypoglycemia caused by insulin–like growth factor
- Clinical
  - Favorable prognosis
- Architecture
  - Lobular mass
  - Alternating hypercellular and hypocellular areas
  - Highly cellular, hyalinized vessels, heterogeneous
  - Patternless pattern
  - Ropey collagen
    - Rare pigment (melanin vs. iron vs. hemosiderin)
- Vasculature
  - Prominent staghorn vessels with variably edematous collagen collars
- Cytology
  - Monotonous plump spindled cells
  - Sheets of blue cells with high nuclear-to-cytoplasmic ratios
- Strong and diffuse for CD34, bcl2+, STAT6+
  - Protein amplification caused by *NAB2-STAT6* fusion by inversion
    - 98% sensitivity, very specific

- ≥4 mitotic figures per 10 hpf has increased metastatic potential (behaves like intermediate grade)
- DDx
    - Synovial sarcoma
    - PEComa—does not show the vessels as much as this, very solid, perivascular in lineage but not morphology
    - Hemangiopericytoma name is retained in central nervous system
    - In sinonasal, *glomangiopericytoma*

Synovial Sarcoma

- Young, deep joint, architecture > cytology
- Architecture
    - Hypercellular, monotonous and blue on low power
    - Fascicular
    - "School of fish" streaming
    - Wiry stromal collagen, stromal mast cells, staghorn (hemangiopericytoma–like) vessels, coarse calcifications
- Cytology
    - Infiltrating bland blue cells
    - Overlapping uniform nuclei
- Gland formation if biphasic
- Immunohistochemistry
    - Expresses (patchy) EMA and keratin (CK8 and CK18)
    - *TLE1* expression is increased on gene–expression profiling or immunohistochemistry
        - Sensitive but not specific
        - 20% of MPNSTs and 5% to 10% of SFTs are also positive
    - S100 is positive in one-third
- t(X;18), *SS18* or *SYT* translocation with *SSX1, SSX2, SSX3,* or *SSX4*
- Use RT-PCR to tell apart

Monophasic Synovial Sarcoma

- Hypercellular, lots of staghorn vessels
- No gland formation
- Areas of keratin+/EMA+ (good supportive evidence)
    - CD99 not really helpful
    - S100+ in 30% with same pattern as MPNST
    - CD34– STAT6–, TLE1+ (not great to confirm)
- DDx: cellular SFT, MPNST

Biphasic Synovial Sarcoma

- Morphology
    - Lobular with large areas of collagen, hypercellular, monotonous and blue
    - Swirling pattern (like a Van Gogh).
    - Both glands and stroma have hyaluronic acid and mucopolysaccharides
    - Psammoma bodies, pigment, **gland–like structures**
        - Only calcifying spindle cell tumors—MPNST and synovial sarcoma
- Vasculature
    - Hemangiopericytoma/staghorn vessels
    - Extravasated red blood cells. Can get myxoid and mast cells
    - Amphophilic cytoplasm, occasional mitoses, monotonous and bland. No atypia, mitoses, etc.

- CD34−, EMA, CD99, **TLE1+** (good for screening)
  - Keratin and EMA stain the glands and some spindle cells
- t(X;18)(p11.2; q11) *SYT-SSX1* is more common than t(X;18)(p11.2;q11) *SYT-SSX2*
  - Rarely *SS18-SSX2* is seen, has a more favorable prognosis
- *p16INK4A* deletion
- DDx: SFT is in the differential but has short fascicles, CD34+, TLE1−

Poorly Differentiated Synovial Sarcoma

- See "Small Round Blue Cell Tumor" section

Adamantinoma
- Rare, low–grade malignancy
- Shaft of tibia +/− fibula
- Classic
  - Older than 20 years of age
  - Epithelial component is prominent
  - Basaloid, tubular, spindle, squamoid
  - Can metastasize
  - Pain is a poor prognostic marker
- Dedifferentiated
  - Younger than 20 years of age
  - *Rare*
  - Looks like osteofibrous dysplasia with woven bone and osteoblast rimming
  - Epithelial component is subtle
- Fibrous component expresses vimentin and epithelial component expresses cytokeratins (CK5, CK14, CK19)

Alveolar Soft Part Sarcoma

- Morphology
  - Low–power impression infiltrative, necrosis, alveolar architecture
  - Dyscohesive epithelioid/rhabdoid cells, eosinophilic bodies, prominent nucleoli
    - Dyscohesion causes an "alveolar" appearance
  - Compartments lined by fibrous septa with delicate vasculature
  - Tightly packed tumor cells
- Tiny rod–shaped crystals, PAS-D+, TFE3+
- DDx: melanoma, renal cell carcinoma in clear cell areas, other carcinomas
  - TFE3+ also in translocation–association renal cell carcinoma
    - But renal cell carcinoma is keratin+
    - Both have t(X;17) *TFE3-ASPL*
- Vimentin+, desmin+, otherwise nonspecific

Epithelioid Sarcoma

- Clinical
  - Classic presentation = distal site in young person
- Architecture
  - Acanthosis, hyperkeratosis in overlying skin
  - Vaguely nodular
  - Infiltrative blue cells, no pattern, perineural invasion
  - Geographic necrosis with palisading histiocyte–like cells
  - Can calcify

- Cytology
  - Can be very bland; be careful!
  - Epithelioid, prominent nucleoli
  - Oval to round, some with clear cytoplasm, nucleoli, bland and uniform
  - Mitoses present
- Patchy keratin, EMA+, SMARC4/INI1 lost
- DDx
  - Atypical fibroxanthoma (uglier than this)
  - Pleomorphic dermal sarcoma (also uglier than this)
  - Rheumatoid arthritis nodules, (xantho)necrobiotic granulomas
    - Younger patient, hands and feet
    - Always get a keratin (EMA)
- Proximal–type epithelioid sarcoma can look like alveolar soft part sarcoma
- Upper thigh, older person

SMALL ROUND BLUE CELL TUMORS (SRBCTS)

General

- See Table 15.1.
- Minimal to no cytoplasm, fine granular chromatin, indistinct nucleolus; no particular architecture, highly proliferative
- Generally in children
- Diagnosis—#1 architecture and morphology, #2 IHC and molecular features
  - Clinical history (e.g., age, presentation) important
- CD99 is positive in Ewing but negative in neuroblastoma
  - Strong membranous staining in all cells
  - If negative, it is *not* Ewing sarcoma
  - If positive, it is *not* neuroblastoma
- WT1 is positive in desmoplastic small round cell tumor (DSRCT) only if it is a C-terminal antibody

Ewing Sarcoma

- Also known as *primitive neuroectodermal tumor* (PNET)
- t(11;22) *EWSR1-FLI1*
- Lots of necrosis and lots of blood
- Hyperchromatic small round blue cells in solid sheets, vague rosetting (not well formed)
- More conspicuous nucleoli than you would typically see in SRBCT
- CD99 strong, membranous

Rhabdomyosarcoma

Botryoid Rhabdomyosarcoma
- Polypoid lesion protruding from the vagina of a young girl
  - Resembling a bunch of grapes
- "Condensation" (more dense cellularity) of tumor cells in subepithelial area—cambium layer

Alveolar Rhabdomyosarcoma
- Younger patients (most common in early to mid-teens, but can happen in all ages)
- Nasal cavity is a classic site
- Large nests of monomorphic cells with some alveolar–type areas

- Falling apart/clefting
- Cells clinging to fibrous septae (alveolar soft parts sarcoma does too)
- Wreath cells (multinucleated giant cells with nuclei in ring)
- Smooth nuclear contours, sparse cytoplasm, open chromatin, rare indistinct nucleoli
- Stains
  - Myogenin nuclear+, desmin+
    - Myogenin staining is a prognostic marker
    - Usually weaker than embryonal
      - Synaptophysin+, chromogranin+, keratin−/+
- 60% *PAX3-FOXO1* (mostly older children/young adults), 20% *PAX7-FOXO1*
  - Embryonal and pleomorphic do not have a specific translocation
- Poorer prognosis than embryonal
  - More solid
  - Weak to heterogeneous myogenin compared with strong homogeneous
- Have strap cells (rhabdomyoblasts) with cross striations

Embryonal Rhabdomyosarcoma
- Densely hypercellular areas, spindle cells and epithelioid cells
- Loose myxoid stroma
- Irregular nuclear contours

Pleomorphic Rhabdomyosarcoma
- Exclusively in soft tissues of adults
- Spindle cells, whorled or storiform pattern
- Enlarged hyperchromatic nuclei

Neuroblastoma

- Arise from parasympathetic chain/adrenal glands
  - Can occur in adrenal medulla (40%, also 15% in retroperitoneum from sympathetic ganglia)
- Very blue, neuropil–like stroma in pseudorosettes (Homer-Wright), some more spindled areas
  - May have ganglion cells
- NSE+, synaptophysin+, CD99−
- *MYCN* amplification (prognostic marker)
- See pediatric chapter for more information

Small Cell Carcinoma

- Spindled (carrot–like) nuclei, indistinct nucleoli, increased mitoses and apoptoses; salt and pepper chromatin
- Should not have prominent nucleoli
- Positive for chromogranin and synaptophysin
- Keratin+ too; be careful!
- All small cell carcinomas (regardless of origin) are positive for TTF1
- DDx: synovial sarcoma is in the differential, but it would be in a younger patient and would not metastasize to adrenal

Merkel Cell Carcinoma

- Nests of cells with slit–like spaces
- Monotonous small blue cells, fine chromatin, indistinct nucleoli
- Numerous mitoses and apoptoses

TABLE 15.1 ■ Small Round Blue Cell Tumors

	CK/EMA	S100	CD45	CD99	DES	MYO	SYN	WT1[a]	TLE1
ES	+	-	-	+++memb	-	-	++	-	-
RMS	-/+[b]	-	-	+	+++	+++nuc	+[c]	-	+
DSRCT	+++	-	-	+	+++dot	-	+	+++	-
NB	-	+	-	-	-	-	+++	-	-
PDSS	+++	+	-	+	-	-	-	-	+++
Lymphoma	-	-	+++	++	-	-	-	-	++
Melanoma	-	+++	-	++	-	-	-	-	-
SmCC	+++	-	-	++	-	-	+++	-	-

[a]also positive in Wilms tumor

[b]30% positive

[c]25% are positive for synapto and chromo; be careful!

CK, Cytokeratin; DES, desmin; DSRCT, desmoplastic small round cell tumor; ES, Ewing sarcoma; memb, membranous; MYO, myogenin; NB, neuroblastoma; nuc, nuclear; PDSS, poorly differentiated synovial sarcoma; RMS, rhabdomyosarcoma; SmCC, small cell carcinoma; SYN, synaptophysin.

- Negative for chromogranin and synaptophysin, positive for CK20 in dot–like pattern (also in small cell carcinoma)—TTF-1
  - Neuroendocrine markers can be positive
  - Polyomavirus positive
- DDx: poorly differentiated synovial sarcoma, Merkel (TTF-1–), small cell carcinoma (TTF-1+)

DESMOPLASTIC SMALL ROUND CELL TUMOR

- Very aggressive, poor prognosis
- Spreads along serosa in abdomen/pelvis
- Usually young men in second and third decade with occasional testicular involvement
- Indistinct and poorly circumscribed nests and cords of very blue cells in a fibrous/desmoplastic stroma, pushing into the fat
- Irregular nest outlines with fibrillary stroma
- Round cells with sparse cytoplasm (some cleared out), open chromatin, single central nucleoli
- Single cell and comedo–like necrosis
- Some cells have more cytoplasm
  - Rosai said it rarely has all the features in its name
- Pink cytoplasmic globules: positive for desmin (dot–like intermediate filaments)
  - Positive for keratin, EMA, MOC31, NSE, CD57, WT1
  - CD99, MyoD1, myogenin—(can gain MyoD1 after radiotherapy)
- *EWSR1-WT1* translocation, t(11;22)(p13;q12)
- DDx: rhabdoid tumor—only found in children, pink cytoplasm, very poor prognosis

POORLY DIFFERENTIATED SYNOVIAL SARCOMA

- Very cellular, very atypical
- Poorest prognosis of all synovial sarcomas
- t(X;18) *SS18-TLE1*

LYMPHOMA

Melanoma

Sinonasal Undifferentiated Carcinoma (SNUC)

Wilms Tumor

EPITHELIOID SARCOMAS

- Epithelioid MPNST
- Epithelioid sarcoma
  - Two types
    - Classic—young, hands and feet
    - Proximal—older, deep soft tissue of trunk
  - Palisading necrosis
  - No specific translocation
  - INI1 loss (*SMARCB1* deletion)
  - High–grade behavior but bland cytology

- CK+, EMA+, vimentin+, CD34+, ERG+/−, FLI1+/−
- DDx includes granuloma annulare (cytokeratin negative)
- Epithelioid angiosarcoma

SYNDROMES AND GENETICS

- See Table 15.2.
- SMARCB1 = INI1
  - Expressed in every normal cell, tumor suppressor
  - Lost in malignant rhabdoid tumor (called *atypical teratoid/rhabdoid tumor* in CNS)
    - Not actually derived from skeletal muscle (do not know origin)

TABLE 15.2 ■ Gene Rearrangements in Soft Tissue and Bone Neoplasms

Gene	Tumor
ALK	Inflammatory myofibroblastic tumor Epithelioid fibrous histiocytoma
CAMTA1	Epithelioid hemangioendothelioma
CCNB3	*BCOR*-rearranged sarcoma Clear cell sarcoma of kidney
CIC	*CIC*-rearranged sarcoma
EWSR1	Ewing sarcoma Clear cell sarcoma Desmoplastic small round cell tumor Angiomatoid fibrous histiocytoma Myoepithelial tumors of soft tissue Extraskeletal myxoid chondrosarcoma Myxoid liposarcoma Sclerosing epithelioid fibrosarcoma
FOXO1	Alveolar rhabdomyosarcoma
FUS	Myxoid liposarcoma Low–grade fibromyxoid sarcoma Sclerosing epithelioid fibrosarcoma Ewing sarcomaAngiomatoid fibrous histiocytoma Extraskeletal myxoid chondrosarcoma
GLI1	Plexiform fibromyxoma Gastroblastoma Pericytoma with t(7;12)
HMGA2	Lipoma Deep angiomyxoma
JAZF1	Endometrial stromal nodule Low–grade stromal sarcoma
MKL2	Chondroid lipoma Ectomesenchymal chondromyxoid tumor
NCOA2	Mesenchymal chondrosarcoma Angiofibroma of soft tissue Uterine tumor resembling ovarian sex cord tumor
NTRK3	Infantile fibrosarcoma Congenital mesoblastic nephroma
PGDFB	Giant cell fibroblastoma Dermatofibrosarcoma protuberans

PLAG1	Lipoblastoma Myoepithelioma of soft tissue Myxoid leiomyosarcoma
ROS1	Inflammatory myofibroblastic tumor
SS18	Synovial sarcoma
STAT6	Solitary fibrous tumor
TFE3	Alveolar soft part sarcoma PEComa Epithelioid hemangioendothelioma Ossifying fibromyxoid tumor
TCF12, TAF15	Extraskeletal myxoid chondrosarcoma
TFG	Extraskeletal myxoid chondrosarcoma Inflammatory myofibroblastic tumor
USP6	Nodular fasciitis Aneurysmal bone cyst Fibro-osseous pseudotumor of digits Myositis ossificans
YWHAE	High–grade endometrial stromal sarcoma YWHAE-rearranged sarcoma

- Also epithelioid sarcoma, renal medullary carcinoma, poorly differentiated chordoma, epithelioid MPNST (lobular, looks like melanoma, S100+, SOX10+, HMB45–, Melan-A–), myoepithelial carcinoma of soft tissue, undifferentiated (rhabdoid) sarcoma, extraskeletal myxoid chondrosarcoma, gastrointestinal rhabdoid sarcoma
  - "Rhabdoid cells"
  - Succinate dehydrogenase
- Syndromes
- Familial paraganglioma syndrome
  - Most common cause for inherited paragangliomas
  - Carney–Stratakis syndrome—paragangliomas and gastric gastrointestinal stromal tumors (GISTs)
- Carney triad—paragangliomas, gastric GISTs, pulmonary chondroma
  - *SDHC* promoter hypermethylation
  - SDHB IHC can detect all of these
- SDH-deficient GISTs (8% of all)
  - Multinodular/plexiform
    - Growth pattern has 99% specificity and sensitivity in detecting SDH deficiency
  - Predominant epithelioid morphology
  - Metastasize to lymph nodes or distant sites but have long overall survival
  - No response to imatinib
  - Risk assessment criteria do not apply
- NKX2.2 = downstream target of EWSR1-ERG product in Ewing sarcoma
- Overexpressed in Ewing sarcoma
- Mesenchymal chondrosarcoma can be positive too
- *CIC-DUX4* sarcomas are negative
- *CIC*-rearrangement sarcomas (round cell)
- Most common Ewing–like sarcoma without *EWSR1* fusion

- Trunk
- Poorer prognosis
- Nuclear ETV4+, WT1+, CD99 patchy
- MUC4+ in low–grade fibromyxoid tumor (>99%)
- *FUS* gene rearrangement
- Also EMA+
- t(12;15) *ETV6-NTRK3*—mammary–analog secretory carcinoma, secretory breast carcinoma, angiomyolipoma, infantile fibrosarcoma, congenital (cellular) mesoblastic nephroma

OTHER

Sarcomatoid Carcinoma

- Spindled, necrosis, mitoses, superficial, entrapping fat, infiltrating, ulcerating skin
- Myxoid stroma
- S100–, keratin+

Mesothelioma

Desmoplastic Melanoma
- Superficial, collagen bundles, some myxoid areas
- Large nuclei, some pleomorphism in papillary dermis
- Diffuse S100+, Melan-A–

Clear Cell Sarcoma

- Also known as *melanoma of soft parts*
- Found at ends of tendons in the second and third decades of life
- Morphology
  - Epithelioid spindled cells, very prominent dark (not cherry) macronucleoli, necrosis and mitosis, sheets
  - Areas of streaming cells with pale amphophilic granular cytoplasm (windswept), no nesting/vague nesting, some have melanin
  - Delicate fibrous septa
  - Often have multinucleated giant cells (nonspecific but can help vs. melanoma)
- Diffuse Melan-A (stains exactly like melanoma)
  - Melanin is present in about one-half
- t(12;22) *EWSR1-ATF1* or t(2;22) *EWSR1-CREB1*
  - Not seen in melanoma; also no connection to epidermis, younger patient, associated with tendon, not *BRAF*-mutated
- Very aggressive, chemotherapy–resistant

Phosphaturic Mesenchymal Tumor

- In response to oncogenic osteomalacia
  - Paraneoplastic syndrome
  - Phosphate wasting
  - FGF-23 production
- 2 to 10 cm, circumscribed, staghorn vessels
- Spindle cells +/– cartilaginous metaplasia (or other metaplasia)
- Grungy pale blue calcification

ODDS AND ENDS

- Synovial cyst (also known as *ganglion cyst*)
  - Dorsal wrist is characteristic
  - Do not sign out as *ganglion cyst—use synovial cyst* or *digital mucous cyst*
  - Description
    - Cyst nearby with necrotic myxoid material in it
    - Bland myxoid stroma interspersed with bland small spindle cells
    - Very little atypia (if any)
    - Small inconspicuous capillaries
    - Stromal muciphages
- Infantile angiosarcoma—GLUT1+
- Follicular dendritic sarcoma—CD21+ and CD35+
- FAT ATROPHY—mucin, signet ring cells floating, delicate vessels
- Sarcomas that are *not* graded
  - Epithelioid (all behave poorly)
  - Well-differentiated liposarcoma/atypical lipomatous tumor (all behave well)
  - Synovial sarcoma
- Fibrosarcoma is very rare, dx of elimination
- Malignant necrosis
  - Ghost cells or sheets of pink, granular debris
  - At margin—mitotic figures, debris, apoptotic cells
- INI-1 negative malignancies
- Mast cells are common in neurofibromas, malignant schwannomas, UPS, leiomyosarcoma, and *synovial sarcoma* (always)
- Most common postradiation sarcoma = UPS ~10 to 12 years (can occur in scars/surgical sites)
- Retroperitoneum in older people—inflammatory and sclerotic liposarcoma
- Sarcomas that can be cytokeratin+
  - DSRCT
  - Epithelioid sarcoma
  - Synovial sarcoma
  - Ewing sarcoma
  - Angiosarcoma
  - Leiomyosarcoma
- Hemosiderin = golden–brown and refractile, melanin = dirty and nonrefractile
  - Sox10 is more specific than S100 for melanoma
- Intranuclear pseudoinclusions
  - PEComa
    - Clear cell sugar tumor
  - Angiomyolipoma
  - Lymphangioleiomyoma
  - Chromophobe
  - Papillary thyroid carcinoma
  - Melanoma
- Diffusely CD34+
  - Dermatofibrosarcoma protuberans (DFSP)
  - Solitary fibrous tumor (SFT)
    - STAT6+ (*NAB2-STAT6* fusion)
    - May be locally destructive, recurrent, metastatic
    - May have hemangiopericytoma–like features, staghorn vessels, coarse collagen

- GIST
- Angiosarcoma
- At least some CD34 positivity
  - Superficial acral fibromyxoma
  - Epithelioid sarcoma
  - Intradermal spindle cell lipoma
- Chemotherapy/radiation effect
  - Necrosis *and* reduction in cellular density
  - Example: 30% of cells are still present (compared with diagnosis) with replacement by hyaline fibrosis/sclerosis

CHAPTER 16

Chemistry, Laboratory Management, and Informatics

Chemistry

PROTEIN ELECTROPHORESIS

- Methods
  - Serum protein electrophoresis (SPEP)—detects proteins in serum
    - Typically performed at pH 8.6
    - Separates proteins by size and charge
    - Must be performed on SERUM instead of plasma so all coagulation factors are consumed and removed
  - Urine protein electrophoresis (UPEP)—detects proteins in urine
  - Immunofixation (IFx)—identifies proteins after SPEP/UPEP
    - Serum added to the plate in six lanes
    - Antisera (antibodies) specific to gamma, alpha, and mu heavy chains and kappa and lambda light chains are added to their respective lanes
      - General fixative added to lane 1
    - Antisera precipitates and fixes protein to gel → wash off all other protein → stain
  - Capillary electrophoresis (CE)—newer, automated, and more sensitive version of gel electrophoresis
    - Has an M-protein detection limit of <0.5 g/L
- Indications
  - Possible myeloma or other B cell disorders
    - Idiopathic Bence Jones proteinuria
      - Urinary monoclonal protein or UPEP ≥500 mg per 24 hours and/or clonal bone marrow plasma cells ≥10%
      - No immunoglobulin (Ig) heavy chain on IFx
      - No CRAB symptoms (hyperCalcemia, Renal insufficiency, Anemia, Bone lesions)
    - AL amyloidosis (primary amyloidosis)
      - Peripheral neuropathy, carpal tunnel, congestive heart failure, nephrotic syndrome, macroglossia, malabsorption
      - Amyloid = unbranched fibrils made of 95% light chains and 5% beta-pleated P-protein
  - Suspected immunodeficiency
  - Possible A1AT deficiency
  - Abnormal serum protein or albumin
  - Inflammation (acute or chronic)
  - Proteinuria or unexplained hypogammaglobulinemia—get UPEP to evaluate for light-chain disease
- Normal constituents
  - Prealbumin = transthyretin
    - Higher concentration in CSF because made by choroid plexus

- Used to monitor nutritional status because it has a shorter half-life than albumin (2 days vs. 3 weeks)
- May be increased in inflammatory bowel disease and Guillain-Barré syndrome
- Albumin
- Alpha 1
  - α_1-lipoprotein (A1LP)—varies considerably in normal adults
  - α_1-antitrypsin (A1AT)—serine protease inhibitor
    - Genetic variants can be absent, decreased, or have abnormal migration
    - Increased in acute inflammation, pregnancy, oral contraceptives (OCP), tamoxifen, tumors, liver disease
      - Hyperestrogenemia
  - α_1-fetoprotein (A1FP)
    - High levels at birth, decreases throughout life
    - Increased at 15 to 22 weeks gestation with open spina bifida, t(21), t(18)
  - α_1-glycoprotein (A1GP)—increased in acute inflammation, end-stage renal disease (ESRD) on dialysis, neonatal sepsis, increased risk for myocardial infarction (MI)
  - α_1-antichymotrypsin—increased in serum and CSF of Alzheimer's, acute-phase reactant
- Alpha 2
  - α_2-microglobulin (A2MG) protease inhibitor and is adjacent or comigrates with haptoglobin
    - Increased in neonates, elderly, hyperestrogen states, nephrotic syndrome, ESRD on dialysis, diabetics, emphysema
  - Haptoglobin—acute-phase reactant that binds free hemoglobin then quickly eliminated through the reticuloendothelial system
    - Genetic polymorphisms cause this region to be complex
    - ↓ in hemolysis (in vitro and in vivo), vitamin B_{12} or folate deficiency, congenital absence, neonates (normally low), OCP use, liver disease
    - ↑ in acute inflammation, burns, corticosteroid therapy, growth hormones, insulin therapy
    - Can be ↑ or ↓ in kidney disease, depending on genotype and degree of renal damage
  - Ceruloplasmin—binds copper (marked decrease in Wilson disease)
  - Fibronectin—prominent in pregnancy or cholestasis
- Beta
  - Transferrin—glycoprotein made in liver that transfers iron from gastrointestinal (GI) tract and reticuloendothelial system to the bone marrow (recycle iron)
    - Total iron-binding capacity (TIBC) is a reflection on amount of transferrin present
      - Think of it as the number of seats on buses that are open for more iron.
      - In iron deficiency, the body really needs more iron for hematopoiesis so it sends a bunch of empty buses to be ready to utilize any available iron.
      - In anemia of chronic disease, the body increases hepcidin to lock the iron away in macrophages. The body does not want any more iron, so it does not send any empty buses to pick up incoming iron.
    - ↑ in iron-deficiency anemia, pregnancy, estrogen therapy, and in CSF (asialo form is also called *tau protein*)
    - ↓ in anemia of chronic disease, cirrhosis, acute inflammation, renal disease, dialysis, burns, congenital absence/decrease
  - C3—complement system
    - In acute phase, initial decrease then increase
  - Fibrinogen—not normally seen here, may be seen if incompletely clotted
  - *IgA M-spikes*

- Gamma
  - C-reactive protein (CRP)—marker of inflammation, low is correlated with higher all-cause mortality (marker of cellular stress)
  - Immunoglobulins
  - *Non-IgA M-spike*
- Serum patterns
  - Acute-phase reactants—α_1-antitrypsin, α_2-microglobulin, fibrinogen, factor VIII, CRP, prothrombin
    - Decreased albumin, transferrin, antithrombin
    - Increased α_1 and α_2, normal gamma globulin
  - Chronic inflammation
    - Including active systemic lupus erythematosus (SLE), infection, cancer
    - Increased gamma globulin, decreased albumin
  - Severe protein loss caused by renal disease (nephrotic syndrome), GI disease (diarrhea), or burns
    - Decreased albumin, transferrin, gamma globulin, α_1-antitrypsin
    - Increased α_2-microglobulin
  - Liver disease
    - Beta-gamma bridging is very suggestive of liver disease
    - Hypoalbuminemia, increased gamma (polyclonal hypergammaglobulinemia)
  - Agammaglobulinemia—decreased gamma
  - Pseudo M-spikes
    - Causes
      - Fibrinogen (incompletely clotted sample)
      - Hemoglobin (hemolyzed sample)
      - ↑ CRP
      - ↑ transferrin
      - Antibiotics
      - Radiocontrast dye (late α_2)
      - Very high serum tumor markers (e.g., CA19-9)
      - Also monoclonal antibody therapies!
    - Some absorb ultraviolet light at 200 nm, some migrate with M-spikes
- Urine patterns
  - Glomerular—strong albumin, α_1, and beta bands
    - Only intermediate-sized proteins left behind (albumin, A1AT, transferrin) because bigger ones are not lost through glomerulus and smaller ones are reabsorbed in the tubules
  - Tubular—weak albumin band, strong α_1 and beta bands
  - Overflow—most commonly monoclonal light chain (Bence Jones protein)
    - Also myoglobin and hemoglobin
- CSF patterns
  - Multiple sclerosis and tertiary/neurosyphilis
    - Increased gamma fraction

CARDIAC BIOMARKERS

- European and American myocardial infarction (MI) definition
  - Detection of the rise and fall of troponin I or T (greater than the 99th percentile), plus at least one of the following:
    - Symptoms of ischemia

- Electrocardiogram (ECG/EKG) changes (ischemia, ST segment changes, bundle branch block)
- New Q wave on ECG
- Imaging: loss of myocardium or wall motion abnormality
- cTnI—reference range = <0.045
  - 99th percentile (different than the usually 95%)
- TnC—not cardiac specific (i.e., cardiac and skeletal troponin C are the same)
- TnI—cardiac specific
  - Cannot compare TnI levels among institutions—different assays detect different forms
- TnT—mostly cardiac specific but increased renal disease (also in skeletal muscle)
- Serial testing
- Concentration is correlated to amount of myocardium necrosis
- More sensitive and specific than CK-MB, which does not add value to troponin
  - CK-B is less specific for the heart
- Chronically increased cTn (cardiac troponin, NOT troponin C) can be secondary to heart failure, renal failure, diabetes, and so on
- Myocarditis increases cTn
  - Infectious, autoimmune, drugs, and so on
  - Acute can resolve or become chronic
  - Diagnostic "gold standard" is endomyocardial biopsy
    - Can do noninvasive clinical diagnosis on signs/symptoms
- Checking for false positive in an immunoassay
  - Heterophile antibody test
    - Can cause false positives and false negatives
  - Dilutions
  - Different assay
- Hemolysis causes false positive in cTnI and false negative in cTnT
  - Do not report results!
- cTn are also measured in acutely decompensated CHF
- Limit of detection (LOD)—1.1 to 1.9 for hs-cTnI (lowest level you can detect)
  - High-sensitivity—measures ng/L (regular is μg/L)
    - Requires CV <20% to report
    - At <6 ng/L, the CV is ~27% (cannot report)
- CV = mean/SD, measures imprecision
- Limit of blank (LOB)—measures baseline "noise" (analytical noise)
- Limit of quantification (LOQ)—lowest level that can be accurately and reliable quantified
  - Usually higher than the LOD
- HyTest—antibodies and where they bind troponin

ELECTROLYTE DISTURBANCES

- Aldosterone
  - Sodium-conservation hormone (and secondary water conservation)
  - ↑ aldosterone → ↑ sodium reabsorption in kidney → ↑ blood pressure
    - ↑ sodium and ↓ potassium in blood
    - Opposite in blood
  - Can measure aldosterone in serum
- Antidiuretic hormone (ADH)
  - Water-conservation hormone
  - Synthesized by hypothalamus
  - Negative regulated by cortisol

- ↑ ADH → ↑ free water
  - ↓ osmolality in serum
  - ↑ osmolality in serum
- Cannot measure directly; use osmolality difference between urine and serum
- Electrolyte exclusion effect
  - 7% of plasma consists of SOLID components
  - When we measure electrolytes, we can use blood gas instruments, vista, or iSTAT
    - Ion-selective electrodes (ISE)
    - Vista dilutes the specimen (indirect ISE)
- Spurious
  - ↑ potassium and ↓ calcium from EDTA contamination
- Calcium aberrations
  - Pseudohypoparathyroidism
    - Resistant to parathyroid hormone (PTH), hereditary mutation in *GNAS*
    - Functional hypoparathyroidism (low calcium, high phosphate) but HIGH PTH
  - Pseudopseudohypoparathyroidism
    - Albright hereditary osteodystrophy
    - Laboratory tests are normal
    - Short stature, round face, brachydactyly, mild mental retardation, subcutaneous ossification, obesity
  - Renal osteodystrophy
    - Renal failure →
    - Cannot make 1-α-hydroxylase, which normally activates vitamin D →
    - Decreased intestinal absorption of calcium and phosphate →
    - Decreased serum calcium →
    - Increased PTH secretion →
    - High serum phosphate and increased bony absorption by osteoblasts
  - Rickets
    - High PTH, low phosphate, low vitamin D, low calcium

LIVER FUNCTION TESTS

- First tier
  - Transaminases—alanine transaminase and aspartate transaminase (ALT and AST)
    - AST = SG<u>P</u>T (*P* is for pyruvate)
      - More abundant and in liver cells, more sensitive
      - Found in muscle and red cells too
      - Higher in alcoholic hepatitis only
    - ALT = SG<u>O</u>T (*O* is for oxaloacetate)
      - More specific for liver disease
      - Longer half-life
      - Higher than AST in all etiologies except alcohol
  - Bilirubin
    - Unconjugated = indirect
      - Insoluble in blood
      - Bound to albumin
      - Increased in hemolysis
    - Conjugated = direct
      - Conjugated to glucuronide
      - Increased in liver disease

- Most comes from heme breakdown (also CYP450)
- Liver conjugates it to make it more soluble, then excretes
  - During biliverdin formation, carbon monoxide forms. During massive hemolysis, can measure carbon monoxide by CO-oximeter.
- Whenever bilirubin forms are found in the urine, it is liver disease
- Alkaline phosphatase (AP)
  - Not specific
  - Isoenzymes: liver, bone, placenta, intestine
    - Bone isoform is heat labile, and others are not—"BONE BURNS"
- Gamma glutamyl transferase (GGT)
  - Most specific for alcohol use
- Albumin and PT/INR
  - Measures production in liver
  - Albumin half-life = 21 days
    - Negative acute-phase reactant, decreased in acute inflammation
- Second tier
  - Hepatitis viral studies and molecular tests
    - HAV, HBV, HCV, HDV, HEV, HSV, EBV, CMV
  - Iron, ferritin, copper
  - α_1-antitrypsin
  - Autoantibody tests
- Patterns of disease
  - Hepatocellular injury or necrosis
    - ALT/AST > AP
  - Cholestatic
    - AP > ALT/AST
    - Microscopic ducts—primary biliary cholangitis (PBC)
      - Middle-aged women
      - Antimitochondrial antibody
      - Granulomatous inflammation
    - Large ducts—carcinoma
    - Both microscopic and large—primary sclerosing cholangitis (PSC)
      - Men, 20 to 50 years of age
      - Ulcerative colitis
      - Cholangiography: beaded string
  - Infiltrative (neoplasm, amyloid)
    - AP > ALT/AST
  - Mixed patterns are common
- Chronic hepatitis defined as >3 months duration
  - Transaminases usually twofold to fivefold elevated
- Autoimmune hepatitis
  - Type I
    - Any age, females > males
    - Antismooth muscle antibody
    - More common
  - Type II
    - 2 to 14 years of age, females > males
    - anti-LKEM antibody
    - Rare

- Environmental toxins
  - Vinyl chloride (plastics manufacturing)
  - Jamaican bush tea
  - Kava kava
  - Amanita phalloides mushroom
    - May need liver transplant
    - Cooking does not help
    - Vomit → feel better → liver failure
- Acetaminophen
  - Rumack–Matthew nomogram
  - Treat with N-acetylcysteine (replenishes glutathione)
- Hereditary hemochromatosis
  - Very high ferritin, genetic testing, liver biopsy
- Wilson disease—*ATP7B* gene
  - Increased urinary copper
  - Low serum ceruloplasmin

RENAL FUNCTION TESTS

- Markers of renal function typically estimate glomerular filtration rate (GFR)
  - Blood urea nitrogen (BUN)
    - Urea is freely filtered in glomerulus; ~40% to 80% reabsorbed
    - Increased in high protein diets, GI bleeds, decreased renal perfusion, loss of renal function (>70% to 80%)
      - Not specific for kidney function
    - Decreased in low-protein diets, overhydration, pregnancy, severe liver disease, anabolic hormones (androgens, growth hormone)
    - *BUN:creatinine ratio*
      - Normal = 12 to 16:1
      - Elevated
        - With normal creatinine—prerenal
        - With high creatinine—postrenal
      - Low—low-protein diet, starvation, severe liver disease, acute tubular necrosis
  - Estimating GFR with creatinine clearance
    - Creatinine clearance = (urine creatinine/plasma creatinine) × (urine volume/time in minutes)
    - Normal is 80 to 120 mL/min
  - Creatinine
    - Produced from muscle creatine
    - Steady rate of production, amount related to muscle mass
    - Freely filtered at glomerulus, actively secreted with high levels
      - Active secretion inhibited by cimetidine, trimethoprim, salicylates, probenecid, dapsone, pyrimethamine
    - Measured by Jaffe method
      - Creatinine + picrate (alkaline solution) → yellow-orange
      - First described in late 1800s, but variations are still used
      - Interference with ketones, hyperglycemia, elevated HbA1c, cephalosporins, high serum proteins
    - Enzymatic methods
      - Can be interfered with by 5-FU and glucose
    - Creatinine clearance = (urine creatinine × volume)/plasma creatinine

- Can lose one-half of glomerular filtration rate (GFR; renal function) and still be within normal limits
  - Older white women are at highest risk for missing early renal disease
- Cystatin C
  - Cysteine protein inhibitor
  - Levels rise in kidney disease
  - Less influenced by age, gender, and race than creatinine
  - Can detect subtle declines in GFR
  - Less available than creatinine
- Proteinuria
  - Normal is <150 mg/day with <30 mg/day of albumin
    - Microalbuminuria = 30 to 300 mg/day
  - Causes: diabetes, hypertension, myeloma, amyloid, hemoglobin (stones, trauma, hemolysis), myoglobin (muscle trauma, rhabdomyolysis), (pre)eclampsia, urinary tract infection, glomerulonephritis, pyelonephritis, vasculitis, connective tissue diseases, congestive cardiac failure, toxic drugs, metals, exercise, orthostatic
  - 24-hour collection is ideal but often unreliable
  - *Albumin:creatinine ratio*
    - Can be performed on a random specimen
    - See Table 16.1
- Chronic kidney disease diagnosis
  - Kidney damage for ≥3 months as defined by structural or functional abnormalities of the kidney (with or without ↓ GFR) that are manifested by *either*:
    - Pathologic abnormalities *or*
    - Markers of kidney damage (imaging, laboratory tests)
  - GFR <60 mL/min for ≥3 months with or without kidney damage
  - 2 main causes = diabetes and hypertension
  - See Table 16.2
  - Risk for cardiovascular disease is increased with creatinine elevations and microalbuminuria
  - 16.8% of patients ≥20 years
  - *Treatment triggers*
    - Diabetics with albumin:creatinine >30 mg/g
    - Nondiabetics with albumin:creatinine >300 mg/g
    - Nondiabetics with estimated GFR <60
- Acute renal failure (ARF)
  - 25% of all hospitalized patients develop ARF
  - Laboratory features
    - Increased BUN and creatinine
    - Hyperkalemia
    - Hyperphosphatemia
      - Hypocalcemia with metastatic calcium deposition can occur
    - Anemia (decreased erythropoietin)
    - Platelet abnormalities

TABLE 16.1 ■ **Categorizing Albuminuria**

	Microalbuminuria	Macroalbuminuria
Males	17–250 mg/g	>250 mg/g
Females	25–355 mg/g	>355 mg/g

TABLE 16.2 ■ **Stages of Chronic Kidney Disease**

Stage	GFR
1	≥90
2	60–89
3	30–59
4	15–29
5	<15

GFR, Glomerular filtration rate.

- Clinical features
  - Azotemia
    - Nausea/vomiting, malaise, abdominal pain, ileus, altered sensorium, asterixis, seizures
    - Pericardial fluid +/− friction rub → cardiac tamponade
    - Platelet dysfunction and clotting abnormalities
  - Hypervolemia
    - Lung rales
    - Hypertension, altered fluid homeostasis
  - Arrhythmia (hyperkalemia)
- Fractional excretion of sodium
  - FENa = sodium clearance/GFR
  - = [(urine sodium) × (plasma creatinine)]/[(urine creatinine) × (plasma sodium)] × 100%
- Prerenal (FENa <1%)
  - Decrease in intravascular volume or changes in vascular resistance
    - Hemorrhage, GI fluid loss, dehydration, excessive diuresis, third-spacing, pancreatitis, burns, trauma, peritonitis
    - Sepsis, anaphylaxis, anesthesia, afterload-reducing drugs, ACE inhibitors
- Intrarenal (FENa >1% to 2%)
  - Acute tubular necrosis—85%
    - Etiologies
      - Ischemia
      - Exogenous toxins
        - Aminoglycosides
        - Amphotericin B
        - Vancomycin
        - Acyclovir
        - Cephalosporins
        - Contrast media
        - Cyclosporine
        - Antineoplastics (cisplatin)
        - Organic solvents
        - Heavy metals (Hg, Cd, As)
      - Endogenous toxins
        - Myoglobin
        - Hemoglobin

- Uric acid crystals (tumor lysis syndrome)
- Bence Jones proteins
- Laboratory features
  - Hyperkalemia, hyperphosphatemia
  - BUN:creatinine <20:1
  - Sediment: muddy casts
  - FENa >3% (kidney cannot hold on to sodium)
- Interstitial nephritis—10% to 15%
  - Etiologies
    - 70% are drug-related
      - Penicillins
      - Cephalosporins
      - Sulfonamides
      - NSAIDs
      - Rifampin
      - Phenytoin
      - Allopurinol
      - Proton pump inhibitors
    - Infections
      - Streptococcal infections
      - Leptospirosis
      - CMV
      - Histoplasmosis
      - Rocky Mountain spotted fever
    - Immunologic
      - Systemic lupus erythematosus (SLE)
      - Sjögren syndrome
      - Sarcoidosis
      - Cryoglobulins
  - Clinical features
    - Fever, rash, arthralgias, eosinophilia
    - Urine: red cells, white cells, white cell casts, proteinuria
- Glomerulonephritis—5%
  - Etiologies
    - Nonproliferative
      - Minimal change
      - Focal segmental glomerulosclerosis
        - HIV, heroin, Alport
      - Membranous glomerulonephritis
      - Thin basement membrane disease
    - Proliferative
      - IgA nephropathy
      - Postinfections
      - Membranoproliferative glomerulonephritis
      - Rapidly progressive glomerulonephritis
  - Clinical features
    - Hypertension, edema
  - Laboratory features
    - Red cell casts, proteinuria (<3 g/dL), FENa low

TUMOR MARKERS

- α-fetoprotein (AFP)
  - Very high in newborns
  - Germ cell tumors
  - Can be ↑ in hepatitis
  - ≥10 or 20 ng/mL can help detect hepatocellular carcinoma in nonpregnant patients
    - Only use in high-risk patients
- Prostate specific antigen (PSA)
  - Screening and staging
    - 4 to 10 = gray zone—suspicious
      - Close follow up, biopsy, or free percentage
    - 10—highly suspicious
      - Obtain biopsy
    - PSA >10 without inflammatory condition upstages
      - Can skip biopsy and treat in some situations
  - Isoforms
    - Total—includes free and complexed
    - Complexed—bound to protease inhibitor
    - Free—low % free PSA = malignant prostatic process
      - *↑ % free PSA = ↓ risk for cancer*
  - Antiandrogens decrease PSA
  - A man's PSA tends to increase with age
  - Assays are not standardized; cannot be used interchangeably among sites
    - Send duplicates to old laboratory and new laboratory if changing care site
- Carcinoembryonic antigen (CEA)
  - Colon, breast, lung, and so on
- CA125
  - Monitoring after debulking surgery
    - Increased/increasing = indication for diagnostic second look procedure
  - Increased in 2% to 5% of healthy females
  - Also increased in cirrhosis, endometriosis, breast cancer, lung cancer, liver cancer, and so on
- CA19-9
  - Pancreatic and GI cancer
- CA15-3/CA27.29
  - Breast cancer
- Thyroglobulin
  - See "Thyroid" section
- Human chorionic gonadotropin (hCG)
  - One component of the quad screen *(see "Prenatal" section)*
  - Exogenous—doping, "hCG diet," Munchausen
  - Classically a dimer—alpha and beta units
    - Alpha unit identical to alpha unit in luteinizing hormone, follicle-stimulating hormone, and thyroid-stimulating hormone
    - 5 bioactive forms
      - Alpha-beta (intact, dimeric)—pregnancy
      - Free beta—tumors
      - Hyperglycosylated alpha-beta—early pregnancy, tumors
        - Some assays do not detect this form
        - Early marker of physiologic invasion of placental tissue into uterine wall

- Hyperglycosylated beta—TUMORS
  - Including any advanced somatic tumors (e.g., breast, lung)
  - Free beta and hyperglycosylated beta are directly synthesized by cancer cells and promote tumor growth
    - Block apoptosis
    - Promote production of metalloproteinases
    - Promote production of collagenases
  - Sulfated alpha-beta—produced by pituitary in low levels in peri-/postmenopausal period
    - <20 in perimenopausal
    - 30 to 40 in postmenopausal
- See Fig. 16.1
- Serum—intact (alpha-beta) > free alpha > nicked > free beta
  - Urine—beta-core fragment (never seen in blood) > free alpha > alpha-beta
  - Tests detect intact only → not as sensitive in urine as serum!!
- Huge range in what can be normal for pregnancy
  - Cannot date a pregnancy based off of hCG levels
- Serum when period is <1 week late, quantitative is most sensitive
- Trends
  - Increases for 10 weeks, then decreases
  - Old adage—doubles every 2 days
  - Should increase 66% or greater in 2 days
- Women with IgA deficiency (up to 30%) can have false-positive serum tests from heterophile antibodies (which do not pass into the urine)
- Multiple gestations and molar pregnancies can have hCG >100,000
- Example reference ranges
  - Nonpregnant 0 to 5 IU/L
  - Pregnant, weeks from last menstrual period
    - 1 to 10 weeks: 64—151,000 IU/L
    - 11 to 15 weeks: 11,800—152,000 IU/L
    - 16 to 22 weeks: 9,380—61,400 IU/L
    - 23 to 40 weeks: 1,740—98,600 IU/L
- Ectopic pregnancy
  - Levels fail to rise ≥66% in 48 hours; nonviable intrauterine or ectopic pregnancy
    - However normal rate of rise can be seen in 20% of ectopics and abnormal can be seen in 20% of normal pregnancies
  - Confirm with pelvic ultrasonography
    - Can see gestational sac or intrauterine fluid at 4 to 5 weeks

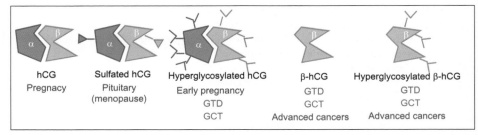

Fig. 16.1   Forms of human chorionic gonadotropin (hCG). *GTD,* Gestational trophoblastic tumor; *GCT,* germ cell tumor.

- After therapeutic removal, remains detectable for 2 to 3 weeks
- Gestational trophoblastic disease (GTD)
  - Usually higher than normal gestations
  - Complete moles hCG > incomplete moles
  - After evacuation, must monitor weekly until undetectable for 3 consecutive weeks (then measured monthly for 1 year)
    - May remain detectable for 10 weeks

VITAMINS

- Methylmalonic acid (MMA) is elevated in patients with vitamin B_{12} deficiency
- Best screening test for vitamin D is 25-hydroxyvitamin D
  - In sarcoidosis, 1-α-hydroxylase is increased, which increases 1,25-dihydroxyvitamin D
- When screening for vitamin D deficiency, do not need to differentiate D2 and D3
  - Only if the patient is being supplemented with D2 (most people get D3)
- MMA is best test to determine tissue B_{12} status (not B_{12} level)
- Whole-blood thiamine test is preferred over serum/plasma thiamine (B_1) test to determine thiamine deficiency
- Vitamin D, 17-hydroxyprogesterone, and estradiol are now mostly done by immunoassay (does have interference)

ENDOCRINE

General

- Heterophile antibodies can falsely increase *or* decrease immunoassays

Pituitary

- Posterior pituitary has axons directly from hypothalamus
  - Antidiuretic hormone and oxytocin
- Anterior pituitary is bathed in hormones in capillary network (from median eminence)
  - Thyroid stimulating hormone, adrenocorticotropin hormone, follicle-stimulating hormone, luteinizing hormone, growth hormone, prolactin

Prolactin

- The only hormone that is *negatively* regulated by hypothalamus
- Macroprolactinemia
  - Immunoglobulin-bound to prolactin, have high prolactin levels but does not actually do anything
    - Not clinically significant
  - Order macroprolactin level to differentiate

Growth Hormone (GH)

- Circulates as multiple isoforms, protein-bound to growth hormone–binding protein
- Assays are incredibly variable
- Must make standards commutable
- Secreted in pulsatile manner, do not use random screen for deficiency
  - Use IGF-1 and IGFBP-3 (random), then GH stim test if positive
  - IGF-1 = longer half-life but can be decreased in malnutrition, diabetes, and so on
  - IGFBP-3 is less influenced by nutritional status
  - GH stimulation test = L-DOPA, clonidine, propranolol, glucagon, arginine, (insulin-induced hypoglycemia)

- Must perform at least twice
- Normal response is >10 μg/L
- GH excess → gigantism (before growth plate fusion) or acromegaly (after)
  - Screen with IGF-1 → if increased or equivocal, do GH suppression test with glucose load (hyperglycemia)
    - Normal response is < 1 μg/L in 2 hours

Luteinizing Hormone (LH) and Follicle-Stimulating Hormone (FSH)

- Follicular phase
  - Starts at start of menses
  - Ends the day before LH surge
- Luteal phase
  - Starts with LH surges (switches to positive feedback)
- Amenorrhea causes
  - ↑ prolactin
  - ↑ TSH (hypothyroidism)
  - ↑ FSH (gonadal failure)
  - ↓ FSH (stress, anorexia, central deficiency from tumor/aneurysm, hemochromatosis)
  - Normal FSH (polycystic ovarian syndrome, testosterone-secreting ovarian tumor, congenital adrenal hyperplasia, or adrenal tumor)
- Testosterone should be measured 8 to 10 a.m. (peak)
  - If low, repeat and get LH/FSH
    - If LH/FSH is elevated, primary gonadal failure
    - If LH/FSH is low, secondary gonadal failure

Antidiuretic Hormone (ADH, Vasopressin)

- Vasoconstriction, free water conservation in collecting tube
- Stimulated by high blood osmolality
- Syndrome of inappropriate antidiuretic hormone (SIADH) = too much ADH
  - Hyponatremia, high urine osmolality (> 100), low blood osmolality
- Diabetes insipidus (DI) = too little ADH
  - Central—hyposecretion of ADH
  - Nephrogenic—kidneys resistant to ADH (lithium)
  - Diagnose with water restriction
    - Normal = increased urine osmolality (should be ≥300)
    - Abnormal = stable urine osmolality (or already elevated) with high plasma osmolality
      - Then give DDAVP
        - Central DI corrects
        - Nephrogenic DI does not

Oxytocin

- Let down reflex in lactating breasts
- Uterine contractions

Thyroid-Stimulating Hormone (TSH)

- Ectopic production of TSH is *extremely* rare (almost never the correct answer)
- Hypothalamus secretes thyroid-releasing hormone (TRH), which stimulates anterior pituitary to secrete TSH, which stimulates thyroid to release T_3 and T_4
- Thyroglobulin (TG)
  - Stored as colloid

- Building block of T_3/T_4
- Use serum TG concentrations to monitor for thyroid cancer recurrence
  - Related to amount of thyroid tissue
  - Anti-TG antibodies can interfere with assay (RIA)
- Thyroxine-binding globulin (TBG)
  - Protein that binds circulating T_3 to T_4
  - 75% of T4 and 80% of T_3
    - Transthyretin (prealbumin) and albumin bind the rest
- Thyroid peroxidase (TPO)
  - Adds iodine to tyrosine moieties
- Thyroid-stimulating hormone (TSH)
  - Shares alpha unit with ACTH and hCG
  - *Single best test for assessing thyroid function*
- Thyroid hormone forms
  - In order of decreasing bioactivity: $rT_3 > T_4 > T_3$ (named for number of iodine residues)
  - rT_3—virtually all from peripheral iodination of T_4, not bioactive
  - T_4—measured, little bioactivity
    - Free T_4 is preferred over free T_3, total T_3, or total T_4 because there is more T_4, and measuring protein-bound hormones can change based on protein levels (without functional changes)
  - T_3—BIOACTIVE
    - 80% from peripheral deiodination
    - Occasional patients can have T_3 toxicosis
    - Low TSH, normal free T_4 → can order T_3 (free < total)
      - Free T_3 is present in tiny amounts, practically unmeasurable
    - Elevation may occur earlier than T_4
- Causes of hyperthyroidism
  - Normal or increased radioactive iodine uptake (RIU, "hot")
    - Graves
    - Hashitoxicosis
    - Toxic adenoma/multinodular goiter
    - Iodine-induced (after deprivation)
    - Secondary to germ cell tumor or trophoblastic disease (hCG cross-reactivity)
    - TSH-producing pituitary adenoma
    - Spurious because of biotin interference
  - Decreased RIU ("cold")
    - Thyroiditis
    - Exogenous hyperthyroidism
    - Ectopic hyperthyroid (struma ovarii, metastatic carcinoma)
- Antibody tests not officially recommended—antithyroid peroxidase (TPO) and antithyroid hormone (formed as a result of thyroid damage in Graves and Hashimoto)
  - Markers of disease, not causative
  - Anti-TSH receptor (thyrotropin) *is* causative
    - "TSI"—thyroid-stimulating immunoglobulin
    - Most specific for Graves! (100%)
    - Stimulating, neutral, or blocking
  - Quantitate levels of TSI in serum
    - Quick, cheap, not specific for stimulating antibodies
  - Bioassay
    - Stimulatory effect of TSI on TSH-responsive cells
    - "TSI index"—reported as ratio (patient:control)

- Subclinical hypothyroidism
  - Normal fT_4 and increased TSH, most commonly in older women
  - Monitor if TSH is 4.5 to 10 mIU/L, and obtain TPO antibody (predicts risk)

Adrenal

Anatomy and Physiology
- Glomerulosa—aldosterone—mineralocorticoids (salt)
- Fasciculata—cortisol—glucocorticoids (sugar)
- Reticularis—androgens (sex)
- Medulla—catecholamines—epinephrine/norepinephrine
- Adrenocorticotropin hormone (ACTH) stimulates cholesterol migration into mitochondria where CYP enzymes do adrenal steroid synthesis
  - Renin-angiotensin system stimulates aldosterone component too

Neuroblastoma
- Diagnosis requires tissue diagnosis or elevated metabolites and metastasis
  - Homovanillic acid (HVA) and vanillylmandelic acid (VMA)
  - HVA is a dopamine metabolite (can become increased in L-DOPA patients)

Pheochromocytoma
- TRIAD: hypertension, headache, sweating
- Diagnosis
  - Low suspicion: 24-hour urine fractionated metanephrines or plasma spot check
  - High suspicion (familial history or syndrome)
1. 24-hour urine fractionated metanephrine
   - Metanephrine and normetanephrine (plus sulfate-conjugates)
2. 24-hour urine catecholamines
3. Plasma fractionated metanephrines
   - Mass on CT/MRI → MIBG
- Norepinephrine and epinephrine are high (*not* HVA or VMA)
  - Metabolized to normetanephrine and metanephrine intratumorally with COMT
    - Levels correlate with tumor size
  - Fractionated means they give you levels for both
  - Vanillylmandelic acid (VMA) is elevated but not specific
    - VMA and homovanillic acid (HVA) are specific for neuroblastoma because norepinephrine and dopamine are metabolized to VMA and HVA, respectively (via MAO)
- Paragangliomas (extra-adrenal pheochromocytomas) can produce dopamine (and therefore HVA)

Hyperaldosteronism
- Hypertension and hyperkalemia
- Aldosterone is still produced in secondary/tertiary adrenal insufficiency (as a result of renin-angiotensin system regulation)
- Plasma renin is decreased in primary hyperaldosteronism

Hypoaldosteronism
- Causes salt-wasting—hyponatremic hypochloremic hyperkalemic

Congenital Adrenal Hyperplasia (CAH)
- Causes

- Number 1: 21-hydroxylase deficiency is the most common cause of CAH (>95%)
    - Associated with increased 17-hydroxyprogesterone
    - Excess ACTH → ↑ DHEAS (androgen) → masculinization
        - Females have ambiguous genitalia
        - Boys more likely to be missed
    - Current newborn screen guidelines only recommend screening for this etiology
    - Number 2: 11-beta-hydroxylase
        - ↑ 11-deoxycortisol (a mineralocorticoid) → hypertension and hypokalemia
- *Partial* deficiency can present with normal cortisol
    - "Simple virilizing"—↑↑↑ ACTH, normal cortisol, normal or minimally ↑ aldosterone
- Salt-losing = severe
    - Low-to-no aldosterone or cortisol
    - 17-OH progesterone usually >10,000
    - Check sodium and potassium to avoid adrenal crisis
        - Hyponatremia, hyperkalemia, acidic, hypochloremia
- Gold standard—ACTH (cosyntropin) stimulation test
    - In reality, use genetics

Cushing Syndrome
- Hypercortisolism
- Centripetal obesity, moon facies, glucose intolerance, hypertension
    - Excess cortisol stimulates mineralocorticoid receptor
- Diagnosis
    - 24-hour urine cortisol
    - Overnight low-dose dexamethasone suppression test
        - No suppression = positive
    - Late-night salivary cortisol
- ACTH-dependent
    - Cushing disease (68%)—↑ ACTH from pituitary
        - Will not suppress at low dose but *will* suppress at high dose
    - Ectopic ACTH (12%)
    - Ectopic corticotrophin–releasing hormone (CRH, hormone from hypothalamus that stimulates ACTH secretion)
- ACTH-independent—all intra-adrenal pathology
    - Adrenal adenoma/carcinoma
    - Micro-/macroglandular hyperplasia
- Pseudo–Cushing—depression and alcoholism

Addison Syndrome
- Chronic adrenal insufficiency—hypocortisolism and hypoaldosteronism
- Acute
    - Altered mental status and hypotension
- Chronic
    - Fatigue, weakness, weight loss, hypotension, hyperpigmentation
- Hypoglycemia, hyponatremia, hyperkalemia, acidosis, hypercalcemia, high BUN, anemia, eosinophilia
- Primary, secondary, tertiary
    - Primary—congenital, CAH, autoimmune, tuberculosis, drugs
        - Acting on adrenal cortex
        - Hyperpigmentation in primary only—↑ ACTH (and ↑ melanocyte stimulating hormone)

- CAH is most common (73%)
- Autoimmune is most common in adults—anti-21-hydroxylase antibody
  - 12% overall, 70% to 90% in adults
- Secondary or tertiary—tumors/surgery/hemorrhage of sella
- Mineralocorticoids are not decreased in secondary or tertiary (because of renin-angiotensin stimulation)
- Diagnosis
  - Random one-time serum cortisol and ACTH
  - If abnormal, ACTH stimulation test

Conn Syndrome
- Hyperaldosteronism
- Hypertension, hypokalemia, alkalosis

Pancreas

Anatomy and Physiology
- Exocrine
  - Bicarbonate and enzymes (amylase, lipase, elastase, trypsin, chymotrypsin)
- Endocrine
  - Beta → insulin
    - See Fig. 16.2
  - Alpha → glucagon
  - Delta → somatostatin (inhibitory)
- Drug that increases insulin secretion without glucose
  - Sulfonylureas and glinides stimulate K_{ATP} channel
  - GLP-1 drugs (exenatide) increase cAMP

Diabetes Mellitus (DM) Criteria
1. Fasting glucose ≥126 mg/dL
2. HbA1c ≥6.5% (best)
   a. HbA1c
      i. Glucose added to N-terminal valine of hemoglobin A beta-chain (nonenzymatically)
      ii. Schiff base—Amadori rearrangement = glycation (not glycosylation)
3. Random ≥200 mg/dL + symptoms
4. 2-hour oral glucose tolerance test ≥200 mg/dL
   a. Pregnant women
   b. Equivocal other results
   c. Cystic fibrosis–related DM
      - If no clear symptoms, must repeat test once for definitive diagnosis

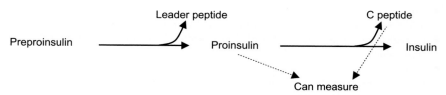

Fig. 16.2 Insulin precursor peptides.

Hypoglycemia
- Definition
  - Diabetics: ≤70 mg/dL
  - Nondiabetics: ≤55 mg/dL and symptoms *or* <40 mg/dL with or without symptoms
    - Insulin should be <3, C-peptide <0.6
- Whipple triad
  - Recognize that symptoms could be caused by hypoglycemia
  - Document that glucose is decreased when symptomatic
  - Show that symptoms go away when glucose is given
- Laboratory testing
  - Order insulin, C-peptide or proinsulin, sulfonylurea and glinide screen, beta-hydroxybutyrate levels
    - Insulin blocks ketosis
  - 72-hour fast (wait for symptoms to recur, and measure again)
  - Glucagon challenge
    - Normal ≤25
    - Hyperinsulinism → increased glycogen sequestration in liver → glucagon releases → >25
  - Average blood glucose = $(28.7 \times HbA1c) - 46.7$
- Differential diagnosis
  - Diabetic on insulin
  - Nondiabetic drug-induced (beta blockers, ACE inhibitors)
  - Alcohol (inhibits gluconeogenesis but not glycogenolysis)
  - Endogenous hyperinsulinism
    - Insulinoma
    - Nesidioblastosis
    - Anti-insulin receptor antibodies
  - Accidental/surreptitious use
  - Pseudo-hypoglycemia (not collected in gray-top tube)
  - Malnourishment
  - Cortisol deficiency
- Osmolality—moles/kg H_2O (preferred)
- Osmolarity—moles/L H_2O (can change with temperature)
- Serum osmolality = $2Na + (glucose/18) + (BUN/2.8)$
  - Normal gap <100 mOsm/kg
  - Would not expect an increase in gap in hyperglycemic hyperosmolar nonketotic syndrome because glucose *is* measured
  - Ethanol, methanol, ethylene glycol, mannitol, acetone, and isopropyl alcohol do

Diabetic Ketoacidosis (DKA)
- See Table 16.3
- Typically only in type 1 DM
- Hyperglycemia (glucose ≥200 mg/dL), ketosis (↑ acetone, acetoacetate, and β-hydroxybutyrate), metabolic acidosis (venous pH <7.3 or bicarbonate <15 mmol/L)
- Increased anion gap
  - AG = $Na - (Cl + HCO_3)$; normal = 10 to 20 mEq/L
- Left-shifted neutrophilia
- High amylase and lipase
- Hyperkalemia initially
  - Life-threatening hypokalemia can occur after treatment

TABLE 16.3 ■ Emergency Syndromes in Diabetes Mellitus

	Diabetic Ketoacidosis	Hyperglycemic Hyperosmolar Nonketotic Syndrome
General	Glucose <800, more common in type I, rapid onset, <65	Glucose >100, more common in type II, insidious onset, >65
pH	↓	↑
Bicarbonate	↓	↑
Ketone (urine/serum)	+	– (or small)[a]
Osmolality	Variable	↑↑ (>320)
Anion gap	↑	Variable
Mental status	Alert → drowsy → coma	Stupor or coma

[a]Because small amounts of endogenous insulin blocks lipolysis → ketones.

Hyperglycemic Hyperosmolar Nonketotic Syndrome (HHNS)

- Altered mental status, extreme hyperglycemia, hyperosmolarity, normal bicarbonate and ketones
- High mortality rate
- Serum osmolality = $(2 \times sodium) + (glucose/18) + (BUN/2.8)$
- Osmolar gap (OG) = (measured osmolality – calculated osmolality)
  - Normal gap <10 mOsm/kg
  - We would not see an increased osmolar gap, but osmolality would be increased
  - Increased OG with ethanol, ethylene glycol, methanol, mannitol, acetone, isopropyl alcohol
- Osmolality vs. osmolarity
  - Osmolality is the number of moles of solute in 1 kg of H_2O (solvent)
  - Osmolarity is the number of moles of solute in 1 L (volume) of H_2O (solvent)
  - Osmolality is preferred as the mass of H_2O is constant, whereas the volume of H_2O can change with temperature
  - However, overall these terms are often used interchangeably because the changes in volume of water with temperature are negligible

Gestational Diabetes Mellitus (GDM)

- World Heath Organization (WHO and American Diabetes Association (ADA) recommend one step
  - 75-g 2-hour oral glucose tolerance test (OGTT)
    - Diagnostic criteria
      - Fasting ≥92 mg/dL
      - 1 hour ≥180 mg/dL
      - 2 hours ≥153 mg/dL
- American College of Obstetricians and Gynecologists (ACOG) recommends two steps
  1. Screening nonfasting glucose challenge → 1-hour, 50-g test
     - Positive screen is ≥135 mg/dL
  2. If step 1 is positive, proceed to 3-hour 100-g test
     - Measure before (fasting) and at each hour. If one or more is increased, positive for GDM
       - Fasting ≥95 mg/dL
       - 1 hour ≥180 mg/dL

- 2 hours ≥155 mg/dL
- 3 hours ≥140 mg/dL
- Why test
  - Relative insulin resistance in third trimester resulting from human placental lactogen
  - Complications in…
    - Mother—preeclampsia, subsequent gestational diabetes
    - Baby—excess growth (necessitating caesarean section), postnatal hypoglycemia, type 2 diabetes mellitus later in life, perinatal death
- When to test
  - If risk factors are present, test at first prenatal visit
    - Family history, weight, inactivity, race, age, polycystic ovarian syndrome (PCOS), hypertension, abnormal lipids
  - If no risk factors, 24 to 28 weeks gestation

Pancreatitis
- Diagnosis
  - Pain—right upper quadrant, back radiation
  - Lipase/amylase three times the upper limit of normal
  - Confirm on imaging
- Poor prognostic markers: hemoconcentration, elevated BUN, hyperglycemia, age >55 years, elevated lactate dehydrogenase, hypocalcemia
- Etiologies: gallstones > alcohol > hypertriglyceridemia (over 100) > post-endoscopic retrograde cholangiopancreatography (ERCP) > trauma
- Lipase assay
  - Increase within 3 to 8 hours of insult; stays elevated for 1 to 2 weeks
  - More specific and sensitive
  - Other causes of high lipase—renal failure, acute cholecystitis, bowel obstruction/infarction, post-ERCP, HIV, DKA, drugs, and so on
- Amylase assay
  - Methods are based on the hydrolysis of starch
  - Increase within 3 to 8 hours of insult, stays elevated for 3 to 6 days
  - Can be normal in 20% of alcohol-related and 50% triglyceride-related
  - Macroamylasemia—high-molecular weight form of amylase in serum (usually immunoglobulin bound to amylase)
    - High serum levels, but low urine levels (amylase-immunoglobulin complex is too large to be filtered in the nephron)
  - Other causes of high amylase—salivary disease, gastrointestinal disorders, hepatitis, cirrhosis, gynecologic disorders, chronic alcoholism, pregnancy, trauma, burns, head injury, renal failure
- Chronic—imaging
  - Calcifications
  - Steatorrhea
    - Gold standard—72-hour quantitative fecal fat
    - Most used—spot fecal elastase
    - Also, secretin stimulation (collect duodenal fluid)
  - Pancreatic insufficiency—decreased fecal elastase

LIPIDS

Lipoprotein Biology

- Structure
  - Outside—cholesterol, phospholipid, and apolipoprotein outside

- Inside—cholesterol ester, free fatty acid, triglyceride in hydrophobic core
- In order of increasing density
  - Chylomicron (less dense than water)—ApoB-48, C, E, lots of triglycerides
  - Very-low-density lipoprotein (VLDL)—ApoB100, C, E
  - Intermediate-density lipoprotein (IDL)—ApoB100, E
  - Low-density lipoprotein (LDL)—ApoB100
    - Most plasma cholesterol is carried by LDL
  - High-density lipoprotein (HDL)—ApoA1, A2, C
- Separate using ultracentrifugation, electrophoresis, liquid chromatography
- Lipoprotein lipase allows for triglycerides to be released into muscle/adipose tissue from lipoproteins
- ApoE interacts with lipoprotein-receptor in liver
- Lipase breaks down chylomicrons into remnants
- Cholesteryl ester transfer proteins exchange triglycerides for cholesteryl esters on ApoB lipoproteins (VLDL, IDL, LDL)
  - Cholesteryl esters are then eliminated through liver (and LDL receptors)
  - Autosomal recessive deficiency leads to very high HDL levels

Assays

- Friedewald equation (mg/dL)
  - LDL = total − (HDL + VLDL)
  - VLDL = triglycerides/5
    - Not always accurate, but a decent estimation
  - Nonfasting samples underestimate LDL
- Cholesterol enzymatic assay measures cholesterol and cholesterol ester
- Triglyceride assay
  - Pseudohypertriglyceridemia can be secondary to increased plasma glycerol
    - Medications, detergents, alcohol
    - X-linked deficiency of glycerol kinase
- HDL assay used to employ polyanion to precipitate out non-HDL
  - *Now* there is a direct automated method
- Fredrickson classification

Pathophysiology

- Cardiovascular risk
  - LDL cholesterol is the dominant form of atherogenic (VLDL is also)
    - Non-HDL-C (LDL + VLDL) is more atherogenic than either VLDL or LDL alone
  - Chylomicrons transport dietary fat (triglycerides), atherogenicity is uncertain
  - Risk factors
    - Cigarette smoking
    - Hypertension
    - Dysglycemia (diabetes)
    - Other lipoprotein abnormalities
    - Age >65 years
  - Lipid level categorization
    - Cholesterol
      - Desirable <200 mg/dL
      - Borderline-high 200 to 239 mg/dL
      - High ≥240 mg/dL

- LDL
  - Optimal <100 mg/dL
  - Near optimal/above optimal 100 to 129 mg/dL
  - Borderline high 130 to 159 mg/dL
  - High 160 to 189 mg/dL
  - Very high ≥190 mg/dL
- Triglycerides
  - Normal <150 mg/dL
  - Borderline high 150 to 199 mg/dL
  - High 200 to 499 mg/dL
  - Very high ≥500 mg/dL
- HDL
  - Low <40 mg/dL
  - High ≥60 mg/dL
- Lecithin-cholesterol acyltransferase (LCAT) deficiency—↓ HDL
- ATP-binding cassette (ABC1) transporter deficiency (Tangier disease)
  - Autosomal recessive, rare
  - *ABCA1* mutated, chromosome 9
  - Unable to transfer cholesterol and phospholipids onto ApoA1
    - Complete absence of HDL
    - Increased cholesterol in cell membranes
  - Hepatosplenomegaly, peripheral neuropathy, orange tonsils, premature coronary artery disease
- Lipoprotein lipase deficiency
  - Autosomal recessive, rare
  - Large chylomicrons and ↑ VLDL
  - Unable to clear chylomicrons → ↑↑ in blood
  - Abdominal pain and pancreatitis
    - No increased risk for coronary artery disease (chylomicrons are not atherogenic)
  - Treatment with low fat diet and fat-soluble vitamin supplement
- LDL receptor mutations—↑ LDL
- Lipoprotein number and ApoE levels can be more useful than genetics for familial hypercholesterolemia

REPRODUCTION AND PREGNANCY

Infertility

- Work up both partners at the same time
- Males
  - Semen analysis—volume, pH, count, concentration, motility, morphology, agglutination, viscosity
- Female
  - Causes—PCOS, tube blockage (pelvic inflammatory disease), hyperprolactinemia, obesity, endometriosis, and so on
  - Menstrual history, serum progesterone, LH surge (OTC); rule out hyperprolactinemia or thyroid disease, FSH, estradiol
    - Progesterone secreted by corpus luteum, measured at day 21
      - If ovulation has occurred, it will be >3
      - See Fig. 16.3
    - FSH and estradiol measured on day 3, measures ovarian reserve

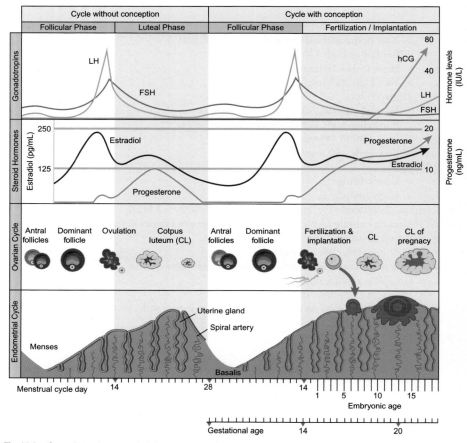

Fig. 16.3 Gonadotropin control of the ovarian and endometrial cycles. *hCG,* Human chorionic gonadotropin; *FSH,* follicle-stimulating hormone; *LH,* luteinizing hormone. (*Reproduced with permission from Mahendroo MS, Cunningham FG. Implantation and placental development. In Cunningham FG, Leveno KJ, Bloom SL, et al (eds): Williams Obstetrics, 25th ed. New York, McGraw-Hill, 2018a*).

- High FSH, low estradiol = primary ovarian failure
- Low FSH, low estradiol = hypopituitarism
- Low FSH, high estradiol = postmenopausal

- Anti-Müllerian hormone (AMH)
    - Secreted by immature testicular Sertoli cells
        - Triggers regression of fetal Müllerian ducts
        - Used as a marker of Sertoli cell function
            - Low in hypogonadotrophic hypogonadism
        - Used as a marker of Sertoli cell tumors
    - Downregulated in puberty by testosterone
    - NHANES study—for each unit increase in serum AMH, 13% lower risk for all-cause mortality
    - Concentration is 5 to 20 times lower in women than in men
    - Secreted by granulosa cells of immature follicles from birth to menopause

- Used as a marker of granulosa cell tumors
- Used as marker of primary ovarian insufficiency (Turner syndrome, status-post gonadotoxic agents)
  - Slowly decreases from third decade to menopause
    - Single measurement "below critical threshold" has 86% to 92% accuracy in predicting time to menopause
- Antral follicle count (via transvaginal ultrasound)
- Clomiphene challenge
- Low ovarian reserve
  - Measure FSH and E2 on cycle day 3
    - FSH > 10 to 20 IU/L: poor response to stimulation (reduced oocytes)
    - FSH normal but E2 > 60 to 80 IU/L: poor response to stimulation (caused by advanced premature follicle recruitment)
  - Anti-Müllerian hormone (<1 ng/mL bad), antral follicle count (US), clomiphene challenge test

Physiologic Changes in Pregnancy

- Estrogen increases transport proteins (e.g., thyroid-binding globulin)
- Relative insulin resistance in third trimester resulting from human placental lactogen
- Decreased albumin (increased free drug fraction and decreased total calcium), increased urine protein, increased blood volume with decreased hematocrit and hemoglobin, lower blood pressure, higher heart rate, higher tidal volume, increased clotting factor

Pathophysiology

Preeclampsia
- ≥140 systolic or ≥90 diastolic after 20 weeks on two occasions and proteinuria
  - *Or* severe features—thrombocytopenia, elevated creatinine, elevated ALT/AST, pulmonary edema, cerebral changes
  - "Proteinuria" = ≥300 mg per 24/hr *or* protein/creatinine ratio ≥0.3 *or* dipstick reading of 1+
- 24-hour urine collection, random urine (protein:creatinine), dipstick
  - Weekly platelet count and ALT/AST
- Eclampsia = previous plus seizures

HELLP Syndrome (Hemolysis, Elevated Liver Enzymes, Low Platelets)
- Diagnostic criteria
  - Microangiopathic hemolytic anemia with schistocytes on blood smear
    - Elevated indirect bilirubin and low serum haptoglobin
  - Platelets ≤100 × 109/L
  - Total bilirubin ≥1.2 mg/dL
  - Serum AST ≥70 U/L
- TREATMENT = DELIVERY

Fetal Lung Maturity (FLM)

- Background
  - FLM achieved at ~37 weeks; testing used between 32 and 38 weeks
  - Stressful pregnancy ↑ corticosteroids early FLM
    - Can utilize for preterm birth—give exogenous steroids
  - Maternal diabetes delayed FLM
  - Optimal specimen = amniotic fluid
  - Must confirm immaturity by second test

- Lecithin/sphingomyelin (L/S) ratio
  - L/S ratio ≥2.5:1 indicates maturity
  - Limitations
    - Not reliable in gestational diabetes
      - High ratio does not always correlate with FLM
      - Phosphatidylglycerol concentration is better
    - Contaminated amniotic fluid introduces false-positive risk
      - Meconium and blood decrease the ratio
- Phosphatidylglycerol (PG) concentration
  - PG concentration indicative of FLM
  - 35 to 36 weeks
  - Blood and meconium do not alter results
  - Limitation: late marker of maturity
- Lamellar body count (LBC)
  - Same size as platelets → can use platelet channel of cell counter to quantify
  - LBC >50, 000/mL is indicative of maturity
  - Limitations
    - Blood contamination decreases LBC
    - Meconium contamination increases LBC
- Fluorescent polarization assay
  - Measures the ratio of surfactant to albumin (S:A ratio)
  - <40 mg/G = immature; >55 mg/G = mature
  - Limitations
    - Results altered by blood and meconium
    - Wide gray zone (40 to 55)
    - No longer available
- Foam stability
  - Not used

Prenatal Screening

- First trimester—PAPP-A, hCG, and nuchal translucency
  - See the "Tumor markers, Serum" section for more on hCG
  - Down syndrome (trisomy 21) will have low PAPP-A, high free β-hCG, and increased nuchal translucency
- Second-trimester quad—inhibin A, unconjugated estriol (uE3), AFP, hCG
  - KNOW THE QUAD SCREEN PATTERNS FOR BOARD EXAMS. See Table 16.4
  - AFP can be increased by incorrect gestational age, neural tube defect, incorrect reporting of race, multiple-gestation pregnancy

TABLE 16.4 ■ **Quad Screen Patterns**

	AFP	uE3	Inhibin	hCG
Tri 21	↓	↓	↑	↑
Tri 18	↓	↓	—	↓
NTD	↑	↓	—	Normal

AFP, Alpha-fetoprotein; *uE*, unconjugated estriol; *hCG*, human chorionic gonadotropin; *Tri*, trisomy; *NTD*, neural tube defects.

- False positives can occur from overestimating gestational age
- hCG is elevated in Down syndrome, decreased in trisomy 18
  - Can be used for doping
  - Can be falsely elevated with heterophile antibodies
- Down syndrome—decreased AFP and uE3, increased hCG and inhibin A
- Amniotic fluid bilirubin
  - Concentration of unconjugated (indirect) bilirubin is a reflection of the severity of fetal hemolysis
  - Obtaining specimen
    - Minimal blood contamination
      - Oxyhemoglobin absorbance can spill over into bilirubin
    - Protect specimen from light by using brown plastic tube
      - UV light rapidly degrades bilirubin
  - Measurement
    - Maximal absorbance at 450 nm (measure 340 to 560 nm)
    - Plot a line for theoretical absorbance of amniotic fluid without pigment
      - Straight line on semilog plot from point at 350 nm to point at 550 nm
    - Measure actual absorbance and compare to previous line
    - Difference = ΔOD 450
  - Interpretation
    - Plot against estimated gestational age on nomogram
    - Queenan or Liley

Newborn Screening

- Heel stick 24 to 48 hours after birth (unless transfusion is planned)
  - And hearing screen at $\geq$12 hours
  - And pulse oxygenation between 24 hours and discharge (to screen for congenital heart disease)
- Newborn screening includes phenylketonuria (PKU), sickle cell, hypothyroidism, congenital adrenal hyperplasia, cystic fibrosis, spinal muscular atrophy (new addition, has a potential treatment), homocystinuria
  - Secondary conditions—can be in the differential of core conditions, unclear sequelae, possible drastic improvement with treatment, and so on

Congenital Disease

- Inborn errors of metabolism
  - Urea cycle disorder
  - PKU
  - Maple syrup urine disease—leucine, isoleucine, alloisoleucine, valine
  - Hyperornithinemia-hyperammonemia-homocitrullinuria
  - Homocystinuria
  - Cystinuria/hyperglycinemia—$\uparrow$ in urine, plasma, CSF
  - Methylmalonic acid—can be B_{12} deficiency or pernicious anemia too
  - Acyl CoA dehydrogenase deficiency—LCAD, MCAD, SCAD (long chain, medium chain, short chain)
  - Tyrosinemia
  - Ornithine transcarbamylase deficiency (OTC)
- Inborn errors of metabolism can present later in life, into adulthood
  - OTC can present after first pregnancy
- Acute metabolic crises tests

- Ammonia, CBC with differential, glucose, arterial blood gases, electrolytes, BUN and creatinine, uric acid
- Specialized
  - Ordered *after* positive newborn screen and genetic referral
  - Plasma amino acids, urine organic acids, plasma acylcarnitine
  - Serum lactate and pyruvate for mitochondrial disorders
- Increased (or rarely decreased) amino acids or organic acids
- Symptoms: none, low birth weight, failure to thrive, mental retardation, coma (caused by hyperammonemia), urinary tract stones, previous sibling death, acid/base disorders, ketones, osteoporosis, ocular degeneration, coarse features
- Sample: plasma, urine, CSF
  - Need to be de-proteinized or frozen quickly to avoid spontaneous deamination
  - Hemolysis—RBC arginase increases ornithine
  - High taurine can be secondary to thrombocytosis
- High-performance liquid chromatography
  - 42 amino acids separated by pK_a (low to high)
  - Buffer—2.3 to 2.8 gradient, temperature gradient
    - Acidic first, basic later
  - Anhydride dyes amino acids → Hitachi spectrometer records on two wavelengths
    - Plot against standard curve
    - One calibrator—arginine
    - Internal standard (example, *N*-acetyl lysine)
      - Neonatal lupus is caused by SS-A and SS-B, most common in mothers with SLE and Sjögren; only happens in 1% to 2%; can be the first indication of mother's autoimmune disease; most common presentation is heart block and rash

CRYOGLOBULINS

- Type I—single monoclonal antibody; associated with plasma cell myeloma, lymphoma, Waldenström macroglobulinemia
  - Does not have rheumatoid factor (RF) activity
- Type II—monoclonal IgM with polyclonal IgG
  - Associated with hepatitis C >>> HBV, HIV, EBV
  - Less frequently
  - Has RF activity (monoclonal)
- Type III—polyclonal IgG
  - Has RF activity (polyclonal)
- Must prewarm to 37°C and run warm

PLEURAL EFFUSIONS

- Transudate—systemic (cirrhosis/left heart failure)
- Exudate—infection, pulmonary emboli, cancer
  - High adenosine deaminase → tuberculosis
- See Table 16.5

ODDS AND ENDS

- Named methods
  - Jaffe—creatinine

TABLE 16.5 ■ Light's Criteria[a]

	Exudate	Transudate
Fluid:serum protein	>0.5	<0.5
Fluid:serum LDH	>0.6	<0.6
Fluid LDH >2/3 ULN	Yes	No

LDH, Lactate dehydrogenase; *ULN,* upper limit of normal.
[a]Only need one for exudate diagnosis.

- Jendrassik–Grof—bilirubin
- Hexokinase—glucose
- Fearon—urea
- Bromocresol purple/green—total protein
- Diazo—conjugated and unconjugated bilirubin
  - Uses caffeine as an accelerant
- Crystals—know coffin-lid for struvite (proteus mirabilis) and envelopes (calcium oxalate)
- Haptoglobins—up to one-third are not resulted because of hemolysis in the tubes
  - H-index = hemolysis index
- Procalcitonin
  - <0.5 → low risk for sepsis
  - 2 → high risk for sepsis
- Polyglandular autoimmune syndrome
  - Autoimmune adrenal insufficiency with other autoimmune endocrine disorders (thyroid, diabetes, parathyroid, pituitary)
- Sweat chloride test for cystic fibrosis (CF)
  - Can only be performed in Cystic Fibrosis Foundation–approved laboratories
  - Positive result is >60 mEq/L
    - Must be positive on two separate occasions
  - False negatives can be caused by low serum protein and edema (such as secondary to nephrotic syndrome)

Toxicology

TUBES

- See Table 16.6
- Royal blue—heavy metals—certified to be free of heavy metals

EQUATIONS

$$\text{Anion gap} = \left[Na^+ \right] - \left(\left[Cl^- + HCO_3^- \right] \right)$$
$$\text{RR: 8–16mmol/L, >20 is significant}$$

$$\text{Osmolal gap} = 2Na + \frac{BUN}{2.8} + \frac{glucose}{18} (\text{OSMg} >10\text{mOsm is significant})$$

TABLE 16.6 ■ **Color Tubes and Their Uses**

Tube	Additive	Type	Uses
Red	None	Serum	Serologies, ANA, CRP, serum toxicology, tumor markers
Green	Heparin sodium or heparin lithium	Plasma	Electrolytes, metabolic panels, LFTs, stat laboratory tests
Blue	Citrate	Plasma	PT/PTT, coagulation factors
Purple	Potassium citrate	Plasma	CBC/diff, T&S, ESR, reticulocyte count
Gray	Sodium fluoride or potassium oxalate (inhibit glycolysis)	Plasma	Glucose, lactate, ethanol, cocaine
Yellow	Citrate dextrose (preserves cells)	Plasma	HLA, DNA-based tests

ANA, Antinuclear antibody; *CBC*, complete blood count; *CRP*, C-reactive protein; *diff*, white blood cell differential; *DNA*, deoxyribonucleic acid; *ESR*, erythrocyte sedimentation rate; *HLA*, human leukocyte antigen; *LFTs*, liver function tests; *PT/PTT*, prothrombin time/partial thromboplastin time; *T&S*, type and screen.

$$\text{Calculated osmolality} = 2\text{Na (mEq/L)} \times \frac{\text{BUN (mg/dL)}}{2.8} + \frac{\text{glucose (mg/dL)}}{18} + \frac{\text{ethanol (mg/dL)} *0.83}{4.6}$$

If osmolal gap is increased but calculating with ethanol dose corrects it, the gap is caused by ethanol. If >10 mOsm gap is still present, suggests presence of isopropanol, methanol, acetone, or ethylene glycol.

$$\text{Vd} = \frac{\text{D}}{\text{C} \times \text{wt}} = \text{D} = \text{dose}, \text{C} = \text{plasma concentration}, \text{wt} = \text{wt in kg}, \text{Vd} = \text{volume of distribution}\left(\text{kg / L}\right)$$

$$\text{Average drug concentration at steady state} = \frac{1.44 \times \text{bioavailability} \times \text{dose}}{\text{Volume of distribution}} \times \frac{\text{half-life}}{\text{time interval}}$$

$$\text{Maintenance dose} = \frac{\text{desired steady-state concentration} \times \text{clearance rate} \times \text{time interval}}{\text{Bioavailability}}$$

$$\text{Half-life} = 0.693 / (\text{elimination rate})$$

$$\text{Blood alcohol content} = \frac{\text{alcohol}\left(\text{oz}\right) \times 5.14}{\text{Weight}\left(\text{lbs}\right) \times r} - \left(0.015 \times \text{hours since last drink}\right)$$

r is a constant. For men, 0.73. For women, 0.66.

GENERAL CONCEPTS

- Zero-order kinetics—no enzyme induction, can be saturated
  - Ethanol, fluoxetine, salicylate, phenytoin, omeprazole
- Some drugs cannot be distinguished by GC/MS or LC/MS-MS because they are isomers
  - Use HLPC instead

- Codeine and hydrocodone
- Morphine and hydromorphone
- Lead assays
  - Do not use EDTA tubes
  - Normal blood levels = 100 to 200 ng/mL
  - Acute poisoning → chelate!!
    - Dimercaptopurine
    - EDTA
    - Succimer
- Aluminum
  - Dialysis with hard water
  - Chronic exposure—bone disease and encephalopathy
  - Acute exposure—seizures, myoclonus, coma, microcytic anemia
  - Use a royal blue tube
  - Atomic absorption spectroscopy (AAS) or inductively coupled plasma mass spectrometry (ICP-MS)
- Aspirin = acetylsalicylic acid
  - Degrades to acetic acid with time—classically an empty bottle next to overdose victim that smells like vinegar
- Standard automated drug immunoassays
  - Can detect: tricyclic antidepressants, barbiturates, amphetamines, methamphetamine, cocaine, cannabinoids, phencyclidine (PCP), morphine, heroin, codeine, ethanol, hydromorphone, hydrocodone
  - Will miss: oxycodone, fentanyl, buprenorphine
- Cyclosporine, tacrolimus, sirolimus, everolimus—whole-blood testing, not temperature dependent, lyse and add internal standards (cyclosporine D)
  - Plus standards and controls bracketing each batch
  - Mycophenolate mofetil is a plasma assay (easier to run)
- Most common mass spectrometry mode is "triple quadrupole" analysis (selected reaction monitoring)

TOXIDROMES

- Anticholinergic
  - Dry as a bone, blind as a bat, red as a beet, hot as a hare
    - Anhidrosis, mydriasis (pupil dilation), flushing, fever, delirium
  - Picking movements, ataxia, agitation, nausea/vomiting, staring into space and muttering, vivid hallucinations, myoclonus, psychosis, seizures, urinary retention, dry mouth, tachycardia
  - Like sympathomimetic, but dry flushed skin instead of sweating
  - Antihistamines, atropine, tricyclic antidepressants, phenothiazines, anti-Parkinson drugs, cyclobenzaprine, scopolamine, Jimson weed
- Cholinergic
  - Watery nasal discharge, diarrhea, urination, miosis (pupil constriction), muscle weakness, tachy- or bradycardia, sweating, emesis, lacrimation, marked salivation, bronchorrhea, bronchoconstriction → wheezing and coughing → respiratory failure
  - DUMB BELSS—diarrhea, urination, miosis, bradycardia, bronchorrhea and -constriction, emesis, lacrimation, sweating, and salivation
  - SLUDGE—salivation, lacrimation, urination, defecation, gastrointestinal distress, emesis/eye miosis

- Organophosphate and carbamate insecticides (cholinesterase inhibitors), certain mushrooms, nicotine, lobeline, coniine (poison hemlock)
- Opioid
  - Coma, <u>central nervous system depression</u>, respiratory depression, bradycardia, hypotension, hypothermia, <u>miosis</u>, pulmonary edema, decreased bowel sounds, decreased reflexes
  - Morphine, codeine, diacetylmorphine, oxycodone, hydrocodone, hydromorphone, methadone
    - Meperidine and propoxyphene causes mydriasis, not miosis
- Sedative-hypnotic
  - Sedation, respiratory depression, hypotension, hyporeflexia, nystagmus, dysarthria, staggering gait, apnea, coma
  - Benzodiazepines, barbiturates, meprobamate, ethchlorvynol, zolpidem
- Sympathomimetic
  - Increased norepinephrine
  - CNS excitation (agitation, anxiety, tremors, delusions, paranoia), tachycardia, hypertension, mydriasis, hyperpyrexia, diaphoresis, seizures, cardiac arrhythmias, coma
  - Like anticholinergic except sweating instead of dry flushed skin
  - Amphetamines, cocaine, PCP, ephedrine, methcathinone, pseudoephedrine
- Hyperthermic syndromes
  - Sympathomimetic toxicity
  - Uncoupling of oxidative phosphorylation (salicylate poisoning and illegal diet pills)
  - Serotonin syndrome
  - Neuroleptic malignant syndrome
  - Malignant hyperthermia
  - Anticholinergic poisoning
  - Withdrawal syndromes (sedative-hypnotic and ethanol)
- Fomepizole or ethanol for methanol or ethylene glycol poisoning

Laboratory Management

CLINICAL LABORATORY IMPROVEMENT ACT (CLIA) 1988

- In response to cytopathology quality issues (pap farms)
- Non-Medicare-affiliated laboratories are still subject to CLIA rules
  - *Research only* laboratories are not
- The Center for Medicare and Medicaid Services (CMS) was responsible for implementing the CLIA
  - Surveys, fee collection, enforcing
- The Food and Drug Administration (FDA) categorizes test complexity
  - Low = waived
  - High or moderate = not waived
- Certificate of…
  - Waiver
  - Provider-performed microscopy
  - Registration → pending survey
  - Compliance → inspected by CMS
  - Accreditation → inspected by accreditation organization (like the College of American Pathologists)
- Waived tests—still need CLIA certificate

- Cleared for home use
- Simple methods (errors are negligibly rare)
- Pose no reasonable harm to the patient if performed incorrectly
- Mostly used in physician office laboratories
- Joint Commission accredits *hospitals* and can be the accrediting agency for laboratories for certificate of accreditation
  - Others for laboratories: American Association of Blood Banks (AABB), American Society for Histocompatibility and Immunogenetics (ASHI), Commission on Office Laboratory Accreditation (COLA)
- CLIA-exempt states—NY and WA
  - Have state-accrediting organizations that are as stringent or more stringent than CMS
- Proficiency testing (PT)—need 80% passing rate *except...*
  - A, B, O, Rh typing and compatibility testing (need 100%)
  - Cytopathology PT (must be performed at least annually)
    - 10 slides with 90% pass rate
      - If failed → another 10 slides (90%)
        - If failed → training and all work reexamined, 20 slides (90%)
- If failed → 35 hours of instruction, no interpretive work, must pass 20-slide test to resume
  - If cytotechnologist routinely screens slides for you, they can screen PT slides
- Always treat PT samples just like patient samples *unless* you would normally send them out to another laboratory (enter that you would send out)
- Regulated analytes
  - Need five challenges per test, three tests per year
  - Example: cholesterol value must be in +/− 30% of the mean of peer group (those with same instrument/methodology)
- Archives
  - Generally—2 years
  - Blood bank—5 years
    - Immunohematology (for FDA)—quality control (QC) data for 10 years
  - Anatomic Pathology
    - Slides—10 years
    - Blocks—10 years
    - Reports—10 years
    - Fine-needle aspiration (FNA) slides—10 years
    - Non-FNA cytology slides—5 years
- Important abbreviations
  - ICD—International Classification of Diseases
    - Set of terms that describe medical conditions
  - CPT—Current Procedural Terminology
    - Medical language used to report procedures and services
  - LOINC—Logical Observation Identifiers Names and Codes
    - Universal language to identify tests and results in a laboratory

LABORATORY AUTOMATION AND INSTRUMENT SELECTION

- Can automate almost any step in testing
  - Barcoding (code 128B symbology for "1D codes")
  - Specimen delivery
  - Task targeted (e.g., uncappers, centrifuges, aliquoters)

- Multifunctional or total laboratory automation
  - Integrate multiple automated modules, typically connected by conveyer belt
  - Most efficient for high-volume laboratories
- Evaluating utility of automation
  - 80% rule
    - If 80% of workload can be standardized and automated, automation is justified
  - Challenges
    - Instrument vendors may not support systems that are not their own brand
    - May ↑ turnaround time (TAT) paradoxically
- Contiguous flow analyzers—inject reagents into stream of patient sample
- Centrifugal flow analyzers—champers → (centrifugal force) → cuvettes
  - Can batch
- Random access analyzers—"selective analyzers"
  - Random orders
  - Multiple channels/wells
  - +/− stat lane
- Selecting new instrument
  1. Asses laboratory needs
  2. "Request for info" from manufacturers (generals)
  3. Prelim cost analysis → "request for proposal" (specifics)
  4. Laboratory grades proposals
  5. Site visit by final candidates (must have at least two)
  6. Final cost analysis
  7. Contract negotiation and budget request from health system
  - Considerations
    - Test menu, anticipated volumes, quality of results (ask other laboratories that are not on the company's list), finances (buy, lease, "free" with X # of reagent purchases), analytical methods used, instrument size/footprints and associated construction cost, maintenance contract (24/7/365 is ideal)

METHOD VALIDATION

- "Measurement procedure" = method
- A lot of guidelines on validation are *recommended*
  - For example, if assay detects very rare condition, you cannot get 40 samples to verify accuracy
- FDA-approved tests come with their own data (sensitivity, specificity, reportable range, reference interval)
  - But they must be *verified* on our machine
  - Laboratory developed tests (LDTs) or a modified version of an FDA-approved test require your laboratory to do *all* of this
- Minimum that needs to be performed for a moderate complexity assay
  - Accuracy
  - Precision
  - Reportable range
  - Confirmation of manufacturer's reference range
- Accuracy—20 to 40 samples (modified FDA tests or LDT, recommended > 40)
  - Compare with standards
  - Compare with another method (in-house or out)

- Compare series from individual patients
- Compare results from PT materials
- Precision
  - FDA approved—5 × 5 × 2
    - 5 days, 5 samples, 2 replicates
  - Modified-FDA and LDT: 20 × 2 × 2
    - 20 days, 2 samples, 2 replicates
  - Levy-Jennings plot
- When establishing specificity, choose drug or substance that *may* interfere logically
- Analytical measurement range (AMR)
  - FDA—5 concentrations, 2 replicates
  - Modified FDA (mFDA) and LDT—7 to 11 concentrations, 2 to 4 replicates
- Reference interval
  - FDA 20 to 40
  - LDT and mFDA—120
    - For rare diseases or tests, can do 40 to 60
  - All are made to capture 95% of *normal* cohort, except for troponin (which is 99%)
  - When non-Gaussian, nonparametric > parametric
- Calibration verification
  - Testing known analyte concentration throughout reportable range and confirming values are within allowable error
  - Perform each 6 months, after major servicing, with new lots, and when performance is questionable
- Delta check—compares current results with previous and flags if outside acceptable limits
  - For example, run patient complete blood count sample on old instrument and new instrument, then compare.

PEDIATRIC LABORATORY MEDICINE

- Collecting samples—heel, finger (capillary blood is different than venous or arterial blood), antecubital, umbilical artery, scalp vein, jugular vein, central vein
- More common to draw off a line to avoid additional sticks
- Smaller blood volumes, tubes, needles
  - No more than 3% to 5% of blood volume can be taken off in a single draw
- Urine collections are difficult
  - Taped bag, catheterize
- Need to have strategies for preparing/comforting while drawing blood
  - Numbing cream, distractions, rewards
  - Infants—breastfeed during draw, Sweet-Ease
- More likely to be hemolyzed
- Some automatic equipment cannot handle small-volume specimens
  - Manual aliquoting introduces time and error
  - Need adapter for centrifuging
- Reference intervals may change with age, weight, pubertal status
  - Example: Alkaline phosphatase has an increased upper limit of normal during ages of bone growth
  - Can adopt published intervals without verification (CLSI approved via "laboratory director .")
    - CALIPER project

- Unique/more common tests in pediatrics: next-generation sequencing (NGS), sweat chloride (can only be performed at Cystic Fibrosis Foundation–approved laboratories only), newborn screening via heel stick, lead screening, respiratory syncytial virus

METRICS

- Reference interval—normal population mean +/− 2 standard deviations
- Normal bell distribution (see Fig. 16.4).
- For skewed distribution, do a log transformation
  - Square root to make normal distribution
  - See Fig. 16.5.
- Normal person's chance that they'll have [X] number of test results abnormal, caused by random chance = $1 - (0.95)^n$
  - $1 \rightarrow 0.05 = 5\%$
  - $2 \rightarrow 1 - (0.95 \times 0.95) = 1 - (0.91) = 0.09 = 9\%$
  - $20 \rightarrow 1 - (0.95)^{20} = 1 - (0.36) = 0.64 = 64\%$
  - Caveat: the tests must be independent (i.e., not Na and Cl)
- Mean +/− 1 SD = 68%
  - Mean +/− 2 SD = 95%
  - Mean +/− 3 SD = 99%
- Can also define reference interval
  - Troponin I and T (different manufacturers) = 99th percentile
    - Arbitrary from committees
    - Decrease false positives and increase specificities
    - Coefficient of variation (CV) *must* be ≤ 10%
      - Tells us how wide the distribution is
      - = SD/mean
  - HbA1c > 6.5% or end-organ damage and glucose ≥ 126 mg/dL = diabetes
    - Retinopathy, nephropathy, neuropathy
    - In International System of Units (SI) units—7 mmol/L
  - Positive/negative
    - Example: pregnancy, microcultures, serology, drug screen
- Performance parameters (see Fig. 16.6).
  - Likelihood ratios

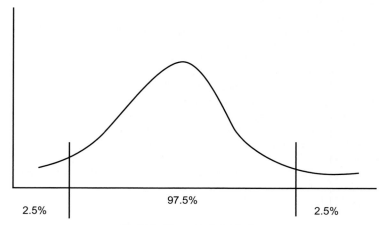

Fig. 16.4 Normal bell distribution.

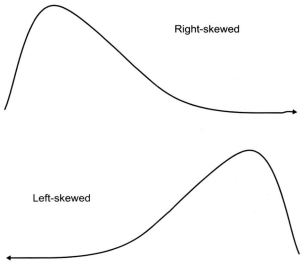

Fig. 16.5   Right- and left-skewed distributions.

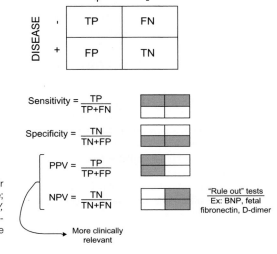

Fig. 16.6   Performance parameters and their relationships. *BNP,* Brain natriuretic peptide; *FN,* false negative; *FP,* false positive; *NPV,* negative predictive value; *PPV,* positive predictive value; *TN,* true negative; *TP,* true positive.

- Positive—odds of getting a positive result in a diseased patient
  - = sensitivity/(1 − specificity)
- Negative—odds of getting a negative result in a healthy patient
  - = (1 − sensitivity)/specificity

BIOLOGIC VARIATION

- Westgard rules website
- Important to understand normal changes versus significant
  - Population-based reference range

- How to determine whether difference is significant or not
  - 1. Calculate reference change value (RCV)
    - Exclude pre-analytical variables (CV_P)

$$RCV = Z + \sqrt{2} + \sqrt{CV_A^2 + CV_I^2}$$

  - Z = Z-score = probability that the assay result is x number of standard deviations away from the mean
    - 1.96 = 95% probability
    - 2.58 = 99% probability
    - Larger Z-score → larger variation → ↑ probability that two numbers are *not* significant if different
  - CV_A = analytical variation = pipetting, machine, reagent issues
  - CV_I = within-subject biologic variation
  - 2. Calculate actual change %
    - Change = 100 × [(higher number − lower number)/lower number]
  - 3. If the actual change is higher than the calculated RCV, then the numbers are significantly different
- Index of individuality = CV_I/CV_G
  - CV = (standard deviation/mean) × 100%
  - CV_I = within-subject biologic variation
  - CV_G = between subject bio variation
  - Higher value (> 1.4) → each patient has wide variation
  - Lower value (< 0.6) → wide variation between patients
    - Do not use population-based reference range; use trends

DIRECTING A CLINICAL LABORATORY

- Costs
  - Capital expenses
    - Lasts longer than 1 year, costs over a set minimum limit, replaces old equipment or supports new products/services
  - Direct costs
    - Traceable to a billable test and end product
  - Indirect costs
    - Not traceable but still necessary to run
    - For example, proficiency testing subscriptions
  - Variable costs
    - Change proportionately with volume of tests
  - Fixed costs
    - Do not change with test volumes
  - Operating expenses
    - Costs incurred to produce a product or service
- Laboratory vendor models
  - Service level agreement (SLA)
    - Outlines responsibility of provider (classically information technology) and client
    - Defines quantifiable metrics and targets of system reliability, response time, and up-time
    - Outlines how technical problems will be addressed
  - Application service provider (ASP)

- Outsources all aspects to a remote location and charges laboratory a fee for use
  - Hardware, software, upgrades, security, data storage
- Advice from Dr. Amy Karger (University of Minnesota)
  - Make an effort to network with or meet clinicians
  - Take some time to observe the status quo before you make wholesale changes
  - Be prepared to deal with a lot of complaints
  - Spend time during the first year familiarizing yourself with the laboratory (tests, instruments)
  - Calls to laboratories are usually not positive feedback
    - Respond promptly and thoroughly with respect for question/request
- Helpful websites
  - http://mayomedicallaboraties.com
  - http://labtestsonline.org
  - http://www.westgard.com
  - www.pubmed.org
  - www.aacc.org
  - https://www.cms.gov/regulations-and-guidance/legislation/CLIA/index.html? redirect = /clia
- CLIA guideline tidbits
  - Exceptions to requiring CLIA certificates
    - Only forensic testing
    - Only research testing that do not report back to patient
    - Only drug of abuse testing (certified by Substance Abuse and Mental Health Services)
    - Washington state or New York state (see earlier)
  - Geographically separated locations in same system/with same director need *different* CLIA certificates

CHAPTER 17

Genetics in Pathology

Basic Molecular and Cell Biology

- Alternative mRNA splicing mechanisms = different "splice acceptor sites"
  - Aberrancy caused by mutation in splice acceptor, splice donor, branch site
- mRNA translation control = miRNA
- Protein structures
  - Primary—amino acid sequence
  - Secondary—alpha-helix or beta-pleated sheet (among others)
  - Tertiary—how secondary structures interact within a polypeptide
  - Quaternary—how secondary and tertiary interact between polypeptides
- See Fig. 17.1.
- Meiosis—only germ cells
  - 1. Replication to 4 N
  - 2. Meiosis I to 2 N
    - Recombination occurs here
    - Nondisjunction most commonly occurs here
    - Oocytes pause at prophase I, restart at ovulation to metaphase II, pause until fertilization
  - 3. Meiosis II to 1 N
- Chromosomes > minibands > chromatin fiber > nucleosomes > DNA + 1 histones
  - 2 H2A, 2 H2B, 2 H3, 2 H4
- Histone modification by...
  - Acetylation, ubiquitination, mono-/di-/trimethylation of lysine (K)
  - Mono-/dimethylation of arginine (R)
  - Phosphorylation of serine (S)
- Epigenetics—cell heritable changes in gene activity not based on DNA sequence differences
  - Creating *permissive* or *repressive* chromatin states/configurations
    - Methylation of cytosine residues
    - Histone modifications
    - Chromatin remodeling
  - *Not* transcriptional regulation (not heritable to daughter cells)
- Alpha satellite or alphoid sequence—major repeat component of centromere DNA
- Telomeres—TTAGGG repeats
- Mitochondria sort randomly during mitosis
  - Daughter cells can get different proportions of affected mitochondria
    - Homoplasy—all mitochondria in a cell are affected
    - Heteroplasmy—*some* are affected
- Classification on genes
  - Protein-coding genes
  - Noncoding, RNA-only genes
  - Regions of transcription regulation
  - Other conserved elements

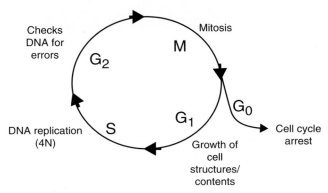

Fig. 17.1 Cell cycle.

- 1qter = terminus of long arm of chromosome 1
- rRNA, tRNA, snRNA, snoRNA, miRNA, lincRNA, others
- CNCs = conserved noncoding DNA sequences (transcription regulation regions)
- LINEs = long interspersed nuclear elements—autonomous transposable nonfunctional insertions
  - Compose 20% of genome
- SINEs = short interspersed nuclear elements, includes Alu repeats
  - Compose 13% of genome

Methods

CYTOGENETICS

- Specimens received include peripheral blood (PB), bone marrow (BM), products of conception, skin, solid tumors
- We can use FISH on interphase cells (do not need to be dividing or cultured, faster)

G-Banding

- Morphology
  - Light (negative) have 45% guanine and cytosine (GC), gene–rich
  - Dark (positive) have 37%, more adenosine and thymine (AT)
  - Chromosomes 17, 19, 22 are gene–rich
  - Chromosomes 13, 18, X are gene–poor
  - Chromosomes 1, 9, 16, and Y are acrocentric
    - Stalks and satellites on acrocentric chromosomes—13, 14, 15, 21, 22
      - Only ones that can have Robertsonian translocations
      - Satellites = nucleolar organizing region (acrocentric attraction)
      - Tandem repeats with hundreds of copies of rRNA genes (deleting is okay because we have backups)
  - Polymorphic regions
    - 1, 9, 16, and Y have heterochromatin regions in proximal Q arm (distal in Y)
      - Constitutive heterochromatin functions to regulate crossing over
        - Consists of alpha satellite DNA, AT-rich
        - Facultative heterochromatin = Barr body
      - Stains darkly
      - C-banding using barium stains heterochromatin
      - Chromosome 1 can get long, banded heterochromatin (just stretched out)

- Use to identify clones
  - Example: The bone marrow transplant recipient had a small heterochromatin region in chromosome 9, where the donor has a large region.
- Alpha satellite (micro- and mini- too) DNA = tandem repeats that separate from other sequences on a gradient → "satellite"
  - Generally not transcribed
  - Repeat of 171 bps, binds with CENP-B, near centromere
    - Mini = repeats of 20 to 70 bps
    - Micro = repeats of 2 to 4 bps
    - Short interspersed elements (SINE-contains Alu family) or LINE
- Media
  - Need green top tube (sodium heparin) and 3 to 5 mL of BM or 5 to 10 mL of PB
  - 0.5 to 1 cm³ in RPMI or saline for lymph node or solid tumor
  - Can use purple top from flow cytometry for FISH and microarray
- Mitogens (used to start mitosis)
  - T cells = PHA
  - B cells = BMA + oligonucleotide
  - Myeloid = 24-hour unstimulated
  - Unknown = 24-hour unstimulated
- Colcemid stops mitotic spindles
- G banding resolutions (400, 550, 850) (metaphase, prometaphase, prophase)
  - Least amount we can detect is 5 Mb
  - Array can see down to 30 kb (cannot see balanced translocations)
- For constitutional karyotype, we use peripheral blood T cells
- Peripheral blood chromosomes are a lot longer (less condensed) than bone marrow
  - Ethidium bromide intercalates and spreads out peripheral blood chromosomes

Fluorescent in Situ Hybridization (FISH)

- Cannot compare G-banding % of abnormal cells to FISH because G-band cells are cultured, which can select for certain clones
- Types of probes (400–600 kb)
  - CEP = centromere enumeration probes
    - Used to count chromosome copies
    - 13 and 22, 14 and 21 cross–react—do not use CEP
  - Locus–specific probe—to a locus other than the centromere
    - Dual fusion probe
      - Normal = 2 red, 2 green
      - Translocation = 2 yellow, 1 green, 1 red
    - Extra signal fusion probe
      - Normal = 2 red, 2 green
      - Translocation = 1 green, 1 big red, 1 tiny red, 1 yellow
    - Break-apart probe—used for promiscuous genes (*KMT2A, IGH*) or that can be seen in multiple abnormalities [t(16;16) or inv(16)]
      - Less likely to see false positives for break–aparts than fusions (which happen from signals overlapping)
      - Normal = 2 yellow
      - Rearranged = 1 yellow, 1 green, 1 red

Products of Conception (Determining Ploidy)

- Partial mole
- Most common cause of triploidy = 1 egg + 2 sperm

- Two copies of father's DNA, one copy of mother's—intrauterine growth restriction, macrocephaly, hydrocephaly, hypotonia, spontaneous abortion (not all show molar features, especially digyny)
- Two copies of mother's DNA, one copy of father's—malformed/degenerative "grape–like" placenta
- P57+ (only expressed in maternal–derived tissue) (p53 can be positive)
- Two populations of villi, not quite as hydropic as complete, can have red blood cells in villi
- Complete mole
  - Cisterns, hydropic villi, one population, uniform cytotrophoblasts, no fetal parts (including red blood cells)
  - Diploid, all genetic material from father
  - No fetal formation, only molar placenta
  - 46, XX >>> anything else (2nd = 46, XY)
- Fertilization of an empty ovum by normal sperm, then DNA duplicated

Other

- MLPA—multiplex ligation–dependent probe amplification
  - Can test for deletions (like *IKAROS*)
  - Not good sensitivity, needs $\geq$ 75% blasts (not good for following minimal residual disease)
  - DNA-based, can test for multiple loci
- We can strip G-banding after identifying chromosomes, then FISH to see where extra DNA (identified on microarray) is inserted
  - "G to FISH"
- DFISH = "snapshot" of what's happening; cells harvested to save for FISH after G-banding culture is finished (5 million cells)
  - G-banding may find aneuploidy we can follow by FISH, but we need baseline
  - G-banding may increase sensitivity

International System for Cytogenetics Nomenclature (ISCN)

- Insertions—recipient first
  - Example: 12 received from 10 = ins(12;10)
- "Inc" = incomplete, cannot tell what's what
- "Proximal" and "distal" are in relation to the centromere
- / separates cell lines (mosaic)
- // separates chimeric DNA (in bone marrow transplant)
  - Recipient // donor
- Idem = "the same as what came before" in Latin
- [#] = how many cells had that karyotype
- Der = derivative, needs more explanation about what's changed, unbalanced!
- FISH—(*ETV6* × 3, *RUNX1* × 1)(*ETV6* con *RUNX1* × 1)

MOLECULAR

- Genome = 3.2 billion base pairs (bp)
- Exome = 30 million bp
  - Only 80% to 95% can be sequenced
- Detect single nucleotide polymorphisms (SNPs) or copy–neutral loss of heterozygosity (LOH), or copy # change
- A … SNP has an minor allele frequency (MAF) of …
  - Common … > 5%

- Near rare ... 1% to 5%
- Rare ... < 1%
- Mixed polymorphisms
  - Combination of repeat size variants and single nucleotide variants
  - "Barcode" of DNA
- Short sequence repeats (SSRs)
  - Microsatellites—2 to 5 bp, 1 to 15 repeats
  - Minisatellites—15 to 500 repeats
- Copy number variants (CNVs)
  - 50 kbp to 5 Mbp, detected by comparative genome hybridization (CGH) array

ACMG Classification

- Pathogenic
  - Very strong PVS1
  - Strong PS1–4
  - Moderate PM1–6
  - Supporting PM1–5
- Benign
  - Stand–alone BA-1
  - Strong BS1–4
  - Supporting BP1–6
- Numbers do not convey changes in importance, just for easier reference

Polymerase Chain Reaction (PCR)

- Extraction
  - 9 mL blood → 300 to 350 µg DNA
  - RNA analysis needs FRESH sample
    - Easily contaminated (RNA is everywhere)
    - 2.5 mL blood → 3 µg RNA
    - Can extract all species (e.g., mRNA, rRNA, tRNA)
  - Isolate cells, lyse cells, remove proteins, isolate DNA, hydrate DNA
- Hybridization
  - Denaturation of DNA, then annealing of primers
- Extension
- Labeling/amplifying/sizing
- Sequencing

Microsatellite Arrays

- Oligonucleotide sequences on solid surface (chip or bead)
- Test 44 to 500 kbp (kilobase pairs, 1000 base pairs; evenly spaced throughout the genome)
- Each spot is known
- Label DNA (or cDNA) from patient with dye then add it to array
  - If using control, use *equal* amounts of DNA
- Can vary on
  - Number of probes
  - Distribution of probes
  - +/− enrichment in genes of interest
- Uses
  - SNP detection

- CGH
- Gene–expression profile (mRNA or DNA)
  - Also can be done by NGS
  - Comparative, not absolute
  - May not reflect actual protein production
- Loss of heterozygosity (LOH; copy neutral)

Comparative Genomic Hybridization (CGH)

- Detects copy number variants (not LOH and not balanced translocations)
- Areas covered by array will affect which CNVs are detected
- Compared with pooled control
  - Yellow—equal amounts
  - Red—higher in patient sample
  - Green—lower in patient sample

Next-Generation Sequencing (NGS)

- Massively parallel, high-throughput sequencing
- Solid tumors and some heme can be done by PCR (smaller area of interest)
- Coverage
  - For inherited conditions—20 to 30× needed for ~99%
    - Test blood
  - For cancer, need even higher
    - May be difficult to get enough sample (fine–needle aspirates, formalin–fixed paraffin–embedded tissue)
- Quality
  - Phred or Q scores
  - Q10—90% accurate
  - Q20—99%
  - Q30—99.9%
  - Q40—99.99%
- Workflow
  - Library prep (amplicon–based library prep captures only regions of interest and avoids pseudogene) and enrichment (amplified with probes specific for region of interest)
  - Sequencing
  - Base calling
  - Sequence alignment
  - Variant calling

Other

- High-sensitivity *BCR-ABL1* PCR = log 4.5 = 1 in 32,000 cells
  - If negative × 3, can come off lifetime tyrosine kinase inhibitor
- Genome-wide association studies (GWAS)
  - SNP array that is cheaper than NGS
  - Must be known SNP → "common variants with small effects"
  - Used in epidemiologic studies
- Sequence capture
  - Large scale
  - Baits bind to DNA, unbound DNA discarded, use magnetic beads to capture, digest baits, amplify, and sequence
  - Versus PCR (smaller with better enrichment of target sequence)

Human Genetic Variation

- "Reference" human genome with one "correct" nucleotide at each position: we all differ from this
  - Reference has errors
  - Reference has disease–causing as alleles (e.g., factor V Leiden)
- Diagnostic testing—find variant to explain phenotype
- Carrier testing
- Predictive testing (e.g., Huntington)
- Precision medicine—guide individual medical management
- "Polymorphism" = more common, not necessarily bad
- "Mutation" = pathogenic connotation, use "variant" instead
- "Standards and Guidelines for the Interpretation of Sequence Variants" paper
  - Pathogenic, likely pathogenic, variant of unknown significance (VUS), likely benign, and benign
- We have 140,000 individual genomes (exac, nomad, 1000 genomes, exome variant server)
  - Not necessarily "healthy"
  - Some races underrepresented (e.g., Hmong)
- Onset, penetrance, and expression variation complicate things
- In silico models predict pathogenicity (e.g., conservation of sequence, splicing)
  - Considered weak evidence

Tumor Syndromes

- Tumor syndromes caused by DNA repair defects
  - *MUTYH*-associated polyposis
  - Xeroderma pigmentosa
  - *BRCA1*
  - *BRCA2*
  - Ataxia telangiectasia
  - Lynch (hereditary nonpolyposis colorectal carcinoma, HNPCC) syndrome
- Tumor (and nontumor) syndromes caused by chromosomal breakage
  - Ataxia telangiectasia
  - Bloom syndrome
  - Fanconi syndrome
  - Xeroderma pigmentosa
  - Nijmegen syndrome
- Syndromes with increased pancreatic adenocarcinoma risk
  - Peutz–Jeghers syndrome—100×
  - Familial atypical mole melanoma—50×
  - Hereditary pancreatitis—50×
  - Familial adenomatous polyposis, *BRCA2*, ataxia telangiectasia, Lynch—2 to 10×
- Syndromes with increased hepatocellular carcinoma risk
  - Hereditary hemochromatosis
  - Tyrosinemia
  - Glycogen storage disease
  - Porphyria cutanea tarda

- Alpha1-antitrypsin deficiency
- Wilson disease
- Galactosemia
- Li-Fraumeni
  - Sarcomas, 500× risk for osteosarcoma
  - Autosomal dominant (AD), *TP53* on 17p13
- Neurofibromatosis type 1 (NF1)
  - Neurofibromas (especially plexiform), malignant peripheral nerve sheath tumors, optic gliomas, rhabdomyosarcomas, pheochromocytomas, carcinoid tumors, café-au-lait, Lisch nodules, axillary freckling, leukemia, medulloblastoma, ampullary adenocarcinoma, breast cancer
    - Bone abnormalities including sphenoid dysplasia, scoliosis, and so on
  - AD, *NF1* gene → neurofibromin, 17q11
    - One-half are sporadic mutations
    - Leads to aberrant RAS signaling
      - Other "RASopathies"
        - Legius syndrome—*SPRED* mutation, café-au-lait spots and macrocephaly
        - Costello syndrome—*HRAS* mutation
        - Cardiofaciocutaneous syndrome
          - Type 1—*BRAF*
          - Type 2—*KRAS*
          - Type 4—*MEK2*
        - Noonan syndrome—*KRAS* or *BRAF* mutations
- Neurofibromatosis type 2 (NF2)
  - Schwannomas (bilateral vestibular nerve schwannomas—pathognomonic), neurofibromas, ependymomas, meningiomas, pilocytic astrocytoma
  - AD, *NF2* gene → merlin, 22q12
    - 30% are sporadic
    - Tumor suppressor
    - Disrupts normal "contact inhibition" of cell cycle
  - See Table 17.1
- Nevoid basal cell carcinoma syndrome (Gorlin syndrome)
  - Odontogenic keratocysts, basal cell carcinomas, bifid ribs, palmoplantar pits, medulloblastoma, rhabdomyosarcoma, meningioma, ovarian fibrothecomas
  - AD, *PTCH1* on 9q22.3
- Maffucci syndrome
  - Cavernous hemangiomas in tissues overlying chondromas
    - Can clot and calcify

TABLE 17.1 ■ **Neurofibromatosis Types 1 and 2**

Neurofibromatosis 1	Neurofibromatosis 2
Common	Rare
Neurofibromas, optic gliomas, iris nodules (Lisch), café-au-lait spots	Eighth nerve schwannomas, meningiomas, gliomas, nonneoplastic Schwann lesions
Lack *NF1* expression (neurofibromin, inhibits RAS)	*NF2* mutations (merlin, membrane receptor signaling)

- Albers–Schönberg syndrome
  - Diffuse radiopacity, persistence of cartilage at growth plates
  - Rare to absent osteoclasts
- Cowden syndrome—*PTEN* mutation on 10q23
  - Intestinal hamartomas, lipomas, fibromas, genitourinary malformations, trichilemmomas, papillomas, palmoplantar hyperkeratosis and pits, macrocephaly, developmental delay and autism, follicular thyroid carcinoma, breast/colon/endometrial carcinomas
  - Lhermitte–Duclos lesion—cerebellar dysplastic gangliocytoma
- Carney complex—*PPKAR1A* gene on 17q22–24
  - Lentiginous nevi, atrial myxomas, blue nevi, myxoid neurofibromas, ephelides (freckles), breast/Müllerian/skin myxomas, endocrine adenomas, of thyroid/pituitary/adrenal glands (including primary pigmented nodular adrenocortical disease), large cell calcifying Sertoli cell tumor of the testis, psammomatous melanotic schwannoma
- Gastrointestinal lesions
  - See Table 17.2
  - Peutz–Jeghers syndrome (PJS)
    - Most frequent genetic cause is AD, mutation in *STK11/LKB1* on 19p
      - Causes loss of regulation on mTOR pathway
    - Mucocutaneous hyperpigmentation
    - Hamartomatous intestinal polyps

TABLE 17.2 ■ **Hereditary Gastrointestinal Lesions**

Syndrome or Disease	Age at Presentation	Gastrointestinal Lesions	Other Lesions
Peutz–Jeghers	10–15 years	Polyps, CRC	Skin macules, lots of carcinoma
Juvenile polyposis	<5 years	Juvenile polyps; carcinomas of stomach, small intestine, colon, pancreas	Pulmonary arteriovenous malformations, digital clubbing
Cowden	<15 years	Hamartomatous polyps, lipomas, ganglioneuromas, inflammatory polyps, CRC	Skin, thyroid, breast tumors
Cronkhite–Canada	>50 years	Hamartomatous polyps	Nail atrophy, hair loss, abnormal skin pigmentation, cachexia, anemia
Tuberous sclerosis	Any	Hamartomatous polyps	Facial angiofibromas, cortical tubers, renal angiomyolipomas
Familial adenomatous polyposis	Any	Multiple adenomas	Congenital retinal pigmented epithelium hypertrophy, osteomas, desmoids, skin cysts, CNS tumors

CRC, Colorectal carcinoma; *CNS*, central nervous system.

- Do not undergo malignant transformation but PJS patients have an underlying increased risk for malignancy
  - Sex cord tumor with annular tubules (SCTAT) in ovary, calcifying Sertoli cell tumor in testis, adenoma malignum in cervix
  - Nasal polyps
  - Increased risk for cancers (including gastrointestinal)
- Juvenile polyposis
  - AD, *SMAD/BNPR1A* mutations
  - Increased colorectal carcinoma (CRC) risk—40% to 70% will get CRC by 60 years of age
  - Juvenile polyps in stomach < small intestine < colon
    - Multiple pedunculated polyps with expanded lamina propria and cystic glands
- Ataxia telangiectasia
  - *ATM* loss-of-function mutation
    - Tumor suppressor, double–stranded DNA repair protein
  - Telangiectasias, seborrheic dermatitis, cutaneous granulomas, café-au-lait spots, gray hair, skin atrophy, hypogammaglobulinemia, leiomyomas and leiomyosarcomas
  - Hematolymphoid, ovarian, breast, thyroid, gastric, salivary, and melanocytic neoplasms
  - Cerebellar atrophy → ataxia
- Multiple endocrine neoplasia syndromes
  - See Table 17.3
- Inherited 13q deletion
  - *RB1* deletion → retinoblastoma
  - Small eyes
  - Dysmorphic features
  - Small for age
  - Developmentally delayed

TABLE 17.3 ■ **Multiple Endocrine Neoplasia Syndromes**

	MEN1 (Wermer syndrome)	MEN2 2A	MEN2 2B
Genetics	Menin (*MEN1* at 11q13)	*RET* proto-oncogene (at 10q) mutation causing constitutively active tyrosine kinase	
Main disease	Primary hyperparathyroidism	Medullary thyroid carcinoma (with background C-cell hyperplasia)	
Additional manifestations	Pancreatic endocrine tumors (gastrinoma) Pituitary adenoma (prolactinoma) Carcinoid tumor	Pheochromocytoma Primary hyperparathyroidism	Pheochromocytoma Multiple neuromas Marfanoid habitus
Mnemonic	3 Ps: Parathyroid Pancreas Pituitary	1 M, 2 Ps: Medullary thyroid carcinoma Pheochromocytoma Parathyroid	2 Ms, 1 P: Medullary thyroid carcinoma Marfanoid/multiple neuromas pheochromocytoma
Rare others	Focal angiofibromas Collagenomas lipomas Meningiomas		

- *RB1* mutation (at 13q14)
  - Retinoblastoma
  - Osteosarcoma
  - Pineal gland tumors
  - Primitive neuroectodermal tumor (PNET)

RENAL CELL CARCINOMA (RCC) SYNDROMES

- Von Hippel–Lindau syndrome, 3p25–26 *(VHL gene)*, AD
  - Clear cell papillary RCC and clear cell papillary–like RCC
  - Central nervous system hemangioblastoma, pheochromocytoma, pancreatic neuroendocrine tumor (islet tumors), pancreatic cysts, cystadenomas of epididymis/broad ligament, papillary tumor of endolymphatic sac origin (temporal bone/inner ear)
- Birt–Hogg–Dubé, 17p11.2 (*BHD/FLCN*), folliculin, AD
  - Mixed chromophobe/oncocytoma
  - Cystic pulmonary lesions with recurrent spontaneous pneumothorax, multiple cutaneous fibrofolliculomas, trichodiscomas, acrochordons
- Familial clear cell RCC
  - Germline 3p ("VHL light"), no other tumors
- Familial papillary RCC
  - Gain of function of *MET* on 7q31
- Tuberous sclerosis
  - AD
    - 80% *TSC1* mutations on 9q34
    - 20% *TSC2* mutations on 16p13
- Features
  - Renal
    - Increased risk for RCCs and angiomyolipomas
  - Skin and soft tissue
    - Facial angiofibromas, ungual fibromas, ash–leaf spots (hypopigmented macules), Shagreen patch
  - Cardiac
    - Rhabdomyomas
  - Pulmonary
    - Lymphangioleiomyomatosis
  - Neural
    - Retinal hamartoma, cortical tubers, subependymal giant cell astrocytoma (SEGA)

Hematolymphoid Neoplasms

LYMPHOBLASTIC LEUKEMIAS/LYMPHOMAS

- Prognosis in B-lymphoblastic leukemia/lymphoma (B-ALL) is worse with…
  - Increased expression of *CRLF2*
  - *IKZF1*
  - *JAK1, 2, 3*
  - *TP53* mutation
- Hyperdiploid B-ALL are sensitive to chemotherapy, good prognosis
- *TCF3-PBX1* translocation—can be balanced or unbalanced
  - 5% to 10% of pediatric B-ALL

- Rare in infants and >18 years of age
- CD10+, CD19+, CD34+
- Most common in African–American children
- Considered standard risk
- Interferes with differentiation of pro-B → pre-B via *Hox* genes
- Mechanism for *more common* unbalanced
    - Trisomy 1 → translocation → loss of der(1)
    - der(19)t(1;19)(q23;p13) (with two normal chromosome 1)

ACUTE MYELOID LEUKEMIA (AML)

- AML with CD19 have t(8;21)
- *CREBBP* fusion—t(8;16) leads to
    - Aberrant histone acetylation → AML
    - Acetylation of lysine moieties → charge change → permissive configuration
- *FLT3*
    - Internal tandem duplication (ITD, >330 bp) in the juxtamembrane region
    - Point mutation Asp835 in the tyrosine kinase domain (TKD)
- Loss of 7 and 7q are common in AML and significant; detect with CEP7 and 7q31 probe

PLASMA CELL NEOPLASMS

- 1q duplications—poor prognosis in multiple myeloma
    - t(14;20) is the most common translocation
- Myeloma—we have a dual probe set
    - Loss of 1p or gain of 1q

OTHERS

- Myeloproliferative neoplasms—*JAK2, CALR, MPL*
- 10% to 15% of follicular lymphomas do not have t(14;18)
    - May have *BCL6* rearrangements (at major or alternative breakpoint regions)
    - May still stain *BCL2* positive (likely caused by upregulation)

Solid Tumors

- Size of alteration
    - DNA sequence alterations
        - Single nucleotide variation
    - Chromosomal alterations
        - Deletion or amplification (copy number change)
        - Rearrangements (interchromosomal or intrachromosomal)
    - In between—insertion/deletions
- Genomic alteration
    - Epigenetics
        - Methylation of specific genes
        - gCIMP (global CpG-island methylator phenotype)
    - mRNA
        - Quantification

- Isoform (alternative splicing)
- Unknown primary (breast, thyroid)
- Considerations—tumor heterogeneity, infiltrating normal components (e.g., inflammatory, stromal), limited samples, genomic clonal evolution (intratumoral, invasive vs. in situ, primary vs. metastasis, primary vs. recurrence)
- Selecting the right test
    - What alteration are you looking for?
        - Rearrangements, gene expression, methylation, sequence mutation, copy number analysis
    - What is the clinical situation?
        - Disease characterization at diagnosis/relapse, monitoring during/post-therapy
    - What are the test requirements?
        - Input type and amount, sample types validated, limit of detection
- Mycancergenome.org
- AMP guidelines
    - Only report tiers I to III

BREAST CANCER

- Gene–expression profiles: Oncotype (21 genes), MammaPrint (70), Prosigna (50)
    - Low risk scores—really good survival with just hormone therapy, avoid chemotherapy in this group
    - High risk scores—supports decision to pursue chemotherapy
    - Do not use core biopsy—need resection specimen to choose highest-grade component (and most mitotically active)
- *HER2*—17q12
    - Array studies show that chromosome 17 tends to be highly rearranged (with gains and losses) in invasive breast cancer
    - Centromere can be amplified with *HER2* (CEP17 increased)
    - Alternative probe set—*RARA* (amplified with *HER2*), on distal 17q; and *SMS* on 17p (does not get amplified)
    - *HER2* to *CEP17* FISH ratio
        - Methods
            - 1. Count all *HER2* signals, and divide by number of cells counted
            - 2. Count all *CEP17* signals, and divide by number of cells counted
            - 3. Divide result of #1 by result of #2
        - Results
            - >2.2 = amplified
            - 1.8 to 2.2 = equivocal (repeat/count more cells)
            - <1.8 = not amplified
    - See Fig. 17.2
- *BRCA* tumor suppressor genes
    - *BRCA1*—17q21; *BRCA2*—13q12–13
    - AD with high penetrance
    - 80% lifetime breast cancer risk (vs. 10% in general population)
    - High risk for cancers in ovary, fallopian tube, colon, uterus, pancreas, prostate
    - 5% of all females with breast cancer have germline *BRCA* mutations
        - 25% of Ashkenazi Jewish women with breast cancer also do

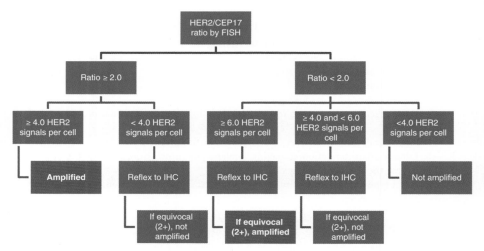

Fig. 17.2 Algorithm for *HER2* testing on breast cancer if fluorescent in situ hybridization (FISH) is performed first. *IHC,* Immunohistochemistry.

- In women with breast cancer who are found to have *BRCA* mutations, there is a 25% chance of developing cancer in the contralateral breast
  - Treated with PARP inhibitors
- Other syndromes that affect breast cancer risk
  - Li–Fraumeni—p53
  - Cowden—*PTEN*
  - Hereditary diffuse gastric cancer—*CDH1* (e-cadherin)
  - Peutz–Jeghers—*STK11*

SPORADIC RCC GENETICS

- Clear cell
  - Aggressive
  - del(3p) = first hit, then additional
    - Where *VHL* is located
  - + for CD10, vimentin, RCC, CAIX (box–like staining)
- Papillary
  - Indolent
  - Loss of Y, gains of 7 and 17
  - Positive for CD10, vimentin, AMACR, CK7
  - Negative for CAIX
- Chromophobe
  - Indolent
  - Hypodiploid (loss of Y, 1, 2, 6, 10, 13, 17, 21)
  - CD10 +/−, vimentin−, CD117+, CK7+
- Collecting duct
  - Aggressive
  - del(1q)
  - HMWK+, CD10−, vimentin−

- Xp11.2 translocation
  - In children, indolent
  - Nuclear TFE3+, CD10+
- Oncocytoma
  - Benign
  - Variable genetics
- Mucinous, tubular, and spindle cell
  - Hypodiploid
  - Indolent
- Angiomyolipoma
  - Benign
  - LOH at *TSC2* (16p)

SOFT TISSUE

- Nodular fasciitis and aneurysmal bone cyst
  - t(17;22)(p13;q13) *MYH9-USB6*
- Ewing family tumors
  - Ewing sarcoma/PNETs
  - Extraskeletal myxoid chondrosarcoma
  - Intra-abdominal desmoplastic small round cell tumors
  - 22q12 (*EWS*) translocation with…
    - 11q24 *(FLI1)*
    - 21q22 *(ERG)*
    - 7p22 *(ETV1)*
    - 17q21 *(ETV4)*
    - 2q33 *(FEV)*
- Chondroid lipoma
  - t(11;16)(q13;p12–13) *C11orf95/MKL2*
- Schwannoma
  - del(22q12) *NF2*
- Neuroblastoma
  - del(1p), +17 *(MYCN)*
- Alveolar rhabdomyosarcoma
  - t(2;13)(q35;q14) *PAX3/FOXO1*
  - t(1;13)(q36;q14) *PAX7/FOXO1*
- Nonossifying fibroma (NOF)
  - Most common benign lesion of the skeletal system
  - Usually spontaneously resolve at skeletal maturity
  - Two sites with different clinical and pathogenic characteristics: mandible and long bone
    - NOF of long bones can have clonal rearrangements of 1, 3, 4, 11, and 14—all in single case reports
    - None reported for mandible
- Low–grade fibromyxoid sarcoma
  - t(7;16)(q34;p11)

PEDIATRIC TUMORS

- Learn to swim
- Lymphoma

- Lymphoblastic leukemia—hyperdiploid is favorable
- Burkitt lymphoma—t(8;14), t(2;8), t(8;22)
- Ewing sarcoma
  - *EWSR1-FLI1*—11;12
  - *EWSR1-ERG*—21;22
- Rhabdomyosarcoma
  - Orbital, genitourinary, parameningeal
  - Alveolar or embryonal types most common
    - Pleomorphic and anaplastic more common in adults
  - Alveolar rhabdomyosarcoma
    - *PAX7-FOX01*—t(1;13)
      - More favorable prognosis
    - *PAX3-FOX01*—t(2;13)
      - More likely to involve the bone marrow
    - t(1;22) *MDM*
  - Embryonal
    - Small round cells, abundant eccentric cytoplasm
    - LOH at 11p15 *(IGF2)* → double minutes
      - Double minutes—tiny doubled chromosomes, not specific for anything (marker of gene amplification)
        - No centromere, do not count in number of chromosomes
- Neuroblastoma
  - Most common extracranial tumor of childhood
  - Prenatal to 4 years, males > females
  - *MYCN* amplification (with CEP2) = high risk
    - Maintains a stem–like state and promotes angiogenesis (potential for VEGF inhibition therapy)
    - Higher expression in neural tissue
    - Also set up CEP4 and 10 to call hyperploidy
    - Need at least 4:1 ratio of *MYCN* signals to CEP2 signals to call amplification
  - Other abnormalities
    - Double minutes
    - Loss of heterozygosity in 1p34 → deletion of *MYCL*
    - Del(1p)
    - Gain of 17q—poor prognosis
    - *ALK* gain-of-function mutation, 2p23 → increased *MYCN* expression
    - *ATRX* deletion in adolescents = chronic progressive
  - Undifferentiated, poorly differentiated, differentiated → based on amount of neuropil and number of neuroblasts
  - PHOX2B+, chromogranin/synaptophysin/CD56+
  - Low, intermediate, and high risk
  - INSS and INRG staging
- Synovial sarcoma
  - t(X;18)—SS18-SSX# or SYT-SSX#
    - # = 1, 2, or 4
  - *TLE1* expression
- Wilms tumor
  - Both ends of *WT1* gene
  - 2 to 5 years of age, abdominal mass
  - 85% survive

- Syndromes—WAGR (microdeletion in 11p13; Wilms tumor, aniridia, genitourinary anomalies retardation), Denys–Drash, Beckwith–Wiedemann
  - *Only 10% are syndromic; most are sporadic*
- Loss of heterozygosity at 1 p and 16q—poor prognosis
- *INI-1* loss
  - Rhabdoid tumor
    - *INI1 (SMARCB1)* deletion
  - Medullary carcinoma
- Miscellaneous
  - MPNST
  - DSRCT
    - *EWSR1-WT1*—t(11;22)
    - "Carcinomatosis" in abdomen of teens to 30 s
    - CD99+
    - Only C terminus of WT-1+
    - Desmin+ (dot–like perinuclear)
  - Melanoma
  - Hepatoblastoma
  - Beta-catenin/Wnt pathway
    - Familial adenomatous polyposis (FAP) syndrome, Beckwith–Wiedemann syndrome
    - Sporadic beta-catenin mutations

GASTROINTESTINAL NEOPLASMS

- Gastric adenocarcinoma
  - *HER2/neu (ERBB2)* amplification in 20% → 50% respond to trastuzumab
  - IHC staining is primary method, followed by FISH in indeterminant
  - MSI status
  - PD-L1
- Pancreatic adenocarcinoma
  - *KRAS* mutation in codon-12
  - *SMAD* mutations
  - Rarely syndromic
    - *BRCA*, PJS, familial atypical mole melanoma syndrome, hereditary pancreatitis, FAP, ataxia telangiectasia, Lynch syndrome
- GISTS
  - 95% *KIT* overexpressed
    - Exon 11—sensitive to tyrosine kinase inhibitors (TKIs)
      - Imatinib, sunitinib, dasatinib
    - Exon 9, 13, 17—somewhat resistant
  - 5% negative or weak for *KIT* will have *PDGFRA* mutation (D842V—complete resistance to TKI)
  - Very rare are negative for *KIT* and *PDGFRA* → *SDH* mutated!
  - Syndromes
    - Carney triad—different than Carney complex
      - Especially *SDH*-mutated
      - GIST, pulmonary chondromas, extra-adrenal paragangliomas
    - NF1—multiple small intestinal GISTs
    - Germline *PDGFR* mutation—multiple GISTs, often epithelioid type
    - Germline *SDH* mutation—multiple GISTs and paragangliomas

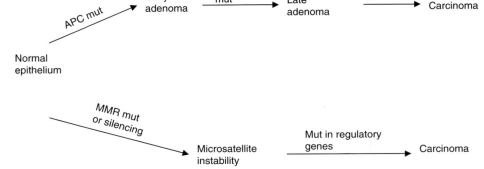

Fig. 17.3   Genetic pathways of colorectal carcinoma. *Mut*, Mutation.

> ▪ Germline *KIT* mutation—multiple GISTs, hyperpigmentation, urticaria pigmentosa, dysphagia

Colorectal Carcinoma

- See Fig. 17.3
- *KRAS/NRAS* do not respond to EGFR inhibitors (cetuximab)
  - Also *BRAF* (nonmicrosatellite instable tumor), *PTEN*, and *PI3K*
- PIK3CA inhibitor trials ongoing
- *BRAF* V600E—if microsatellite stable, bad prognosis and poor response to EGFR inhibition
- Microsatellite instability
  - Acquired
    - Inherited
- No role for staining CRC for PD-L1 (dictated by microsatellite status)

APC Gene Mutation (85% of Cases)

- *APC* mutation (5q) early
  - Second hit (LOH or *KRAS* mutation)
- Germline = familial adenomatous polyposis (FAP)
  - >100 polyps by 35 years of age
  - Adenocarcinoma by 50 years of age
  - Fundic gland polyp
  - Ampullary adenoma/adenocarcinoma
  - Thyroid carcinoma
  - Fibromatosis
- Tubular adenoma → cancer (left–sided with dirty necrosis)
- Gardner syndrome = FAP + epidermal cysts, jaw osteomas, fibromatoses, congenital hypertrophy of retinal pigmented epithelium
- Turcot syndrome = (FAP or MMR) + CNS tumors

Mismatch Repair Deficient (MMR; 15% of Cases)

- Microsatellite instability (MSI)
  - Do not benefit from 5-fluorouracil
  - Get tumors in tissues with high mitotic rate (skin, colon, lung, endometrium)

- Acquired
  - *MLH1* hypermethylation
    - 50% to 70% of patient's also have *BRAF* V600E, essentially rules out Lynch syndrome
  - *BRAF* V600E
- Inherited
  - Germline → inactivating mutation
    - = Lynch (HNPCC)
      - Lifetime risk for CRC—50% to 70%
      - *MLH1* and *MSH2*—80% to 90% of cases
        - *EPCAM* deletion leads to silencing of *MSH2*
      - *PMS2* and *MSH6*—10% to 15% of cases
    - Muir–Torre = Lynch + genitourinary cancers + keratoacanthomas + sebaceous tumors
- Events
  - First hit—mutation in mismatch repair genes → MSI and allowance of further mutations
    - MSI is a result of MMR dysfunction
    - *MSH6* loss doesn't cause MSI, it causes increased SNPs
  - Number two—*BRAF, KRAS, p16INK4a*
- Morphology is typically sessile serrated adenoma that progresses to cancer with mucinous or medullary differentiation, no dirty necrosis, prominent tumor–infiltrating lymphocytes

Other Syndromes
- Juvenile polyposis
- Peutz–Jeghers syndrome

LUNG NEOPLASMS
- Non-small cell lung carcinoma (NSCLC)
  - EGFR therapy (cetuximab, erlotinib, gefitinib)
    - Resistance is caused by *KRAS* mutation (codon 12/13), *BRAF* V600E, *BRAF* exon 20 deletions, or *EGFR* p.T790M
    - Susceptibility caused by *EGFR* L858R and exon 19/21 mutations
  - Emerging: *BRAF, HER2, MET, RET, ROS1*
  - Mutually exclusive mutations—*KRAS, EGFR, ALK, BRAF, PIK3CA*
  - Lung adenocarcinoma
    - Essentially required panel at diagnosis: *EGFR, ALK, ROS1*
    - One-third have unknown genetic driver
    - 20% have *EGFR* mutation, exon 19 and 21
      - Some mutations confer sensitivity to EGFR inhibitors
    - *ALK* rearrangement—resistant to EGFR inhibitors
      - Targetable by crizotinib (ALK and ROS inhibitor)
      - Also ALK+ anaplastic large cell lymphomas in trials
    - *KRAS*—resistant to EGFR inhibitors (25%)
    - *ALK* rearrangement and *KRAS* mutations → resistance to TKIs
    - Variants
      - Cribriform mucinous and signet ring adenocarcinoma—*EML4-ALK*
      - Very rare morphology
      - Well–differentiated fetal–type adenocarcinoma—beta-catenin mutations
      - Mucinous adenocarcinoma—*KRAS* mutations
  - Squamous cell carcinoma
    - *FGFR1, PIK3CA, PTEN*, 3q amplifications *(SOX2)*

- Clinical trials ongoing
- Small cell and large cell lung carcinoma have *TP53* mutations
- Sarcomatoid, high–grade lung tumors
  - 20% have *MET* splice abnormality
    - Targetable
    - *MET*—mesenchymal to epithelial transition
      - Fibroblast growth factor
      - NSCLC with *MET* exon 14 mutation may respond to crizotinib or cabozantinib
- Pulmonary hamartomas are neoplasms (and not malformations) with consistent cytogenetic abnormalities in chromosomes 6 and 12
- Pleuropulmonary blastomas
  - Germline *DICER1* mutations
  - Also Sertoli–Leydig tumors, cystic nephromas, nodular thyroid hyperplasia

NEURAL TUMORS

- Gliomas
  - Pilocytic astrocytoma
    - *BRAF* (17q) rearrangements, use FISH
  - Astrocytoma, oligodendroglioma
    - *IDH*, 1p/19q codeletion
      - High–grade = no *IDH* mutation
      - Intermediate = *IDH* mutation without 1p/19q codeletion
      - Lowest–grade = *IDH* mutation with 1p19q codeletion
    - Can also have *TERT* promoter or *ATRX* inactivating mutations
    - *MGMT* methylation and *IDH* mutations are associated with a more favorable prognosis with temozolomide therapy (which is standard of care)
  - Glioblastoma multiforme can have lots of copy number changes
    - Primary tumors—7p12 amplification *(EGFR)* and *PTEN* mutation
    - Secondary tumors (lower–grade glial tumor that has transformed)—10q23 deletion *(PTEN)*
- Other neural tumors
  - NF2 schwannomas and meningiomas—chromosome 22 deletion (22q12)
    - Larger deletions → milder phenotype (can be LOH)
  - Ependymomas—+19
  - Medulloblastoma—i(17q10) or –17p or +17q *(TP53)*
  - Neuroblastoma—2p24 amplification *(MYCN)*
  - Retinoblastoma—*RB1* on 13q14
  - Atypical teratoid and rhabdoid tumors (ATRTs)—*SMARCB1* loss, 22q11.2, encodes *INI1*

OTHERS

- Desmoplastic small round cell tumor
  - t(11;22)
- Melanoma
  - *BRAF* > *NRAS* > *KIT* (*GNA11* and *GNAQ* in uveal) > *NF1* and *TERT*
  - Anti-*BRAF* treatment (TKI), imatinib for *KIT*, high dose IL-2, cytotoxic regimens
- Thyroid
  - *BRAF* (papillary thyroid carcinoma), *RAS* (follicular thyroid carcinoma and noninvasive follicular thyroid neoplasm with papillary–like nuclear features), *PTEN PIK3CA*

- Endometrial
  - Universal testing for Lynch syndrome → follow with *MLH1* promoter methylation test
- Ovarian
  - Germline *BRCA1* and *BRCA2* (PARP inhibitor sensitivity)
    - Germline negative patients → tumor testing
- Head and neck
  - Squamous cell carcinoma—human papillomavirus (HPV) status is most important (p16 immunohistochemistry is a good surrogate)
  - Salivary gland tumors
    - Salivary duct carcinoma—*HER2* amplification
    - Mucoepidermoid carcinoma—*MECT1-MAML2*
    - Mammary–analog secretory carcinoma—*ETV6-NTRK*
    - Adenoid cystic carcinoma—*MYB*
    - Hyalinizing clear cell carcinoma—*EWSR1*
    - Pleomorphic adenoma—*PLAG1*
- Sarcomas with MSI or MMR deficiency have higher rates of copy number variation and aneuploidy
  - Lynch syndrome can get rhabdomyosarcoma
  - Malignant PEComas
  - About 10% of unclassifiable pleomorphic sarcomas are mismatch repair deficient (MSI)
    - May not predict response to immunotherapy
- Cardiac
  - Myxomas—*PPKAR1*-alpha (17q24)—protein kinase A
  - Rhabdomyomas
    - *TSC1* (9q34)—hamartin
    - *TSC2* (16p13.3)—tuberin
    - Fibromas—*PTC* (9q22.3)—transmembrane protein
- Hepatocellular carcinoma
  - Hemochromatosis, tyrosinemia, glycogen storage disease, alpha1-antitrypsin deficiency, Wilson disease, galactosemia
- Prostate adenocarcinoma
  - 50% have *TMPRSS2-ERG* functional rearrangements
    - Both are on 21q
      - Most common mechanism is interstitial deletion
    - May be associated with progressive cancer
- Myxomas
  - Mazabraud syndrome—multiple myxomas and fibrous dysplasia
  - McCune–Albright syndrome—multiple myxomas, hyperpigmentation, endocrine abnormalities
  - *GNAS1* mutation—intramuscular myxomas and fibrous dysplasia

Hereditary Nonneoplastic Disease
STORAGE/METABOLISM DISORDERS

- Hurler disease
  - Increased glycosaminoglycans that accumulate in heart and neural tissue
  - Can have zebra bodies on electron microscopy (EM)
  - Alder–Reilly inclusions (many large blue granules in all white blood cells)
- Farber disease
  - Ceramide accumulation

- Banana and zebra bodies
- Krabbe disease
  - Galactocerebroside beta-galactosidase deficiency
  - Globoid cells
  - Rapid neurologic degeneration
- Fabry disease
  - X-linked, alpha-galactosidase A (AGA) deficiency
  - *GLA* gene, Xp22.1
    - Accumulation of neutral glycosphingolipids (especially globotriaosylceramide)
      - Endothelium, myocardium, renal tubules
      - Foamy/vacuolated
      - Zebra bodies
    - Heterozygous females may have some symptoms caused by skewed lyonization
  - Present in childhood
    - Acroparesthesias, angiokeratomas, hypohidrosis, corneal and lenticular opacities
    - With age, develop progressive renal, cardiac, and cerebrovascular disease
  - Diagnosed by absent AGA in white blood cells, confirmed by genetics
- Gaucher disease
  - Beta-glucocerebrosidase deficiency
  - Accumulation of glucosylceramide in macrophages
  - Kidneys: PAS+ "crinkled paper" macrophages in gloms and interstitium
  - EM: intracytoplasmic membrane–bound lysosomal inclusions with characteristic tubules
- Niemann–Pick disease
  - NP cells—foamy histiocytes with uniform vacuoles
  - Sea blue histiocytes
- *MTHFR* (methylenetetrahydrofolate reductase)
  - 1p36, C677T (p.A1298C)
  - Homocystinuria—lens displacement, marfanoid habitus, pes excavatum, developmental delay, strokes
  - Age–related hearing loss
  - Alopecia areata
  - Anencephaly and spina bifida (neural tube defects)
- Glycogen storage diseases
  - Type I (von Gierke)—glucose-6-phosphatase—75%
  - Type II—lysosomal acid maltase (Pompe disease)—15%
  - Type II—debranching enzyme—25%
  - Type IV—branching enzyme
  - Type VII—phosphofructokinase

LIVER DISEASE

- Alagille syndrome/syndromic paucity of bile ducts/arteriohepatic dysplasia—*JAG1*
  - Neonatal jaundice, characteristic facies, cardiac defects, vertebral and eye anomalies
- A1AT deficiency
  - *SERPINA1* on 14q31–32.3, AR
    - Most healthy—PiMM
    - Most deficient—PiZZ (<1% of population) or PIZS (<1%)
  - Neonatal hepatitis, early onset panacinar emphysema, cirrhosis, hepatocellular carcinoma, panniculitis
- Bilirubin conjugation disorders—*UGT1A1*
  - Unconjugated bilirubinemia

- Gilbert (mildly decreased) or Crigler–Najjar (severe)
- Bilirubin secretion disorders
  - Mild conjugated bilirubinemia
  - Dubin–Johnson—*MRP2* (pigmented but undamaged liver)
  - Rotor—no liver pigmentation
- Wilson disease (hepatolenticular degeneration)
  - ↑ Oxidative stress
  - Presents as liver disease, neuropsychiatric disease, hemolysis, Kayser–Fleisher rings
    - Kayser–Fleisher rings are generally a predictor of neuropsychiatric disease
  - Liver biopsy
    - Glycogenated nuclei, steatosis, inflammation → cirrhosis
  - Autosomal recessive (AR), *ATP7B*
    - Encodes a copper–binding ATPase
  - Expressed in hepatocytes
  - Used for biliary copper excretion and copper incorporation into ceruloplasmin
    - In 40,000
- Hemochromatosis
  - ↓ hepcidin → ↑ iron absorption in gastrointestinal tract → ↑ iron in liver, pancreas, pituitary, synovium, heart skin
  - Cirrhosis, pancreatic fibrosis with diabetes, hypogonadism, infertility (caused by hypopituitarism), osteoarthritis, cardiomyopathy, bronze skin
  - AR with variable penetrance → females are one-half as likely to develop complications as men (possibly due to blood loss during menstruation)
  - *HFE* within major histocompatibility region on 6p21.3
    - Most common—C282Y
    - Second—H63D
    - Others
      - F65C
      - Compound heterozygotes (C282Y and H63D): ~2% of general population; most have no symptoms
  - Other genes: *HFE2* (1q21), *HAMP* (19q13), *TFR2* (7q22), *FTH1* (11p13)
  - Iron in liver is in hepatocytes (not Kupffer cells like in secondary siderosis)
- Caroli disease and congenital hepatic fibrosis—*PKHD1*, 6p

GASTROINTESTINAL AND PANCREATIC DISEASE

- Microvillus inclusion disease
  - Most common cause of neonatal malabsorption, AR
  - Grossly paper–thin small intestine
  - Villous blunting, mucosal atrophy, apical intracellular inclusions (PAS+, CD10+, CEA+)
- 90% of esophageal atresia part of larger syndrome, like VACTERL
  - Vertebral, anal, cardiac, tracheal, esophageal, renal, limb
  - Present with polyhydramnios and feeding difficulty
  - Associated with distal tracheoesophageal fistula
- Cystic fibrosis
  - *CFTR* on 7q31.2, F508 (66%)
    - Most common mutation in Caucasians is delta-F508
  - Most common autosomal recessive condition in Caucasians (1 in 2000)
  - Meconium ileus, nasal polyps (children), male infertility caused by congenital bilateral absence of the vas deferens, liver disease, recurrent lung infections → bronchiectasis
    - *Staphylococcus aureus, Burkholderia cepacia, Pseudomonas aeruginosa*

HEART DISEASE

- Dilated cardiomyopathy
  - X-linked—dystrophin , *DMD* gene (Xp21)
  - AD—*MYH7* (14q12) gene
- Hypertrophic cardiomyopathy
  - 1 in 500, AD
  - *MYH7* (14q12)—myosin heavy chain
  - *MYBPC3* (11p11.2)—myosin binding protein C
  - *TNNT2* (1q32)—troponin T
- Arrhythmogenic right ventricular cardiomyopathy
  - Type 1—14q23-q24
  - Type 2—*RyR2* (1q42–43)
- Naxos syndrome
  - Plakoglobin, *JUP* gene (17q21)
- Long QT syndrome (sodium/potassium channels)
  - Type 1—*KCNQ1* (11p15.5)
  - Type 2—7q35-q36
- Familial isolated cardiac amyloidosis
  - *TTR* gene (transthyretin), AD
- Trisomy 21
  - Endocardial cushion defects → membranous ventricular septal defect (VSD), patent ductus arteriosus, atrial septal defect, atrioventricular septal defect
- Turner syndrome (45X)
  - Bicuspid aortic valve, coarctation, aortic root dilation → dissection
- 22q11 deletion—DiGeorge (velocardiofacial syndrome)
  - Conotruncal malformations (tetralogy of Fallot, interrupted aortic arch, VSD, truncus arteriosus)
- 7q11.23 deletion—Williams disease
  - Dysmorphic facies, developmental delay, short stature, hypercalcemia, abnormal connective tissue, supravalvular aortic stenosis (hourglass stenosis)

KIDNEY DISEASE

- Alport syndrome
  - Type IV collagen
  - Triad
    - Glomerulonephritis → hematuria → kidney failure
    - Sensorineural hearing loss
    - Ocular lesions
  - Mostly X-linked recessive
    - Female carriers may have asymptomatic hematuria
  - Diagnose with skin or kidney biopsy—absent type IV collagen (alpha-5 chain)
  - EM: basement membrane thinned, split/splintered, and/or disrupted
    - "Basketweave" on EM
  - *COL4A5* gene on Xp22.3
- Autosomal recessive polycystic kidney disease
  - Cystic collecting ducts, biliary plate malformations, *PKHD* (6p)
- Autosomal dominant polycystic kidney disease

- 100% penetrance by 40 s, 1 in 500 live births, hypertension, cortical and medullary cysts, hepatic cysts, berry aneurysm, mitral valve prolapse, pancreatic cysts
- Congenital nephrotic syndrome
  - <3 months of age
  - DDx
    - Perinatal infectious
      - Rubella
      - Toxoplasmosis
      - Syphilis
      - CMV
    - Inherited disorders
      - Congenital nephrotic syndrome, Finnish type—nephrin (*NPHS1* gene, 19q) large placenta, abnormal foot processes
      - Pierson syndrome—beta-2 laminin (*LAMB2* gene, 3p), associated with fixed small pupils
      - Nail–patella syndrome—*COL4A3* (9q)
      - Denys–Drash/Frasier—*WT1* (11p) mutations—Wilms tumor, male pseudohermaphrodites, gonadoblastoma (sex cord cells and germ cells)
      - Familial AD focal segmental glomerulosclerosis (FSGS)—*ACTN4* (alpha actin) or *TRPC5* (cation channel), onset in adolescence or early adulthood
      - Familial AR corticosteroid–resistant nephrosclerosis—podocin (*NPHS2*), early childhood onset
        - Biopsy initially minimal change, eventually FSGS
- Denys–Drash syndrome
  - Diffuse mesangial sclerosis
- Renal Fanconi syndrome
  - Proximal tube dysfunction caused by...
    - Inherited—cystinosis, tyrosinemia, galactosemia, glycogen storage disease, hereditary fructose intolerance, Wilson disease, idiopathic renal Fanconi syndrome, Dent disease
    - Acquired—myeloma, urate, heavy metal, amyloid, collagen vascular disorder, renal transplant rejection, medication (antineoplastic, antiretroviral, aminoglycosides)
- Cystic renal dysplasia—usually sporadic from ureteral obstruction, usually unilateral, cystic kidneys with loose stroma +/− cartilage formation
  - Can be associated with Meckel–Gruber syndrome—kidney disease, polydactyly, occipital encephalocele

MOVEMENT DISORDERS

- Huntington disease
  - CAG repeats in *HTT*, 4p
    - <28 normal
    - 28 to 35 premutation
    - 36 to 40 reduced penetrance
    - >40 always fully penetrant
- Spinal muscle atrophy—AR, *SMN1*
- Duchenne and Becker muscular dystrophy
  - Xp21.2, *DMD*, X-linked recessive
  - Biopsies show variation in fiber size, increased endomysial connective tissue, fatty infiltration, regenerating fibers (large nuclei)
- Myotonic muscular dystrophy—AD, triple nucleotide repeat

OTHER GENETIC COMPLEXES

- Dyskeratosis congenita
    - Many mutations, typically proteins that stabilize telomerase
        - Anticipation can occur (especially with *TERC* mutations)
    - Presentation triad: reticular hyperpigmentation, oral leukoplakia, nail dystrophy
    - Other findings: infection susceptibility, short stature, hypogonadism, cerebellar hypoplasia, ataxia, lymphopenia, hypogammaglobulinemia, premature gray hair
        - Most can also be seen in ataxia telangiectasia
    - Treat with bone marrow transplant, G-CSF, skin cancer surveillance
        - ***Do not*** give busulfan—patients develop pulmonary fibrosis
- Klinefelter syndrome
    - XXY
    - Very high follicle–stimulating hormone (FSH) and normal to slightly increased luteinizing hormone (LH)
    - Tall, abnormal proportions, small testes
        - Sclerosis of seminiferous tubules
        - Nodular hyperplasia of Leydig cells
        - Decreased spermatogenesis
    - Increased breast cancer risk
    - No change in germ cell tumor risk
- Sturge–Weber syndrome
    - *GNAQ* p.R183Q
    - Eye enlargement, glaucoma, port-wine stains in trigeminal distribution, hemangiomas
- Charge sequence
    - Coloboma, heart malformations, choanal atresia, developmental delay, genital hypoplasia, deafness
- Williams syndrome
    - 7q11.23
    - Elf–like facies, growth retardation, cardiac abnormalities, developmental delay, hypercalcemia
- Wolf
    - 4p del
    - Intrauterine growth restriction, cardiac abnormalities, microcephaly, cleft lip/palate
- Miller–Dieker syndrome
    - 17p13
    - Microcephaly, lissencephaly, cardiac and renal abnormalities, seizures, prominent forehead, vertical furrowing of brow
- Shwachman–Diamond syndrome
    - *SBDS* gene
    - Bone marrow failure and exocrine pancreatic insufficiency with fatty metaplasia
- Johanson–Blizzard
    - Hypoplasia of nasal alae, exocrine pancreatic insufficiency and pancreatic lipomatosis, hypothyroidism, deafness
- Congenital adrenal hyperplasia
    - Number one—21-hydroxylase deficiency (*CYP21* at 6p21) → salt wasting, no hypertension
        - Increased serum 17-OH progesterone
    - Number two—11-hydroxylase deficiency → non-salt wasting, hypertension

- Cerebral autosomal dominant arteriopathy with subcortical infarcts and leukoencephalopathy (CADASIL)—*NOTCH3*
  - Migraines, transient ischemic attacks → dementia
  - Skin biopsy: granular eosinophilic medial deposits in vessels
- McCune–Albright syndrome
  - Gain-of-function mutation of *GNAS1*
  - All cases are somatic mosaics
    - Germline = incompatible with life
  - Polyostotic fibrous dysplasia ("shepherd crook" hips)
  - Café-au-lait spots
  - Endocrine hyperfunction
    - Precocious puberty
  - Myxomas
- Cystathione beta-synthase deficiency
  - Homocystinuria, thrombosis, developmental delay, lens dislocation, long slender fingers
- Osler–Weber–Rendu syndrome (hereditary hemorrhagic telangiectasia)
  - AD, *ENG* or *ACVRL1* mutation
  - Vascular fragility
    - Hemorrhagic telangiectasia, "platelet–type" bleeding
    - Symptoms change with age
      - Child—epistaxis
      - Adolescents—skin lesions
      - Adult—GI bleeding

INCREASED SUSCEPTIBILITY

- Type 1 DM—HLA-DR3 and HLA-DR4
  - Siblings 5% to 10%, identical twins 60%
  - Heterozygotes have 2 to 3× risk, homozygotes have 10× risk
- Alzheimer disease
  - Early onset—*APP*—chromosome 21
  - Late onset—*APOE*, E4 allele
- Pick disease (frontotemporal dementia and Parkinsonism)—*MAPT* (encodes tau protein)
- Familial Parkinson *or* Lewy body dementia—*PARK1-PARK8*
- Celiac sprue
  - HLA-DQ2 in ~95% of patients but only ~1% of HLA-DQ2 patients have celiac sprue

INTERCHROMOSOMAL DUPLICONS/SEGMENTAL DUPLICATIONS

- Large, ~1 Kbp
- Caused by unequal crossing over in meiosis
- Examples
  - 7q—Williams–Beuren syndrome
  - 16p—alpha-thalassemia
  - 17p
    - Charcot–Marie–Tooth
      - AD, duplication on 17p12, *PMP22*
    - Smith-Magenis syndrome
      - del(17)(p11.2p11.2)

- Developmental delay, prominent forehead, self–mutilation, disturbed rapid eye movement cycles
  - Brachycephaly, macrocephaly, flattened facies, frontal bossing, developmental delays, cognitive disabilities, executive function issues, decreased self–control, temper tantrums, self–mutilation and picking, pull out nails, reverse circadian rhythms (melatonin secreted during day instead of at night)
  - Most symptoms secondary to *RAI1* deletion (retinoic acid inducer)
    - Evidence: smaller deletions, point mutations, and knockout mouse
  - 1:250,000
  - Breakpoints flanked by LCR (low copy repeats)
- 22q—velocardiofacial syndrome

MICRODELETION DISORDERS

- DiGeorge—22q11.2—thymic and parathyroid hypoplasia, developmental delay, cardiac abnormalities
- Cri du chat—5p15.2—microcephaly and developmental delay
- Kallman—Xp22.3—anosmia, hypogonadism
- Pearson syndrome
  - AD, pancreatitis and bone marrow failure
- Microdeletion in mitochondrial DNA

MITOCHONDRIAL DISORDERS

- Kearns–Sayre—salt-and-pepper retinopathy, ataxia, ophthalmoplegia, deafness, diabetes mellitus, and so on
  - Major structural mitochondrial DNA rearrangements
- Pearson—sideroblastic anemia → pancytopenia, pancreatic exocrine insufficiency
  - Major structural mitochondrial DNA rearrangements
- Mitochondrial encephalopathy, lactic acidosis, and stroke–like episodes (MELAS)
  - *MT-TL1* (on mitochondrial DNA)
- Myoclonic epilepsy with ragged red fibers (MERRF)
- Mitochondrial neurogastrointestinal encephalomyopathy (MNGIE)

EPIGENETIC MUTATION DISEASE

- Genomic imprinting
  - Shortly after fertilization, paternal DNA is DEmethylated (actively)
  - ICF syndrome—*DNMT3B*
  - Rett syndrome—*MECP2*
  - Rubinstein-Taybi syndrome—*CREBBP*
  - 9q34 subtelomeric deletion—*EHTM1*
  - Coffin-Lowry syndrome—*RSK2*
  - X-linked alpha-thalassemia—*MRATRX*

Disease Caused by "Epimutation" of a Specific Gene

- 15q11–13
  - Normal
    - Several centromeric genes paternally expressed, including *MAGEL2*
      - Controlled by *SNRDN* promoter

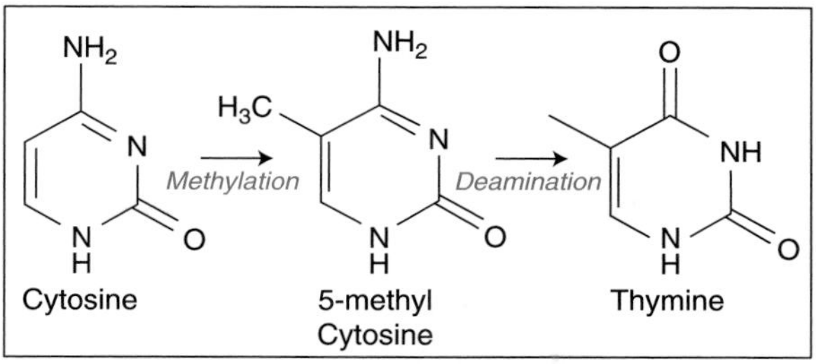

Fig. 17.4 Spontaneous deamination of cytosine.

- Two telomeric genes maternally expressed, including *UBE3A*
- Disease
  - Prader–Willi—paternal deletion of this locus; only maternal genes present
  - Angelman—maternal deletion
  - *Rare other causes:* uniparental disomy or maternal inactivating mutation in *UBE3A*
- 11p15.5
  - Beckwith-Wiedemann—both imprinted like father—*IGF2, CDKN1C*
    - Normally only mother's genes here are expressed
    - Large for gestational age, polyhydramnios, large placenta with long cord, macrosomia, macroglossia, hemihypertrophy, omphalocele, ear pits, renal/adrenal anomalies, Wilms tumors, hepatoblastomas
  - Silver-Russell—both imprinted like mother—*IGF2*, others
- Fragile X mental retardation—*FMR1*
- Facioscapulohumeral muscular dystrophy—*D4Z4*
- CpG = dinucleotide palindrome with phosphate sugar between (normal)
  - 80% of cytosines are methylated, can undergo spontaneous deamination to thymine
    - Increased mutation rate, slowly being weeded out by evolution
    - See Fig. 17.4

Pharmacogenetics

- Methotrexate (MTX) mechanism
  - Inhibits dihydrofolate reductase (DHFR), which catalyzes DHF → THF, and thymidylate synthetase (TS, production of nucleotide thymidine) → decreased DNA synthesis and replication
  - Polymorphism in *RFC* → decreased MTX (and folate) entrance into nucleus → poorer prognosis and more side effects
  - Polymorphism in *TS* → no upstream transcription factors → lower survival
  - *CCND1* releases transcription factors
    - Polymorphism = lower survival
  - 5, 10-methylene THF → 5-methyl THF (with 5, 10-methylene THF reductase [MTHFR])
  - Polymorphisms (frequency >1%) or mutations (frequency <1%, permanent change) → decreased activity, increased serum homocysteine
- CYP enzymes
  - CYP1A2—induced by smoking, caffeine, theophylline, St. John's wort
  - CYP2D6—codeine (to morphine), tricyclic antidepressants

TABLE 17.4 ■ **Tumor Markers with Specific Drug Therapy**

Gene/Biomarker	Therapy
ALK	Crizotinib
BRAF	Trametinib, dabrafenib
BRCA1/2	Olaparib
CTLA4	Ipilimumab
EGFR	Erlotinib, osimertinib, afatinib, gefitinib
EGFR	Cetuximab, panitumumab
ER and *PR*	Hormonal therapy
HER2/neu	Trastuzumab, pertuzumab, ado-trastuzumab
KIT	Imatinib mesylate
KRAS	Cetuximab, panitumumab
PD-1	Pembrolizumab, nivolumab
PD-L1	Atezolizumab, avelumab, durvalumab

- CYP2C9—warfarin, phenytoin
- CYP2C19—omeprazole, phenytoin, diazepam, clopidogrel
- Vitamin K epoxide reductase (*VKORC1*)—inhibited by warfarin
- N-acetyltransferase—metabolism of isoniazid, polymorphisms cause increased or decreased activity
- Malignant hyperthermia (hypercarbia under anesthesia)—*RYR1*, calcium channel
- Actionable mutations
  - Therapeutic (e.g., *JAK2* inhibition)
    - Sensitivity and resistance to therapy
      - *BTK* and *PLCG2* → resistant to some therapies
  - Prognostic
  - Diagnostic
  - Reproductive
- Immuno-oncology
  - Rapidly changing field
  - See Table 17.4

Odds and Ends

- *WRN* gene
  - Helicase—separates DNA strands for replication
  - Werner disease—accelerated cell aging
- Gain of 1q (usually on chromosome 16) can be seen in multiple hematolymphoid and solid tumors (Wilms)
  - der(16)t(1;16)(q12;q11.2)—a derivative chromosome 16 is present that has part of the long arm of chromosome 1 in place of it's own long arm
- Women can be affected by X-linked recessive disorders if…
  - Homozygous (usually caused by really high mutant gene frequency)
  - Asymmetric lyonization

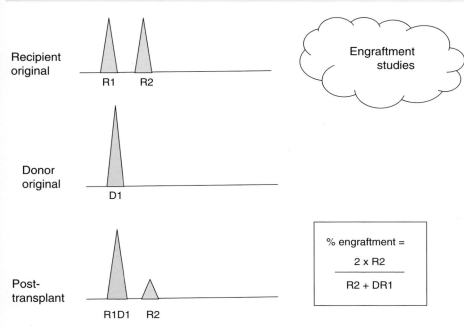

Fig. 17.5 Engraftment studies. *D1,* Donor peak 1; *R1,* recipient peak 1; *R2,* recipient peak 2.

- Turner syndrome
- PCR inhibitors: melanin, heparin, collagen, hematin, calcium, bile, urea
- Post–stem cell transplant engraftment studies—see Fig. 17.5
- Important autosomal dominant conditions
  - Huntington
  - Neurofibromatosis
  - Hereditary spherocytosis
  - Marfan syndrome
  - Osteogenesis imperfecta
  - Autosomal dominant polycystic kidney disease
  - Familial adenomatous polyposis
  - Von Willebrand disease
  - Ehlers–Danlos syndrome
  - Achondroplasia

CHAPTER 18

Immunology

Cellular Biology Basis of Immunology

INNATE IMMUNE SYSTEM

- Barriers
- Phagocytic cells—neutrophils and macrophages
  - M1 macrophages = proinflammatory (IL-2, IL-6)
  - M2 = anti-inflammatory and profibrotic (IL-10, TGF-β), promotes tumor growth
  - Leukocyte diapedesis
    - Injury/infection
      - Increased TNF and IL-1 cause endothelial cells to express E-selectin and B-selectin ligands
      - Histamine secretion causes Weibel–Palade bodies release P-selectin to the endothelial surface
      - L-selectin and ligands for E- and P-selectins on neutrophils bind to their components on neutrophils
    - Rolling and loose adhesion
      - Selectins
    - Firm adhesion
      - Integrins (CD11a + CD18 = LFA-1) and ICAM-1
      - Leukocyte adhesion deficiency
        - Autosomal recessive (AR)
        - Decreased neutrophil adhesion and motility
    - Transmigration
      - PECAM1
  - Chemotaxis
    - Chemotactic agents
      - Endotoxin lipopolysaccharide and fMLP (fML-3H-P)
      - Complement—C3a, C4a, C5a
      - Thrombin
      - Fibrinolytic breakdown products
      - Leukotrienes
    - Inhibitors of chemotaxis—CF1 and prostaglandin A
  - Histamine
    - ↑ Arteriolar dilation
    - ↑ Vascular permeability
    - Stored in mast cells and platelets
- Dendritic cells
- Complement (see Fig. 18.1)
- Pattern recognition receptors
  - Toll–like receptors (TLRs)
    - On antigen–presenting cells (APCs) and some epithelial cells (e.g., collecting duct)

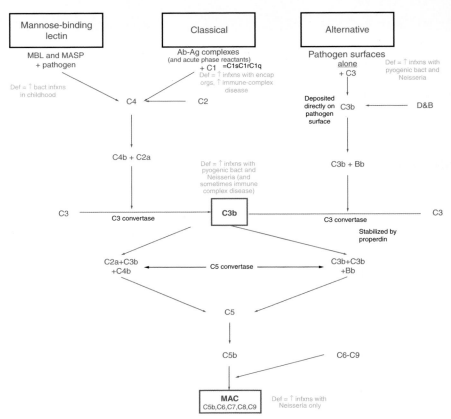

Fig. 18.1 Complement pathways. *Ab Ag,* Antibody, antigen; *bact,* bacteria; *def,* deficiency; *infxns,* infections; *MAC,* membrane attack complex; *MBL,* mannose-binding lectin; *orgs, organisms.*

- Recognize carbohydrates on bacterial surface
- Influence transcription on phagocytes
- Leucine–rich repeats
- 1, 2, 4, 5, 6 on membrane
  - In general, lower numbers
- 3, 7, 9 in cytoplasm (higher numbers)
- Signal through MYD88 to nuclear factor-κB (NF-κB)
  - *Congenital MYD88 deficiency*
    - AR
    - Severe pyogenic bacterial infections (strep and pseudomonas)
    - Resistance to other microbes
    - Improves with age
- Nucleotide oligomerization domain–like receptors (NODs)
  - Expressed on APCs and some epithelium
  - Leucine–rich repeats
  - All intracellular
  - Sense peptidoglycan breakdown products (bacteria)
  - NF-κB

- NOD1 important for protection against *H. pylori*, *C. difficile*, and *Listeria*
- Induces cytokine release
- Frameshift in NOD2 (expressed on epithelium and Paneth cells) leads to increased risk for *Crohn's disease*
- IL1, IL6, TNF-α, IFN-α (from phagocytes)

Complement System

Normal Function

- Adaptive (classical pathway) *and* innate immune systems (alternative pathway)
- Classical and alternative (micro-organisms can activate) pathways are analogous and both converge on C3 → C3b → → C5 convertase
- Requires two immunoglobulins bound to membrane antigens to activate complement
  - See Fig. 18.2.
- Amplification loop: C3bBb and release of H
- Alternative pathway and T cell immunity linked
  - C5a and C3a bind to T cell receptor and major histocompatibility complex (TCR-MHC) bound complex and increase proliferation/decrease apoptosis
- C3b can be inactivated by tryptic enzymes into C3c and C3d (the latter stays on membranes!)
- C4d is analogous, measured to test for antibody–mediated rejection
- Activators of alternative pathway
  - Lipopolysaccharides
  - Fungal cell wall
  - Snake venom
  - Viruses
  - Aggregated Ig
  - Necrotic cells
- Inhibitors
  - Membrane–bound regulators—typically inhibit C3 and C5 convertases
    - CR1 (CD35)
    - DAF (CD55)
    - MCP (CD46)
    - Thrombomodulin—enhances factor I, activates fibrinolysis
    - CD59—main membrane attack complex (MAC) regulator
      - Attached by phosphatidylinositol glycan
      - Loss → paroxysmal nocturnal hemoglobinuria
  - Unbound (plasma–bound) regulators
    - C1 esterase inhibitor
      - ↓ C1r, C1s, MASP1, and MASP2 (also deactivates kallikrein → bradykinin)
      - ↓ C3 and normal C4
      - C1 esterase inhibitor deficiency = hereditary angioedema

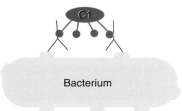

Fig. 18.2 Activation of the complement system.

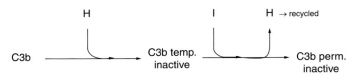

Fig. 18.3 Inactivation of C3b. *Temp,* Temporarily; *perm,* permanently.

- C4-binding protein
- Factor H (competes with factor B for C3b binding)
    - ↓ C3b, destabilizes C5 convertase
    - Protects endothelium
    - Can have congenital deficiency *or* acquired inhibiting antibody
    - Made in liver
    - See Fig. 18.3.
- Factor I—↓ C3b and C4b
- Protein S—↓ C9 binding to C7
- Clusterin—prevents MAC insertion, apolipoprotein
- Complement testing
    - If classical pathway (CP) is activated, C3 and C4 are ↓
        - If kidney transplant biopsy has C4d + IF, you know the classical pathway has been activated and inactivated
    - If alternative pathway (AP) is activated, C4 is normal and C3 is ↓
        - AP is constantly activated at low level (C3 → C3a + C3b)
        - Loss of inhibition on first step (C1 esterase), C4 ↓, C2 ↓, C3 close to normal

Abnormal Structure/Function

- Dysregulation of alternative pathway
    - Paroxysmal nocturnal hemoglobinuria (PNH) = acquired mutations in hematopoietic stem cells in *PIGA* gene so glycosylphosphatidylinositol (GPI) cannot anchor CD55 and CD59 (regulate complement)
        - MAC formation on red blood cell → hemolytic anemia, hemoglobinuria, +/− myelodysplastic syndrome
        - Responds to eculizumab
        - ↓ CD59 → intravascular hemolysis
        - ↓ CD55 → extravascular hemolysis
    - Atypical hemolytic uremic syndrome (aHUS) = acquired or genetic (usually against factor H) → kidney failure (from hemoglobinuria)
        - MAC formation on endothelial cells
        - Also CD46 (MCP), factor I, factor B (gain of function), DGKE, plasminogen
        - Responds to eculizumab (and plasma exchange if acquired)
        - ↑ C3 levels and normal C4 levels
        - May be related to HELLP syndrome (hemolysis, elevated liver enzymes, low platelets) because CD46, CD66, and CD59 are expressed on trophoblastic membranes
    - Fluid phase
        - C3 nephritic factor (↑ C3 convertase)
        - C3 glomerulopathy (also known as *dense deposit disease*)
- Age–related macular degeneration
    - Dry (atrophic) or wet (neovascular)
    - Wet: vascular endothelial growth factor, genetic (complement—CFH mutation, lipid metabolism, other immune)

- CHAPLE syndrome: complement hyperactivation, angiopathic thrombosis, and protein–losing enteropathy
  - Sort of PNH + aHUS
  - Loss-of-function mutation in *CD55*
  - T cells—↑ C activation → soluble C5a
- Anaphylaxis
  - C5a and C3a are anaphylatoxins (C5a is more powerful)
  - C5a-mediated and histamine (from mast cells)
- HELLP—likely endothelial damage in liver similar to kidney in aHUS
  - Dysregulation of alternative pathway, mutation in *CD46, CD46/55/59* expressed on tro-phoblasts, ↑ in patients with systemic lupus erythematosus (SLE)
- Deficiencies
  - *In general, complement deficiencies can lead to increased incidence of SLE because…*
    - Decreased clearance of immune complex
    - Inability to maintain self–tolerance
    - Inability to clear apoptotic cells
  - C1, C4 = rare, lupus–like disease
  - C2 = 1:10, 000, "waste disposal hypothesis" → faulty clearing of apoptotic cells → autoantigens
  - C5 = severe *Neisseria* infections
  - C6 = 1:10, 000, severe *Neisseria* infections
  - C9 = common in Japan (1:260), severe *Neisseria* infections
  - Properdin = X-linked, severe *Neisseria* infections

Interleukins (ILs)

- Innate immune system—IL-1, IL-6, TNF-α, IFN (from phagocytes), IL-12, IL-17
  - Stimulate macrophages and NK cells
  - IL-1 and TNF—fever, inflammation, and tissue destruction
- Adaptive immune system—IL-2, IL-4, IL-5, IFN-γ, IL-5, IL-17
- Stimulates T cells
- Proinflammatory ILs
  - IL-1, IL-6, IL-10, IL-23, TNF-α→ increases vascular permeability
  - IFN-γ→ attracts and stimulates macrophages
    - Increases TNF and nitric oxide
  - TGF-β→ activates fibroblasts (stops inflammatory process)
- IL-8
  - Secreted by monocytes, macrophages, fibroblasts, keratinocytes, endothelium
  - Neutrophil chemotaxis and degranulation
  - Chemotaxis of naïve T cells
  - ↑ Angiogenesis
- RANTES
  - Stands for "regulated on activation, normal T cell expressed and secreted"
  - Secreted by T cells, endothelium, platelets
  - Attracts monocytes, NK cells, T cells, basophils, dendritic cells (DCs)
  - Stimulates basophil degranulation and activates T cells
- MCP-1
  - Secreted by monocytes, macrophages, T cells, basophils, and DCs
  - Activates macrophages, ↑ histamine release from basophils, ↑ Th2
- MIP-1α
  - Secreted by monocytes, macrophages, T cells, mast cells, fibroblasts

- Attracts monocytes, NK cells, T cells, basophils, DCs
- ↑ Th1 immune response, competes with HIV-1
- MIP-1β = same as MIP-1α *except...*
  - Only secreted by monocytes, macrophages, neutrophils, and endothelium
  - Does not attract basophils
- IL-3—↑ granulopoiesis and megakaryopoiesis

Cytokine Receptor Families

1. Immunoglobulin family
   a. Used by IL-1, M-CSF
2. Class I cytokine receptor family
   a. Hematopoietin, GM-CSF, G-CSF
   b. α and β chains, sometimes γ
   c. IL-2 through IL-15 (minus 3, 8, 10, 14)
3. Class II cytokine receptor family/interferon receptor family
   a. IFN α, β, γ
   b. IL-10
4. TNF receptor family
   a. Death, decoy, and activating receptors
   b. TNF-α/β/γ, CD30L, CD40L, FasL
5. Chemokine receptor family
   a. Serpentine G-protein–coupled receptors
   b. CC, CXC, CXCR4, CC5
   c. Used by IL-8, RANTES, MIP-1, PF4, MCAF
6. Inhibitors of acute inflammation
   a. PGE1
   b. Bacterial leukocidin
   c. α₁-antitrypsin
   d. COX1 inhibitors and lipoxins

ADAPTIVE IMMUNITY

T Cell Immunity

- CD4+ T cells differentiate through IL-2R stimulation into:
  - Th1 (IFN-γ and IL2)
    - Promotes cellular immunity
    - Also induced by IL-12, IL-13, IL-23, IL-27
    - Secretes IFN-γ, which inhibits Th2
  - Th2 (IL-4, IL-5, IL-13, B cells)
    - Promotes humoral immunity (and atopic disorders)
    - Induced by IL-4
    - Secretes IL-10 and TGF-β, which inhibits Th1
  - Th17 (IL-17)
    - Innate–adaptive system overlap here
    - Protects against some extracellular bacteria and some fungi
    - Inverse relationship with Treg
  - Tfh (IL-21)
  - Tregs

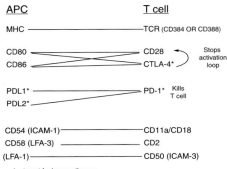

Fig. 18.4 Binding antigens on antigen–presenting cells (APC) and T cells.

* = target for immunotherapy
Anti-PD1 and anti-PDL1 are better together in melanoma

- CD4+, CD8–, low CD127+, CD25+ (also known as IL-2 receptor α chain)
- Only compose ~5% to 10% of CD4+ T cells
- If depleted → autoimmunity
- FOXP3 required for regulation
  - X-chromosome forkhead transcription factor
  - Mutation = *IPEX* (polyendocrinopathy and enteropathy)
- See Fig. 18.4.
- Nonprofessional APCs present *own* antigens on MHC to T cells but *lack* CD80/CD86–CD28 costimulation → anergy (does not die, but not activated)
  - Anergy can be reversed by really high levels of IL2
- CD8+ T cells need (1) TCR-MHC interaction, (2) CD28-CD50 stimulation, and (3) IL12 or IFN-α/β (perforin and granzyme)
- T cell receptor genes
  - α and γ = V and J (like light chains)
  - β and δ = VDJ (like heavy chains)
  - CD3 = γ-ε + δ-ε *or* α-ε + β-ε
- α β T cells
  - CD3 + ζ, CD4+ *or* CD8+
  - Has memory
  - Positive selection (thymic education—CD4+ CD8+) then negative selection (central tolerance—CD4– CD8–)
- γ δ T cells
  - CD3 and ζ (CD4– and CD8–)
  - Mucosal sites
    - ~10% of all intraepithelial lymphocytes
  - Bridge innate and adaptive
    - Innate—cytotoxic function within hours against malaria, CMV, mycobacteria *without* previous exposure
    - Adaptive—antigen–specific surface receptor
      - No memory though!!
- NK cells
  - No T cell receptor
  - No memory

Major Histocompatibility Complex (MHC) Molecules

- Class I MHC
  - Endogenous antigens

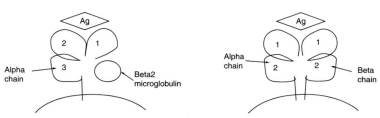

Fig. 18.5 Major histocompatibility complex (MHC) structure. *Ag,* Antigen.

- Recognized by CD8+ T cells
- Class II MHC
  - Exogenous antigens
  - Recognized by CD4+ T cells
- See Fig. 18.5.
- >200 genes code for MHC molecules on chromosome 6
- Codominant
  - Each person has 2 HLA-A, 2 HLA-B, 2 HLA-C, 2 HLA-DP, 2 HLA-DQ, 2 HLA-DR

Human Leukocyte Antigens (HLA)

- Genes
  - Class I
    - A, B, C
    - Expressed on all nucleated cells
  - Class II
    - DP, DQ, DR
    - Expressed on B cells, monocytes, macrophages, dendritic cells (DCs), and *activated* T cells
  - Class III
    - NOTCH4, complement, TNF, hereditary hemochromatosis, 21-hydroxylase
- Virtual crossmatch
  - Interfering or sensitizing substances
    - Antithymoglobulin
      - Rabbit—used after solid organ transplant, can be adsorbed out
      - Equine—used after bone marrow transplant, cannot be adsorbed
    - Pregnancy
      - *Strongest and most sustainable sensitization*
    - Intravenous immunoglobulin (IVIG)
    - Transfusions
  - Bead counts—want ≥40 beads to be confident
  - Raw values—reaction sum without subtracting background
    - "Normal"—reaction sum with normalization for background
    - Units = MFI (mean fluorescent intensities)
  - Positive: ≥500 MFI (moderate risk)
    - 3000 = high risk
- Final crossmatch

TABLE 18.1 ■ **Crossmatching for Transplant**

T cell XM	B cell XM	Antibody Class
+	+	Class I
+	–	Class I but at low levels
–	+	Class II

XM, Crossmatch.

- Allo and auto (used to differentiate clinically significant)
- Flow cytometry
- Gives DSAs (donor–specific antibodies)
- T cells—class I only
- B cells—class I and II
- See Table 18.1.
- HLA associations
  - B27—reactive arthropathy with *C. jejuni*
  - Ankylosing spondylitis
  - DQ2—celiac disease
    - Also DQ8, DQB1*06
  - DQ6—narcolepsy
  - B35—subacute thyroiditis
  - DQ8—type 1 diabetes
  - DR15 and DQ6—multiple sclerosis
  - DR4—rheumatoid arthritis
  - DR8—juvenile rheumatoid arthritis
  - DR17—Graves' disease
  - B51—Behçet's disease
- Ancestral haplotype A1, B8, DR17, DQ2
  - Northern Europeans
  - Type 1 diabetes mellitus, systemic lupus erythematosus, celiac disease, common variable immunodeficiency, IgA deficiency, myasthenia gravis, accelerated HIV course
- Public epitopes
  - Epitopes common to many HLA alleles
  - Examples: Bw4, Bw6

Immunoglobulins (and B Cell Immunity)

- B cell maturation
  - Pro-B—D-J rearrangement (CD10+ CD19+)
  - Pre-B—V-DJ rearrangement → 2 heavy chains (CD19+ CD79+)
  - Immature B cell—light–chain rearrangement (CD10– CD19+ CD20+)
  - Mature naive B cell—IgM and IgD on surface
  - Memory B cell—CD19+ CD20+ CD27+; IgA, IgE, or IgG on surface
  - Plasma cells—CD27+ CD19– CD20–; *secrete* IgA/E/G
- Immunoglobulin functions
  - Opsonize—Fc receptor on macrophages and neutrophils
  - Antibody–dependent cellular cytotoxicity—NK cells with Fc receptor
  - Activate complement—IgG and IgM

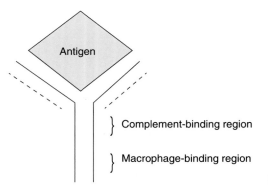

Fig. 18.6   Immunoglobulin structure.

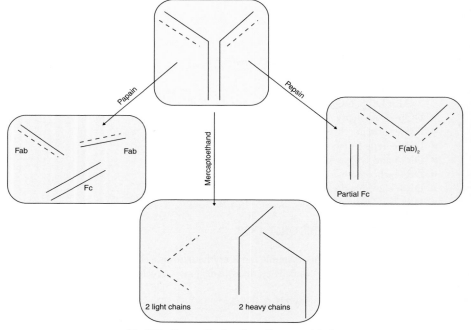

Fig. 18.7   Enzymatic digestion of immunoglobulin.

- ■ Agglutination and precipitation of microbes
- ■ Toxin and viral neutralization
- ■ Prevents penetration of epithelium—only IgA
- ■ Degranulation of eosinophils, basophils, mast cells—IgE
- ■ Circulate in T shape and conform to and shape when bound to antigen
  - ■ Opens up complement–binding region
  - ■ See Figs. 18.6 and 18.7.
- ■ IgM is great at identifying polysaccharide and repetitive antigens
- ■ IgG half–life is 23 days
- ■ IgG1, 3, and 4 can cross the placenta (not IgG2)

- Starts in third or fourth month of gestation
- IgG4 does not fix complement
- Process of creating monoclonal antibodies
  - Give animal an antigen intravenously
  - Collect plasma cells (PCs) from mouse
    - Each PC has specificity for a different epitope of the antigen
  - Mix with myeloma cells without HGPRT activity
  - Hybrid cells are formed and selected for in HAT medium
  - Separate all hybrid cells into 1 cell per well
    - Presumably with different epitope specificity
    - Grow in bulk

IMMUNOGENIC COMPONENTS OF AND DEFENSE AGAINST PATHOGENS

- Bacteria
  - Gram positive—teichoic acid
    - Alternative complement system and antibodies
    - Resistant to lysis (thick wall)
  - Gram negative—lipopolysaccharide
    - Classic and alternative complement, antibodies, and phagocytes
    - Sensitive to lysis (thin wall)
  - Mycobacteria
    - Macrophages and cell–mediated
    - Strong humoral response but ineffective (because it is intracellular)
  - Spirochetes
    - Complement, antibodies, cell–mediated
    - Outer membrane
  - Infections lead to increased IL6, which leads to increased C-reactive protein
- Viruses
  - IFN α/β/γ → ↑ NK-mediated killing of infected cells
  - Complement damages envelope of some viruses
  - Humoral
  - MAIN: cytotoxic T cells
- Fungi
  - Intracellular—Th17 CD4+ T cells
  - Cross–linked polysaccharide wall → resistant to lysis
- Protozoa
  - Alternative complement
  - Neutrophil/macrophage phagocytosis
  - Humoral for malaria, amebiasis, and trypanosomiasis
  - Cell–mediated for leishmania and toxoplasma
- Helminths
  - Eosinophils and mast cells
  - IgE → antibody–dependent cellular cytotoxicity

Autoimmune Clinical Syndromes

HYPERSENSITIVITY REACTIONS

- Type I

- IgE binding to mast cells (FcεR)
- Release histamine, heparin, serotonin arachidonic acid
- Anaphylaxis (urine histamine is elevated for ~24 hours)
- Type II—antibody–mediated cellular cytotoxicity
  - Antigen–antibody → opsonization → tissue damage
  - Example: Goodpasture, myasthenia gravis, immune hemolysis, erythroblastosis fetalis, hyperacute graft rejection
- Type III—immune complex
  - Antigen–antibody → activation of complement
  - Example: systemic lupus erythematosus (SLE), Henoch–Schönlein purpura, serum sickness, poststreptococcal glomerulonephritis, membranous glomerulonephritis, Arthus reaction (edema in vessel walls → fibrinoid necrosis and thrombosis)
- Type IV—delayed–type
  - T cell antigen interaction +/− granulomas
  - Example: tuberculin skin test, poison ivy

SPECIFIC AUTOANTIBODIES

- Antinuclear antibodies (ANA)
  - Use indirect immunofluorescence on HEp2 cells (human epithelial cell tumor line)
  - ≥1:80 considered significant
  - Patterns
    - Homogenous
      - Bright nucleus and mitotic bars
      - +/− nuclear membrane accentuation
      - +/− minimal cytoplasmic background stain
      - Drug–induced lupus–like syndrome (procainamide/hydralazine)
      - SLE
    - Course speckled
      - Extractable nuclear antigens (ENAs) including Sm proteins (snRNP—small nuclear ribonucleoproteins); SLE, Sjögren syndrome (SS), mixed connective tissue disease (MCTD)
      - Nonspecific!
    - Centromere (fine nuclear dots)
      - CREST (calcinosis, Raynaud's esophageal dysmotility, sclerodactyly, telangiectasia)
    - Nucleolar
      - Raynaud's and scleroderma
    - Other less common
      - Nuclear envelope (extremely diagnostic for SLE, but very rare), dense fine speckled (anti-LEDGF), proliferating cell nuclear antigen (PCNA), clumpy nucleolar, few nuclear dots, centromere/centriole, mitotic spindle apparatus (MSA), peripheral (SLE)
- Antineutrophil cytoplasmic antibodies (ANCA)
  - Negative does not rule out vasculitis
  - ANCA types
    - p-ANCA = antimyeloperoxidase (MPO)
      - Ulcerative colitis, primary sclerosing cholangitis, microscopic polyangiitis, polyarteritis nodosa
    - c-ANCA = antiproteinase 3 (PR3)
      - Wegener's, microscopic polyangiitis

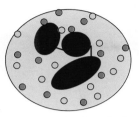

Ethanol-fixed   Formalin-fixed

O = p-ANCA (MPO)
● = c-ANCA (PR3)

Fig. 18.8 Antineutrophil cytoplasmic antibodies.

- Distinguished on ethanol–fixed neutrophils (must also perform on formalin–fixed cells to rule out ANA)
- See Fig. 18.8.
- Antimitochondrial—primary biliary cholangitis
  - Cytoplasmic reticular pattern
- Anti-smooth muscle—autoimmune hepatitis
- Antiliver kidney microsomal—autoimmune hepatitis
- Antiparietal cell—pernicious anemia
- anti-dsDNA—SLE
  - Use *Crithidia luciliae* to detect them
  - Circular dsDNA genome which is *way* more stable than linear dsDNA
  - ssDNA antibodies are not clinically relevant
  - Only high–affinity dsDNA antibodies are diagnostic for SLE
  - See Fig. 18.9.
- Anti-Jo1—polymyositis and dermatomyositis
  - Multiple cytoplasmic dots
- Antihistone—drug–induced lupus
- RF—rheumatoid arthritis (RA)
- Anti-CCP—RA
- Extractable nuclear antigens
  - Smith—SLE
  - RNP—MCTD
  - Nucleolar—scleroderma
  - SS-A/SS-B (Ro/La)—SS, SLE
    - Ro/SS-A—neonatal lupus → complete congenital heart block
  - Microsomal—Hashimoto
  - Endomysial—celiac sprue and dermatitis herpetiformis
  - Gliadin and transglutaminase—celiac sprue
  - GBM—Goodpasture
  - IF (intermediate filament)—polymyositis/dermatomyositis (PM/DM)
  - Scl-70—scleroderma
    - Also known as *antitopoisomerase*
  - PM1—scleroderma/dermatomyositis overlap syndrome
  - Thyroglobulin—Hashimoto
  - Thyroid–stimulating antibody (LATS)—Graves'
  - RNA-pol 3—scleroderma

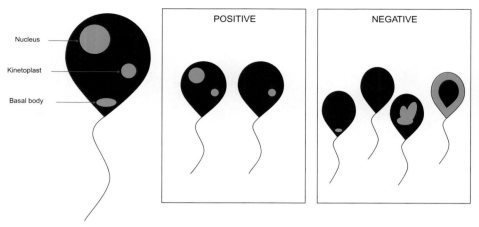

Fig. 18.9 Antidouble–stranded DNA using *Crithidia luciliae*.

- Ribosomal P—PM/DM
- PCNA—specific for SLE (but only seen in 2% to 10% of SLE patients)

AUTOIMMUNE DISORDERS

Autoimmune Encephalitis

- Anti-NMDA receptor (allows calcium to flow in)
  - Can test for antibodies in serum or CSF (more sensitive)
  - Use rat brain (hippocampus) cross–sections and/or cultures
  - Clinical findings—behavior changes, psychosis, seizures, memory and cognitive deficits, abnormal movements, dysautonomia, and decreased Glasgow Coma Scale
  - May be paraneoplastic (usually ovarian teratoma)
  - Ketamine blocks pore (so does magnesium)
    - Glycine and glutamate bind
    - Magnesium must be removed before activation
  - Lymphocytes in CSF +/− oligoclonal bands
- The limbic system
  - Includes corpus callosum, fornix, pineal gland, anterior thalamus, hypothalamus, mamillary body, amygdala, cingulate gyrus, parahippocampal gyrus, hippocampus
  - Limbic encephalitis—*memory loss*, irritability, sleep changes, delusions/hallucinations, seizures, psychosis
    - Caused by antibodies against:
      - Surface antigens: AMPAR (associated with thymomas), LGI1 (thymoma), CASPR2, GABAb (small cell carcinoma of lung)
      - Intracellular antigens: Hu (small cell carcinoma of lung), Ma2 (testicular seminoma)
        - Mediated by cytotoxic T cells
        - Harder to treat than antibodies to surface antigens
- Therapy: remove tumor if present, steroids, plasma exchange, IVIG
  - Second line: CellCept, rituximab, Cytoxan
- Aquaporin 4 receptor—neuromyelitis optica, acute myelitis

TABLE 18.2 ■ Primary Biliary Cholangitis vs. Primary Sclerosing Cholangitis

Primary Biliary Cholangitis	Primary Sclerosing Cholangitis
Female, middle–aged (30–65 years)	Male (20–40 years)
Pruritus and fatigue, xanthelasmas, hyperpigmentation, arthropathy	Progressive obstructive jaundice
Laboratory tests: cholestatic	Laboratory tests: cholestatic
Intrahepatic	Intra- and extrahepatic
Granulomas, inflammation and duct destruction, most common cause of progressive ductopenia	Inflammation and "onion skinning fibrosis"
No specific imaging	"Beads on a string" ductogram
Associated with other autoimmune disorders	Associated with ulcerative colitis (70%)
Cirrhosis	Cirrhosis, cholangiocarcinoma, and hepatocellular carcinoma
Early treatment with ursodeoxycholic acid can help	Increased T cells, anti-smooth muscle antibody, antinuclear antibody, rheumatoid factor, p-ANCA
	High alkaline phosphatase

TABLE 18.3 ■ Autoimmune Hepatitis

	Type 1	Type 2
Antibodies	ANA, smooth muscle, soluble liver protein, Saccharomyces	Liver–kidney microsomal 1 (LKM1)
Age of onset	10–20, 45–70	2–14, girls
IgG	↑ ↑ ↑	↑
IgA	Normal	Normal / ↓
HLA associations	B8 DR3, DR4	B14 DR3

ANA, Antinuclear antibodies; *HLA*, human leukocyte antigen.

Autoimmune Liver and Biliary Disease

- Can get "atypical pANCA" in autoimmune hepatitis
  - Not anti-MPO but antinuclear envelope protein
- Primary biliary cholangitis and primary sclerosing cholangitis
  - See Table 18.2.
- Autoimmune hepatitis
  - See Table 18.3.

Celiac Disease

- Dermatitis herpetiformis
  - Immunofluorescence (IF) = IgA+ granular, basement membrane

- Celiac disease has a direct effect on the CNS → neuropsychiatric symptoms
  - Incidence of celiac = 1:100
  - α-gliadin
  - CD4+ T cells → damaged epithelium
- FLA-DQ2 (95%) or DQ8 (5%)
  - If patient is negative, they *cannot* get celiac (but + does not guarantee disease)
- Tissue transglutaminases deaminates α-gliadin
- IgA and other peptides → ↑ immunogenicity
- Antiendomysial IgA = highly specific
  - Indirect IF
  - Equivalent to antitissue transglutaminase IgA or IgG (ELISA)
- Antigliadin has a lot of false positives
- IgA deficiency is 10 to 15 × more common in celiac than general population

Other Autoimmune Disorders

- Polymyositis/dermatomyositis (PM/DM)
  - Antibodies
    - Jo1—histidyl-tRNA synthetase
    - PL7—threonyl-tRNA synthetase
    - PL12—alanyl-tRNA synthetase
  - Antisynthetase syndrome = variant of PM/DM
    - Interstitial fibrotic lung disease, mechanic's hands, myositis

Immunodeficiency Disorders

GENERAL

- Antibody formation against carbohydrates requires B cell function only
  - Antibody formation against proteins requires *B cell and T cell function*
- Assess delayed–type hypersensitivity for T cell function
  - Tuberculin skin test
- Chromium release assay for NK cell function

TABLE 18.4 ■ **Classic Clinical Presentations of Immunodeficiency Disorders**

Clinical Presentation	Syndrome
Enteroviral encephalitis	X-linked (Bruton) agammaglobulinemia
Pneumocystis jirovecii	Severe combined immunodeficiency, Hyper IgM
N. meningitidis	Terminal complement
HSV encephalitis	TLR3 signaling
Alopecia	Omenn (RAG1/2)
Thrombocytopenia	CD40, CD40L
Eczema	Wiskott-Aldrich Syndrome, DOCK8
Kaposi	OX40
Endocrinopathy	IPEX, APECED

- Oxidative burst assay (yellow → blue) for neutrophil functions
- TLR, MYD88, or IRAK4 pathway deficiencies → bacterial infections
  - TLR3 deficiency → increased susceptibility to herpes encephalitis
- Classic clinical presentations. See Table 18.4.

B CELL DEFECTS

- Pulmonary and gastrointestinal infections (especially bronchiectasis and giardia), small lymph nodes
- Bruton (X-linked) agammaglobulinemia
  - Recurrent bacterial infections beginning ~6 months
    - Encapsulated bacteria = yes, some killer bacteria have pretty nice capsules
      - *Yersinia pestis*
      - *Streptococcus pneumoniae*
      - *Klebsiella pneumoniae*
      - *Bacillus anthracis*
      - *Haemophilus influenzae*
      - *Pseudomonas aeruginosa*
      - *Neisseria meningitidis*
      - *Cryptococcus*
  - ↑ Susceptibility to polio, hepatitis, and enteroviruses
  - ↓↓↓ IgG, IgA, IgM, CD19+ B cells
  - Tonsils and lymph nodes are rudimentary
  - Treat with IVIG; do *not* give live vaccines
- Common variable immunodeficiency (CVID)
  - Onset in second or third decade
  - Recurrent upper and lower respiratory infections, intestinal bacterial overgrowth, Giardiasis, bronchiectasis
  - Low IgG, IgA, IgM
  - B cells cannot become plasma cells
    - Germinal centers = hyperplastic
    - Pronounced reactive follicular lymphoid hyperplasia (with germinal centers) and no plasma cells
- Selective IgA deficiency
  - Most common immunodeficiency
  - Associated with autoimmune disorders (like celiac)
- Hyper IgE (Job) syndrome
  - Recurrent staph infections, coarse facies, ↑ IgE
    - Leads to increased abnormal T cell activation
    - *STAT3* mutations, autosomal dominant

TABLE 18.5 ■ Immunodeficiencies with Abnormal IgE Levels	
High IgE	Job syndrome
	Wiskott–Aldrich syndrome
	Nezelof syndrome
Low IgE	Bruton agammaglobulinemia
	Ataxia telangiectasia

- Eosinophilia and eczema
- See Table 18.5.

T CELL DEFECTS

- Viral and fungal infections (especially mucocutaneous candidiasis)
- DiGeorge syndrome
  - Third and fourth pharyngeal pouches
  - Hypoplastic thymus → ↓ T cells → ↑ risk for *Pneumocystis jirovecii* pneumonia (PCP), transfusion–associated graft-versus-host disease (TA-GVHD)
  - Hypoplastic parathyroid → neonatal hypocalcemic tetany
  - Great vessel anomalies, facies (hypertelorism, low set ears, small jaw), bifid uvula, esophageal atresia
  - *Partial* is more common than complete
    - May present with CHARGE sequence
      - Coloboma
      - Heart defect
      - Atresia (choanal)
      - Retardation of development
      - Genital hypoplasia
      - Ear anomalies
  - Lymph nodes = ↓ paracortical areas
  - Spleen = ↓ periarteriolar lymphatic sheaths (PALS)
  - Microdeletions in 22q11.2
  - Some sporadic from in utero exposure to Accutane
- Severe combined immunodeficiency (SCID)
  - Multiple subtypes, see Table 18.6.
  - Decreased or no T cell function, decreased or no immunoglobulin, thymic dysplasia
  - Life–threatening, ↑ risk for TA-GVHD
  - T cell receptor excision circles (TRECs)
    - If absent (or nearly absent), indicate T cell immunodeficiency
      - Most frequently SCID and DiGeorge
  - Atypical SCID
    - Instead of no γ constant chain (which makes an integral part of many interleukin receptors), has truncated γ chain or *JAK3* mutations (which is a common pathway midpoint for IL receptors)
- Omenn syndrome

TABLE 18.6 ■ **Subtypes of Severe Combined Immunodeficiency (SCID)**

Types of SCID	T Cells	B Cells	NK Cells
γ chain deficiency JAK3 deficiency	−	+	−
IL-7R-α deficiency CD3ε or CD45 deficiency	−	+	+
Adenosine deaminase (ADA) deficiency	−	−	−
RAG1 or 2 deficiency Artemis deficiency	−	−	+

- SCID + diffuse erythroderma, alopecia, protracted diarrhea, eosinophilia, hepatospleno-megaly, lymphadenopathy, lymphocytosis
  - No circulating B cells
- T cell infiltration of skin and gut
  - Mostly Th2
  - Increased γδ T cells during infections (especially in CMV)
- No germinal centers in lymph nodes
- Hypoplastic thymus
- ↑ IgE, other immunoglobulins are absent
- *RAG1/2* mutations
  - Peripheral expansion of autoimmune clones to epithelial antigens (↓ autoimmune regulator—AIRE)
- Fatal without bone marrow transplant
- Hyper IgM syndrome (X-linked immunodeficiency with hyper IgM)
  - Impaired isotype switching
    - ↑ IgM, ↓ IgA/IgG/IgE
    - Clinically similar to Bruton
    - CD154 defect (T cell ligand for B cell receptor–associated CD40 , also called CD40 ligand or CD40L)
- Wiskott–Aldrich syndrome
  - *WAS* gene on X chromosome, encodes WASP
  - (1) eczema, (2) thrombocytopenia, (3) immunodeficiency
  - ↑ risk for *Streptococcus pneumoniae* (and other encapsulated bacteria), PCP, and herpesvirus
- Ataxia telangiectasia (Louis Bar syndrome)
  - (1) Cerebellar ataxia, (2) oculocutaneous telangiectasia, (3) recurrent sinopulmonary infections, (4) ↑ risk for malignancies
  - Combined B and T defect, autosomal recessive, *ATM* gene on 11q22.3
    - Many mutations
  - ↓ IgA (and IgE and IgG2), ↑↑↑ serum AFP and CEA
  - ↑ DNA fragility
  - No thymic epithelial components (Hassall's corpuscles)
- Chronic mucocutaneous candidiasis
  - Selective T cell defect against *Candida*
  - Associated with endocrinopathies and autoimmune disorders
  - Mutation in autoimmune regulator (AIRE) gene on 21q22.3
- Duncan disease (X-linked lymphoproliferative disease)
  - Fulminant or fatal immune response to EBV
  - Immune dysfunction like CVID
  - Inverted CD4:CD8 in blood, ↓ immunoglobulin
  - *SH2D1A* on Xq25
    - SH2 domain on signal–transducing protein SLAM-associated protein (SAP)
- T cell immunodeficiency with detectable T cells
  - ZAP70 deficiency, ↑↑ immunoglobulin
  - Neonatal diarrhea, autoimmune disorders
  - Normal CD4, absent CD8

NEUTROPHIL/PHAGOCYTIC DEFECTS

- Staphylococcal and other catalase–positive infections (campylobacter, listeria, bacillus)
- Chronic granulomatous disease

- X-linked, gp91phox
- Deficiency of NADPH oxidase (most commonly) → ↓ *intracellular oxidative killing of engulfed microorganisms*
  - Other conditions that lead to impaired phagocytosis and intracellular killing: myeloperoxidase deficiency, glutathione reductase deficiency, Chediak-Higashi syndrome
- Chronic catalase + infections (staphylococcus, Enterobacter, aspergillus)
  - *Not streptococcus!*
- Extensive granulomas
- Diagnose with NBT test
- Leukocytes lack C3b receptors; erythrocytes have null Kell (Kx), or MacLeod phenotype
- Chediak-Higashi syndrome
  - Lysosomal trafficking regulator *(LYST/CHS1)* mutation at 1q42.1
  - Autosomal recessive
  - (1) Neutropenia with chunky granules, (2) oculocutaneous albinism, (3) thrombocytopenia, (4) recurrent infections
- May-Hegglin anomaly
  - *MYH9* mutation
  - Autosomal dominant, Dohle–like bodies in granulocytes and monocytes, variably sized platelets, thrombocytopenia
  - Dohle–like bodies can be digested by ribonuclease
- Alder–Reilly anomaly
  - No functional impact
  - Large blue granules in all leukocytes
  - Associated with mucopolysaccharidoses
- Pelger-Huet anomaly
  - No functional impact
  - Autosomal dominant, bilobed or monolobated nuclei (Stodtmeister cells)
- Jordan anomaly
  - Fat vacuoles in leukocytes
- Severe congenital neutropenia (Kostmann syndrome)
  - Multiple mutations include *ELANE, HAX2, SBDS,* and so on
    - Autosomal recessive or dominant inheritance
  - Rare, Caucasian children, equal sex distribution
  - Intermittent diarrhea, ear infections, staphylococcal skin infections
  - Low absolute neutrophil count, increased monocyte count, normal morphology

COMPLEMENT DEFECTS

- Classical pathway deficiency (C1q, C2, C3)
  - Autoimmune disorders
- C2 and C3 deficiencies
  - Gram–positive encapsulated bacterial infections
- MAC deficiencies (terminal complement)
  - *N. meningitidis* and *N. gonorrhoeae* infections
- C1 esterase inhibitor (C1Inh) deficiency (hereditary angioedema)
  - Autosomal dominant
  - During attacks

- ↑ Urine histamine
- ↑ Serum C1
- ↓ CH50, C4, C2
- Between attacks
  - ↓ C4
  - C2 = normal
- Treatment = recombinant C1Inh, plasma, kallikrein inhibitors, and so on
- Prophylaxis = androgenic drugs (danazol, oxandrolone, methyltestosterone)

Other Clinical Syndromes/Disorders

VASCULITIDES

- Without serology markers—use demographics and clinical presentation
  - Giant cell arteritis (GCA)
    - Older adults
    - Temporal vision problems, jaw claudication, polymyalgia rheumatica
    - Most common vasculitis in adults
    - Large and medium aortic branches
    - Transmural inflammation, lymphocytes and multinucleated giant cells
      - Fragmentation of the internal elastic lamina with intimal hyperplasia
      - No thrombi usually
  - Takayasu arteritis
    - Children and teens
    - Pulseless extremities, blood pressure difference between extremities
    - Major branches of aorta (like GCA)
    - Looks histologically like GCA (difference in patient characteristics)
    - Japan, China, India, Mexico
    - Diagnosis = angiography
  - Kawasaki syndrome
    - Children (usually 2 or 3 years of age)
    - Fever ≥4 days, erythema of palms and soles, desquamation, bilateral conjunctivitis, cracked lips and strawberry tongue, cervical lymphadenopathy
    - *Mucocutaneous lymph node syndrome*
    - Can lead to coronary artery aneurysm
  - Henoch-Schönlein syndrome
    - Children
    - Palpable purpura of the lower extremities, abdominal pain, glomerulonephritis
      - Kidney biopsy looks similar to IgA nephropathy with mesangial IgA deposits
  - Buerger syndrome (thromboangiitis obliterans)
    - Young male smokers
    - Arterial insufficiency affecting hands and feet
- Behçet syndrome
  - Oral and genital aphthous ulcers and uveitis
    - Middle East, Far East, Mediterranean
    - Pathergy test (erythema and pustule at site of needle stick at ~48 hours)
  - Cogan syndrome
    - Rare, young adults
    - Keratitis and vestibulo–auditory
- With serology markers—use vessel size and serologies

- Polyarteritis nodosa
  - Medium–sized arteries
  - Involves kidneys, nerves (mononeuritis multiplex), mesenteric vessels, and skin
    - Spares lungs
  - Biopsy shows segmental fibrinoid necrosis (segmental active lesions, healing lesions, and normal next to each other) of vessels
  - Likes vessel branch points
  - **+/– HBV or HCV seropositivity**
- Microscopic polyangiitis
  - Small arteries and venules
  - Lungs, kidneys (looks like focal segmental necrotizing glomerulonephritis—FSNGN), and others
  - **+ pANCA (or anti-MPO)**
- Churg–Strauss syndrome
  - "Allergic angiitis and granulomatosis" or "eosinophilic granulomatosis with polyangiitis"
  - Adult–onset asthma → fulminant vasculitis
  - Widespread effects + peripheral eosinophilia
  - Death from cardiac involvement
  - **+ pANCA (or anti-MPO)**
- Wegener's granulomatosis
  - *Granulomatosis with polyangiitis*
  - Widespread effects
    - Upper respiratory tract, lower respiratory tract, kidney (focal segmental glomerulosclerosis, pauci–immune type)
  - **+ cANCA (or anti-PR3)**
- Goodpasture syndrome
  - Lungs and kidneys
  - **+ Anti-GBM**
- Cryoglobulinemia
  - Widespread
  - **+ Cryoglobulins**
- Syphilis
  - Widespread
  - Can mimic Takayasu arteritis
  - **+ RPR**
- Rheumatoid arthritis (and other collagen vascular disorders)
  - Widespread
  - **+ RF, ANA, RPR, and so on**

ALLOGRAFT REJECTION

- Hyperacute
  - Preformed donor–specific antibodies to MHC antigens that cause complement fixation
  - Minutes to hours
  - Thrombosis and fibrinoid necrosis
- Acute
  - Antibody–mediated
    - Donor specific antibodies → complement activated

- 3 months
- Treat with anti–B cell drugs (e.g., rituximab)
- Cell–mediated
  - Intense infiltration of lymphocytes and macrophages
  - Weeks to years
  - Treat with immunosuppression
- Chronic
  - Both humoral and cell–mediated
  - Microvasculature changes
  - Months to years

Odds and Ends

- Normal κ-to-λ; ratio = 0.26 to 1.65
- T cells must be activated to express MHC class II
- Class II MHC can be abnormal on non–antigen–presenting cells in autoimmune disorders and malignancies
- Plasmablasts—halfway between activated B cell and plasma cell
  - CD19+, CD20–, CD38+
  - ↑ Circulating plasmablasts in IgG4-related–disease
- IgG4 class antibodies have a serine instead of proline at hinge disulfide region

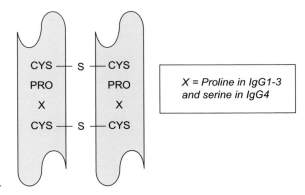

Fig. 18.10 IgG antibody structures.

- This allows the sides to dissociate and reassociate with other antibodies → BISPECIFIC
- See Fig. 18.10.
- Poststreptococcal glomerulonephritis
  1. Complement deposition in capillary loops
  2. Neutrophils are recruited
  3. Glomerulonephritis

CHAPTER 19

Coagulation

Normal Coagulation

PRIMARY HEMOSTASIS

- Platelets
  - Adhere to site of injury
    - GPIa/IIa + collagen
    - GPIb/IX/V + von Willebrand factor (VWF)
  - Release granule contents
    - Dense and alpha
  - Form plug
    - GPIIb/IIIa + fibrin
    - GPIb + VWF
  - Provide a substrate for the coagulation cascade
- Most potent platelet activators are protease–activated receptor 1 and interaction with thrombin

SECONDARY HEMOSTASIS

See Fig. 19.1.
- In vitro
  - Extrinsic pathway is started by tissue factor activating factor VII (FVII)
  - Intrinsic pathway is started by high-molecular weight kininogen (HMWK) and prekallikrein (PK) activating FXII (and driven by thrombin from extrinsic pathway)
- In vivo, the extrinsic pathway is activated, then thrombin activates factors XI, VIII, and V

Normal Thrombolysis

- See Fig. 19.2.
- See Fig. 19.3.
- Protein C
  - Serine protease (made in liver)
  - Thrombomodulin and protein C receptor required for thrombin activation of protein C
  - Degrades FVa and FVIIIa
  - Cofactor protein S is crucial for its function
  - Vitamin K-dependent factor
  - Blocks plasminogen activator inhibitor 1 (PAI1) and blocks tissue plasminogen activator (tPA) receptor → increased fibrinolysis
  - *PROC* gene on chromosome 2q14.3
  - Levels
    - Lower in neonates and infants (reaches normal at puberty)
    - Secondary decrease
      - Warfarin

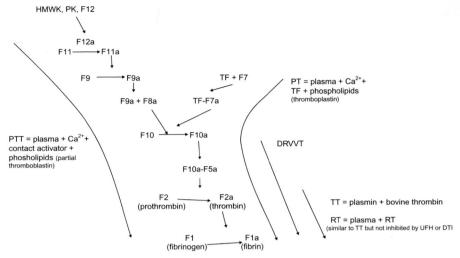

Fig. 19.1   Coagulation cascade. *DTI,* Direct thrombin inhibitors; *HMWK,* high-molecular-weight kininogen; *PK,* prekallikrein; *PT,* prothrombin time; *PTT,* partial thromboplastin time; *RT,* reptilase time; *TF,* tissue factor; *TT,* thrombin time; *UFH,* unfractionated heparin.

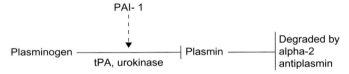

Fig. 19.2   Thrombolysis regulation. *PAI,* Plasminogen activator inhibitor; *tPA,* tissue plasminogen activator. PAI-1 suppresses plasminogen activation.

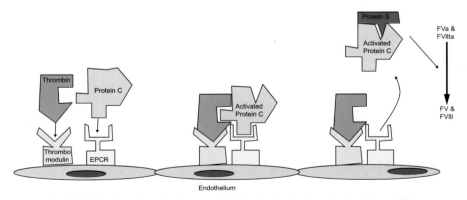

Fig. 19.3   Function of protein C and protein S in the inactivation of factors Va and VIIa.

- Vitamin K deficiency
- Consumptive (disseminated intravascular coagulopathy—DIC, acute thrombosis, and so on)
- Liver disease
- L-asparaginase therapy
- False low—elevated FVIII, factor V Leiden

- Protein S
  - Vitamin K dependent
  - Cofactor for protein C
  - Circulates bound (60%) and free (40%)
    - Binds to C4b binding protein
- Antithrombin
  - Natural anticoagulant that inactivates thrombin (factor IIa) and factors IXa, Xa, XIa, XIIa
  - Unfractionated heparin potentiates 1000-fold
  - Levels
    - Secondary decrease
      - Liver disease
      - Consumptive (DIC, active thrombosis, and so on)
      - Surgery
      - Sepsis
      - Inflammatory bowel disease
      - L-asparaginase therapy
      - Nephrotic syndrome
      - High estrogen states
    - Secondary increase
      - Menopause
      - High heparin cofactor II levels
    - False increase by warfarin and argatroban

Basic Coagulation Assays

- See Table 19.1.

PROTHROMBIN TIME/INTERNATIONAL NORMALIZED RATIO (PT/INR)

- Sodium citrate tube
- Plasma (centrifuge whole blood)

TABLE 19.1 ■ Coagulation Assay Patterns

PT/INR	PTT	TT	Causes
↑	–	–	F7 deficiency or inhibitor, Vitamin K antagonist or deficiency, liver disease, +/– anti-Xa, factor deficiency or inhibitor (FX, V, II), LAC
–	↑	–	Factor deficiency (VIII, IX, XI, XII, HMWK, PK), DTI, VWD, LAC
–	–	↑	Heparin, LMWH, low or very high fibrinogen, DTI, LAC
↑	↑	–	Factor deficiency (X, V, II), vitamin K antagonist or deficiency, liver disease, anti-Xa
–	↑	↑	Heparin (UFH) and multifactor deficiency
↑	↑	↑	Low-quality sample, DIC, liver disease, low fibrinogen, dysfibrinogenemia, DTI, bridging, high UFH

DIC, Disseminated intravascular coagulopathy; DTI, direct thrombin inhibitor; HMWK, highmolecular–weight kininogen; INR, international normalized ratio; LAC, lupus anticoagulant; LMWH, low-molecular–weight heparin; PK, prekallikrein; PT, prothrombin time; PTT, partial thromboplastin time; TT, thrombin time; VWD, von Willebrand disease; UFH, unfractionated heparin.

- Plasma + calcium + thromboplastin (tissue factor + phospholipid)

$$INR = \left(\frac{PT\,mean}{PT\,geometric\,mean} \right)^{ISI}$$

  - ISI of the test reagent = ISI reference preparation × slope of regression line
- INR factor sensitivities
  - Regulation agencies require laboratories to determine the amount of factor deficiency triggers an increase in INR
- Alternatives to INR: chromogenic factor 10, clot-based factor 2
  - Do not always agree with each other and do not agree with INR → different therapeutic ranges
    - Especially at low INRs (early in anticoagulation)
- Decreased by hemolyzed/contaminated samples or increased factor VII
- Prolonged by...
  - Vitamin K antagonists
  - Vitamin K deficiency
  - Liver disease
  - Direct thrombin inhibitors (DTIs)
  - Consumption (clotting, bleeding)
  - Factor deficiency = II, V, VII, X, fibrinogen
  - Factor inhibitor (and lupus anticoagulants)
  - Paraproteinemia
  - Low quality sample
    - Under-/overfilled tube
    - Contamination
    - Polycythemia
  - Anti-Xa drugs
  - Dysfibrinogenemia
  - Unfractionated heparin (UFH; but most laboratories have heparin neutralizer)
    - Neutralizer can be overcome with a *lot* of UFH

PARTIAL THROMBOPLASTIN TIME (PTT)

- Prolonged by...
  - Vitamin K antagonists
  - Vitamin K deficiency
  - Liver disease
  - DTIs
  - Consumption
  - Factor deficiency (XII, XI, IX, VIII, X, IV, II, I, HMWK, PK)
    - XII, HMWK, and PK deficiencies prolong PTT but do not make you bleed
  - Factor inhibitor (and lupus anticoagulants)
  - Paraproteinemia
  - Low-quality sample
    - Under-/overfilled tube
    - Contamination
    - Polycythemia
  - Anti-Xa drugs
  - Dysfibrinogenemia

- UFH—Brill–Edwards for monitoring, better than PTT
  - Compares PTT and anti-Xa
- High levels of low-molecular-weight heparin (LMWH)
- von Willebrand disease (VWD; because of FVIII deficiency—see later)

THROMBIN TIME (TT)

- Low or very high fibrinogen
- Dysfibrinogenemia
- Consumption
- Low quality sample
- Liver disease
- UFH and LMWH at high levels
- Factor inhibitors and lupus anticoagulants
- DTIs (and factor II auto-antibodies)

OTHERS

- Activated clotting time (ACT) = whole blood + contact activator + calcium
  - "Whole-blood PTT"
  - Can be done bedside with a syringe
    - Used for ECMO, dialysis, point-of-care monitoring of UFH and DTI
  - Sensitive to decreased platelet number or function
- Dilute Russell viper venom time (DRVVT)
  - Tests common pathway, alternative to thrombin time
  - Factors X, V, II, and fibrinogen (factor I)
- Anti-Xa assay
  - Can use for direct FXa inhibitors
  - Must use for...
    - LMWH monitoring
    - Heparin monitoring when at extremes of age, extremes of weight, renal impairment, pregnant
      - Looks for heparin effect first, then runs chromogenic assay
      - Patient plasma + heparin + antithrombin (AT) + factor Xa → [Heparin-AT-FXa] complex + free FXa
    - Then add a chromogenic substrate for FXa
    - If there is more heparin on board, there is less FXa to cleave, there is less color change
  - Interference
    - Falsely increased—lipemia, renal impairment (that is not recognized/taken into account)
    - Falsely decreased—hemolysis, hyperbilirubinemia, delay in sample analysis

Anticoagulants

- See Fig. 19.4.

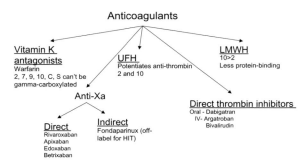

Fig. 19.4 Types of anticoagulants. *HIT*, Heparin–induced thrombocytopenia; *IV*, intravenous; *LMWH*, low-molecular-weight heparin; *PCI*, percutaneous coronary intervention; *UFH*, unfractionated heparin; *w/o*, without.

WARFARIN

- Effects factors II, VI, IX, X, C, S, Z
- ↓ Vitamin K oxide reductase → ↓γ-carboxylation of factors
  - Decreased *activity* of factors II, VII, IX, X, C, and S
  - Decreased free S *antigen*
- P450 system—genetic mutations (*CYP2C9*2*, *CYP2C9*3*, *VKORC1*) and so on
- Reversal
  - Chest guidelines
    - See Table 19.2.
  - Nonbleeding
    - <4.5—↓ or hold next dose
    - 4.5 to 10—hold
    - >10—hold and give vitamin K orally
  - Bleeding—hold and give IV vitamin K +/− 4 factor prothrombin complex concentrate (PCC)
    - PCC has heparin contamination (contraindicated in heparin–induced thrombocytopenia)

UNFRACTIONATED HEPARIN (UFH)

- Pork–derived (patient may have religious objections)
- Complex clearing
  - Rapidly saturable (bound to proteins)
  - Slow first order through kidney
- Monitoring
  - aPTT monitoring (1.5 to 2.5 × normal)
    - Na citrate tube
    - Centrifuge → platelet–poor plasma
    - Plasma + surface activator + phospholipid + Ca
    - ↑ FVIII → ↑aPTT
    - Activated clotting time is similar to aPTT, but with whole blood
  - Heparin–specific assays = anti-IIa or anti-Xa based
    - ↑ pNA (reaction product) = ↓ heparin
  - PTT therapeutic range—use Brill–Edwards method
  - Thrombin time is very sensitive
- Monitoring troubleshooting

TABLE 19.2 ■ **Warfarin Reversal Guidelines Based on INR**

INR	Clinical Scenario	Management
<4.5	No bleeding	Hold warfarin until INR in therapeutic range
	Rapid reversal required	Hold warfarin Give oral vitamin K
4.5–10	No bleeding	Hold warfarin until INR in therapeutic range Give oral vitamin K
	Rapid reversal required	Hold warfarin Give oral vitamin K or low-dose IV vitamin K
>10	No bleeding	Hold warfarin until INR in therapeutic range Give low-dose IV vitamin K
	Rapid reversal required	Hold warfarin Give low-dose IV vitamin K, and repeat as needed
Any INR	Serious or life–threatening bleeding	Hold warfarin Give high-dose IV vitamin K Give 4 units FFP/plasma *or* PCC

FFP, Fresh–frozen plasma; *INR,* international normalized ratio; *IV,* intravenous; *PCC,* prothrombin complex concentrate.

- PTT ↑↑ and anti-Xa therapeutic
  - Factor deficiency or inhibitor, liver disease, warfarin, vitamin K deficiency, LAC, direct thrombin inhibitor, low-quality specimen, amyloidosis
- PTT therapeutic, anti-Xa ↑↑
  - ↑FVIII (e.g., others, stress, sepsis), fondaparinux, rivaroxaban, apixaban, enoxaparin
- PTT ↑↑, anti-Xa ↑↑
  - Too much UFH, heparin contamination
- PTT ↓↓, anti-Xa ↓↓
  - Not enough UFH, saline draw, antithrombin deficiency (depending on assay methodology), heparin–induce thrombocytopenia (HIT)
  - Causes of heparin resistance (subtherapeutic PTT)
- Antithrombin III deficiency
  - Unable to inhibit factor IIa, Xa (and others)
  - Congenital—autosomal dominant, rare
    - Types I (low antigen and activity) and II (low activity, normal antigen)
    - Homozygous—incompatible with life
    - Heterozygous—increased risk of venous thromboembolism (VTE)
  - Acquired
    - DIC, liver disease, nephrotic syndrome, heparin therapy
  - Antithrombin concentrates can be used to treat hereditary deficiency
  - High factor VIII or fibrinogen (acute phase reactants)
- Heparin reversal
  - Protamine sulfate
    - Dosed based on time since last dose
    - 1 mg neutralizes 100 units of heparin

LOW-MOLECULAR-WEIGHT HEPARIN (LMWH)

- Enoxaparin (Lovenox)
- Also pork derived
- Anti-Xa > anti-IIa activity
- Still requires patient to have functional antithrombin for drug to work
- Renal, predictable clearance
- Monitor with anti-Xa
- Reversal
  - Protamine sulfate (not 100% effective)
  - Time

FONDAPARINUX (Arixtra)

- *Indirect* anti-Xa activity only, *no* anti-IIa
  - = miniheparin
  - *(X for 10!)*
- Synthetic, not pork–derived
- Used off-label to treat HIT
- Does not affect PT/PTT/INR
- No therapeutic range
- Not routinely monitored, can use anti-Xa with specific calibrator
- No reversal agent
  - Can try recombinant factor VIIa (but anti-Xa activity will not be removed)

DIRECT XA INHIBITORS (ORAL)

- Rivaroxaban (XARELTO), apixaban (ELIQUIS), edoxaban (EAVAYSA)
  - (X for 10!)
- Used for atrial fibrillation and venous thromboembolism prophylaxis
- PT/PTT/INR not reliable
- Monitoring
  - Anti-Xa activity
  - Antithrombin assays helpful if they are factor Xa-based, not thrombin-based
- Reversal
  - Activated charcoal if ingested recently
  - Andexanet Alfa—decoy Xa

DIRECT THROMBIN INHIBITORS

- Argatroban, bivalirudin, dabigatran
- Bind and block thrombin's active site
- Will give long R on thromboelastography
- When checking factor levels, DTIs look like inhibitor
- Used for HIT and percutaneous coronary intervention
- Monitor with PTT (goal = 1.5 to 3 × baseline)
- When bridging argatroban to warfarin, stop argatroban when INR >4 *or* chromogenic 10 is 20% to 40%
- Argatroban
  - Intravenous

- Cleared by liver
- Monitor with PTT or with antithrombin assays if thrombin-based, not Xa
- No reversal agent, turn off infusion (short half-life)
- Bivalirudin (Angiomax)
    - Intravenous
    - Cleared by kidneys
    - Monitor with plasma–diluted TT or with antithrombin assays if thrombin-based, not Xa
    - No reversal agent, turn off infusion (short half-life)
- Dabigatran (PRADAXA)
    - Oral
    - Cleared by kidneys
    - Monitor with PTT (or creatinine clearance)
    - Reversal
        - Idarucizumab—monoclonal antibody that binds the drug
        - Activated charcoal if ingested recently
        - +/− hemodialysis
        - +/− PCC

ANTIPLATELET DRUGS

- Aspirin—irreversible platelet inactivation
- Clopidogrel
    - Blocks ADP from binding to P2Y12 receptor, which suppresses GpIIb/IIa from binding, leading to decreased platelet aggregation
    - Two-step activation in liver
        - Prasugrel = 1 step activation
        - Ticagrelor = no steps, already active!
    - Polymorphisms in *CYP2C19* (*2 and *3 are associated with a slower metabolism of clopidogrel)
- NSAIDs
- Abciximab (GpIIb/IIIa inhibitor)

Disorders of Primary Hemostasis

INTRODUCTION

General Categories

- Disorders of blood vessels
- Von Willebrand disease
- Thrombocytopenias (↓ quantity)
- Platelet dysfunction (↓ quality)
    - Platelets turn over in 7 days

Workup for Patient with Platelet Disorder

1. History and physical
    - Old vs. new
    - Demographics and family history
    - Mucosal vs. deep soft tissue and joints
    - Severity

- Previous therapy
- Medications
  - Selective serotonin reuptake inhibitors, heart drugs, oral contraceptives/hormonal therapy, over-the-counter or herbal drugs
  - Antiplatelet drugs
  - Anticoagulants
- Liver and kidney function
- Syndromic features
  - Absent radii
  - Albinism
  - Cataracts

2. Complete blood count (CBC) with differential and smear
   - White blood cells—number and differential, left shift, leukemia, inclusions
   - Red blood cells—schistocytes, sickling, target cells, hemoglobin/hematocrit, MCV, MCHC
   - Platelets—number, MPV, granules
     - Pseudothrombocytopenia
       - Clumping/satellitosis—can be secondary to autoantibodies that recognize platelet antigens in combination with EDTA hapten
         - Use sodium citrate or heparin tubes instead
     - Size
       - Micro—Wiskott–Aldrich
       - Macro—Bernard–Soulier and MYH9 disorders

3. INR/PTT/TT, fibrinogen, D-dimer
4. Bleeding time
5. Thromboelastography and platelet mapping
6. Platelet aggregation (gold standard)
7. PFA-100
8. Electron microscopy
9. Von Willebrand studies (antigen levels, activity, factor VIII levels)
   - Collagen–binding assay
10. Antiphospholipid antibody (LAC)
11. Flow cytometry
12. Verify now/platelet works (anticoagulant testing)
13. Secretion studies
14. Liver and kidney function tests
    - Chronic kidney insufficiency causes bleeding diathesis through...
      - Anemia (low erythropoietin production)
        - Normally red blood cells flow in the center of vessel and platelets move to the outside
        - In anemia, the platelets are no longer pushed to the sides by red cells → platelet-type bleeding
      - Platelet dysfunction
        - Decreased platelet adhesion and decreased synthesis of thromboxane A2
        - Dialysis *may* improve bleeding; DDAVP is known to improve hemostasis in uremic patients
15. Platelet antibody screen and platelet–associated antibodies (like direct antiglobin test [DAT] for platelets) (ITP)

Platelet Count in Bleeding

- High—reactive thrombocytosis (illness, anemia, postsplenectomy), myeloproliferative neoplasms (platelets do not work well)
- Normal
  - Medications—aspirin, antiplatelets, penicillin, cephalosporins, amphotericin, antidepressants, nitrofurantoin, hydroxychloroquine, beta blockers
  - Uremia
  - Congenital
    - Glanzmann thrombasthenia
      - Do not give platelets! The patient will make antibodies against GpIIb/IIIa
    - Signal transduction disorder
    - Platelet storage pool disorders
  - VWD
  - Extracorporeal membrane oxygenation (ECMO), left ventricular assistance device (LVAD), intra-aortic balloon pump (IABP), dialysis
    - Exhausted platelets
- Low (increased destruction or decreased production)
  - Splenomegaly
  - Congenital—Bernard–Soulier, Wiskott–Aldrich syndrome (WAS), Fechtner, Gray platelet, MYH9, Hermansky–Pudlak
  - Malignancy
  - Infection/sepsis
  - Consumptive—bleeding, DIC, thrombocytopenic thrombotic purpura (TTP)
  - Type 2B VWD/platelet type
  - Immune—HIT, immune thrombocytopenic purpura (ITP), TTP, post-transfusion purpura, antiphospholipid antibodies
    - ITP treatment
      - First line
        - Corticosteroids, IVIG, Rhimmunoglobulin (in Rh-positive patients)
      - Second line
        - Rituximab, dapsone, splenectomy
      - Pregnant patients treated the same as nonpregnant adults
        - Neonates born to mothers with ITP may be thrombocytopenic
          - Neonatal alloimmune thrombocytopenia (NAIT)
          - Can occur in first pregnancy
          - Anti-HPA-1a
  - Drugs—clopidogrel, gemcitabine, vancomycin, spironolactone
  - Hemolysis, elevated liver enzymes, low platelets (HELLP) syndrome in pregnancy
  - Liver disease (↓ thrombopoietin)
  - Lupus anticoagulant
  - ECMO/LVAD/IABP/dialysis
  - Production—aplastic, myelophthisic, infection

PLATELET FUNCTION TESTING

Platelet Aggregometry

- Gold standard

- Time and resource intensive (though can do secretion studies at same time)
- Impedance aggregometry
  - Whole blood alternative to standard aggregation studies
  - Saves ~2 hour of specimen prep
- Platelet–rich plasma (slow spin) + activators (epinephrine, ADP, collagen, ristocetin, arachidonic acid) → measure absorbance (now we can do impedance aggregometry instead of absorbance)
  - Ristocetin (RCo) measures GpIb-VWF interaction
  - Epinephrine has 2 bumps of aggregation—primary and secondary
  - Collagen binds GpVI and GpIa–IIa
  - ADP binds P2Y12 and P2Y1
  - GpIIb/IIIa is tested by ADP, epinephrine, and collagen (and second phase of ristocetin)
- Patterns
  - See Table 19.3.
  - Aspirin (inhibits cyclooxygenase)
    - Primary epinephrine wave, no secondary
    - ADP drifts up (unstable, de-aggregates); no arachidonic wave
    - Shaggy RCo pattern
  - Bernard–Soulier—no response to RCo (GpIb-IX binds to VWF)
  - Glanzmann thrombasthenia or abciximab
    - Barely any response to anything (afibrinogenemia can too) because GpIIb/IIIa not there
      - Afibrinogenemia and dysfibrinogenemia too

TABLE 19.3 ■ Platelet Aggregometry Patterns

	ADP	Arachidonic Acid	Epinephrine	Collagen	Ristocetin
VWD	N	N	N	N	↑/N/↓
GT	↓/0	↓/0	↓/0	↓/0	N
BS	N	N	N	N	↓/0
Aspirin	↓/0	↓/0	↓	↓/0	N
Clopidogrel	N/↓	N	N/↓	N	N
Abciximab (GpIIb/ IIIa inhibitor)	↓/0	↓/0	↓/0	↓/0	N

0, Absent; *BS,* Bernard–Soulier; *GT,* Glanzmann thrombasthenia; *N,* normal; *VWD,* von Willebrand disease.

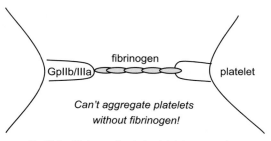

Fig. 19.5 Fibrinogen's role in platelet aggregation.

- See Fig. 19.5.
- Except 1st phase of RCo, but not stabilized (drifts/de-aggregates)
- Thrombocytopenia shifts everything up a little
- VWD 2B/platelet type
  - RCo-induced platelet aggregation (RIPA) shows too much aggregation at lowest RCo concentration
- Dense granule disorders—complex pattern, hypogranular platelets
  - Hermansky–Pudlak
    - Oculocutaneous albinism
    - Puerto Rico
- We can do serotonin release assay on same machine/at the same time as platelet aggregometry

PFA-100

- Replaced bleeding time and reptilase time
- Simulates capillary flow with "injury" to create platelet plug
- Whole blood test (may be abnormal in thrombocytopenia or anemia)
- Stimulate with collagen and epinephrine (more sensitive)
  - If abnormal, run collagen and ADP
- Patterns
  - Prolonged aggregation in collagen/epinephrine, normal in collagen/ADP = aspirin–like
  - Prolonged aggregation with both—VWD, GPIIb/IIIa inhibitor (abciximab), Glanzmann thrombasthenia, Bernard–Soulier, gray platelet disorder
  - Normal aggregation with both—clopidogrel*, dense granule disorder, primary secretion disorder
    - *or normal epinephrine and ↑ with ADP
- Useful for von Willebrand disease (VWD) screening
  - Cannot detect some mild VWD cases and mild platelet function disorders (like Scott syndrome)

Thromboelastography (TEG)

- Whole blood + activator (kaolin) → cup spins around pin on wire; if clot forms, tugs on pin
- With or without heparinase
- Cannot see aspirin and clopidogrel effect; need platelet mapping
- ROTEM is similar to TEG but vibration effect taken care off (pin on wire spins instead, light detector)
- Variables
  - R—reaction time—factor deficiencies, factor inhibitors, LAC, anticoagulants
  - K—time for 2 to 20 mm change
  - Alpha—slope of clot formation
    - Decreased in thrombocytopenia
    - MA—max amplitude—how strong is the clot?
    - Platelet count (not function, so aspirin has no effect) and fibrinogen amount affect height
  - LY30, LY60—amount of lysis in 30 or 60 minutes

Platelet Mapping (PM)

- Platelet function
- Reptilase (fibrinogen → fibrin without coagulation cascade) and factor XIII
- Test with thrombin, fibrin, and ADP

Verify Now/Plateletworks

- Cartridge based, fibrinogen coated beads + blood (blue-topped tube) + activator
- Like mini-aggregometry (light transmittance); determine platelet count on impedance platelet counter
- Used to check drug effect—aspirin (waived CLIA test), P2Y12, GpIIb/IIIa
  - If you are on a drug and not responding, these check if you are resistant *or* confirm compliance *or* tell when okay to go to surgery
  - up to 55% of people are resistant to standard therapy
  - ~45% for P2Y12 inhibitors (clopidogrel)
- Similar to platelet mapping
- EDTA baseline tubes and arachidonic acid agonist
  - Impedance
  - Must be run right away
- Gives % inhibition
- Not affected by hematocrit

PRIMARY PLATELET DISORDERS

- Platelet granule disorders
  - Alpha bodies contain:
    - Platelet–derived growth factor
    - Beta-thromboglobulin
    - Factor V
    - P-selectin
    - Fibrinogen
    - VWF
      - Also in Weibel–Palade bodies of endothelial cells with P-selectin
    - Platelet factor IV
    - TGF-beta
    - Fibronectin
  - Alpha-granule disorders
    - Gray platelet syndrome
    - Paris–Trousseau or Jacobsen syndrome
      - Mild bleeding diathesis, mental retardation, cardiac and craniofacial abnormalities
      - Less than 100 cases worldwide
      - 11q23 deletion
    - Quebec platelet syndrome
      - Increased urokinase
    - Arthrogryposis (with renal dysfunction and cholestasis)
  - Dense (or delta) bodies contain:
    - ADP
    - ATP
    - Serotonin
    - Calcium
    - Magnesium
    - Pyrophosphate
    - Epinephrine
  - Dense body disorders
    - Chediak–Higashi syndrome

- Hermansky–Pudlak syndrome
- Griscelli syndrome
    - Hypopigmented skin, silver hair, developmental delay, seizures, hypotonia, immunodeficiency
        - HIGH RISK FOR HEMOPHAGOCYTIC LYMPHOHISTIOCYTOSIS
- Glanzmann thrombasthenia = deficient or defective GPIIb/IIIa (CD41 and CD61 respectively)
    - Normal platelet count
    - No aggregation with ADP, collagen, epinephrine, arachidonic acid
        - Only ristocetin
- Bernard-Griscelli Soulier = GPib/IX/V receptor (VWF receptor) deficiency, autosomal recessive, severe bleeding
    - Big Suckers
    - Low platelet count
    - Opposite aggregation as GT
        - Normal with ADP, collagen, epinephrine, AA
        - Absent with ristocetin

VON WILLEBRAND DISEASE (VWD)

- Von Willebrand factor (VWF)—largest soluble protein in blood
    - Functions
        - Carry inactive factor VIII
        - Binds GpIb (congenital lack in Bernard–Griscelli Soulier)
        - Bind collagen
        - Multimerize (have the right size)
    - Can be increased in
        - Endothelial damage—stress, sepsis, crying, exercise
        - Estrogen—oral contraceptives, hormonal replacement therapy, pregnancy, menses except first 3 days of cycle
        - Medications—vasopressin/DDAVP
        - Transfusions
        - Blood groups—O < A, B < AB
        - Age—↑ in newborns, then ↓, then normal
        - Hyperthyroidism
        - Race
        - Secreters
    - Gets glycosylated (ABO blood type)
        - Type O people can have normal levels that are below the reference range (for both antigen and activity)
    - Suggested screening panel: factor VIII, Ag (ELISA or latex immunoassay), ristocetin cofactor activity
        - "Activity" assay—GpIb antibody
            - Actually structure for platelet binding site
            - Gets around RCo site mutations that are not clinically significant
            - ELISA with GpIb in wells
        - RCo activity—sometimes done with platelet aggregometry; add ristocetin cofactor and cause (measure) interaction between VWF and platelets
            - Patient plasma + donor platelets + ristocetin → *rate* of aggregation (aggregometry)
                - *Or* patient plasma + ristocetin + fixed platelet reagent → automated (rocking cup)

- RIPA is the same but with *patient* platelets
- True aggregation assay (+/− 30%)
- Activity assays are really automated with high reproducibility
- Collagen binding—measures VWF ability to bind collagen
  - Type of collagen and concentration can highly vary results
- Factor VIII—one stage, look at PTT with patient plasma (and at dilutions)
  - Levels decrease in tubes over time, can get falsely low levels with heparin
- RCo assay looks at rate, RIPA looks at maximum (on platelet aggregometer, +/− 30%)
- ISHT bleeding assessment tool—pretest probability
- Multimers—western blot, takes 4 days
- Autosomal recessive or dominant
  - Hemophilia A is X-linked

Von Willebrand Subtypes

- See Table 19.4.
- See Table 19.5 and Fig. 19.6.
1. Partial quantitative deficiency of VWF (<30%, maybe 30% to 50%)
2. Qualitative VWF deficiency
   a. ↓ VWF-dependent platelet adhesion with selective deficiency in high molecular weight (HMW) multimers
   b. ↑ affinity for platelet GpIb (associated with ↓ platelet count)
   m. ↓ VWF-dependent platelet adhesion without selective deficiency in HMW multimers
   n. Markedly ↓ binding affinity for FVIII (must be ruled out in hemophilia A), cannot protect FVIII (low FVIII)
3. Virtually complete deficiency of VWF
   a. May be type 1 + type 2 (or another combination)
- "Platelet-type VWD"—Gp1b is hyper-responsive and overbinds VWF; treat with platelet transfusions

TABLE 19.4 ■ **Von Willebrand Disease Subtypes**

	VWF Ag	RCo	FVIII	RCo/Ag (activity)	FVIII/Ag	Multimers	Other
1	↓	↓	n/↓	N	N	^	
2a	↓/n	↓↓	n/↓	↓	N	↓HMW	RIPA↓
2b†	↓/n	↓↓	n/↓	↓	N	↓HMW	↓plt ct RIPA↑~
2m	↓/n	↓↓	n/↓	↓	N	n/↑ HMW	Genetics*
2n	n/↓	n/↓	↓	N	↓		**
3	↓↓	↓↓	↓↓				

^Normal multimer distribution but fainter than normal.
†May be associated with low platelet count.
~Hyper-responsive at low-doses (0.5) must rule out platelet type with mixing study (patient platelets + donor plasma). if long = platelet–type, if normal type 2b.
*May get ↑ HMW in sepsis/trauma/and so on. Must exclude allele variants in RCo binding site if RCo-based activity assay (by genetics). Allele variants are benign/irrelevant mutations that changes RCo's binding site—no bleeding risk (do collagen-binding test).
**Must rule out hemophilia A. FVIII-binding study or genetics.
Ag, Antigen; *FVIII,* factor VIII; *HMW,* high molecular weight; *n,* normal; *RIPA,* ristocetin–induced platelet aggregation; *plt ct,* platelet count; *RCo,* ristocetin; *VWF,* von Willebrand factor.

TABLE 19.5 ■ Protein S Deficiencies

Type	Q/Q	Functional Protein S	Free Protein S	Total Protein S
I	Quantitative	Decreased	Decreased	Decreased
II	Qualitative	Decreased	Normal	Normal
III	Quantitative	Decreased	Decreased	Normal

Q/Q, Quantitative/qualitative.

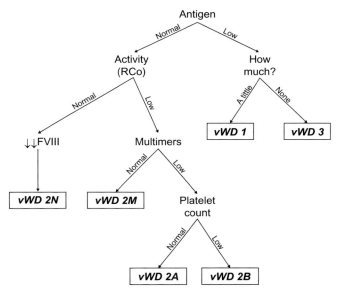

Fig. 19.6 Differentiating subtypes of von Willebrand disease. *FVIII*, Factor VIII; *RCo*, ristocetin.

- Acquired VWD
  - Shear—↓ RCo:Ag and ↓ HMW; LVAD, ECMO, aortic stenosis, balloon pump
    - Lose highest-molecular-weight multimers first
    - Can have normal or increased antigen
  - "Sticky"—↑ platelets—essential thrombocythemia and other myeloproliferative neoplasms, reactive thrombocytosis, pediatric tumors
    - VWF gets bound up by ↑↑↑ GPIb available
    - Can have normal or increased antigen
  - Antibody inhibitor—use ELISA-based test instead of mixing, *or* compare levels of propeptide and VWF (secondary to autoimmune disease, solid tumor, pregnancy, myelodysplastic syndrome, chronic lymphocytic leukemia, myeloproliferative neoplasm)

Treatment

- DDAVP is most useful in type 1, contraindicated in type 2B, and variable with other type 2 subtypes

HEPARIN-INDUCED THROMBOCYTOPENIA (HIT)

- Two types
  - Type I—nonimmune

- Transient, mild thrombocytopenia
- 1 to 2 days of heparin therapy
- Heparin binds to platelets
- Type II—immune
  - Severe, possibly life–threatening
  - 5 to 10 days after heparin exposure
  - Antibody formation against heparin-platelet factor 4 complex
  - Mostly UFH but can be with LMWHs
- Hepatic necrosis/limb necrosis syndrome
  - ↓ production of protein C and antithrombin due to liver dysfunction
- HIT has venous and arterial thromboses
  - Can get thrombotic event before the platelets drop or after has been stopped (up to 3 weeks)
  - Can have anaphylactoid reaction of your recent exposure was <90 days ago
- 4T score
  - Thrombocytopenia
    - Platelet count fall <30% *or* platelet nadir <10:—0 points
    - Platelet count fall 30% to 50% *or* platelet nadir 10 to 19—1 point
    - Platelet count fall >50% *and* platelet nadir ≥20—2 points
  - Timing of platelet count fall
    - Platelet count fall <4 days without recent exposure—0 points
    - Consistent with days 5 to 10 fall, but not clear; onset after day 10 *or* fall ≤1 day (prior heparin exposure 30 to 100 days ago)—1 point
    - Clear onset between days 5 to 10 *or* platelet fall ≤1 day (prior heparin exposure within 30 days)—2 points
  - Thrombosis or other sequelae
    - None—0 points
    - Progressive *or* recurrent thrombosis; non-necrotizing skin lesions; suspected thrombosis (not proven)—1 point
    - New thrombosis *or* skin necrosis; acute systemic reaction post-IV heparin bolus—2 points
  - Other causes for thrombocytopenia
    - Definite—0 points
    - Possible—1 point
    - None apparent—2 points
  - Critical actions
    - ≤3 points: low probability of HIT (<1% to 5%)
    - 4 to 5 points: intermediate probability (14%)
    - 6 to 8 points: high probability (64%)
  - There is an alternative to 4T score for patients on ECMO
- Diagnosis
  - Serotonin release assay is gold standard
  - Donor platelets (with radio–labeled serotonin) + patient plasma
    - Positive is >20% at low-dose heparin (therapeutic) and <20% at high-dose heparin (supratherapeutic)
  - Heparin–induced platelet activation (HIPA)
    - Donor platelets + patient plasma + low-/high-dose heparin
    - Measure light transmission
  - Immunoassays—"screening assay"

- ELISA with platelet factor 4 and heparin bound to the well
- ↓ specificity from clinically insignificant anti-PF4 antibodies
    - Can ↑ specificity by using IgG-only assays, or increasing the OD cutoff for positivity
- In the United States: screen with ELISA, confirm with SRA
    - Only if 4T score is ≥4
- Therapy
    - STOP HEPARIN, STOP WARFARIN, give vitamin K, start argatroban
        - Even if therapeutic on warfarin
        - Warfarin decreases protein C, increasing risk for skin necrosis
    - HIT + clot—anticoagulation for at least 3 months
        - No clot—at least 4 weeks
    - Bivalirudin can be used instead of argatroban (direct thrombin inhibitors) or fondaparinux (can be discharged on it, anti-Xa inhibitor)
    - Total plasma exchange is category III (see "Transfusion Medicine" chapter)
    - No platelet transfusions unless life threatening or severe bleeding

Disorders of Secondary Hemostasis

- Platelet aggregation works well, coagulation cascade does not
- No mucosal bleeding (platelet-type bleeding), more deep soft tissue or joint bleeds

DIAGNOSIS OF SECONDARY HEMOSTATIC DISORDERS

1. Basic coagulation studies (PT/PTT/INR)
2. Mixing studies
    a. ↑ PTT
        i. 1:1 to 1:4 mix
    1. Corrects = factor deficiency (could have diluted out inhibitor)
    2. Still long = factor inhibitor (could be multifactor severe deficiency)
    b. Do incubated studies to look for time–dependent inhibitor (classical FVIII inhibitor)
    c. Do not do mixing studies upfront because it increases false positives
        i. A borderline prolonged PTT may actually "correct" with dilution
3. If factor deficiency, first do qualitative (functional) factor testing
    a. For example, chromogenic or clot-based
    b. Next step = quantitative
        i. ELISA or LIA
4. If mixing study does not correct, assess for lupus anticoagulant, drug effect, or factor-specific inhibitor antibody (see later)

FACTOR TESTING

- One stage—patient plasma + factor deficient plasma (in multiple dilutions) → time to clot (PTT or PT)
    - See Fig. 19.7.
- Two stage—similar to one stage—adds complexity without much value
- Chromogenic—non-clot–based pathway
    - Factor X + cleave-able target that looks like prothrombin, but has chromogenic properties so we can detect color change (rivaroxaban inhibits factor X cleavage)

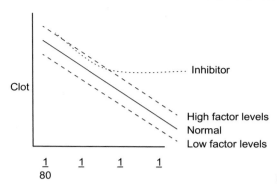

Fig. 19.7 Disorders in secondary hemostasis.

- ■ Can also do factor VIII
    - ■ Can use to monitor warfarin, can lag behind INR change (factor VIII has shorter half-life than factor X)
    - ■ Can use for argatroban to warfarin bridge
- ■ Antigen (does not really help tell you how much is there *and* functional)
- ■ Fibrinogen—routine assay is activity (not antigen)
    - ■ Claus method—dilute pat sample and run a TT, then plot on calibration curve
- ■ Factor specific assays
    - ■ FX activity—looks for deficiency, routine (PT/PTT, whole pathway)
    - ■ FX chromogenic—looks at FX ability to cleave one product, not whole pathway less interference (by rivaroxaban)
    - ■ Factor VIII–binding study (ELISA)
        - ▪ Well with anti-VWF bound to bottom, add patient plasma, wash, add reagent factor VIII
        - ▪ <100% = 2 N; 100% = hemophilia A
- ■ Normal variation of clotting factor levels based on age
    - ■ Lower in children
        - ▪ Vitamin K–dependent factors (II, VII, IX, X), V, XI, XII, prekallikrein, HMWK
    - ■ Normal or higher in children than adults
        - ▪ Fibrinogen, factor VIII, VWF
- ■ Half-life of factors
    - ■ FI—90 hours
    - ■ FII—65 hours
    - ■ FV—15 to 36 hours
    - ■ FVII—5 hours
        - ▪ Recombinant factor VII has a very short half-life
        - ▪ FVIII—10 to 12 hours
        - ▪ FIX—18 to 24 hours
        - ▪ FX—40 hours
        - ▪ FXI—50 hours
        - ▪ FXII—50 to 70 hours
        - ▪ FXIII—200 hours
        - ▪ Fibrinogen—4 days (96 hours)

FACTOR DEFICIENCIES

- Prekallikrein deficiency
  - Really long PTT that corrects on mixing study
  - On incubated mixing study, elongates slightly with time (autoactivation)
- Dysfibrinogenemia
  - Prolonged INR, PTT, long or normal thrombin time
  - Can clot or bleed or both
    - Clotting mechanism—abnormal thrombin binding sites → increased clot formation
      - Abnormal fibrinogen → fibrin clot resistant to plasmin degradation
  - Get fibrinogen activity levels and fibrinogen antigen levels
  - Thrombin time is the best screening test
- Factor XII deficiency causes delayed arterial THROMBOSIS (not bleeding)
  - Hereditary angioedema
  - Prolonged PTT (very high), INR is not prolonged
- Hemophilia B
  - Factor IX deficiency
  - High-end normal PTT/INR and soft bleeding history
    - INR and PTT are least sensitive for FIX levels
  - When replacing with recombinant factor IX, give loading dose then maintenance dose every 24 hours
    - Need circulating factor IX levels to be 50 to 100 IU/dL before surgery (loading dose of 4000 to 8000 IU). Repeat dosing every 12 to 24 hours for 7 to 10 days
    - Maintenance dose = ½ of loading dose
  - Calculated dose in units = % change in factor desired * body weight (kg) * 1.0 IU/kg
  - Target goal for hemarthrosis = 50%
  - Target goal for major surgery = 100%
- Hemophilia A
  - Factor VIII deficiency
  - When replacing, give loading dose then maintenance dose every 12 hours
  - Calculated dose in units = % change in factor desired * body weight (kg) * 0.5 IU/kg
    - Target goal for hemarthrosis = 50%
    - Target goal for major surgery = 100%
- Congenital factor VII deficiency
  - Rare complication is thrombosis, usually secondary to recombinant therapy or surgery
- FXIII deficiency
  - "Fibrin–stabilizing factor"—crosslinks fibrin through peptide bonds
  - INR, PTT, TT are all normal
    - The factor acts too late in the cascade to affect these assays
  - Rare autosomal recessive disorder
  - Features
    - Bleeds—delayed/rebleeds, umbilical stump bleeding, circumcision bleeding, hematomas, soft tissue bleeding, intracranial hemorrhages
    - Poor wound healing
    - Recurrent spontaneous abortions in the first trimester
  - Testing
    - Historic test: clot solubility; low sensitivity, need ≤2% to have positive test
      - Clots from patients rapidly dissolve in urea or monochloroacetic acid
    - Better: FXIII activity (not FDA-approved) or F14 antigen (FDA-approved, may miss those with normal levels but ↓ function)

- Treatment: FXIII concentrate or cryoprecipitate
- DDx includes α_2-antiplasmin deficiency
  - Solubility in urea is *normal* but euglobin lysis time is shortened
- Secondary factor deficiencies
  - Decreased FV from bovine thrombin exposure (antibovine antibody)
  - Decreased FX from amyloidosis (possible antiamyloid antibody)
  - End-stage liver disease
    - Decreases all clotting (and anticoagulation factors) except FVI and VWF
      - FV most sensitive
    - Decreased platelets from splenic sequestration and decreased thrombopoietin

FACTOR INHIBITORS

- Typically an antibody against a specific factor
- Can caused acquired hemophilia A or B, acquired VWD
- Factor VIII inhibitor
  - Bethesda assay
    - Antifactor VIII assay
    - Dilutional series that determines strength of inhibitor antibody
  - Most frequently caused by alloantibodies against exogenous FVIII in those with hemophilia A
  - Classically TIME-dependent
    - Gets stronger with time
    - May be missed if measured right away

Thrombophilia
WORKUP

- Venous thromboemboli (VTE)
  - Over 100,000 deaths per year
  - 25% to 40% are unprovoked
  - Hereditary thrombophilia—4% to 10% of population
    - ~50% of patients with VTE
- When to workup patient for thrombophilia
  - Spontaneous thrombosis in a young patient (<50 years of age)
  - Recurrent VTE
  - First-degree relatives with recurrent VTE
  - Thrombosis at unusual sites
    - Mesenteric veins, portal veins, splenic veins, renal veins, cerebral sinus
      - Paroxysmal nocturnal hemoglobinuria classically causes clots in splenic vein or other unusual spots
  - Without other risk factors
    - BMI >30, smoking, immobilization, trauma, surgery, age >65 years, myeloproliferative neoplasm, sepsis, and so on
1. History and physical
   - Clotting history
     - i. Where? Provoked? First or recurrent? Family history?
   - Liver disease, renal disease, autoimmune, infection, pregnancy

- Meds: oral contraceptives/hormone replacement therapy, anticoagulants, antiplatelets, antidepressants, cardiac
2. CBC
   - RBC—high or low, sickle, fragments
   - WBC—high or low, left shift, leukemia
   - Platelets—high or low, baseline
3. INR/PTT/TT
   - Baseline
   - Already on drug and subtherapeutic
4. Fibrinogen
5. Mixing studies
6. Protein C and S
7. Antithrombin
8. Factor V Leiden/activated protein C resistance studies
9. G20210A prothrombin
10. Paroxysmal nocturnal hemoglobinuria
    - 7 × thrombotic risk
    - Treated with eculizumab and/or bone marrow transplant
11. Antiphospholipid syndrome
12. D-dimer
    - Used to rule OUT pulmonary embolism (PE)
    - i. High D-dimer in trauma, thromboembolism, surgery, DIC
    - ii. Do not use Weiss criteria (for PE) in inpatient setting
       1. Odds of D-dimer being elevated are high
       2. Just go straight to imaging if worried

ETIOLOGIES

- Protein C pathologies
  - Deficiency (quantitative or qualitative)
    - Autosomal dominant, 0.5% of population
    - Leads to decreased degradation of procoagulation factors
    - Types
      - Quantitative (more frequent)
      - Qualitative
    - Clinical features
      - Increased risk for VTE (not arterial)
      - Homozygous is rare—neonatal purpura fulminans
        - Severe DIC in infants
      - Initiation of warfarin may induce thrombosis and skin necrosis because of short half-life (shorter than other vitamin K dependent factors)
        - "Warfarin–induced skin necrosis"
      - Pregnancy complications
    - Treatment—protein C concentrate
    - Testing
      - Rule out secondary—warfarin, vitamin K deficiency, liver disease, inhibitor, acute clot, L-asparaginase, age <15 years, DIC
      - Antigen—ELISA or Laurell rocket (rare)
      - Activity—clot-based < chromogenic
        - Clot based

- PT < aPTT based
- Plasma + phospholipid + contact activator + protein C activator (Protac—copperhead snake venom) → incubation → add CA++ → time to clot
- Result influenced by protein C, Va, and VIIIa levels
  - Factor VIII is an acute phase reactant
- Less protein C → shorter clot time
  - Because no inhibition of factor V and VIII
- INTERFERENCE
  - False increase
    - Anticoagulants—anti-Xa inhibitor, direct thrombin inhibitor, UFH, warfarin
    - Factor deficiencies, LAC
  - False decrease
    - Increased FVIII
    - Factor V Leiden
- Chromogenic
  - Plasma + protac → incubation → add chromogenic substrate → measure a color change by optical density
  - No interference by the aforementioned
- Icterus, lipemia, hemolysis interferes somewhat with optical read
- ■ Activated protein C (APC) resistance
  - ■ Factor V Leiden (FVL)
    - Most common cause of APC resistance (90% to 95%)
      - Prevalence is dependent on race
        - Asian Americans—0.5%
        - Blacks and Native Americans—1%
        - Whites—5%
        - Greeks/other Europeans—15%
    - One protein C cut sites on factor 5 is mutated/lost
      - Other 10% are other factor 5 mutations
    - G1691A mutation in factor V gene that messes up APC's arginine cleavage site (R506Q)
      - Heterozygous—3 to 7 × risk of VTE (not arterial)
      - Homozygous—80 × risk
    - 10-fold lower cleavage (and inactivation) rate of FVa by APC and protein S
    - Testing
      - Genetic is most common
      - Functional
        - aPTT
          - Compare aPTT of patient plasma with and without added protein C
          - Normal—2 to 3.5 × prolonged
          - Heterozygote—1.6 × prolonged
          - Homozygote—1.2 × prolonged
      - INR, modified aPTT with predilution with factor V deficient plasma, chromogenic (not clot-based, no interference), DRVVT (activates FX)
  - ■ Other causes of APC resistance:
    - Autoimmune inhibitor
    - Other FV mutations
    - Spurious (caused by inappropriate testing modality)
- ■ Protein S Deficiency

- Prevents APC from inactivating FVa and FVIIIa
- Three general subtypes, see Table 19.5
  - Type I—do not make it—quantitative
  - Type II—does not work—qualitative
  - Type III—not enough free, too much bound
- Clinical features
  - Homozygote—neonatal purpura fulminans (less rare than in protein C)
  - Heterozygote—pregnancy complications, increased VTEs, warfarin–induced skin necrosis
- Testing
  - Rule out secondary—warfarin, vitamin K deficiency, hormone therapy, high estrogen states, nephrotic syndrome, acute thrombosis, liver disease, females < males, inflammation, age <6 months
  - Total S—ELISA > radioimmunoassays
    - Detects epitope away from C4bBP binding site
    - Not recommended
  - Functional—clot based
    - Increased clot time—increased protein S activity
    - False decrease—FVL, activated protein C resistance, elevated FVIII (antigen or activity)
    - False increase—anti-Xa and direct thrombin inhibitors
  - Free protein S
- Antithrombin deficiency
  - Congenital deficiency occurs in ~0.10% of population
  - Heterozygous—heparin resistance and clots
  - Homozygous = not compatible with life
  - Can be qualitative or quantitative; see Table 19.6
  - Testing
    - Rule out secondary—heparin, liver disease, nephrotic syndrome, protein-losing enteropathy, acute clot (including DIC, TTP, and so on), age <3 months, dialysis/extracorporeal membranous oxygenation,
    - Chromogenic—based on inhibition of factor IIa or Xa in the presence of heparin
      - More AT shows more chromogenic substrate cleavage (less color)
      - Less AT shows less chromogenic substrate cleavage (more color)
- Tissue plasminogen activator (tPA) deficiency
  - Leads of failure to activate plasminogen to plasmin, leading to increased clot stability
  - Hypofibrinolysis and risk for thrombosis
  - tPA activity can be inhibited by excess plasminogen activator inhibitor 1 activity (PAI-1)

TABLE 19.6 ■ **Antithrombin Deficiencies**

Type	Q/Q	Functional AT	AT antigen	Site
I	quantitative	decreased	decreased	–
II	qualitative	decreased	normal	reactive site
			normal	heparin-binding site
			Normal or decreased	pleiotropic

AT, antithrombin; Q/Q, Quantitative/qualitative.

- PAI-1 deficiency → excess fibrinolysis and mild-to-moderate risk of bleeding
- Hyperhomocysteinemia
  - Inherited thrombotic disorder caused by a metabolic defect
  - Causes endothelial cell toxicity and disruption of vascular hemostatic mechanisms
  - Next-generation sequencing for methylenetetrahydrofolate reductase (MTHFR)
- Prothrombin gene mutation G20210A
  - Guanine to adenine substitution in 3' untranslated region
  - Leads to increased FIIa
  - Need genetics to identified
- Tissue factor pathway inhibitor
  - Rare, not routinely tested for
  - Binds to factor Xa and inactivates the TF/VIIa complex
  - Can also inhibit free Xa in plasma
- Factor XII deficiency—delayed arterial thrombosis
- Lupus anticoagulant (LAC) can be factor-specific (usually to FII)—check factor levels
  - "Anticoagulant" in tube but prothrombotic in vivo
  - Clinical signs
    - Clots (arterial and venous), pregnancy complications
    - Not necessarily associated with systemic lupus erythematosus
  - IgG or IgM
  - LAC ISTH diagnostic criteria:
    - Prolonged phospholipid-based clotting assay (INR, PTT, DRVVT)
    - Mixing study does *not* correct
    - Excess phospholipid + PTT → shortened PTT (saturate inhibiting antibody)
    - Rule out other causes (especially rivaroxaban and apixaban)
      - Direct thrombin inhibitors can cause false negatives
- Antiphospholipid antibodies
  - Detect cardiolipin and β_2 glycoprotein with ELISA titers
    - IgG and IgM
  - Detect LAC with clot-based assays
    - INR = tissue factor + phospholipid + Ca
    - PTT = phospholipid + contact agent + Ca
    - Get LONG results because the antibody blocks phospholipid
  - Antiphospholipid syndrome
    - Acquired
    - Need one clinical (clot/miscarriage) and one laboratory criteria (cardiolipin, beta-2 glycoprotein, lupus anticoagulant) with at least one repeat 6 to 12 weeks later

Odds and Ends

- Tubes
  - Red—serum—chemistry and antibodies
  - Lavender—EDTA—blood bank and CBCs
  - Green—lithium/sodium heparin—chemistries
  - Yellow—ADCA (citrate)—special coagulation tests
  - Blue—Na citrate—most coagulation tests
    - We need to add back calcium after centrifuged to get only plasma
- Drug–induced TTP causes

- Cyclosporine
- Tacrolimus
- Clopidogrel
- Mitomycin C
- Gemcitabine
- Tranexamic acid is an antifibrinolytic
  - High LY30 by TEG/ROTEM
- Stages of liver transplantation and hemostatic changes
  - Preanhepatic—surgical dissection and mobilization
    - Prohemorrhagic
  - Anhepatic to reperfusion—from occlusion of hepatic vasculature to reperfusion
    - Prohemorrhagic (loss of coagulation factor synthesis and clearance, hyperfibrinolysis)
  - Postreperfusion
    - Prohemorrhagic (resolution of fibrinolysis, restoration of coagulation factor synthesis and clearance, heparin-like effect from donor liver)
  - Postoperative
    - Hypercoagulable (early recovery of procoagulants; elevated factor; delayed recovery of AT, protein C, and protein S)
    - Also thrombocytopenic
- There is no good evidence to support the use of routine coagulation tests for predicting bleeding or thrombotic risk in liver disease
  - Poor predictors!
- Thrombopoietin mimetics may increase the risk or progression of bone marrow reticulin deposition.
  - Receptor = CD110 (encoded by gene *c-mpl*)
  - Mainly produced in liver and endothelium
  - No risk of autoantibodies
  - Risk of VTE, hepatic toxicity, bone marrow reticulin fibrosis
- Disseminated intravascular coagulopathy (DIC) mechanism
  - Elevated thrombin → clots
  - Elevated plasmin → bleeds
- Aortic stenosis and left ventricular assist devices are associated with gastrointestinal bleeds
  - Arteriovenous malformations from low pulse pressure causing low intestinal perfusion causing increased vascular endothelial growth factor
  - Plus acquired VWD
    - High-molecular weight multimers are chopped up going through LVAD or stenotic valve → more likely to bleed
- MYH9 platelet disorders
  - May-Hegglin
  - Sebastian
  - Fechtner
  - Epstein

CHAPTER 20

Transfusion Medicine

Laboratory Methods

- Forward typing—what antigens are on the patient's red cells?
  - Patient cells + known antisera
- Reverse typing—what antibodies are in the patient's serum?
  - Patient serum + known cells
- Number of units that must be screened to find a negative unit for any given antigen:

$$\frac{\text{= \# of units desired}}{\text{\% donors negative for antigen}}$$

- "Type and screen" (T&S)—determine patient's blood type (forward and back typing) and screen for antibodies (small panel)
  - T&S expire at 3 days in pregnant and transfused patients because of the higher likelihood of alloimmunization (developing antibodies against allogeneic red cells)
    - Can be extended in other patients
- Elution direct antiglobulin test (DAT)—best chance at concentrating antibodies
- Immediate spin (IS) phase—cold antibodies = IgM (usually clinically insignificant)
- Antihuman globlulin (AHG) phase—IgG
- Potentiators increase sensitivity of antibody screens
  - LISS = low ionic-strength saline
    - Lower salt concentration than normal saline
  - PEG = polyethylene glycol
- Adsorption—remove nonspecific autoantibodies (usually warm autoantibodies) to find significant allogeneic antibodies
  - Treat patients red blood cells (RBCs) with ZZAP (DTT and papain) to remove autoantibodies already bound
  - Incubate with patient's serum (autoantibodies should bind RBCs and be removed)
  - Treat *same* plasma several times with ZZAP-treated patient RBCs to remove all autoantibodies
  - Complete antibody panel with patient's adsorbed serum
- Buffy coat—layer containing white blood cells and platelets after centrifuging anticoagulated whole blood at high speed
- Must confirm tests in same media as screening
- "HLA+" under "special antigen typing" = has remnant of white blood cell marker that was not completely removed during cell maturation
- Able to rule out all antibodies on one panel? Do another panel.
  - Ruled out again? "Unidentified antibody with no specific reactivity"
- Separating out cells
  - If you are unable to differentiate between two or three antibodies, look back at cells in which one of the antigens is positive but the other(s) are negative
  - Must find to such cells with positive reaction to rule in
- Evaluating for blood type change after stem cell transplant

- Requirements
  - Only donor RBCs (front type)
  - Back type does not have to match but must be compatible
  - No transfusions in 120 days
  - 95% chimerism in marrow and/or CD15 fraction of blood
  - Monitor chimerism with CD3 (T cell) and CD15 (myeloid) markers
    - T cell conversion lags behind myeloid conversion
  - *Cannot* have relapsed disease
- Rh immunoglobulin (RhIg) should be given to prevent sensitization
  - Must be given within 72 hours!
  - RhIg dose = KB% × (mother's blood volume)/30
    - If #.5 to #.9 → round up two vials (if less, round up one)
    - Blood volume = weight in kg × 70 mL/kg
      - If unavailable, estimate as 5000 mL
    - KB% is the percent fetal cells by Kleihauer-Betke assay
- Labeling of blood products should only occur after
  - Donation records have been reviewed
  - All holds are resolved
  - Infectious disease testing is negative
  - Quality control has passed

Blood Products

RED BLOOD CELLS (RBCS)

- Additive solution = adenine, saline, phosphate, glucose, bicarbonate, mannitol (in addition to citrate)
  - CPD and CPD-A for children—less mannitol
- Storage
  - Stored at 1° to 6°C
    - Transported at 1° to 10°C
  - Storage life
    - CPDA-1 + additive solution-3 (AS-3)—42 days
      - 28 days (if irradiated)
    - CPDA-1 only—35 days
    - CPD or CP2D—21 days
  - Storage lesion
    - ↓ ATP, ↓ 2, 3-DPG (BPG), ↓ nitric oxide, pH changes, sodium changes, potassium changes, ↑ lysis
  - Can freeze with glycerol (cryoprotectant)
    - Typically used if someone is storing their own red cells prior to a procedure
- Contains 150 to 250 mg of iron
- Hematocrit
  - If with additive solution: ~60%
  - If without additive solution: 70% to 80%
- Prestorage leukoreduction
  - Decreases risk for CMV infection, HLA alloimmunization, febrile nonhemolytic transfusion reactions
  - Better than bedside leukoreduction (via filter) because white cells do not have time to release cytokines into product during storage (which are thought to cause many of the aseptic febrile nonhemolytic transfusion reactions)

- Give washed cells for IgA-deficiency and severe allergic reactions
- The only fluid that can be given at the same time and in the same line as RBC is saline

PLATELETS

- Do not need to be ABO or Rh matched
  - Platelets contain <2 mL RBC/unit
    - If giving a lot of Rh+ platelets to Rh− patient, can give Rh immunoglobulin (like RhoGAM, Rhophylac, WinRho, etc.)
- Immune refractoriness shows bump, then decrease
  - Most common causes are HLA-A, HLA-B, and HPA antibodies
  - Nonimmune shows almost no bump
    - Examples: hypersplenism, graft-versus-host disease, disseminated intravascular coagulopathy, bone marrow transplant, veno-occlusive disease
  - CCI = [BSA × (increase in platelet count)]/4
    - <5000 × 2 consecutive → refractory
    - Measure "post-transfusion" 30 minutes to 4 hours after completion
- Antigens (human platelet antigens, HPA) include GpIa, GpIIb/IIIa
- Platelet crossmatch
  - Detects HLA, HPA, ABO incompatibility
  - Uses solid-phase red cell agglutination (SPRCA)
    - Plate with wells coated with known-type platelets
    - Patient's serum added to wells
    - anti-IgG coated red cells added
    - NO agglutination if positive
- Antiplatelet antibody test
  - ELISA to detect HPA and HLA antibodies
  - See Fig. 20.1.
- Antihuman globulin lymphocyte cytotoxicity test (AHG-LCT)—tests for anti-HLA antibodies (not HPA)
  - Patient's serum + panel of lymphs → analyzed for complement–mediated cellular toxicity
    - Acridine orange and ethidium bromide added → dead = green; alive = orange
  - Detects IgG and IgM

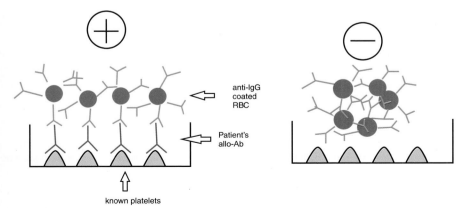

Fig. 20.1 Enzyme–linked immunosorbent assay (ELISA) for detecting antiplatelet antibodies. *Allo-Ab,* alloantibody; *RBC,* red blood cell.

- AHG increases sensitivity
- Stored and transported at 20° to 24°C
  - Cold platelets
    - Refrigerated after collection
    - "Activated"
    - Do not give good bump in platelet count, but function increases a lot
      - May be useful in trauma

FRESH-FROZEN PLASMA (FFP)

- Freeze within 8 hours of collection
  - If 8 to 25 hours—*frozen plasma*
- Must be transfused within 24 hours of thawing
  - If more than 24 hours—*thawed plasma*

CRYOPRECIPITATE ("Cryo")

- Contents
  - Must have 80 IU factor VIII and 150 mg fibrinogen
  - Also contains von Willebrand factor (VWF)
- How to make cryo
  - Thaw FFP and centrifuge at 1° to 6°C
  - Freeze precipitate within 1 hour at −18°C
  - Can be stored for up to 1 year
- Must be thawed before transfusion, usually pooled
  - If thawed and *not* pooled, can store at 20° to 24°C for up to 6 hours
  - If thawed and pooled, can store at 20° to 24°C for up to 4 hours
- Cryo calculation

  $$\text{Dose} = \frac{(\textit{goal fibrinogen} - \textit{current fibronogen}) \times PV}{100} \div 250$$

  - 250 mg/unit = amount of fibrinogen in bag of cryo
  - PV = plasma volume = (70 mL/kg × weight) × (1-hct)

Antigens and Antibodies

- Carbohydrate antigens are more antigenic
- Type 1 chains in secretions (glycolipid), *FUT2*
- Type 2 chains on RBCs (glycoproteins), *FUT1*

ABO Blood Group

- A1 (80% of all A) blood type is agglutinated by *Dolichos biflorus* lectin; A2 (20%) is not
- H = precursor to A and B, only antigen on type O unless they are the very rare Bombay type (no A, B, or H)
  - Detected with *Ulex europaeus* lectin
  - Receptor for Norwalk virus and Candida
- Type 1 H and Leb chains = receptors for *H. pylori*
- A1 type has much more antigens on surface than A2
  - 80% are A1, aggregates with *Dolichos biflorus*

- 20% are A2, no aggregation with *Dolichos biflorus*, some make anti-A1
  - More A2B make anti-A1!
- Bombay → typing looks like O, all screen cells are 4+
  - Lacks *FUT* gene to add fucose to galactose
- ABO hemolytic disease of the fetus/newborn (HDFN) is less severe than Rh because…
  - Anti-ABO antibodies are not fully developed until 3 to 6 months of age
  - A and B antigens in plasma neutralize anti-A and anti-B

RH BLOOD GROUP

- DCcEe
- D is most immunogenic; significant extravascular hemolysis and severe HDFN
- Rh null: no Rh antigens → hemolytic anemia with stomatocytes
- Two genes—*RHCE* (CcEe) and *RHD* (D)
- Haplotypes and their prevalence
  - See Table 20.1.
  - White—R1 > r > R2 > R0
  - Black—R0 > r > R1 > R2
- Genotypes
  - R1R1 (DCe/DCe)—30% to 50% risk for anti-E or anti-c after exposure to E+ blood because 98% of E+ donors are c+
  - Anti-E, give R_zR_z (DcE/DcE)—2%
  - See Table 20.2.
  - Platelets with anti-c or anti-e should not get Rh– (D–) blood because highly likely to get rr (dce/dce) blood
- G = either C or D
- f = c and e in cis (on same gene)
- 99% of Rh– are E– and C–
  - If you are in a pinch and need E– or C– blood, grab Rh–!
- C+e– are 1/40, 000 (R2 and r")
  - Cannot always tell between C antibody (Ab) and e Ab; usually honor both

OTHER ANTIGEN GROUPS

- Lewis
  - You cannot be Lewis B (Le^b) if you are not a secretor

TABLE 20.1 ■ Rh Group Haplotypes

Fisher-Race	Weiner	Prevalence
Dce	R0	Common in Black Americans
DCe	R1	Very common
DcE	R2	Common
DCE	Rz	Very rare
dce	r	Common
dCe	r'	Rare
dcE	r"	Rare
dCE	Ry	Almost never happens

TABLE 20.2 ■ Rh Group Genotypes

Fisher-Race Genotype	Prevalence in White Americans
Rh-positive	
CDe/cde	31%
CDe/CDe	19%
CDe/cDE	12%
cDE/cde	10%
cDe/cde	3%; 22% in Black Americans!
CDE/cDE	2%
CDE/CDE	<1%
Rh-negative	
cde/cde	15%
CdE/CdE	<1%

- *FUT2* gene
- Le^b does not make anti-Le^a
- We only see antibodies against Le in pregnant women
  - Antigen expression is usually lost in pregnancy
  - They are cold antibodies, not clinically significant
  - Neutralize with saliva
- Secretors = Le(a–b+)
- Nonsecretors = Le(a+b–)
- Anti-Le does not cross the placenta
- Le(a+b+) not possible, but Le(a–b–) is
- Kell = five sets of antigens
  - K ("kell") and k ("cellano"); Kpa, Kpb, Kpc; Jsa and Jsb; K11 and K17; K14 and K24
  - K$_{null}$ lacks all except Kx protein and develops anti-Ku (universal) after exposure
  - Kx protein—linked by disulfide bond to Kell antigens
    - McLeod phenotype—lacks Kx
      - ↓ Kell Ags, acanthocytosis, hemolytic anemia, associated with X-linked chronic granulomatous disease
        - Lack NADPH oxidase → ↑ *Staphylococcus aureus* infections
      - Anti-KL antibodies (against K and XK) = neuromuscular acanthocytosis
- Anti-K is not uncommon, but >90% of Ig donors are negative
  - IgG, warm–reacting, exposure required
  - Can cause HTR, HDN, neonatal anemia
    - *"Kell kills, Lewis lives"*
- Anti-k uncommon
- Second most antigenic after Rh—"Kell kills"
- Rarely shows dosage
- 9% of people are K+, 99.8% are k+
- Kidd (Jka and Jkb)
  - Displays dosage
    - Anti-Jka reacts stronger with homozygous Jka/Jka than with Jka/Jkb
  - Reactivity waxes and wanes—"Kidd hides"

- Antibody quickly fades then responds to second exposure with anamnestic response (stronger than first reaction)
- Panel can be negative when the patient is actually positive!
  - "Anamnestic response"
    - Check previous blood bank records before transfusing! Can cause severe hemolysis!
- Most common antibody associated with hemolytic transfusion reactions
  - Fix complement but IgG (usually IgM fixes it) → intravascular hemolysis
- Jk(a–b–) cells are resistant to urea lysis
- Duffy (Fya and Fyb)
  - Fy(a+b–) most common, Fy(a–b–) more common in Black people (gives resistance to *Plasmodium vivax*)
    - Fyb is present on endothelial cells → Fyb– patients do not usually form Abs
    - Receptor for *Plasmodium vivax*
  - Displays dosage, can fade, can be severe (like Kidd)
  - Fyb and Jkb not strongly antigenic but dirty (cross–react)
  - Fya is on DARC receptor that absorbs chemokines and decreases cancer risk
  - Those with a mutation in transcription factor *GATA1* **lack** Duffy antigens on red cells, but retain them on endothelial cells
    - Type as Fy(a–b–), but do not form anti-Duffy antibodies
- MNSsU
  - Displays dosage
  - M and N are on glycophorin A and S, s and U are on glycophorin B
    - A is receptor for *Escherichia coli* in urinary bladder
    - B is absent in most Black people
    - Both may be *Plasmodium falciparum* receptors
      - Patients negative for M and N are resistant to *P. falciparum*
  - Antibodies
    - M and N antibodies are naturally occurring and clinically insignificant
    - Anti-N is associated with dialysis (when machines are sterilized with formaldehyde)
    - S, s, U antibodies require exposure and are clinically significant
  - *Vicea graminea* agglutinates with N
- P1/P/Pk
  - P = parvovirus receptor
  - Naturally occurring cold IgM
    - Neutralized by *Echinococcus* (hydatid cyst fluid) and pigeon egg fluid
  - Associated with paroxysmal cold hemoglobinuria
    - Polyclonal IgG 2/2 microorganism
    - Donath-Landsteiner test
      - Tube 1—0 °C—no hemolysis
      - Tube 2—37 °C—no hemolysis
      - Tube 3—0 °C → 37 °C—hemolysis!
      - Biphasic antibody: binds in cold, hemolyzes in warm
- I/i—expression is age–dependent (see Fig. 20.2), cold IgM, anti-I associated *with Mycoplasma pneumoniae*, anti-i associated with EBV

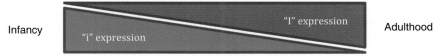

Fig. 20.2 Age–dependent expression of I/i antigens.

Antigen Properties

- "Dosage"
  - If test RBCs have both antigens (heterozygous), they mask each other and patient's serum may not react
  - Duffy (Fya, Fyb), Kidd (Jka, Jkb), MNS, Cc
- Enzyme sensitive antigens—"Duffy men's choir"
  - Fy, MNSs, Cc, Rh
  - ↑—ABO family (ABO, Lewis, I/i, P), Rh, Kidd
  - ↓—MnSsU, Duffy
  - ↔—Kell
- DTT gets rid of Kell, Lutheran, and IgM because it's a thiol and both are anchored with sulfhydryl groups
- Do not worry about finding homozygous Kell cells on antibody panel
  - 1/1000 are KK, K is extremely antigenic, no worries about dosage
- Cw and V are low–frequency antigens
  - V has slightly higher allele frequency in Black communities
- Neutralization
  - ABO: saliva (secretor)
  - Lewis: saliva (secretor)
  - P: hydatid cyst fluid or pigeon egg fluid
  - Sd^a: urine
  - Chido/Rodgers: serum
- *Vicea graminea* agglutinates with N

ANTIBODIES

- Passive anti-D usually secondary to RhIg
- IgM can cause agglutination by themselves ("complete" Abs) but are only active at temps <37°C (in vitro usually, not clinically relevant)
- U—uncommon but clinically significant antibody
- Do not worry about Cw, V, Kpa, Jsa, Lea, N, Lua
- Anti-Kpa, Jsa, Lua are usually insignificant
- Warm autoantibodies tend to have anti-e specificity
- Anti-Lua or Lub show loose mixed field aggregation patterns
- High–titer low–affinity (HTLA) antibodies
  - Weak AHG reaction, variable, difficult to reproduce
  - Rarely react at room temperature or body temperature
  - IgG, noncomplement binding
  - Difficult to adsorb or do elutions, easily washed away
    - Do not react with own cells

Apheresis

- Leukoreduction—need symptoms and high WBC
  - Symptoms
    - Lungs—shortness of breath
    - Brain—altered mental status
    - Retina—visual disturbances
    - Kidney—acute kidney injury

- White blood cell counts are not strict cutoffs
  - Acute myeloid leukemia >100,000
  - Acute lymphoblastic leukemia >400,000
  - Chronic myeloid leukemia >20, 000
  - Chronic lymphocytic leukemia >50,000
- *Or* pregnant with CML or CLL
- Typically 1.5 to 2 × the patient's blood volume is processed (7.5 to 10 L in an adult)
- Hyperhemolysis syndrome—lots of hemolysis in sickle cell patient after transfusion
  - RBC transfusions are contraindicated!
  - May need plasmapheresis +/- dialysis for free hemoglobin
- Replacement fluids for plasmapheresis
  - Thrombotic thrombocytopenic purpura (TTP)—FFP
  - Most—albumin and normal saline
    - If effective, fibrinogen levels will decrease by 70% (can use as marker of effectiveness)
    - If performed daily or fibrinogen getting too low, switch to FFP after a few days
- Red blood cell exchange
  - Important numbers for automated exchanges
    - Target hematocrit ≤30%, hemoglobin ≤10
  - Sickle cell anemia—target hct = 21%
    - Exchange fluid hct—55% to 60% (ACD-A, CPD is about 70)
    - FCR (fraction of cells remaining)—30
      - Also considered "fraction of hemoglobin S" remaining
    - We match all blood with Rh and Kell
    - Fy^b does not show up on phenotypes (silenced on RBCs)
      - Receptor for *P. vivax* and *P. knowlesi*
- Peripheral blood stem cell transplant (PBSCT) mobilization
  - G-CSF
  - Plerixafor (prevents SDF-1 from binding to CXCR4)
    - Only approved for myeloma and non-Hodgkin lymphoma

Transfusion Reactions

- Febrile non-hemolytic transfusion reactions (FNHTR) can be caused by leukocyte cytokines or recipient HLA/HNA (human neutrophil antibodies) antibodies against transfused WBCs (in nonleukoreduced or bedside leukoreduction after storage)
  - Unclear in prestorage leukoreduced blood
- Irradiation is performed to prevent GVHD
- Coagulopathy of trauma
  - 25% of trauma patients
  - Most have PT increasing > PTT increase (but PTT predicts better than PT)
  - Dilutional, hypothermia, acidosis, consumption, hypoperfusion
    - Thrombomodulin + thrombin → increased protein C → decreased Factors V and VIII
  - Massive transfusion can lead to hypocalcemia and hyperkalemia
  - TRIM—transfusion–related immune modulation
  - 1:1 or 1:2 plasma:RBC ratio (start plasma early)
  - Colloids inhibit VWF
- Transfusion transmitted diseases
  - Syphilis, HepB, HepC, HIV, WNV, Chagas, malaria, babesia, prions, zika, HTLV 1 and 2, chikungunya, dengue
  - NAT tested in pools of 16 to 24 donors. If positive, broken out and tested individually
  - Only test for CMV in granulocyte donors or for intrauterine transfusions

- Antineutrophil antibodies (HNAs) can cause...
  - Neonatal alloimmune neutropenia
  - FNHTR
  - TRALI—needs predisposing condition + biologically active lipids transferred in stored blood components
  - Transfusion–related alloimmune neutropenia
  - Autoimmune neutropenia
  - Persistent post-bone marrow transplant neutropenia
- Bacteremia
  - 1 in 60, 000 platelet transfusions
  - Coagulase–negative *Staphylococcus, Streptococcus, Bacillus cereus*
- Risk for transmitting infectious disease
  - Hepatitis B—1 in 80, 000 to 100, 000
  - HIV—1 in 2 million

TRANSFUSION–RELATED COAGULATION TOPICS

- Acquired factor deficiencies
  - Decreased factor V (F5)—bovine thrombin exposure (Ab production)
  - Decreased F10—amyloidosis (Ab production?)
  - End–stage liver disease decreases all clotting (and anticoagulation factors) except F8 and VWF; decreased platelets—splenic sequestration and decreased thrombopoietin; F5 most sensitive
  - Acquired VWD—aortic stenosis and LVAD
- Antiphospholipid Abs
  - Detect cardiolipin and β_2 glycoprotein with ELISA titers
  - Detect lupus anticoagulants with clot–based assays
    - INR = tissue factor + phospholipid + Ca
    - PTT = phospholipid + contact agent + Ca
    - Get LONG results because the Ab blocks phospholipid
  - LAC ISTH diagnostic criteria
    1. Prolonged phospholipid–based clotting assay (INR, PTT, DRVVT)
    2. Mixing study does *not* correct
    3. Excess phospholipid + PTT → shortened PTT (saturate Ab)
    4. Rule out other causes (especially rivaroxaban)
  - Clinical signs = clots (arterial and venous), pregnancy complications
  - Laboratory signs = +LAC, cardiolipin, β_2 glycoprotein; repeat + 6 to 12 weeks later
  - Lupus anticoagulant (LAC) can be factor–specific (usually to F2)—check factor levels
- Prothrombin mutation = G→A at 20210 (leads to increased F2a)
- Dysfibrinogenemia—can clot or bleed or both; get fibrinogen activity levels and fibrinogen antigen levels
- Activated protein C (APC) resistance
  - F5 Leiden = 90%
  - F5 does not get inactivated by APC and protein S
  - Diagnostic by genetic testing or coagulation testing
    - Pt plasma + F5 def plasma → (PTT) → A
    - Pt plasma + F5 def plasma + APC → (PTT) → B
      - Normal—A = normal, B = 2 to 3.5 × prolonged
      - Heterozygote—A = normal, B = 1.6 × prolonged
      - Homozygote—A = normal, B = 1.2 × prolonged

- Protein C problems—decreased antigen or decreased function
  - Get activity levels to assess both
  - Caused by warfarin, vitamin K deficiency, liver disease, inhibitor Ab, acute clot, L-asparaginase, age <15 years, diffuse intravascular coagulopathy (DIC)
- Protein S problems—low Ag, low activity, or low free antigen (not bound to C4b-binding protein)
  - Caused by everything that causes protein C deficiency + age <6 months, pregnancy, oral contraceptives, hormone replacement therapy, inflammation
- Protein C & S problems—cause clots, pregnancy complications, neonatal purpura fulminans (bad DIC in babies), warfarin–induced skin necrosis
- Antithrombin problems—get activity level in F2- or F10-based assays (to avoid effect of any anticoagulants)
  - Decrease caused by heparin, DIC, acute clot, liver disease, nephrotic syndrome, congenital, age <3 months, TTP/hemolytic uremic syndrome (HUS), plasma exchange
  - Can cause clots or heparin resistance
- Those with type O blood have less circulating von Willebrand factor than non-O blood types

DONOR SELECTION

- Medications, must off for...
  - Finasteride—1 month
  - Dutasteride—6 months
  - Isotretinoin—1 month
  - Acitretin—3 years
  - Etretinate—indefinite
- Must wait 4 weeks after MMR, chickenpox, or shingles vaccine
  - 21 days for Hepatitis B vaccine and 1 year for immunoglobulin
- Deferment periods
  - Babesiosis—indefinitely
  - Travel to a malaria–endemic area—12 months
  - *Received* a transfusion—12 months
  - Vaccines
    - None (if symptom free)—influenza, Hepatitis A, Hepatitis B, diphtheria, tetanus, pertussis, pneumococcal, polio (Salk), HPV
    - 2 weeks—measles, mumps, oral polio (Sabin), typhoid, yellow fever
    - 4 weeks—rubella, varicella
    - Smallpox
      - No complications—until scab separates spontaneous *and* it has been at least 21 days
      - If complications are present—14 days after resolution of symptoms
  - Postdonation intervals
    - Double red cell donation to any other donation—16 weeks
    - Whole–blood donation (to whole–blood donation or platelet donation)—8 weeks
    - Platelet donation to whole-blood donation—2 days
    - Plasma donation to plasma donation—2 days, no more than twice a week
- For donated blood products, the Food and Drug Administration requires testing for...
  - Each time: HbsAg, HbcAb, HBV DNA, anti–Hepatitis C antibodies, HCV RNA, anti-HIV antibodies, HIV RNA, anti-HTLV antibodies, syphilis serologies, West Nile RNA

- One time (for the donor): *Trypanosoma cruzi*
- State–dependent: *Babesia*
- Best HIV screening method has the shortest window period (10 to 11 days)
  - Nucleic acid testing for HIV!
  - Performed on minipools of donor samples (8 to 24)
    - If a minipool is positive, all samples in minipool are individually tested

STEM CELL TRANSPLANTS AND CELL PRODUCTS

- Cryopreservation
  - Not needed for peripheral blood stem cell transplants (PBSCTs) if they will be infused in less than 48 hours
    - Just store at 4° to 15°C
  - Hematopoietic precursor cell (HPC) cryoprotectant = DMSO and autologous plasma
  - Controlled rate freezing
  - –70 degrees, can store for several years
- Mismatch
  - "Major"—recipient antibodies against donor cells
    - Can cause delayed red blood cell engraftment (caused by residual recipient plasma cells)
  - "Minor"—donor antibodies against recipient cells
    - Passenger lymphocyte syndrome
- PBSCTs engraft faster than HPCs harvested from bone marrow or umbilical cord blood
  - Especially granulocytes and platelets
  - Decreased risk for graft-versus-host disease
- HPCs must be tested for HIV1, HIV2, Hepatitis C, Hepatitis B, HTLV1, HTLV2, CMV, syphilis
  - +/– West Nile and Chagas (depending on location)
- Minimum number of stem cells for one transplant—2×10^6 CD34+ cells per kilogram
- Liquid nitrogen dry shippers must be maintained at –150°C or less for at least 48 hours past delivery time
  - Continuous temperature monitoring is required
- Give IL-2 with NK cell products
  - But this increases T regulatory cells, which kill NK cells
  - IL-diphtheria toxin fusion protein can deplete Tregs!

Odds and Ends

- Chromosome 9 → glycosyltransferases for A (NAG), B (Gal), or O (null, stop codon)
- Blood banks are regulated by the Food and Drug Administration
  - They can be accredited by the American Association of Blood Banks (AABB), the College of American Pathologists (CAP), or the Joint Commission
- Adult blood volume = 5 L
- Thrombopoietin agonists—romiplostim and eltrombopag

CHAPTER 21

Hematopathology

Introduction and Hematopathology Basics

STEPS TO EVALUATING BONE MARROW

1. Adequacy
2. Bony trabeculae
3. Cellularity
4. Myeloid lineages
5. Lymphs and plasma cells
6. Vessels and stroma
7. Abnormal infiltrates

IMMUNOPHENOTYPE

By Cell Line

- Remember that blasts can aberrantly express anything
- Myeloid
  - Myeloperoxidase (MPO), CD13, CD33, CD117
  - Maturation process
    - Lose CD13, then gain back, then gain CD16
    - CD64 gets brighter
    - CD38 gets dimmer
- Myeloblast
  - Surface: CD34, CD33, CD13, DR
  - Cytoplasm: MPO
- Monocytes
  - CD11c, CD14, CD36 (also erythroids), CD64, lysozyme, non-specific esterase (NSE)
  - May fall into blast gate
- T cells
  - sCD3 or cCD3
  - Alpha/beta—CD2, CD3, CD5, CD7, CD4 or CD8, CD56+/−, CD57+/−, cCD3
    - Follicular-helper T cells and large granular lymphocytes (LGLs)
    - Normal CD4:CD8—>10 or <0.1 requires reporting
  - Gamma/delta—CD2, CD3, CD7, partial CD56, CD3, CD5 dim-to-negative, CD8 dim-to-negative
  - See Fig. 21.1.
  - Tregs—CD4+, CD25+
  - Follicular helper T cells—CD4+, CD10+, CD57+
- T lymphoblast
  - Surface: CD4, CD8, CD7, CD5, CD2
  - Cytoplasm: cCD3

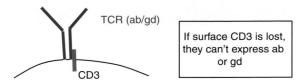

Fig. 21.1   T cell receptor (TCR) structure. *ab*, alpha/beta; *gd*, gamma/delta.

TABLE 21.1 ■ **Differentiating T Cells and NK Cells**

	T cells	NK cells
CD3 (surface)	+	−
CD8	+/−	+/−
CD56	−	+
CD16	−	+

- Nucleus: TdT
- NK cells
  - CD2, CD7, CD8 +/−, CD16, CD56, CD57+/−, sCD3−, partial CD161, partial CD94
    - Uniform CD94 is aberrant
    - Use KIRs (CD158 a/b/c) for clonality
    - May fall into blast gate
    - See Table 21.1.
- Hematogones
  - CD10+, CD38+, CD20−, kappa/lambda−
- B cells
  - CD19 → if strong, need one more B cell antigen. If weak, need two more
    - Most commonly used: CD10 and CD22, also CD20, kappa and lambda, cCD22, cCD79a
  - CD22 is positive in basophils
- B lymphoblast
  - Surface: CD10, HLA-DR, CD19, CD20, CD22
  - Cytoplasm: Mu, cCD22, cCD79a
  - Nucleus: terminal deoxynucleotidyl terminase (TdT)
- Plasma cells
  - IgG/IgA/IgM (most frequently)
  - Surface immunoglobulin (sIg)−, CD20−, MUM1+, CD79a+, CD38+, CD138+
- Megakaryocytes
  - CD61
- Megakaryoblasts
  - CD61, CD41a
- Erythroids
  - CD36 (also monocytes), glycophorin A (CD235a)
- Basophils
  - CD13+, CD33+, HLA-DR−
  - May fall into blast gate
- Eosinophils
  - CD16−, CD13+, CD15 dimmer than myeloids, brighter CD45, mostly CD10−

By Marker

- CD2 smears in T-lymphoblastic leukemia (T-ALL) flow cytometry
- CD4 is positive in histiocytes!
- CD5—small resting lymphs in peripheral blood (PB), primary follicles, and follicular mantle zones; mantle cell lymphoma (MCL) and chronic lymphocytic leukemia/small lymphocytic lymphoma (CLL/SLL)
  - In T cells, correlates with alpha-beta T cell receptor (TCR) status (i.e., gamma–deltas are CD5–)
- CD8—T cells, histiocytes, dendritic cells
- CD10—normal (not neoplastic) B cells, reactive germinal centers (clonal or not), hematogones, in situ follicular neoplasm, follicular lymphoma
- CD14—germinal–center B cells
- CD21 and CD23—follicular dendritic network (to see follicular structure better)
  - Not positive in primary follicles (only secondary)
- CD30—normal immunoblasts and plasma cells
- CD34—hematopoietic progenitors, early lymphoid progenitors (hematogones), and leukemic blasts
  - Can be positive in normal eosinophils
- CD57—follicular–helper T cells, NK cells, LGLs
- CD68—histiocytes
  - PGM1 in bone marrow
  - KP1 in tissues
- CD117 is bright on mast cells and dim on erythroid precursors
  - Also expressed on myeloblasts and promyelocytes
  - Indicative of c-KIT mutation
- CD49d and CD38 are poor prognostic markers in CLL/SLL
- BCL2 –/+ in marginal zone lymphoma (MZL) and follicular lymphoma (FL)
  - Negative in normal germinal centers and Burkitt lymphoma (BL)
- OCT and BOB are B cell transcription factors (so stains are nuclear)
  - B cell lymphomas are positive for both; classic Hodgkin lymphoma (CHL) is negative for one or both
- CyclinD1 is positive in plasma cells and occasional nonspecific stromal cells
- T cell disorders
  - CD10—angioimmunoblastic T cell lymphoma (AITL)
  - CD25—adult T cell leukemia (ATLL)
  - CD30—anaplastic large cell lymphoma (ALCL, big cells typically do not survive flow cytometry)
  - CD52—T cell prolymphocytic leukemia (T-PLL, theoretically), in CAMPATH tube
- FMC7 is positive when CD20 is bright and negative when CD20 is negative or dim
  - Positive in mantle cell lymphoma; negative in CLL

By Indication

- Rule out post-transplant lymphoproliferative disorder (PTLD) on tissue
  - CD3, CD20, EBV-encoding RNA (EBER)
- Hodgkin
  - CD15, CD30, PAX-5, CD20, CD3, CD45
- Large cell panel
  - CD10, CD5, CD3, CD2, MYC, BCL2, BCL6, MUM1, Ki67
  - If blastic morphology—CD34 and TdT to rule out acute leukemia

- Myelodysplastic syndrome (MDS) bone marrow
  - CD34, CD61, reticulin, +/− trichrome

Small B Cell Lymphoma Immunophenotypes

- CLL
  - Positive: CD4, CD23, CD27, CD43, BCL2, dim CD20, dim light chains
  - Negative: FMC7, CD20, CD79b
- Mantle cell lymphoma
  - Positive: CD5, CD43, BCL2, cyclin D1
  - Negative: CD10, CD23
- Follicular lymphoma: CD5−, CD10+, BCL2+
- Hairy cell leukemia
  - CD11c, CD25, CD103, and CD123+
  - CD27−
  - Variant—CD11c+, <u>CD25−</u>, <u>CD27</u>+, CD103+, <u>CD123−</u>
  - PITFALL—may fall into monocyte gate (and there is usually monocytopenia)

CYTOCHEMICAL STAINS

- MPO (myeloperoxidase)—myeloblasts positive, monoblasts faint, lymphoblast and mega-karyocytes negative, mature neutrophils and monocytes positive
  - Count 100 blasts
- NSE (nonspecific esterase, usually naphthyl acetate esterase)—monoblasts and promono-cytes positive
  - Count 100 cells
- PAS (periodic acid Schiff)—erythroblasts in acute erythroid leukemia
- NAP (neutrophil alkaline phosphatase) or LAP (leukocyte alkaline phosphatase)—chronic myeloid leukemia CML has low NAP/LAP score
- TRAP (tartrate resistant acid phosphatase)—hairy cell leukemia positive
- NBT (nitroblue–tetrazolium)—phagocytes (granulocytes and monocytes/macrophages)
- Sudan back—myeloblasts through myelocytes
- Chloracetate esterase—specific for granulocytes

See Table 21.2.

TABLE 21.2 ■ **Immunophenotype of Thymocytes According to Their Maturity**

Stage	Positive Markers	Negative Markers
Least mature	Dim CD45 Dim CD2 Dim CD3 Bright CD7 CD10 CD34	CD3 CD4 *and* CD 8 (heterogeneous)
Immature (cortical)	Intermediate CD45 CD1a CD2 CD5 CD7 CD99 CD4 *and* CD8	CD10 CD34
Mature (medullary)	CD2 CD3 CD5 CD7 CD4 *or* CD8	CD1a CD10 CD34 CD99 CD4 *or* CD8

FLOW CYTOMETRY

General Principles

- Analysis of cells using laser beams
  - Red laser (633 nm)—APC and APC-Cy7
  - Blue laser (488 nm)—FITC, PE, PE-Cy5, PerCP, PerCP-Cy5.5, PE-Cy7
- Separate cells based on physical properties, antigen expression, DNA content, metabolic activity, viability
- Specimen processing—suspend WBCs, lyse RBCs and precursors, +/– weight gradient; run specimen; analyze results
  - Optional to add permeability agent to assess cell contents
- Forward scatter (FSC) depends on *size;* side scatter (SSC) depends on *complexity* (e.g., multiple nuclear lobes, cytoplasmic granulation)
  - No stains needed for these
  - See Fig. 21.2.
- Can separate initially be FSC vs. SSC or CD45 vs. SSC
  - CD45 = common leukocyte antigen (LCA)
    - Negative or dim on plasma cells, dim on blasts
    - CD = clusters of differentiation
- "Monotypic" is a surrogate for monoclonal
  - Kappa-to-lambda ratio for B cell monotypia
    - normal kappa-to-lambda = 0.26 to 1
    - Flow cytometry only assesses for surface immunoglobulin unless a permeability agent is added. Immunohistochemical (IHC) on paraffin–embedded sections assess surface and cytoplasmic because individual cells are sectioned through, revealing cytoplasmic (and nuclear) antigens
    - Absence of both or presence of both on individual cells = abnormal (though could be a technical problem)
  - T cells
    - Alpha/beta vs. gamma/delta
      - All undergo delta and gamma rearrangement (see "Molecular" section of this chapter)
      - Most T cells in blood are alpha/beta
      - T cells in skin, gastrointestinal (GI) tract, and spleen are gamma/delta
    - V betas
      - Use antibodies to 24 possible antigens on V portion of TCR protein
      - Normal should have mixture
      - Need difference in 50% *or* >10 × upper limit of normal (%)
        - If >70% is negative for all tested, we can assume they are monoclonal for a V-beta not tested
    - TCR cB1

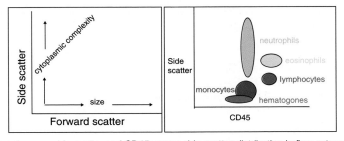

Fig. 21.2 Forward versus side scatter and CD45 versus side scatter distribution in flow cytometry.

- KIRS—Killer immunoglobulin–like receptors
  - Normal on NK cells and some cytotoxic T cells
  - CD158 a, b, e—normal is a mixture
  - CD94 and CD161—normal is partial
  - Useful on sCD3—and gamma-delta cells (cannot do V-betas)
    - PITFALL—some T-NK neoplasms are not KIRS-restricted
- Compensation—adjustment for signals from other fluorochromes that "bleed into" fluorochrome of interest
  - Example: FITC is green, PE is yellow. When PE is attached to a highly expressed antigen, it can look like FITC is also slightly positive
  - Proper compensation lines up middle of populations (though compensation does cause some widening errors)
- BV605 and FITC are relatively weak fluorochromes; PE is bright
- Can use flow to monitor immunosuppression in solid organ transplant patient
- Fluorescent antibodies use stokes shift
- Must subtract overlapping spectrum = "compensation"
  - Some stains cannot be used together because there is too much overlap
- When describing expression, first is positive/negative/partial
  - Partial is events on both sides of axis
  - Next description is dim, bright, heterogeneous, bimodal
- CD4:CD8 T cell ratio can be useful
  - Increased in nodular lymphocyte–predominant Hodgkin lymphoma (NLPHD)
  - Decreased in T cell/histiocyte–rich B cell lymphoma (THRBCL)
- Hematogones
  - Stage 1 can lose a little CD10 (that is okay)
  - Stage 3 coexpress CD5 (usually dim) and CD10—PITFALL
  - See Fig. 21.3

Pitfalls

- Hematogones with surface light–chain restriction can be mistaken for marrow involvement by lymphoma
  - Hematogones—CD10+, CD19+, bright CD38+, CD200+, CD43+, CD20 smear
  - Hematogones differ from lymphoma cells by CD45 expression and side scatter
  - Hematogones are usually persistent
  - Follicular lymphoma has dimmer CD10 than background B cells
  - False surface light chain restriction from daratumumab or alemtuzumab
    - Both are kappa
    - See Fig. 21.4.
- Many myeloid sarcomas are CD34–
  - Try CD117, CD56, lysozyme
  - Eosinophils are only present in a subset
- Normal plasma cells and immunoblasts are CD30+
- Hairy cell leukemia may fall into monocyte gate (and there is usually monocytopenia)
- LGL expansion can occur after bone marrow transplant (BMT), immunosuppression, or autoimmune
  - CD57+, CD3+
  - Abnormal if alpha-beta LGLs are CD16+ or dim
- Platelets can express CD34!
  - Should have dim CD45, low forward scatter, low side scatter
- NK cells can fall into the basophil/hematogone area on CD45 × SSC
- Blasts can be CD45–

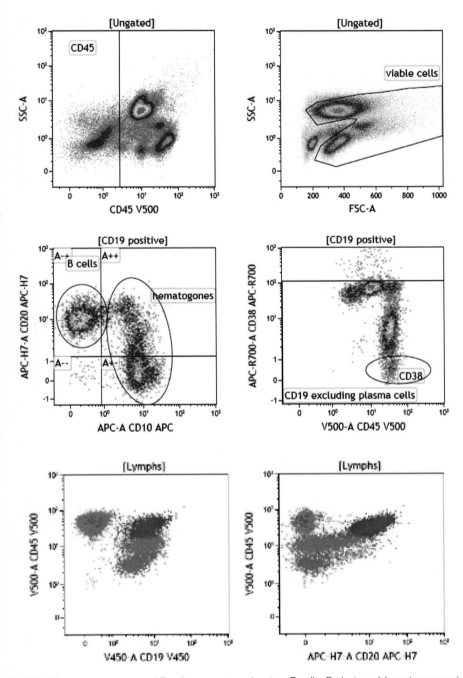

Fig. 21.3 Hematogones or normal B cell precursors and mature B cells. *Red,* stage 1 hematogones; *pink,* stage 2 hematogones; *purple,* stage 3 hematogones; *blue,* mature B cells.

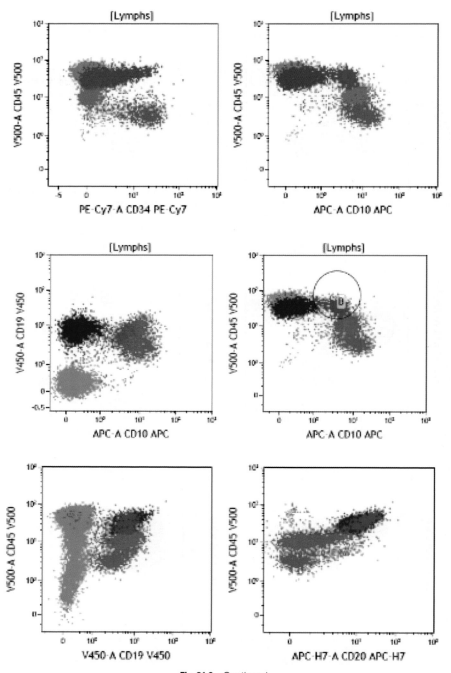

Fig. 21.3 Continued

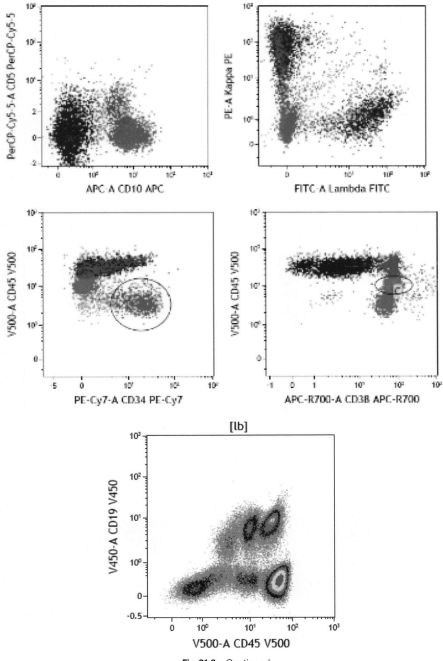

Fig. 21.3 Continued

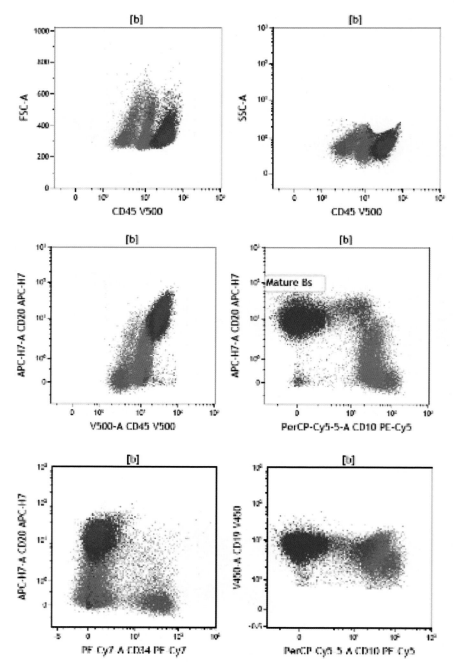

Fig. 21.3 Continued

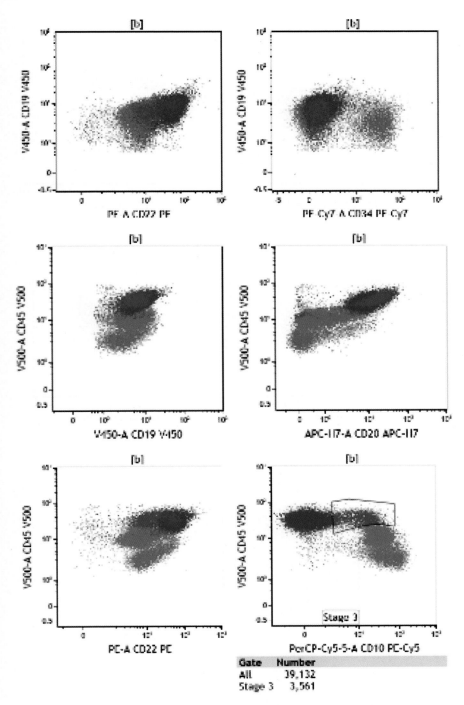

Gate	Number
All	39,132
Stage 3	3,561

Fig. 21.3 Continued

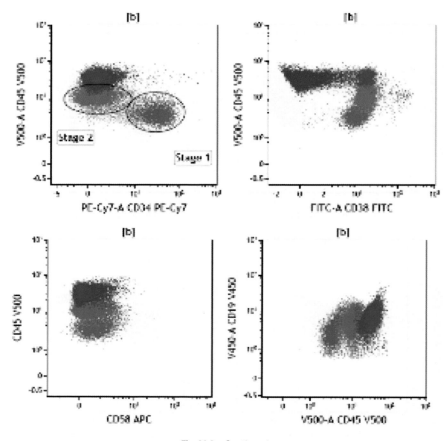

Fig. 21.3 Continued

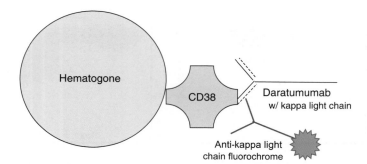

Fig. 21.4 False light chain restriction on hematogones caused by daratumumab.

Nonneoplastic

PLATELET ABNORMALITIES

- Giant platelets
  - MDS
  - Bernard–Soulier
  - Postsplenectomy
  - Immune thrombocytopenia (ITP), other hemolysis, hemorrhage
  - May–Hegglin
  - Familial macrothrombocytopenia
- Small platelets
  - Wiskott–Aldrich
  - Glanzmann thrombasthenia
  - X-linked immunodeficiency with eczema and thrombocytopenia

WHITE CELL ABNORMALITIES

- Pelger–Huët anomaly—hyposegmented granulocytes, asymptomatic (uni- or bilobed)
  - May be associated with developmental delays, epilepsy, and skeletal abnormalities
  - Pseudo-Pelger–Huët—MDS and left–shift
- May–Hegglin anomaly—distinctive, prominent, large, blue, crescent–shaped cytoplasmic inclusions; large platelets that are decreased in number; most asymptomatic
- Chediak–Higashi syndrome—abnormal fusion of lysosomal granules, autosomal recessive
  - Large, irregular gray-green to gray–orange granules in neutrophils
  - Granules in eosinophils and basophils are large and irregular too
  - Partial albinism, photophobia, infections, early death
- Mucopolysaccharidoses (with Alder–Reilly anomaly)
- Vacuolated lymphocytes (Wolman disease and ceroid lipofuscinoses)
- Gaucher disease (glucocerebroside)
- Niemann–Pick disease (sphingomyelin)

ERYTHROCYTIC ABNORMALITIES

Common Changes in Complete Blood Counts

- Anemia
  - Microcytic (decreased hemoglobin production)
    - Iron–deficiency anemia (ICD)
      - Microcytic hypochromic anemia with insufficient reticulocytosis and sometimes reactive thrombocytosis
      - Low iron, low iron saturation, high total iron–binding capacity (TIBC), low ferritin
    - Anemia of chronic disease (ACD)
      - Iron is locked away in macrophages by hepcidin
        - Iron may promote microorganism or tumor cell growth
        - Hepcidin prevents bone marrow macrophages from passing iron to erythroid precursors
      - High ferritin (storage form of iron), low TIBC, low serum iron, low iron saturation

- Total iron–binding capacity (TIBC) is a reflection on amount of transferrin present
  - Think of it as the number of seats on buses that are open for more iron
  - In iron deficiency, the body really needs more iron for hematopoiesis, so it sends a bunch of empty buses to be ready to use any available iron
  - In anemia of chronic disease, the body increases hepcidin to lock the iron away in macrophages. The body does not want any more iron, so it does not send any empty buses to pick up incoming iron
- Sideroblastic anemia
  - Normal sideroblast range: 20% to 50% (⅓ to ⅔)
    - Can take iron studies into account → if they are normal, sideroblast percentage is probably normal
  - Inherited or acquired defective heme synthesis
  - Dimorphic population on peripheral blood smear (microcytic hypochromic and normocytic normochromic) with anisopoikilocytosis and basophilic stippling
  - Iron stain on bone marrow (BM): nucleated red blood cells (nRBCs) with blue granules around nucleus (≥5 granules, >⅓ around the nucleus) = ring sideroblasts
- Thalassemia (see later)
- Normocytic
  - Peripheral destruction
    - Hemolysis
      - Intravascular
        - Destroyed in blood vessels
          - Disseminated intravascular coagulopathy (DIC), thrombotic thrombocytopenia purpura (TTP), hemolytic uremic syndrome (HUS), immune hemolytic anemia, paroxysmal nocturnal hemoglobinuria, malaria
          - Low haptoglobin (scavenges free hemoglobin), high free hemoglobin, hemoglobinuria Extravascular
          - Related to reticuloendothelial system
          - Something is wrong with the structure of the red cells, so the macrophages in the spleen and liver try to "clean them up" by taking bites and recycling the hemoglobin
          - Hereditary spherocytosis, glucose-6-phosphate dehydrogenase (G6PD) deficiency (Heinz bodies), pyruvate kinase deficiency (echinocytes), sickle cell anemia
          - High unconjugated bilirubinemia, normal haptoglobin, no free hemoglobin
          - Note: most are not solely intra- or extravascular. G6PD deficiency has a significant intravascular component, and malaria may have a significant extravascular component.
      - Blood loss
        - Trauma, gastrointestinal, menorrhagia, post–blood donation
        - After acute blood loss, it takes 5 days to produce reticulocytosis
  - Decreased production
    - Toxins, infections (parvovirus B19), end–stage renal disease (low erythropoietin production), aplastic anemia (e.g., congenital, acquired, toxin), myelophthisic process
- Macrocytic
  - Enough hemoglobin, not enough DNA
  - Folate or B_{12} deficiency
    - Megaloblastic—large red cells, hypersegmented neutrophils
    - Folate—high serum homocysteine, normal methylmalonic acid
    - B_{12}—high serum homocysteine, high methylmalonic acid

- □ Alcoholism
- □ Liver disease
- □ Drugs that interfere with DNA synthesis (e.g., 5-fluorouracil, methotrexate)
- ■ Acanthocytosis of >10% can be associated with...
  - ■ McLeod blood group phenotype
  - ■ Abetalipoproteinemia, homozygous hypobetalipoproteinemia, and advanced liver disease
- ■ Echinocytes are associated with uremia, burns, and old sample
- ■ If (hemoglobin * 3)—hematocrit > +2, then think that something is interfering with the measurement → red cell clumping or opacification of the plasma (by free hemoglobin, triglycerides, or bilirubin) (or very rarely high MCHC)
- ■ Always compare MCV with baseline for patient
  - ■ MCV of reticulocytes = 140
  - ■ Physiologic MCV changes:
    - □ Neonate—high (105)
      - ▫ Neonatal microcytosis is most commonly caused by transfusion with adult RBCs
    - ■ Infant ~6 months—low (76)
    - ■ Remain small through childhood
    - ▫ Pregnancy—slightly high in third trimester (100 to 105)
  - ■ See Fig. 21.5.
- ■ MCHC can be artifactually increased but *not* decreased
- ■ Reticulocyte index = reticulocytes × (HCT/normal HCT)
  - ■ "Normal HCT" used = 45
- ■ Point of care (POC) devices that measure hemoglobin use conductivity–based methods
  - ■ Conduction of whole blood decreases with increasing cellular elements
- ■ If conjugated bilirubin is higher than unconjugated, it can be hemolysis, Crigler–Najjar, or Gilbert
- ■ B_{12} deficiency
  - ■ Low B_{12}, high homocysteine, high A2

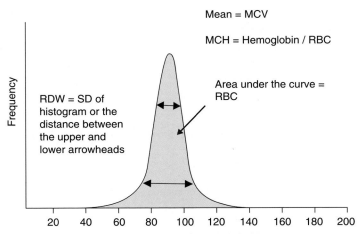

Fig. 21.5 Hemogram values. *MCH*, Mean corpuscular hemoglobin; *MCV*, mean corpuscular volume; *RBC*, red blood cell count; *RDW*, red cell distribution of width; *SD*, standard deviation.

Erythrocyte Inclusions

- Howell–Jolly bodies—nuclear fragments (DNA), seen in asplenia
- Basophilic stippling
  - Fine = unstable RNA in young erythrocyte
  - Course = heavy metal poisoning, decreased hemoglobin synthesis, megaloblastic anemia
- Siderotic granules (Pappenheimer bodies)—irregular, blue, peripheral inclusions. Prussian blue+, iron. Seen in iron overload, some anemias, asplenia
- Cabot rings—thin circular or figure–eight strands; can be seen in association with basophilic stippling; megaloblastic anemia; heavy metal poisoning; asplenia
- Heinz bodies—invisible on Wright–Giemsa; use methylene blue; G6PD deficiency, some thalassemias, unstable hemoglobins, oxidant exposure
  - Usually cleared by splenic macrophages → bite cells and veil cells
- POST-SPLENECTOMY BLOOD PICTURE—siderotic granules, Howell–Jolly bodies, target cells, +/– acanthocytes and fragments, large platelets
  - Loss of reticuloendothelial system's ability to "clean up" blood components

Hemoglobin Genetics

- Alpha globin is encoded on chromosome 16
- Beta and beta–like genes (gamma and delta) encoded on chromosome 11
  - Epsilon is beta–like and zeta is alpha–like embryonic genes, only transcribed first 8 weeks of gestation
  - Delta is not transcribed as well as beta (if beta gene is there and functional, it will predominate)
- All hemoglobin (Hb) variants are tetramers
  - HbA = 2 alpha, 2 beta; 98% of normal people's Hb (>2 years)
  - HbA2 = 2 alpha, 2 delta (2%)
    - Delta is not as stable or efficiently transcribed as beta
  - HbF = 2 alpha, 2 gamma (both have 4 genes!)
    - Gamma has G-gamma and A-gamma, alpha has alpha1 and alpha2
    - Normally only seen in fetuses and babies up to 2 years
    - Elevated in juvenile myelomonocytic leukemia (JMML)

Hemoglobin Electrophoresis

- However, label intensive, requires experience for interpretation, densitometry scanning may be less accurate for small differences in % Hb
- Fast–moving hemoglobin variants
  - Hemoglobin H
    - Loss of three alpha genes
  - Hemoglobin Barts
    - Absence of all four alpha genes—also fast migrating, but fetus dies in utero or shortly after birth
    - Low-to-normal Hb, severe microcytosis and hypochromia
  - Hemoglobin J
    - Not associated with microcytosis or anemia
  - Hemoglobin N—Baltimore trait
    - Beta–chain variant
    - Not associated with microcytosis or anemia
- High–performance liquid chromatography is also used (glycosylation causes interferences, but can measure A_2 down to low percentages)
- Capillary electrophoresis is now the standard of care

- Fully automated, separates and identifies nearly all hemoglobins, accurate measurement of small percentages
- Requires some experience to interpret percentages

Thalassemia

- Inherited decrease or absence of transcription of one or more globin genes
  - Quantitative globin defect → hemolytic anemia
- First microcytic nonanemic, then microcytic anemia
- Iron–deficiency can decrease HA_2—replete before making thalassemia diagnosis
- *Alpha thalassemia*
  - Gamma tetramer = Hb Barts, tells you there is some kind of alpha thalassemia going on at birth!
  - Common in Africans and Asians
  - Four genes (two on each copy of chromosome 16), pathology from DELETIONS
  - *One gene deleted—silent carrier with no symptoms*
    - Alpha thalassemia trait (only *one* gene missing)—silent carrier trait
    - Normal CBC and normal electrophoresis after 1 year of life (no beta–tetramers)
    - Excess gamma, Barts at birth but *not* after 2 to 4 weeks of life
      - Newborn screen is important to catch this for future family planning
  - *Two—most common, "trait" or minor*
    - Alpha thalassemia minor (*two* alpha genes affected)
    - Microcytic nonanemic (at birth), Barts at birth (on newborn screen), normal electrophoresis
    - Cannot really tell one or two genes deleted based on newborn screen
    - Will decrease MCV (72 to 78 fL) with higher RBC count (>6 million cells/μL)—different "normal" range!
    - Sometimes erroneously treated with iron, which can lead to iron overload
    - Can be cis or trans
  - *Three—HbH disease; major*
    - HbH disease or alpha thalassemia major (*three* alpha genes affected)
    - Extra beta tetramers precipitate and form intracellular inclusions, leading to increased extravascular hemolysis in the reticuloendothelial system
    - Microcytic anemia, Barts at birth, HbH (beta tetramer) on electrophoresis
  - *Four—fatal (hydrops fetalis)*
- Beta thalassemia
  - Common in Mediterraneans
  - Two genes (1 on each copy of chromosome 11), pathology from *mutations*
  - *Minor—heterozygote, often asymptomatic; increased HbA2 (>3%), looks like iron deficiency anemia (IDA)*
    - Trait = 1 beta gene deleted (or poorly transcribed—"intermedia")
    - Lifelong mild hemolytic anemia
      - Usually clinically silent
    - Microcytic slight anemia (11 to 11.5 with MCV in mid 60 s) with increased RBCs (6 to 7 million)
      - *Normal newborn screen*, may be microcytic in first few weeks, but fetal Hb compensates; may be jaundiced
    - Increased HbA_2 on adult electrophoresis (ELP; "adult" = older than 6 months of age), sometimes *increased HbF* (delta-delta-alpha-alpha)
      - 5% A_2 (compared with normal 1% to 2%)
      - 2% to 5% HbF (normal is none as adult)

- Increased HbA_2 in beta thalassemia trait, beta thalassemia + hemoglobinopathy *and* double heterozygotes for hemoglobinopathies (e.g., HbSC)
  - Iron and folate therapy (and deficiency?) can suppress delta transcription *(masking thalassemia)*
- Beta0 = absence of beta gene
- Beta+ = impaired/diminished beta globin transcription
  - Beta+ and sickle cell trait → sickling disease
- Delta-beta-thalassemia trait is clinically silent but resembles beta-thalassemia
  - Has microcytosis, elevated F, normal A_2
  - Beta thalassemia has microcytosis, normal F, high A_2
- Major—severe hemolytic anemia, excess alpha precipitates out and damages cell, increased HbF
  - Beta thalassemia major—no HbA on newborn screen, microcytic anemia on CBC (Cooley anemia)
  - Lifelong severe anemia—should be managed by clinical hematologist

Hemoglobinopathy

- Mutation that causes translation of abnormal globin genes (leading to production of a novel/abnormal hemoglobin)
- HbS—African
  - Heterozygous—normal CBC, HbS on ELP; only sickling in exceptional circumstances
    - Normal Hb, NCH, RBC, MCV, RDW
  - Homozygous—sickling disease
    - Sickled red cells (two sharp points at either end, no pallor) with asplenic blood picture
      - Precipitated HbS
      - Irreversibly deformed
      - "Boat cells" are plumper than sickle cells and their deformation is reversible
    - Sickle crisis is a clinical diagnosis, there is no laboratory test
    - Hgb ELP or HPLC
  - Other sickling diseases include one Hb beta-S combined with…
    - Bc, Be, B-null, B+, Bo-Arab
      - Beta-null—abnormal gene that is not expressed or deleted
      - Beta+—reduced but not absent expression of abnormal gene
    - BsBc and BsB-null are bad sickling disease
- HbC—African—mild hemolytic anemia as heterozygote and homozygote
  - Heterozygote usually clinically silent
- HbE—Asian (and all over)—microcytic nonanemic as heterozygote, microcytic anemia as homozygote
  - No A
  - Elutes at A_2 window on HPLC
  - HbEE—numerous codocytes (target cells)

Combinations of Hemoglobinopathies and Thalassemias

- HbC/alpha-thalassemia
  - Microcytosis, lower C than expected (<35%), increased A_2 (3% to 5%)
- HbC/beta-thalassemia
  - Microcytosis, target cells, crystals
  - High C! (>60%, higher than A), elevated A_2 and F
- HbE/beta-thalassemia

- Microcytic hypochromic anemia, ↑ RBC
- Seen in those from Southeast Asia
- HbC/HbS (SC disease)
    - Folded (taco) cells, target cells, boat cells, +/− HbC crystals
    - Hb > 10, MCV minimally decreased

Newborn Screen Patterns

- FAS—sickle trait (rule out beta+/S, which can have clinically variable course)
- FAC—HbC trait (rule out beta+/S)
- FAE—HbE trait (rule out beta+/S)
- FS—sickling disease (rule out beta-null/S)
- FC—HbC disease (rule out beta-null/S)
- FE—HbE disease (rule out beta-null/S)
- FSC—SC disease
- *For all, get an ELP at 1 year to rule out double heterozygosity for beta-plus or beta-null*

Porphyrias

- Inherited or acquired disorders of heme synthesis
- Almost all inherited are autosomal dominant AD
- Those that lead to tetrapyrrole ring accumulation are photosensitive
    - Hereditary coproporphyria—coproporphyrinogen oxidase
    - Erythropoietic protoporphyria—ferrochelatase
        - Pruritic urticarial swelling and redness on sun–exposed skin, unbearable burning sensation, mild microcytic anemia, liver failure
        - Porphyria cutanea tarda—uroporphyrinogen decarboxylase
        - Bullous dermatitis on sun–exposed skin, milia, hypertrichosis
        - Differential diagnosis (DDx) includes pseudoporphyria (photosensitivity secondary to tetracyclines)
    - Congenital (erythropoietic) porphyria—uroporphyrinogen III cosynthase
        - Extremely rare, autosomal recessive
        - Severe blistering and fragility on sun–exposed skin, severe scarring, hemolytic anemia, brown teeth, blindness
- Acute intermediate porphyria is not photosensitive
    - Uroporphyrinogen I synthetase deficiency → buildup of delta-ALA (aminolevulinic acid) and porphobilinogen
    - Neuropsychiatric symptoms and abdominal pain/vomiting
    - Most severe form, female predominance

Hemolysis

- Hepcidin
    - Mechanism of action
    - Regulates the amount of iron that enters the circulation from the gut by degrading the iron channel
        - High hepcidin decreases iron absorption
    - Prevents macrophages in spleen and bone marrow from releasing salvaged Fe to recycle
    - Suppresses erythropoietin production
    - Low hepcidin levels
        - Nutritional iron deficiency
        - Hemochromatosis
            - Mutations in the *HFE* gene cause inappropriately low hepcidin expression → too much iron absorption

- High hepcidin levels
  - Transfusion–induced iron overload
  - Infections
  - Chronic inflammatory states → anemia of chronic disease
    - IL-6 is increased, which triggers the liver to produce more hepcidin

Miscellaneous Nonneoplastic RBCs

- RBCs use glycolysis for energy
  - Embden–Meyerhof pathway (10%) anaerobic
  - Hexose-monophosphate pathway (90%) aerobic, produces antioxidants
    - Glucose-6-phosphate dehydrogenase (G6PD) deficiency (Heinz bodies) and pyruvate kinase deficiency (echinocytes) → hemolysis with oxidant exposure and shortened lifespan, respectively
- Massively burned patient
  - Spherocytosis, fragmentation, and vesiculation
  - Contribute to renal failure
  - Can cause pseudothrombocytosis (small fragments counted as platelets)
  - "Pyro-poikilocytosis"
- Causes of basophilic stippling
  - Defective or accelerated heme synthesis (such as leukoerythroblastic reaction)
  - Thalassemia
  - Lead intoxication
  - Structural hemoglobinopathies
  - Myelodysplasia
  - Severe megaloblastic anemia
  - Congenital erythropoietic anemia

BONE MARROW FAILURE DISORDERS

General

- Severe aplastic anemia is defined as <30% marrow cellularity, no other hematologic malignancy (especially hairy cell leukemia and large granular lymphocytic leukemia), and at least two of the following:
  - Absolute neutrophil count <500
  - Reticulocyte <1%
  - Platelets <20,000
- Long–term survivors are at risk for paroxysmal nocturnal hemoglobinuria (PNH), MDS, and acute myeloid leukemia (AML)
- Single lineage aplasias
  - Red cell aplasia—pure red cell aplasia, transient aplastic crisis (parvovirus), transient erythroblastopenia of childhood (likely infectious but no organism yet discovered), Diamond–Blackfan
  - Granulocyte aplasia—immune mediated >> direct toxicity
    - >90% fatal if untreated
- Megakaryocyte aplasia—amegakaryocytic thrombocytopenic purpura (very, very rare)

Causes

- Inherited
  - Fanconi anemia

- Pancytopenia, hyper- or hypopigmented cutaneous lesions, skeletal defects, short stature, and many other abnormalities have been reported, but 30% have none!
  - Median presentation at 5 to 10 years, but can present as an adult
  - Increased MDS/AML risk (>5000 × the general population), solid tumors
  - Chromosomes break with DEB or mitomycin C
  - Heterogeneous genetics, mostly autosomal dominant, mostly *FANCA* mutations
- Diamond–Blackfan
- Kostmann
- Shwachman–Diamond
  - Autosomal recessive
  - Severe neutropenia, malabsorption, skeletal abnormalities
  - Increased risk for AML and MDS
  - *SBDS* gene mutation in 90%
  - Bone marrow biopsy shows granulocytic hypoplasia and left–shifted myeloids
- Dyskeratosis congenita
- Pearson (ring sideroblasts)
- Secondary
  - Radiation
  - Drugs—e.g., chemotherapy, benzene, chloramphenicol, NSAIDS, antiepileptics, gold
  - Viruses—hepatitis viruses, EBV, parvovirus, HIV
  - Autoimmune—thymoma, eosinophilic fasciitis, hypogammaglobulinemia
  - Pregnancy
  - Paroxysmal nocturnal hemoglobinuria (PNH)
    - Acquired clonal disease that affects males and females, median onset at 40 years
    - GPI glycolipid is abnormal, leading to decreased surface expression of several antigens
      - CD55 (DAF), CD59 (MIRL), CD16, CD14, LAP, folate receptor, urokinase receptor
        - Decreased CD55 and CD59 expression leads to lysis of red cells, activation of platelets, and decreased in vitro colony formation
      - *PIG-A* gene on Xp22.1
      - Binds directly with fluorescein aerolysin (FLAER)
    - Causes intravascular hemolytic anemia with normal RBC morphology
    - Thrombosis in 20% of patients—hepatic and cerebral veins are classic
    - CAN lead to bone marrow failure
      - One-third have previously diagnosed aplastic anemia, one-third will develop it, and one-third will stay purely hemolytic without bone marrow failure
    - Bone marrow biopsy shows hyper- or hypocellularity, dyserythropoiesis (with no dysplasia in megakaryocytes or granulocyte precursors)
- Idiopathic—most common cause, 70% to 80% of all aplastic anemias

MEDICATION/DRUG EFFECTS

- Hydroxyurea
  - Used in myeloperoxidase neoplasms (MPNs), causes neutropenia and anemia with high MCV (megaloblastic features)
  - Acts on ribonucleotide reductase, mimics B_{12}/folate deficiency
- Absolute lymphopenia
  - Steroids (and other meds), zinc deficiency, autoimmune disease, sarcoid, viral infection (HIV), malignancies (including lymphomas)
- Paracortical expansion can happen with phenytoin

- Drug–induced thrombocytopenia: furosemide, tacrolimus, amphotericin, pipercillin/tazobactam
- Drug–induced thrombotic thrombocytopenia (TTP) can be caused by cyclosporine, tacrolimus, clopidogrel, mitomycin C, and gemcitabine
- Levamisole
  - Cutting agent in cocaine
  - Can develop an atypical pANCA and peripheral vasculitis, especially on the ears
  - Can also get agranulocytosis

INFECTIOUS ETIOLOGIES FOR BLOOD SMEAR CHANGES

- Pertussis can cause striking peripheral leukocytosis with abnormal–looking cells.
- *Plasmodium vivax* life cycle: ring form, double ring form, trophozoites, mature schizont, free merozoites, gametocytes
- *Borrelia recurrentis* = relapsing fever, large numbers of many loosely coiled spirochetes
- *Clostridium perfringens* produces a lecithinase that dissolves RBC membrane, looks like hereditary pyropoikilocytosis

REACTIVE LYMPHADENOPATHY

- Immunoblast
  - Intermediate between lymphocyte and plasma cell
  - One prominent nucleoli
  - CD30+
  - Can be B lineage (CD20) or T lineage (CD3)
  - Tend to be ↑ in mononucleosis
- Centroblast
  - Activated B cell
  - CD10+, BCL6+, BCL2–
  - Multiple nucleoli attached to nuclear membrane
- Centrocytes
  - Cleaved, small with compact chromatin
- Secondary follicles have germinal centers (GCs); primary follicles do not
  - Predominantly B cells (some T cells and dendritic cells)
- Post-germinal–center B cells
  - In peripheral blood and marginal zone
  - Pan-B markers +
  - sIgM+, CD5–, CD10–
- Interfollicular space and paracortex—mostly T cells >> plasma cells and histocytes
- Medullary cords— plasma cell (PC) rich
- GROSSING LYMPHOMA SPECIMENS
  - Cut perpendicular to long axis
  - Keep a light touch
  - Cut thin
  - Sit in formalin for a long time
- REASSURING SIGNS OF FOLLICLE CENTERS
  - No extension into fat/capsule
  - Normal architecture
  - Primary and secondary follicles

- Follicles respect each other (intact mantle zones)
- GCs of different sizes and shapes
- Polarized (light side has less mantle zone and more tingible body macrophages)
- Mixture of cells (centrocytes and centroblasts)
- BCL2–, CD10+, BCL6+, high Ki-67
  - BCL2 will be positive in follicular lymphoma, non-GC B cells, and some T cells
- "Follicular hyperplasia. No evidence of lymphoma"

Lots of Follicles

- DDx = FL, MZL, SLL, follicular hyperplasia, other reactive
- Follicular hyperplasia is the most common pattern
  - Nonspecific, usually cannot find out etiology
- SLL has proliferation centers (follicles implies benign)

Lots of plasma Cells

- MALIGNANT—MZL, LPL, plasmacytoma
- REACTIVE
  - Castleman, plasma cell variant (systemic HHV8)
  - Lymph node (LN) involved by nonhematologic malignancy
  - HIV/AIDS
  - Syphilis
  - "Luetic lymphadenopathies" near genitals, primary syphilis, follicular hyperplasia, capsule fibrosis and infiltration by plasma cells, granulomas, +/– vasculitis
  - Use Steiner or IHC or Warthin–Starry
  - Autoimmune— systemic lupus erythematosus (SLE), rheumatoid arthritis (RA), juvenile RA, Sjögren
    - Follicular hyperplasia, neutrophils in sinuses, lots of centrocytes in GC, thickened capsule but not infiltrated by plasma cells

Expanded Sinuses

- Malignant— Langerhans cell histiocytosis (LCH), ALCL, carcinoma, melanoma, sarcoma
  - LCH—Langerhans cells with eosinophils, rarely presents in lymph nodes without bony lesions
- Reactive
  - Sinus histiocytosis +/– histiocytes with included material
    - Niemann–Pick, Gaucher, Whipple, prosthesis/breast implant/replaced joints/tattoos, bacteria, other foreign material
    - Vascular transformation of sinuses—upstream of lymph blockage
  - Rosai–Dorfman
  - Sinus histiocytosis with massive lymphadenopathy
  - Young (~20), male > female
  - Massive bilateral cervical lymphadenopathy + B symptoms (fever, weight loss)
    - May have extranodal involvement in 25% to 40% including skin, upper respiratory tract, soft tissue, bone, salivary, CNS, breast, pancreas
  - Self–limited disease course
    - Lasts 3 to 9 months before spontaneous regression
  - Large histiocytes with round nuclei with dispersed chromatin, prominent nuclei, abundant pale cytoplasm with emperipolesis (of plasma cells and neutrophils)
  - S100+, CD1a–

Reed–Sternberg–like Cells

- Malignant—CHL, dffuse large B cell lymphoma (DLBCL)
- Reactive
  - Viral inclusions
    - Cytomegalovirus (CMV)—monocytoid B cells with abundant cytoplasm with viral inclusions
    - Herpes simple virus (HSV)—viral inclusions
    - Toxoplasma—inclusions
    - Epstein–Barr virus (EBV)
      - Not real inclusions
      - Reactive binucleated immunoblasts (both B and T)
      - Expanding paracortex
      - Early: follicular hyperplasia, monocytoid B cell aggregates, epithelioid histiocytes
      - Late: paracortical expansion, mottled pattern, increased immunoblasts, +/− distended sinuses with monocytoid cells

Granulomas

- Malignant—CHL, other lymphomas, some carcinomas
- Reactive
  - Necrotizing—mycobacterial vs. fungal (AFB-Fite and GMS)
  - Nonnecrotizing—malignant vs. sarcoid
    - Sarcoidosis–compact confluent noncaseating; Hamazaki–Wesenberg bodies (PAS/AFB+)
    - Suppurative—cat scratch (Warthin–Starry, serologies, necrotic), lymphogranuloma venereum, tularemia, *Yersinia*, listeria
    - Eosinophilic—Kimura, drug reaction, parasites, allergy
      - Kimura—florid follicular hyperplasia, acellular proteinaceous debris, Caucasians and Asians, peripheral eosinophilia, head and neck mass

Castleman Disease (See Later)

Monocytoid B Cell Proliferation

- Mantle zone lymphs *not* in the mantle zone
- Larger than background B cells and with irregular nuclear contour
- Nonspecific
- Infection—HIV, CMV, cat–scratch, EBV
- Toxoplasma—monocytoid B cells, follicular hyperplasia, epithelioid histiocytes that encroach on and invade GCs, *no* granulomas

Other Patterns

- Progressive transformation of GCs (PTGC)
  - Macronodules 2 to 3 × GC size made of small lymphs with mantle zone B cell immunophenotype
  - 1 to 2 per LN = normal; all of 1 LN = PTGC
  - Associated with NLPHL (concurrently or subsequently)
  - Expansion of mantle zone lymphs into adjacent sinusoids and germinal centers
  - Mostly B with some T
  - Follicles are 3 to 5 × normal diameter
  - Small, round-to-oval, no atypical features, no invasion into extranodal tissues
  - Within follicles, larger immunoblasts remain (EMA−, BCL6−, no T cell rosette)

- Resemble popcorn cells in NLPHL (EMA+, BCL6+, T cell rosette)
  - Must rule out NLPHL and FL
- Usually occurs in association with reactive follicular hyperplasia; not premalignant
  - Asymptomatic persistent lymphadenopathy
- Dermatopathic lymphadenitis/changes
  - Lymphadenopathy in area draining chronic dermatitis
  - Mottled/moth–eaten at low power
  - Histiocytes/Langerhans cells/dendritic cells containing melanin > iron (in interfollicular paracortex)
  - CD68-PGM1 is more specific
- Toxoplasmic lymphadenitis
  - Follicular hyperplasia, monocytoid B cells, clusters of epithelioid histiocytes in paracortex and GCs, no multinucleated giant cells or granulomas
- Kikuchi disease
  - See below.

HEMATOLYMPHOID MANIFESTATIONS OF SYSTEMIC DISEASE

Systemic Lupus Erythematosus

- SLE lesion
  - Coagulative necrosis (rule out lymphoma and Kikuchi), follicular hyperplasia, neutrophils scant but present, hematoxylin bodies (degenerative nuclear fragments that aggregate together, dark blue)
- LE cell
  - Cytoplasmic inclusion in neutrophil, nucleus of a dead cell with attached antibodies against DNA + histone
  - Seen primarily in SLE

Marrow Trabeculae Changes in Renal Failure

- Incursions of osteoclasts (moth–eaten)
- ↑ Bone turnover, irregular trabeculae
- ↓ Albumin, ↓ ability to bind calcium, ↑ calcium lost in urine → ↑ PTH production
- In multiple myeloma, plasma cells release RANKL and DKK1 which create more osteoclasts and activate them, respectively

Causes of Functional Asplenia

- Infarcts
- Acute graft versus host disease (GVHD)
- Celiac sprue "exacerbation"

INFECTIOUS DISEASE

Babesia

- Sit at periphery of red cell (platelets sit in center)
- Asplenic, may get falsely high automated count as a result of Heinz bodies
- When do count, it is number of parasitized red cells, *not* parasites
  - Example: one RBC with three parasites = 1

HHV-8–Associated Entities

- Castleman
- Primary effusion lymphoma
- Plasmablastic lymphoma
- Infectious mononucleosis (see "EBV-related Diseases" later)

HISTIOCYTIC/FUNCTIONAL DISORDERS

Rosai–Dorfman Disease

- Sinus histiocytosis with massive lymphadenopathy
- Has emperipolesis (other white blood cells travel through histiocyte cytoplasm without being damaged)

Kikuchi Disease

- "Histiocytic necrotizing lymphadenitis"
- Female > male, young, Asian, cervical lymphadenopathy with leukopenia
- Must rule out SLE
- Early proliferating—lots of immunoblasts mixed with large mononuclear cells (including histiocytes with twisted nuclei)
  - Plasmacytoid—CD123+
- Necrotizing—patch paracortical coagulative necrosis, lots of karyorrhectic debris surrounded by mononuclear cells
- Xanthomatous/healing—many foamy histiocytes (CD163+), fewer immunoblasts (CD30+), +/– necrosis
- No neutrophils!

Castleman Disease

- Hyaline–vascular variant—(most common)
  - Usually localized ("unicentric"), broad age range, males and females, some associated with HIV
  - No systemic symptoms, favorable prognosis
  - Morphology
    - Increased follicles of same size scattered throughout the cortex and medulla
    - Lollipop atrophic/sclerotic GCs with vessel
      - With onion–skinning (CD21 highlights)
    - Twinning (one follicle with two GCs)
    - EXPANDING mantle zone, vascular proliferation (hyaline vascular)
    - HHV8–, unicentric (1 to 3 LNs)
    - GCs contain little to no small lymphocytes
    - Increased hyaline deposits
- Plasma cell variant
  - AKA "multicentric," involves multiple lymph node chain, poor prognosis
  - Rarely, multicentric Castleman can have hyaline vascular morphology
  - HIV+, HHV-8+
  - PC hyperplasia *plus* hyaline vascular morphology, systemic symptoms
    - Lymphadenopathy, B symptoms, hepatosplenomegaly (HSM), edema, effusions, rashes, neurological changes
    - Anemia, thrombocytopenia, polyclonal hypergammaglobulinemia, and elevated IL-6 lactate dehydrogenase (LDH), C-reactive protein (CRP), and erythrocyte sedimentation rate (ESR)

- Glomeruloid hemangioma of the skin can occur in patients with multicentric disease and POEMS syndrome (see below)
  - Requires chemotherapy or rituximab!
- Can be associated with paraneoplastic syndrome due to elevated IL-8
- Associated with…
  - Hodgkin lymphoma
  - Vascular stuff
    - Vascular neoplasms—e.g., angiosarcoma, hemangioma
    - Angiomyoid proliferative lesions
    - Angiomatous hamartomas
    - Kaposi sarcoma

Langerhans Cell Histiocytosis

- Elongated oval/reniform nuclei with longitudinal groves, delicate nuclear membrane, clear chromatin, no nucleoli, abundant eosinophilic cytoplasm
  - Indented, notched, lobulated, folded, grooved, coffee bean
- Eosinophils, epidermotropism
- Skull, long bones, organs (spleen, liver, lung), ear, eye
- CD1a and S100+ (CD68+ is variable), langerin+
- Birbeck granules (tennis rackets) on electron microscopy (EM)
- Hand–Schüller–Christian
  - Form of LCH, also called *multifocal unisystem LCH*
  - Infants and children
  - Classic triad: exophthalmos, diabetes insipidus, and lytic skull lesions
  - Additional symptoms: fever, skin eruptions

Hemophagocytic Lymphohistiocytosis (HLH)

- Uncontrolled histiocyte activation and cytokine storm
- Commonly fatal
- Diagnosis (need 5 of 8)
  - Fever
  - Splenomegaly
  - 2 to 3 cytopenias
  - High triglycerides or low fibrinogen
  - Hemophagocytosis on biopsy
  - Low or absent NK-cell activity
  - Ferritin >500
  - Increased soluble CD25 receptor
- Primary
  - Familial—usually caused by a mutation in the NK/T cell cytotoxic pathway (like perforin), autosomal recessive
- Secondary
  - Infection—EBV, histoplasma, other rare infections
  - Malignancy—especially T cell malignancies
    - Most frequent is subcutaneous panniculitis–like T cell lymphoma
- Autoimmunn

OTHER NONNEOPLASTIC DISEASE

Autoimmune Lymphoproliferative Syndrome (ALPS)

- Children; chronic lymphadenopathy, splenomegaly, cytopenias
- Increased risk for B cell lymphomas
- Mutation in death receptor (FAS family) → accumulation of alpha/beta CD4– CD8–T cells
  - \> 1% of lymphs or > 2.5% of CD3+

Neoplastic

MYELOID NEOPLASM OVERVIEW

Ten Rules for Myeloid Maturation

1. Cells become smaller in size
   a. Exception—promyelocytes are larger than myeloblasts; megakaryocytes get larger as they mature until platelets are released
2. N:C ratio decreases
   a. Exception—megakaryocytes get more cytoplasm
3. Nucleus becomes more irregular in shape
   a. Exception—erythroids stay small and round until expelled
4. Nucleus stains more intensely
5. Chromatin becomes more condensed and clumped
6. Parachromatin becomes more distinct
7. Nucleoli disappear
   a. Exception—nucleoli okay in normal mature monocytes
8. Cytoplasm becomes less basophilic (because RNA decreases)
9. Cytoplasm acquires cell line's characteristic color
10. In cells with granules, they appear and increase in number

MYELOPROLIFERATIVE NEOPLASMS

See Fig. 21.6.

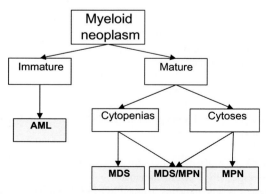

Fig. 21.6 Myeloid neoplasms. *AML*, acute myeloid leukemia; *MDS*, myelodysplastic syndrome; *MPN*, myelo-proliferative neoplasm.

Chronic Myeloid Leukemia (CML)

- Clinical
  - Accounts for 15% to 20% of leukemias
  - Median fifth to sixth decade
  - Often asymptomatic or nonspecific/B symptoms and picked up on routine CBC
  - Most important prognostic marker is response to tyrosine kinase inhibitor (TKI) treatment
  - Others include age, fibrosis extent
    - National Comprehensive Cancer Network (NCCN) guidelines for hematologic, cytogenetic, and molecular responses
    - Also mutation–based therapy
    - Imatinib, nilotinib (more potent), dasatinib (binds active and inactive, resistant to p-loop mutations)
      - Can acquire resistance
        - 50% clonal evolution, 50% *BCR-ABL*-related changes
        - Can be treated by increasing TKI dosage or changing TKI
- Genetics
  - Philadelphia (Ph) chromosome = der(22), caused by t(9;22) that has the *BCR-ABL1*
    - Gene product has cytoplasmic localization
    - 90% will show translocation on G bands, but 10% are cryptic
  - *ABL1-BCR* on chromosome9 (der(9)) not important
  - *BCL* breakpoints
    - P210 is most common (60%) breakpoint in CML
      - Most common in Ph+ ALL
        - 90% of children
        - 60% of adults
      - "Major breakpoint"
    - P190 is second most common breakpoint in ALL, but not common in CML; looks like CMML
      - "Minor breakpoint"
    - P230 is least common, "microbreakpoint"—mature neutrophilia or high platelets in CML (looks like essential thrombocythemia or chronic neutrophilic leukemia—rule out with CG)
      - Called CML-N or CML-increased platelets
  - Causes tyrosine kinase to be auto-phosphorylated and constitutively activated
- Peripheral blood of chronic phase (CP)
  - Myelocyte bulge (infection has more mature granulocytes)
  - Neutrophilia
    - Can be marginally increased or hugely (>200,000)
  - Basophilia
  - Normal monocyte count (except with minor breakpoint) (<3%)
  - +/– Eosinophilia
  - +/– Anemia
  - +/– Thrombocytopenia or thrombocytosis
- Bone marrow of CP
  - Hypercellular with high myeloid-to-erythroid ratio
  - Dwarf megakaryocytes with hypolobation
  - Pseudo-Gaucher cells, sea-blue histiocytes
  - Fibrosis
    - May be a poor prognostic marker

- Accelerated phase (AP)
  - Unresponsive to treatment *and*
    - Persistent high WBC (>10)
    - Splenomegaly
    - Persistent high platelets (>1000)
    - Persistent low platelets (<100)
  - Clonal cytogenetic evolution
    - +8, +Ph, iso(17q), +19, complex, 3q26.2 abnormalities—consistent with accelerated phase
    - –Y, +21, +17, –7—if absent at diagnosis but present later, consistent with evolution
  - 10% to 19% blasts in bone marrow (BM)/peripheral blood (PB)
  - PB basophils >20%
  - Myelodysplasia, clusters/sheets of megakaryocytes, fibrosis
- Blast phase (BP)—meets criteria for AML, myeloid sarcoma, or ALL
  - More rarely, megakaryocytic or erythroid leukemia
  - Large focus of blasts on bone marrow biopsy is enough
  - 70% AML (through AP) and 20% to 30% ALL (mostly B-lymphoblasts, develop abruptly from CP)
    - Up to 25% can have mixed phenotype

Polycythemia Vera (PV)

- Large megakaryocytes
- Prepolycythemic phase → polycythemic → spent phase
  - Cannot diagnose spent phase without previous diagnosis of PV, no longer requiring phlebotomy
    - Looks exactly like primary myelofibrosis (PMF) with leukoerythroblastic reaction (LEBR)
- Need both major criteria or 1st major plus any 2 minor
  - Major criteria
    - Increased hemoglobin (>18.5 g/dL in male, >16/5 g/dL in female)
      - Normochromic, normocytic
    - *JAK2* V617F mutation (85% to 97%)
      - Or functionally similar, like *JAK2* exon 12
  - Minor criteria
    - Bone marrow biopsy showing hypercellularity for age with trilineage growth (panmyelosis)
    - Serum erythropoieitin level below the reference range for normal
    - Endogenous erythroid colony (EEC) formation in vivo
- Low risk for transformation, increased with chemotherapy treatment
  - Do not treat!!
- Do not give iron → can precipitate thrombosis
- Other symptoms: bleeding *or* clotting, pruritus, erythromelalgia, gout, hepatosplenomegaly

Other Erythroid MPNs

- Acute erythroleukemia (both erythroid and myeloid lines) is now called *MDS with erythroid hyperplasia*
- Pure erythroid leukemia
  - CD117+, CD34–, CD71+, e-cad+, glycophorin+, Hb+
  - Karyotype: complex (–7, –5, –17)

Primary Myelofibrosis (PMF)

- Large megakaryocytes
  - Tight clusters
  - Cloud–like nuclei
- Prefibrotic → fibrotic
  - Fibrotic phase—often osteomyelosclerosis, dacryocytes
    - New WHO recommendation for collagen stain (such as trichrome, positive in grade 3 fibrosis)
- Rule out essential thrombocythemia (ET) in prefibrotic phase
  - PMF has increased proliferation in other cell lines (in addition to megakaryocytes, usually granulocytic hyperplasia) and LEBR in peripheral blood; ET only has increased megakaryocytes
- Rule out secondary fibrosis (e.g., radiation, chemotherapy)
- 5% to 30% risk for transformation to acute leukemia
- Megakaryocytes in sinusoids and naked megakaryocyte nuclei
- Need all 3 major and 2 minor
  - Major criteria
    - Megakaryocyte proliferation and atypia with either reticulin and/ or collagen fibrosis
      - Or if negative, megakaryocyte changes with increased marrow cellularity 2/2 increased granulopoiesis and decreased erythropoiesis (like in prefibrotic cellular phase)
    - Not meeting criteria for PV, CML, MDS, or other myeloid neoplasm
    - *JAK2* V617F (50%), *MPL* W515K/L (thrombopoietin receptor), or calreticulin (*CAL-R*)
      - All increase JAK-STAT pathway signaling
      - OR if negative, no evidence that findings are secondary to other causes
  - Minor criteria
    - LEBR
    - Increase in serum LDH
    - Anemia
    - Splenomegaly

Essential Thrombocythemia (ET)

- Large megakaryocytes
  - Loose clusters
  - Staghorn nuclei
- Lower risk for acute leukemia (<5% risk)
- Fibrosis is rare (usually grade 0 to 1)
- Usually only increased megakaryocytes/platelets, no leukoerythroblastic reaction (LEBR/ leukemoid reaction)
- Prefibrotic → fibrotic
  - Takes one to two decades to get end–stage fibrosis (slower than PML)
- Need all four criteria
  - Sustained platelet count ≥450
  - Bone marrow biopsy showing proliferation of mainly megakaryocytes with increased numbers of enlarged, mature megakaryocytes. No significant increase or left–shift of granulopoiesis or erythropoiesis
  - Not meeting criteria for PV, PMF, CML, MDS, or other myeloid neoplasm
  - + *JAK2* V617F (50% to 60%) or other clonal marker (*MPL, CAL-R*)

- OR if negative, no evidence of reactive thrombocytosis (iron deficiency, splenectomy, surgery, infection, inflammation, connective tissue disease, metastatic cancer, lympho-proliferative disease)

Chronic Neutrophilic Leukemia (CNL)

- Rare, neutrophilia with *minimal* left–shift, hepatosplenomegaly
  - $>25 \times 10^9/L$, 80% of WBCs are neutrophils
- Hypercellular marrow only caused by neutrophilia
  - No dysplasia, BM blasts <5%, PB immature granulocytes <10%
- *CSF3R* (T618I) mutation
- Must rule out other diseases including plasma cell neoplasms (PCNs)
  - 2% of CNL cases have underlying PCNs, it is unclear whether CNL is the primary malignancy or is secondary to cytokines

Chronic Eosinophilic Leukemia, Not Otherwise Specified (CEL)

- Eosinophilia (≥1.5)
- No other disease, especially AML with inv(16)
- Blasts <20%
- Clonal/molecular evidence of clonality *or* blasts >2% in PB or >5% in BM (implied clonality)
- If last point cannot be proven → "hypereosinophilic syndrome"
  - Usually a syndrome secondary to other disease
  - Lymphocytic variant of hypereosinophilic syndrome
    - Eosinophilia driven by abnormal T cell clone
    - T-cell immunophenotype is abnormal but not enough for a pripheral T cell lym-phoma (PTCL) diagnosis

Myeloproliferative Neoplasm, Unclassifiable

MYELOID AND LYMPHOID NEOPLASMS WITH EOSINOPHILIA AND GENE REARRANGEMENT

- Secondary to a rearrangement in a pluripotent stem cell
- Can lead to myeloid or lymphoid neoplasms
- Consider especially when patient has eosinophilia
- FISH for *PDGFRA* (karyotype for others)
  - *PDGFRA* cannot be seen on routine G-banding/karyotype
- *PDGFRA*
  - CEL > AML, T-ALL, MPAL (T and myeloid)
  - With *FIP1L1* on 4q12 (*CHIC2* deletion bringing them together)
  - Sensitive to TKIs
  - Increased mast cells and increased serum tryptase
- *PDGFRB*
  - Looks like CMML > aCML > CEL
  - t(5;12) *ETV6-PDGFRB*
  - Sensitive to TKIs
- *FGFR1*
  - T-lymphoblastic lymphoma (T-LBL > AML)
  - 8p11 translocation with multiple partners
  - 90% have eosinophilia, tissue-based leukemia, and BM with MPN
  - Poor prognosis—resistant to TKIs

- *PCM1-JAK2*
  - New in 2016
  - Mimics PMF or ALL (B or T)
  - Eosinophilia with lymphoid aggregates
  - t(8;9) *PCM1-JAK2*
  - Treat with JAK2 inhibition
- Report as: [MPN/leukemia/lymphoma] with [mutated gene]/[specific entity]
  - Example: leukemia with *PDGFRA*/chronic myelomonocytic leukemia

MASTOCYTOSIS

- Abnormal mast cells (MCs) can be hypogranular, atypical nuclear forms, spindled
- *KIT* D816V mutation can treat with TKIs
- B findings—"Burden of disease"
  - High mast cell burden (>30% on bone marrow biopsy and serum tryptase > 200 ng/mL)
  - Signs of dysplasia of non-mast cell lineages (but no criteria met)
  - Hepatomegaly without impairment of function
  - Splenomegaly without hypersplenism
  - Lymphadenopathy
- C findings—"cytoreduction–requiring"
  - Bone marrow dysfunction caused by mast cell infiltration
    - At least one cytopenia
  - Hepatomegaly with impairment of function, ascites, and/or portal hypertension
  - Osteolytic lesions with or without pathologic fractures
  - Palpable splenomegaly with hypersplenism
  - Malabsorption with weight loss caused by GI mast cell infiltrates

Cutaneous Mastocytosis

- Urticaria pigmentosa (maculopapular cutaneous mastocytosis)
  - Multiple pigmented lesions in a child
  - Darier sign
- Diffuse cutaneous mastocytosis
- Mastocytoma of skin

Systemic Mastocytosis

- Indolent mastocytosis
  - Meets criteria for systemic mastocytosis
  - No "C findings"
  - No associated hematologic neoplasm
  - Low mast cell burden
  - Skin lesions
- Smoldering systemic mastocytosis
  - Meets criteria for SM
  - ≥ B findings; No "C findings"
  - No AHN
  - High mast cell burden
  - Does not meet criteria for mast cell leukemia
- Systemic mastocytosis with associated hematologic neoplasm
  - Meets criteria for SM
  - Also meets criteria for MDS, MPN, AML, lymphoma, or other distinct entity
    - CMML is most common (cannot use serum tryptase criterion)

- Aggressive systemic mastocytosis
  - Meets criteria for SM
  - ≥ 1 C finding
  - Does not meet criteria for mast cell leukemia
  - Usually no skin lesions
- Mast cell leukemia
  - Meets criteria for SM
  - Bone marrow biopsy: diffuse infiltrate of atypical immature mast cells
- Aspirates: $\geq 20\%$ mast cells
  - Classic: $\geq 10\%$ mast cells in peripheral blood
    - Aleukemic variant is *more* common ($<10\%$ in PB)
  - Usually no skin lesions
- Bone marrow mastocytosis
  - (The default one when other criteria are not met)
- Requires the major criterion and 1 minor or ≥ 3 minor criteria
  - MAJOR
    - Multifocal, dense infiltrates of mast cells (≥ 15 mast cells in aggregates) in bone marrow or extracutaneous organ (ECO) sections
  - MINOR
  - In BM or ECO sections, $>25\%$ of mast cells are spindled or atypical
    - *Or* in BM aspirate smear, $>25\%$ of MCs are immature/atypical
  - Activating point mutation at codon 816 of *KIT* in BM, blood, or ECO
  - Mast cells in BM, blood, or ECO = CD2+ +/− CD25+
    - In addition to normal mast cell markers (CCD117, IgE, CD203c, mast cell tryptase)
  - Serum tryptase persistently $>20\,\text{ng/mL}$
    - *Without* associated myeloid neoplasm
    - Sidebar: beta-tryptase is released in anaphylaxis and can be useful in forensics

Mast Cell Sarcoma

MYELODYSPLASTIC SYNDROMES

General

- Ineffective hematopoiesis (cytopenias) with hypercellular marrow caused by increased apoptosis from genetic abnormalities
  - Hb <10, ANC <1.8, platelets <100
  - Disorganized hematopoiesis
  - Immature myeloids away from trabeculae
    - Abnormal localization of immature precursors (ALIP)—associated with poorer prognosis even in low–grade MDS
      - Normal = least mature next to trabeculae, and more mature further out
  - Erythroids do not form clusters/islands
  - Megakaryocytes do cluster
- Features of dyspoiesis in each cell line composing $\geq 10\%$ of line
  - Dysgranulopoiesis
    - Hypogranular to agranular cytoplasm
    - Small size
    - Hyposegmentation (pseudo-Pelger–Huet) or hypersegmentation (less commonly), abnormal shapes
    - Abnormal chromatin (block clumping and/or nuclear projections/"sticks")

- Coalescing salmon granules without purple granules, uneven granulation
  - *Mimics:* drugs (trimethoprim/sulfamethoxazole → nonlobulated nucleus)
- Dyserythropoiesis
  - Irregular nuclear contours
  - Nuclear budding
  - Bridging
  - Karyorrhexis
  - Megaloblastoid changes (nuclear-to-cytoplasmic dyssynchrony)
  - Ring sideroblasts—≥5 iron particles and ≥ one-third of nuclear circumference
  - PAS+ coalescing vacuoles in pronormoblasts
    - *Not* seen in vitamin B_{12}/folate deficiency—useful in differential diagnosis
  - *Mimics:* zinc toxicity → copper deficiency, lead poisoning, alcohol, isoniazid
- Dysmegakaryopoiesis
  - Hypolobulated or nonlobulated nucleus
  - Micromegakaryocytes
  - Multiple widely separated nuclear lobes (true multinucleation)
- Children with MDS, think Fanconi anemia (they frequently develop MDS)
- Organomegaly not uncommon (but raises possibility of MDS/MPN or MPN)
- Genetics
  - Cytogenetics
    - G bands—used in prognostication (IPSS-R, Greenberg et al, 2012, Blood)
    - FISH (lower yield)
    - 50% have a normal karyotype
  - Molecular
    - *SF3B1* mutation can help diagnose MDS with ring sideroblasts (favorable prognosis)
  - 50% have normal karyotype
  - MDS-defining aberrations: *del(5q) or -7*
    - –Y, +8, or del(20q) as sole abnormality is not diagnostic without morphology
  - Prognostication
    - Favorable prognosis: normal karyotype, –Y, del(5q), del(20q)
    - Poor prognosis: chromosome 7 abnormalities, complex karyotypes
    - Intermediate prognosis: not fitting "good" or "poor" criteria
- Exposures that increase risk: benzene, agricultural solvents, cigarettes
- Role of flow cytometry in MDS
  - Quantify blasts
  - Determine abnormal immunophenotype on blasts
  - ↓ side scatter on granulocytes
  - Ogata criteria (scoring system)
- PITFALL: avoid MDS diagnosis if secondary cause is present
  - Drugs/toxins—chemotherapy, radiation, heavy metals, arsenic, alcoholism
  - Deficiencies of vitamin B_{12}, copper, folate
  - AIDS, autoimmune
  - Neoplasms (hematologic or solid tumor)

MDS with Single–Lineage Dysplasia (MDS-SLD)

- Formerly refractory cytopenia with unilineage dysplasia (RCUD)
  - The cytopenia does not have to be in the same lineage as dysplastic cells!
- Low risk for transformation
- Refractory anemia, refractory neutropenia, refractory thrombocytopenia
- PB: unicytopenia > bicytopenia, <1% blasts (if pancytopenic—MDS-U)
  - Hb <10, ANC <1.8, platelets <100

- ≥10% dysplastic cells in one myeloid lineage, <5% blasts, <15% of erythroid precursors are ring sideroblasts

MDS with Ring Sideroblasts and Single–Lineage Dysplasia (MDS-RS-SLD)

- Formerly RARS (refractory anemia with ring sideroblasts)
- Low risk for transformation
- PB: anemia, no blasts
    - Can get dimorphic RBC population—normochromic normocytic and hypochromic macrocytic
- BM: ≥15% of erythroid precursors are ring sideroblasts, single–lineage dysplasia only, <5% blasts
    - Only need ≥5% ring sideroblasts if *SF3B1* mutation is present
- *MDS-RS-T* = RARS plus thrombocytosis and *JAK2* mutation

MDS with Multilineage Dysplasia (MDS-MLD)

- RCMD (refractory cytopenia with multilineage dysplasia)
- 10% transform to AML
- Median survival = 20 months
- PB: cytopenia(s), <1% blasts, no Auer rods, <1 × 10⁹/L monocytes
    - Must exclude CMML
- BM: dysplasia in ≥10% in ≥2 myeloid lineages, 5% blasts, no Auer rods
- *MDS-MLD-RS* = RCMD + ≥15% ring sideroblasts

MDS with Excess Blasts-1 (MDS-EB-1)

- RAEB-1 (refractory anemia with excess blasts-1)
- 25% transform to AML
- PB: cytopenia(s), 2% to 4% blasts, no Auer rods, <1 × 10⁹/L monocytes
- BM: uni- or multilineage dysplasia, 5% to 9% blasts, no Auer rods

MDS with Excess Blasts-2 (MDS-EB-2)

- RAEB-2 (refractory anemia with excess blasts-2)
- Highest risk for transformation to AML (33%)
- 9-month survival
- PB: cytopenia(s), 5% to 19% blasts, no Auer rods, <1 × 10⁹/L monocytes
- BM: uni- or multilineage dysplasia, 10% to 19% blasts, +/− Auer rods
- **Any cases with Auer rods and <20% blast = RAEB-2

MDS Associated with Isolated Del(5q)

- Female, favorable prognosis, good response to lenalidomide
- Survival >5 years
- Isolated del(5q)
    - Can (oddly) have one other cytogenetic abnormality that is *not* monosomy 7 or del(7q)
- PITFALL: MPN and MDS/MPN may have del(5q) and thrombocytosis → check megakaryocyte morphology
- PB: anemia, normal or increased platelets, <5% blasts
    - Often macrocytic
- BM: normal or ↑ megakaryocytes with hypolobated nuclei, ↓ erythroids, <5% blasts, no Auer rods

Myelodysplastic Syndrome, Unclassifiable (MDS-U)

- Several possibilities

- PB: cytopenia(s), ≤1% blasts, dysplasia in <10% in ≥1 myeloid lineages + MDS-defining cytogenetic abnormality
- Pancytopenia with only one dysplastic lineage
- Clonal cytogenetic abnormality and no dysplasia
- Exactly 1% blood blasts and <5% marrow blasts

Therapy–Related Myeloid Neoplasms

- No strict blast count (see section below)

Refractory cytopenia of childhood

- Prominent dyserythropoiesis and dysmegakaryopoiesis, slightly increased blasts
- Monosomy 7
- Must work up for Fanconi anemia!

MYELODYSPLASTIC/MYELOPROLIFERATIVE NEOPLASMS

Chronic Myelomonocytic Leukemia (CMML)

- Persistent monocytosis—>1,000 (can be within normal range) and ≥10% of WBCs
- No Ph chromosome, no *BCR-ABL1*, no *PDGFRA/B*
- < 20% blasts
  - CMML 0, 1, or 2 (based on blast count, which includes promonocytes)
- *With* dysplasia and acquired clonal cytogenetic changes *or* present for >3 months
  - *ASXL1, SETBP1, SRSF2, TET*
- Characteristically has nodules of CD123+ mature plasmacytoid dendritic cells in bone marrow

Atypical CML

- Leukocytosis (>13,000) with left–shifted neutrophilia
- Dysgranulopoiesis
- No Ph chromosome/*BCR-ABL1*
- No basophilia, no monocytosis (<1,000)
- <20% blasts
- Hypercellular marrow with increased grans
- *CSF3R* mutation (receptor for G-CSF) (like CNL)
- *SETBP1* mutation in ~ one-third

Juvenile Myelomonocytic Leukemia (JMML)

- See JMML symposium guidelines, Atlanta, GA, 2008.
- Splenomegaly, no *BCR-ABL1*, >1000 monos, <20% blasts, mutation (*RAS, PTPNI1, NF1,* monosomy 7)
- Juvenile xanthogranulomas

Myelodysplastic Syndrome/Myeloproliferative Neoplasm with Ring Sideroblasts and Thrombocytosis (MDS/MPN-RS-T)

- No longer provisional
- Dysplasia (typically erythrodysplasia, ≥15% ring sideroblasts, and thrombocytosis (>450,000)
- Large and lobulated megakaryocytes
- Frequent *JAK2* mutation (rarely *MPL*)

MDS/MPN-U

- Sufficient material, but does not fit any category

Bonus point: Splanchnic vein thrombosis patients have an increased risk for *JAK2* mutation. Some have MPN, some will develop one, and some never will

ACUTE MYELOID LEUKEMIA

General

- Two-hit hypothesis
  - It cannot differentiate past myeloblast
  - Primitive cells self–replicate
- Definition—>20% blasts in BM or PB *or* if they have certain genetic abnormalities *or* if they have a myeloid sarcoma
  - Blasts should be positive for MPO, NSE, or have an Auer rod
- Prognosis in general
  - Poor with *FLT3* mutation

AML with Recurrent Genetic Abnormalities

- General
  - By FISH, conventional karyotyping, or PCR
  - Do not need >20% blasts!
  - 50% to 60% of cells must have karyotypic abnormality
- *RUNX1/RUN1T1*, t(8;21)(q22;q22)
  - Core–binding factor
  - Morphology
    - Salmon–colored granules (less commonly azurophilic)
    - Perinuclear hof
    - Chediak–Higashi granules (chunky, shiny)
      - "RUNX has rocks"
    - Long slender Auer rods
    - *Dysgranulopoiesis* (homogenous pink cytoplasm and pseudo-Pelger–Hüet)
      - No dyserythropoiesis or dysmegakaryopoiesis
  - Immunophenotype
    - bright CD34, HLA-DR, MPO, and CD13
    - dim B cell markers (CD19, CD79a, PAX-5+), dim CD33
    - +/– CD15
  - Secondary abnormalities
    - *c-Kit* mutation
      - Poor prognosis
      - Associated with CD56 and CD117 expression
    - –X, –Y, del(9q), *KRAS/NRAS* mutations, *ASXL2* mutations
- Acute promyelocytic leukemia (APL)
  - *PML-RARA* t(15;17)(q22;q12)
    - Variants (from common to rare), all resistant to tretinoin
      - t(11;17)—*ZBTB16-RARA*—regular nuclei, hypergranulated, rare Auer rods, pel-geroid neutrophils, MPO++
      - t(11;17)—*NUMA1-RARA*

- t(5;17)—*NPM1-RARA*—major population is hypergranular, minor population is hypogranular, no Auer rods
  - t(17;17)—*STAT5B-RARA*
- Abnormal promyelocytes with reniform or bilobed nucleus, abundant azurophilic primary granules, and abundant Auer rods
- Favorable prognosis, treated with all-trans retinoic acid (tretinoin) and arsenic
  - Risk for DIC, leukopenia
- CD34–, HLA-DR–, CD64+, CD117+, CD33 bright, high side scatter (merges with granulocyte gate), heterogeneous CD13+, CD11b+
  - CD2 expression associated with *FLT3*-ITD
- Hypo-/microgranular variant
  - May have Auer rods
  - Will have butterfly nucleus
  - Leukocytosis
  - CD34+, HLA-DR+
- Inv(16) or t(16;16)(q22;p13.1)—*CBFB-MYH1*
  - Myelomonocytic blasts
    - May have multiple blast populations
  - Hypereosinophilia with red and blue granules (harlequin eosinophils), very high WBC
  - Core–binding factor
  - Aberrant CD2+, bright CD34, CD117
  - Favorable prognosis, especially with cytarabine
  - Secondary abnormalities:
    - Trisomy 22 (favorable prognosis, characteristic!), trisomy 21, gains in 22 (favorable prognosis), gains 8 (poor prognosis), del(7q)
    - *KIT* mutations (poor prognosis, but not as drastic as *RUNX* translocated AML with *KIT* mutation), *NRAS* mutation, *FLT3*-ITD (poor prognosis), no *ASXL2* mutations
- t(9;11)—*KMT2A-MLLT3*
  - Myelomonocytic or monocytic blasts
  - Can present with myeloid sarcoma or gingival infiltration
  - Abnormalities with *KMT2A* (11q23) also seen in
    - Therapy–related myeloid neoplasms, specifically after topoisomerase II inhibitors
    - Infantile subset of B-ALL
  - Variant rearrangement partners—*KMT2A* with *AFF1* (previously *MLLT2*) or *MLLT1*
  - CD34–, CD64+, CD4+, CD11b+, CD33+, HLA-DR+, CD13 dim or negative
    - CD14 tends to be negative in children and positive in adults
  - Poor prognosis
    - Intermediate prognosis if no *c-KIT* mutation
  - Secondary abnormalities: +8, *MECOM* overexpression
- Inv(3) or t(3;3)—*GATA-MECOM*
  - De novo or from MDS
  - Thrombocytosis, megakaryocytic dysplasia and hyperplasia
  - CD38+, CD7+, CD61 +/–
  - Secondary abnormalities: monosomy 7, del(5q)
  - Aggressive
- t(6;9)—*DEK-NUP214*
  - Low leukocytosis (~12,000), basophilia, dysplasia
  - Sole abnormality

- Young, <2 years of age
- Looks like AML with maturation or myelomonocytic blasts
- Poor prognosis
- t(1;22)—*RBM15-MKL1*
  - Myelofibrosis (cause dry taps), hepatosplenomegaly
  - Sole abnormality
  - Infants <18 months
  - Most common in patients without tri(21)
  - Megakaryocytic differentiation (CD61+), CD34–
  - Poor prognosis
- Provisional: AML with t(8;22) *BCR-ABL1*
  - Poor prognosis
  - No specific morphology

AML with Myelodysplasia–Related Changes

- Poor prognosis
- >20% blasts with one of the following
  - Personal history of MDS or MDS/MPN
  - MDS-related cytogenetics
    - Del(7q), –7, del(5q), –5, i(17q), t(17p), –13, del(13q), del(11q), del(12p), t(12p), del(9q), idic(x)(q13)
      - Should be MPO+
      - Balanced translocation: 11/16, 3/21, 1/3, 2/11, 5/12, 5/7, 5/17, 5/10, 3/5
  - Multilineage dysplasia
- And with no history of cytotoxic therapy or recurrent cytogenetic abnormalities!

Therapy–Related Myeloid Neoplasm

- Poor prognosis
- Can be MDS or AML in morphology
- Etiologies
- Topoisomerase II inhibitors
  - Daunorubicin, doxorubicin, epirubicin, etoposide, teniposide, amsacrine, mitoxantrone
  - AML > MDS
  - t(11q23.3) (*KMT2A* rearrangements), t(21q22.1)
  - Compose about 30%
  - 2- to 3-year latency
- Alkylating agents
  - Bendamustine, busulfan, chlorambucil, cyclophosphamide, melphalan, mitomycin C, nitrogen mustard, procarbazine, cisplatin, carboplatin, azathioprine, fludarabine, carmustine, lomustine, thiotepa
  - MDS > AML
  - Del(5q), monosomy 7, del(7q), del(17p)
  - Compose about 70%
  - 5- to 7-year latency
- Radiation
- 5 to 9 years

Myeloid Sarcoma

- Extramedullary AML with blasts replacing normal tissue and forming a mass
- Skin, CNS, testicles, female reproductive tract
- CD45 +/–, CD117, MPO, lysozyme
- Can occur before or after diagnosis of AML

AML-NOS

- Does not meet criteria for any other category but has >20% blasts
- No recurrent genetic abnormalities
  - Trisomy 8 associated with monocytosis
- Not arising in a setting of previous MDS or after cytotoxic therapy (see "Therapy–Related Myeloid Neoplasm")
- Characterized by degree of differentiation, usually recapitulating M0, M1, or M2
  - Old classification system—less commonly used in diagnosis now
    - M0—minimally differentiated
      - Can lack myeloperoxidase expression
    - M1—without maturation
    - M2—with maturation, most commonly seen with t(8;21), favorable prognosis
    - M3—promyelocytic, virtually always seen with t(15;17), favorable prognosis
    - M4—myelomonocytic (inv(16), favorable prognosis, 11q23 translocation, poor prognosis
    - M5—monocytic or monoblastic, 11q23 translocation, poor prognosis
    - M6—erythroblastic differentiation
    - M7—megakaryoblastic differentiation
- *FLT3*
  - Point mutation of activating loop domain is most common
  - Internal tandem duplication (ITD) → poor prognosis
- *NPM1* mutation
  - Favorable prognosis, but only important in a normal karyotype
    - If *FLT3*-ITD is present, intermediate prognosis
  - Myelomonocytic or monocytic blasts
  - Fishmouth/nuclear cup
  - Extramedullary disease, multilineage dysplasia
  - CD34–, HLA-DR–, CD56+, CD117+ (similar to APL)
- Provisional entity: AML with *RUNX1* mutation
  - Some have germline mutations
  - Thrombocytopenias and abnormal platelet function
  - Poor prognosis, especially with *ASXL1* comutation
- Biallelic *CEBPA* mutations
  - Young adults, may be germline
  - CD7+, HLA-DR+, CD56–, CD15+
  - Typically favorable prognosis
  - FLT3-ITD in about 25%, associated with intermediate prognosis
- Monocytic differentiation (M4 and M5)
  - Bright CD64+, CD11c+, HLA-DR+, lysozyme+, CD163+, CD68+ (PGM1 is better for monos than KP-1), dim CD4+, CD36+, NSE+, CD14+/–, cd34–, MPO– (may be weakly positive in promonocytes), CD117–

- Often CD56+ and CD7+
- *KMT2A* translocation, *NPM1* or *CEPBA* mutations, inv(16), t(8;16)
- M4—acute myelomonocytic leukemia (can have more granulocytes than monocytes)
- M5—acute monocytic and monoblastic leukemia (need ≥80% monocytic)
- If ≥80% are blasts = AML
- See Fig. 21.7.

Other

- Transient abnormal myelopoiesis (TAM) in Down syndrome
  - May persist to AML associated with Down syndrome, or may spontaneously regress
  - Abnormal myeloid blasts in peripheral blood
  - Megakaryoblastic differentiation (CD61+, CD41a+)
  - Associated with *GATA1* mutation
- See Table 21.3.

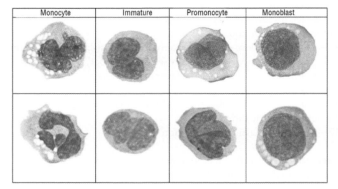

Fig. 21.7 Acute myeloid leukemia with monocytic or monoblastic differentiation can be challenging. Monoblasts and promonocytes are blast equivalents. The bottom-left cell is a monoblast with rounded nuclear contours and multiple prominent nucleoli. The cell on the right is likely a promonocyte with a delicately folded nucleus with tissue paper-like chromatin. *From: Arber DA*. Chapter 46: *Acute myeloid leukemia. In Jaffe ES, Arber DA, Campo E, et al (eds): Hematopathology, 2nd ed. Elsevier, 2017: 817–845.e11.*

TABLE 21.3 ■ **Clues to Acute Leukemia Lineage**

	AML	ALL
Blast size	Large, uniform	Small to intermediate, variable
Chromatin	Fine, dispersed	Coarse
Nucleoli	1–4, may be prominent	0 or 1–2, indistinct
Cytoplasm	Abundant	Scant
Granules	Often	Rarely
Auer rods	~ two-thirds	Never
Myelodysplasia	Often	Never (unless concurrent myeloid neoplasm)

AML, Acute myeloid leukemia; *ALL*, acute lymphoblastic leukemia.

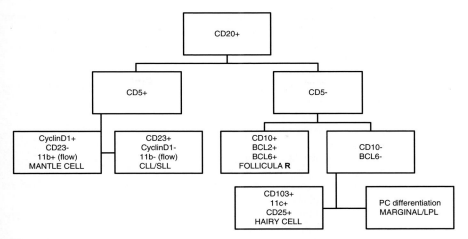

Fig. 21.8 Small B cell lymphoma diagnostic algorithm. *CLL/SLL*, Chronic lymphocytic leukemia/small lymphocytic lymphoma; *LPL*, lymphoplasmacytic lymphoma.

CHRONIC B CELL LYMPHOPROLIFERATIVE NEOPLASMS

General

- See Fig. 21.8.
- Older patients are more likely to have involved marrow
- B cell maturation
  - Precursor B cells—B-ALL (dim CD45, no surface immunoglobulin, CD34, TdT, no surface CD20, morphology)
    - No rearrangement of immunoglobulin
  - Pre–germinal–center (GC) B cells—mantle cell
  - GC B cells—FL, BL, DLBCL (some), Hodgkin
  - Post-GC B cells—MZL (MALT), LPL, CLL/SLL, DLBCL (some), plasma cell neoplasms (MUM1 [IRF4], cytoplasmic Ig, no CD20 or PAX5, CD138 and bright CD38)
    - Activated B cell phenotype
  - Splenic MZL centroblast–like cells = para-immunoblasts

Chronic Lymphocytic Leukemia/Small Lymphocytic Lymphoma (CLL/SLL)

- General
  - Most common leukemia
  - WBC <5,000 of clone
  - Richter transformation = CLL/SLL → DLBCL
- Clinical
  - Can have hypogammaglobulinemia or M spike (IGM), rarely autoimmune hemolysis
- Morphology
  - Snicker doodle cookie or soccer ball–like clumped chromatin
  - Monotonous with some prolymphocytes (2 × normal lymph size with central nucleoli)
    - If >55% prolymphocytes → PLL

- Lymph nodes can have "proliferation centers"—slightly lighter areas with more prolymphocytes
- BM pattern: interstitial, nodular, mixed, diffuse
- Immunophenotype
  - Positive for: 19 dim, 22, 20 dim, sIg dim, 5, 43, 23
  - Negative for: FMC7, 79b, 10, 39 variable (+ = bad prog), cyclin D1 (dim in prolif centers)
  - LEF1 expression is almost pathognomonic for CLL/SLL
- Genetics
  - Rearrangements involving 13q, 11q, 12q, 17p, 6q (in decreasing frequency)
- Genetics and prognosis
  - Immunoglobulin variable heavy chain (*IGHV*) somatic hypermutation
    - Hypermutation present = better prognosis, more mature clone
    - Unmutated clones tend to have CD49d and CD38 expression, therefore these are poor prognostic markers
      - ZAP70 was used for the same reason, but has since decreased in popularity because of quick breakdown in samples
      - Cutoff = 30% positivity
- Poor prognosis
  - Del(17p) involving *TP53*
  - *TP53* mutations
    - Associated with fludarabine resistance and high–risk disease
  - Del(11q22) involving *ATM*
  - *NOTCH1* mutations
  - Unmutated immunoglobulin heavy chain
    - Associated with CD38 and CD49d expression
  - *SF3B1* mutations
    - Associated with 11q22 deletions, fludarabine resistance, faster progression, and poor overall survival
- Intermediate prognosis
  - Trisomy 12
- Favorable prognosis:
  - *BIRC3* mutations
  - 13q deletions

Monoclonal B cell Lymphocytosis (MBLs)
- Precursor to CLL, 5% of older adults have it
- Like CLL but WBC $<5 \times 10^9$/L
- Separated into groups based on immunophenotype (IP)
  - CLL—CD5+, CD19+, CD23+, dim CD20, dim-to-negative monotypic surface light chains, dim-to-negative CD79b and FMC7
  - Low count with CLL IP ($< 0.5/\mu$L)—virtually benign, no follow-up
  - High count with CLL IP (0.5–$5/\mu$L)—behaves like stage 0; needs follow-up
- Atypical CLL IP—CD5+, CD19+, CD20 bright, moderate-to-bright monotypic surface light chains, variable CD23
- Non-CLL IP—dim-to-negative CD5+, CD19+, CD20 bright, moderate-to-bright monotypic surface light chains

Follicular Lymphoma (FL)
- t(14;18)
  - Does not define FL (can have point mutations)

- Follicular (only primary follicles) on low power
  - Back-to-back monotonous follicles
  - If diffuse, consider transformation to DLBCL
- Centrocytes
  - Twisted, raisinoid, or cleft nuclei with compact chromatin
- Centroblasts
  - Larger, open chromatin, multiple small nucleoli
  - Do not confuse with follicular dendritic cells (look like snowmen with only two balls, very fine chromatin, small nucleoli)
  - Graded by amount of centroblasts per high–power field
- CD10+, CD5–, BCL2+, BCL6+, low Ki67
  - Mutated *BCL2* stops apoptosis, so the neoplastic cells slowly build up
- Bone marrow involvement is classically paratrabecular

In situ Follicular Neoplasm
Leukemic Follicular Lymphoma
- BM: paratrabecular aggregates
- Small cleaved cells on smear (buttock cells), angulated centrocytes that look like raisins
- t(14;18)—*IGH-BCL2*

Marginal Zone Lymphoma (MZL)
- Monocytoid lymphocytes
  - Small nucleus, abundant cytoplasm
- Variable amounts of larger cells
- CD5–, CD10–
- *MYD88* mutations are rare (but can happen)
  - Presence favors lymphoplasmacytic lymphoma (LPL), as does M protein presence

Nodal Marginal Zone Lymphoma (NMZL)
- Expanded marginal zone around reactive follicles
- Gains of chromosomes 3 and 18; no translocations

Splenic Marginal Zone Lymphoma (SMZL)
- Indolent, frequently involves the blood
- Polar lymph projections
- BM: CD20+ cells filling the sinusoids
- Surface Ig+, cytoplasmic Ig +/–, CD5/CD10–, FMC-7–, negative/dim HCL markers
- Loss of 7q > trisomy 3
- 300 × more likely to get SMZL if hepatitis C+
  - Some cases will resolve with hepatitis treatment
- *All splenic lymphomas, by definition, require a spleen sample. Splenectomies are now rare for lymphomas*

Extranodal Marginal Zone Lymphoma (MALT Lymphoma or MALToma)
- Inciting organisms/conditions
  - Stomach—*H. pylori* gastritis
  - Salivary—Sjögren's syndrome
  - Thyroid—Hashimoto syndrome
  - Lacrimal—*Chlamydia psittaci*
  - Skin—*Borrelia burgdorferi*

- Immunoproliferative small intestine—*Campylobacter jejuni*
- CGA: t(11;18), t(14;18)(*IGH-MALT1*), t(1;14), t(3;14)
  - >>> trisomies 3, 8, 18
- Lymphoepithelial lesions (cytokeratin stains can help show them) with centrocyte–like cells (may differentiate to plasma cells—rule out LPL) and/or centroblasts and/or immunoblasts, reactive germinal centers

Mantle Cell Lymphoma (MCL)

- t(11;14)
- Morphology
  - Vaguely nodular in lymph nodes, around follicles, diffuse
    - rule out lighter areas as CLL proliferative centers (neoplastic follicles)
  - Can cause polyposis coli
  - Notched nuclei
  - Epithelioid histiocytes in background
- Immunophenotype
  - CD20 bright, CD5+, CyclinD1+, CD23–, CD79b+, FMC7+ (cousin of CD20, they go together), CD200–
    - CD5 can rarely be negative
  - Unmutated IgH = positive staining for SOX11 = more aggressive
    - More likely to be in LN or extranodal (not PB, BM, or spleen)
    - "Classic" → blastoid or pleomorphic (not leukemic)
  - CCND1– MCLs are positive for SOX11 (and CCND2)
    - CCND1 and CCND2– are MOST aggressive
    - Extremely rare triple negatives have cryptic t(11;14)
  - CCND1+ and SOX11– are virtually all leukemic MCL

Leukemic Mantle Cell Lymphoma

- LN, spleen, GI tract
- FISH t(11;14) involving *BCL-1*
- Moderately aggressive
- Immunophenotype
  - Nuclear cyclin D1 with negative SOX11
  - Positive for 4, 43, sIg, 79b, FMC-7, cyclin D1
  - Negative for 10 and 23
- PITFALL: myeloma can have t(11;14) and positive cyclin D1

B cell Prolymphocytic Leukemia (B-PLL)

- Very rare
- Must exclude CLL and circulating mantle cells; no t(11;14)
- Prolymphocytes >55% of circulating WBCs
- Bright surface Ig, CD19+, CD20+, CD22+ CD5 +/–, CD23 +/–, CD10–, cyclin D1–
- Del(17q), del(13q14)

Splenic B Cell Leukemia/Lymphoma, Unclassifiable

- Splenic diffuse red pulp
- HCL variant (looks like HCL with different nuclear qualities and slightly different immunophenotype)

Lymphoplasmacytic Leukemia (LPL)

- "Waldenstrom macroglobulinemia" if symptoms of hyperviscosity are present
- Russell bodies or Dutcher bodies, Mott cells
- Immunophenotype
  - Positive: surface immunoglobulin, CD19, CD20, CD22
  - Negative: CD10, CD23, CD103
  - Cyclin D1 is negative always
    - If positive, consider IgM plasma cell myeloma
  - B cell clone and PC clone
  - *MYD88 (L265P)* mutation

Hairy Cell Leukemia

- Clinical
  - Median age of 50 years, M > F
  - Splenomegaly, pancytopenia, monocytopenia, (lymphadenopathy, leukocytosis)
  - At diagnosis, may have lymphocytopenia with very rare hairy cells
  - Treat with cladribine (can get very long-term remissions)
- Morphology
  - Villous projections all the way around the cell
  - Reniform nucleus, can lose some cytoplasm (light blue)
  - BM—widely spaced lymphs with lots of red cell lakes and increased reticulin, +/− emperipolesis
- Immunophenotype
  - Bright CD22, CD20, surface light chains, CD11c/CD25
  - Positive TRAP, DBA-44 (best for MRD), CD103, CD123, annexin A1 (most specific), FMC7
  - Weak cyclin D1
  - Negative CD5, CD10
  - Variable CD23
- *BRAF* V600E mutation in ~100%

Hairy Cell Leukemia Variant
- No *BRAF* mutation
- Immunophenotype
  - Bright CD11c, surface light chains
  - Positive/variable CD19, CD20, CD22, CD103, FMC7
  - Negative CD5, CD10, CD25, CD123, CD200

Burkitt Lymphoma (BL)

- Cell of origin is likely centroblasts
  - Mutated IgH
- Types
  - Endemic—children, classically African, always EBV+
  - Sporadic—children and young adults, EBV+ in 30%
  - Immunodeficiency–related—HIV
- Morphology
  - Intermediate sized cells with finely distributed (pale and powdery on smears) chromatin
    - Smaller than DLBCL

- One to two nucleoli (less than DLBCL)
- More monotonous than DLBCL
- Retraction artifact → cobblestone look
- Smears: deeply basophilic cytoplasm with cytoplasmic vacuoles
- Starry sky
- Immunophenotype
  - CD20+, CD19+, CD10+, BCL2–, BCL6+
  - *Slightly* larger by FSC, dim CD19, CD10+, CD5–
    - Can also be seen in follicular lymphoma
  - Bright CD20, bright CD38 (resulting from *MYC* translocation)
  - Ki67 near 100%!
    - Compared with variable ~40% in comparable DLBCL
- t(2;8) or t(8;22)—involves *MYC*
- Treatment
  - High risk for tumor lysis syndrome
    - Allopurinol and lots of fluids
    - Start with prephase chemotherapy (low dose)
      - Cyclophosphamide, steroid, rituximab
  - 60% to 90% cure rate
    - R-CODOX-M/IVAC for 12 weeks (modified Magraff)
    - DA-EPOCH-R—less aggressive, better tolerated, 6 to 7 months
    - HyperCVAD—less commonly used
  - Needs CNS prophylaxis!

Diffuse Large B Cell Lymphoma (DLBCL)

- Most common non-Hodgkin lymphoma
- Germinal center versus non-GC (HANS ALGORITHM)
  - See Fig. 21.9.
  - CD10+, BCL6+, MUM1+, DLBCLs are a heterogeneous group and are enriched for *IRF4* mutations or rearrangements
    - They are mostly GCB type, but 34% are misclassified by Hans algorithm (gold standard is gene expression profiling)
- *MYC* mutations are frequently seen in transformed FL (with *BCL2* translocation)
- Background T cells are predominantly CD8

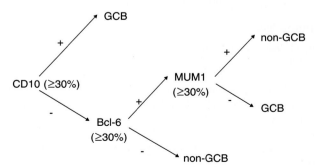

Fig. 21.9 Hans algorithm for classifying large B cell lymphomas. *GCB*, germinal–center B cell.

Intravascular/Intrasinusoidal DLBCL

- BM involvement is sinusoidal/serpiginous, large blastoid cells
- In young males with same pattern but CD3+, think hepatosplenic γ/Δ lymphoma

High–Grade B Cell Lymphoma

- … With *MYC* and *BCL2* and/or *BCL6* rearrangements
  - New category for "double/triple hit lymphomas" that are morphologically DLBCLs
  - Currently, only counts if translocated/rearranged, not if there are increased copies/expression, though amplifications may be prognostic/predictive as well
- … With features between DLBCL and BL
- … With features between DLBCL and CHL
- … NOS

EBV+ DLBCL

- >50 years of age, secondary to immunosenescence
  - Age and prognosis inversely related
- Transformed immunoblasts +/– reactive background
- Activated B cell type (MUM1+, CD10–, BCL6––)
- CD30+, sometimes CD15+
- DDx: if *IGH-MYC* rearrangement is present, consider plasmablastic lymphoma

B Cell Lymphoma, Intermediate Between DLBCL and CHL

- CHL morphology with strong CD20+/79a+ and CD15–
- PMBL morphology with 15+ or EBER+ and 20–

T Cell Rich/Histiocyte Rich B Cell Lymphoma

- Diffuse architecture
- CD45+
- 10% of all cells are B cells (no small B cells present)

Plasmablastic Lymphoma

- Usually associated with HIV
  - Can be immunocompetent though
- *MYC* rearranged
- Large B cell lymphoma with plasmablastic features can be product of transformed small B cell lymphomas

Posttransplant Lymphoproliferative Disorders

- Usually presents within 1 year of transplant
- Solid organ or stem cell
  - Highest risk with heart or lung transplant
- Usually associated with EBV (not always)
- Types
  - CHL
  - Monomorphic
    - DLBCL
    - Burkitt lymphoma
    - Plasma cell myeloma
    - PTCL NOS
    - Hepatosplenic T cell lymphoma

- Polymorphic
- Nondestructive
  - Plasmacytic hyperplasia
  - Infectious mononucleosis
  - Florid follicular hyperplasia

HODGKIN LYMPHOMA (HL)

General

- Lymphadenopathy, especially cervical
- Contiguous lymphatic spread
- Young adults
- Prognosis most strongly correlated with clinical stage
- Subtypes (most favorable to poorest prognosis): NLPHL > CHL

Nodular Lymphocyte Predominant Hodgkin Lymphoma (NLPHL)

- Clinical:
  - Approximately 5% of all HL
  - 30- to 50-year-old males, presents as lymphadenopathy, usually low stage
    - Only very rarely involves the bone marrow
  - Increased risk with autoimmune lymphoproliferative syndrome (ALPS)
  - Favorable prognosis even with frequent relapses, slowly progressive, rarely fatal
    - may transform to DLBCL
  - May be preceded by, coexist with, or follow progressive transformation of germinal centers
    - Mantle cells invade germinal centers
    - <5% of follicles involved
- Morphology
  - LN effaced by nodular (or nodular and diffuse) infiltrate
    - If all diffuse, rule out T cell/histiocyte rich DLBCL (which is CD8 > CD4)
    - MOTH EATEN
  - L & H ("lymphocytic and/or histiocytic Reed-Sternberg variants") or LP (lymphocyte predominant) cells
    - GC B cell at centroblast stage
    - Popcorn cells/elephant feet
    - Immunophenotype
      - CD20/79a+
      - CD45+
      - BCL6+
      - EMA 50%+
      - Oct-2/BOB.1+ (stronger than background normal B cells)
      - CD30/15−
      - Bright PAX-5
    - Rearranged Ig genes, aberrant somatic hypermutation, *BCL6* rearrangement
    - May be indistinguishable from RS cells
  - Background: small lymphs (Bs and Ts), rare histiocytes, rare plasma cells
    - No eosinophils, neutrophils, fibrosis, or necrosis
    - Rosette of CD4 > CD8 T cells
      - CD3+, CD57+, CD279+

- Expanded follicular dendritic network
- Patterns: classic nodular, serpiginous, extranodular, T cell rich nodular, diffuse T cells

Classic Hodgkin lymphoma

- Clinical
  - Bimodal age distribution (15 to 35 years of age, then older adults), increased risk with HIV or allogeneic BMT
  - 75% involve cervical LNs, 20% spleen, 5% BM
    - Extranodal and mesenteric involvement is rare
  - B symptoms in 40% to 50%
  - Favorable prognosis overall (80% to 85% cure with chemotherapy/radiotherapy)
    - Some difference in subtype, but small
      - Nodular sclerosing > mixed cellularity/lymphocyte rich > lymphocyte deplete
    - Radiation and ABVD
- All subtypes
  - Morphology
    - Effaced architectures with rare RS cells (≤2 nucleoli) and low CD8+ cells (except in HIV)
    - Malignant cells (Hodgkin/Reed–Sternberg, HRS cells)
      - Reed–Sternberg cells—≥2 nuclear lobes/nuclei, rounded with prominent nuclear membranes
        - Mature germinal–center B cells (have already gone through somatic hypermutation)
      - Hodgkin cell—mononuclear RS cell
      - Mummified cell—pyknotic RS
      - Lacunar cell—highly lobulated RS with smaller nucleoli, NS CHL, formalin fixation artifact
    - Immunophenotype
      - CD30+ (membranous/golgi), 15+ (golgi/membranous, depends on antibody clone), +/– CD79a (< CD20 staining), dim Pax-5, MUM1+ (CD138–), fascin+
        - CD15 may be very faint
        - CD20 in 30% to 40% (when positive, dim/variable), CD79a in less than that
        - CD45 (LCA) –, (one or both) OCT-2/BOB.1 –, PU.1 nuclear negative
        - <2% have T cell IP
    - Background: reactive lymphs (CD4 > CD8), neutrophils, and histiocytes
    - BM involvement
      - Classic RS cells not required if patient has previous diagnosis, the morphology of the background cells are correct, and variant cells are present
  - Recurrent gains by array comparative genome hybridization
  - See Table 21.4.

PLASMA CELL

Monoclonal Gammopathy of Uncertain Significance (MGUS)

- Criteria
  - Serum M protein <3 g/dL
  - Clonal plasma cells in bone marrow <10%
  - No end organ (CRAB) symptoms or amyloidosis
- Predictive/prognostic
  - Size of M-spike
  - Type of M-protein
    - IgM MGUS usually transforms to lymphoplasmacytic lymphoma

TABLE 21.4 ■ Classic Hodgkin Subtypes (Most Common to Least Common)

Subtype	Morphology	EBV+ HRS Cells
Nodular sclerosis Most common, M = F, mediastinal, favorable prognosis, may have cellular phase without fibrosis	Nodular with broad bands of collagen fibrosis (+/– lacunar cells), variable background cells	10%–40%
Mixed cellularity Males in 30s, HIV, spleen and BM more commonly involved	Mixed background (eosinophils, plasma cells, histiocytes, neutrophils, lymphocytes), may have some fibrosis but not broad like NS	~75%
Lymphocyte rich Older age, without bulky disease, more favorable prognosis, rare B symptoms, rule out NLPHL stains	Nodular/diffuse, rare–absent eosinophils and neutrophils; looks like NLPHL but IP = CHL	Between NS and MC
Lymphocyte deplete Least common (<1%), males in 30s, HIV, deep organs, higher stage, B symptoms	Predominant RS cells, diffuse fibrosis (not broad bands), RS cells may be very pleomorphic	Between NS to MC

BM, Bone marrow; *CHL,* classic Hodgkin lymphoma; *EBV,* Epstein–Barr virus; *F,* female; *HIV,* human immunodeficiency virus; *HRS,* Hodgkin/Reed–Sternberg; *IP,* immunophenotype; *M,* male; *MC,* mixed cellularity; *NLPHL,* nodular lymphocyte–predominant Hodgkin lymphoma; *NS,* nodular sclerosis; *RS,* Reed–Sternberg.

- Serum free light chain (SFLC) ratio
- *MYC* rearrangement can cause progression of MGUS to PCM, means more aggressive disease

Smoldering Myeloma

- Serum M protein >3 g/dL and/or >10% clonal PCs in BM
- Still no CRAB symptoms or amyloidosis

Myeloma

- Number one cause for BMT (usually autologous)
- Clinical
  - Can get anemia secondary to myelophthisis or immunomodulatory of processes of myeloma
  - CRAB + (new myeloma-defining events)
    - ≥60% plasma cells on BM
    - Involved-to-uninvolved SFLC >100
    - MRI lesion(s) >5 mm
    - Hypercalcemia
    - Renal dysfunction
    - Anemia
    - Bone lesions
- Russell bodies—intracytoplasmic inclusions in plasma cells
  - Mott cell—cell filled with Russell bodies
- Dutcher bodies—intranuclear inclusions in plasma cells
- Laboratory testing
  - Protein electrophoresis and immunofixation
    - 3% have no M protein on immunofixation
      - Light chain only or very little secreted

- ~85% nonsecretors
- ~15% nonproducers
- To quantify M spike: quantitate all protein (turbidimetry), then take area-under-the-curve
  - Example: total protein = 9 g/dL, M-spike = 30% = 3 g/dL
- Immunophenotype
  - CD138+, but some carcinomas and normal tissues also express
  - CD38 not lineage-specific but BRIGHT on plasma cells
  - CD56 aberrantly positive
  - CD19 aberrantly—(and CD45 usually dim-to-negative)
  - CD20+ myelomas
    - Associated with small mature plasma cells
    - Associated with t(11;14) *IGH-CCND1*
      - + Cyclin D1 (associated with longer survival)
      - Found in 35% to 50% of light chain only myeloma (overrepresented in light chain, nonsecretory, and IgD myelomas)
    - Higher degree of bone marrow involvement
    - Lymphoplasmacytic morphology
    - Can use rituximab
- Cytogenetics
  - FISH > G-banding
  - Early events
    - Hyperdiploidy with gains in odd-numbered chromosomes
    - Lots of rearrangements with IgH (chromosome 14)
      - t(4;14), t(14;16), t(14;20)(q32;q11.2) (last one only recurrently found in myeloma—specific!)
    - del(17p13) *TP53*
  - t(4;14) in PCM is susceptible to bortezomib
  - *MYC* rearrangements
    - FISH positive for *MYC* rearrangement was seen in ~0% MGUS, 15% untreated PCM, 50% of relapsed/refractory PCM, and >90% of PCM cell lines
    - Associated with increased MYC expression (by IHC), and decreased PFS and OS
      - Median survival is 20 months!
      - Higher incidence of plasma cell leukemia or extramedullary disease

Plasmacytoma

- Can be osseous (if solitary) or extraosseous
- Most common extraosseous location is in the upper respiratory tract

TEMPI Syndrome

- Telangiectasia
- ↑ EPO → ↑ RBC
- Monoclonal gammopathy (usually at MGUS level)
- Perinephric fluid collection
- Intrapulmonary shunting
- **There have only been about 15 cases reported**

POEMS Syndrome

- Polyneuropathy, organomegaly, endocrinopathy, monoclonal protein, skin changes
- Mandatory
  - Polyneuropathy
  - Monoclonal PC disorder (almost always lambda)

- Major (need one)
  - Castleman, plasma cell variant
  - Sclerotic bone lesions
  - ↑ VEGF
- Minor (need one)
  - Organomegaly
  - Extravascular volume overload
  - Endocrinopathy (adrenal, thyroid, pituitary, gonadal, parathyroid, pancreatic)
  - Skin changes (hyperpigmentation, hypertrichosis, glomeruloid hemangiomata, plethora, acrocyanosis, flushing, white nails)
  - Papilledema
  - Thrombocytosis or polycythemia

AL Amyloidosis

- Acquired factor 10 deficiency
- 70% lambda light chain

Plasma Cell Leukemia

- >2000 absolute or >20% in blood
- More frequently CD20+, CD56–
- t(11;14) overrepresented

T and NK Cell

General

- More rare than B cell lymphomas
- NK cells are part of innate immune system
- Originate in BM, mature in thymus
- Helper T (CD4) and cytotoxic (CD8)
- TCR components–Alpha-beta (helper and cytotoxic)—98%
  - Gamma-delta (neither helper or cytotoxic; 4–/8–; innate immunity)—2%

- Mature T cells—CD3 (surface and cytoplasmic; + by flow and IHC), 2, 5, 7 and 4 or 8, some 56/57, +TCR
- Mature NK cells—CD3 (only cytoplasmic——by flow, positive by IHC), 2, 7, 56, 16, some 57, –TCR, –5
- By flow → look for aberrant markers or size of population
  - No clonal marker for T/NK cells, like for B cells with lambda/kappa
- Prevalence of subtype varies by geography (associated with viruses)
  - North America—PTCL > angioimmunoblastic > ALK + ALCL > ALK—ALCL
- Prognosis is poor for most (except ALK + ALCL: ~70% 5-year survival)
- See Table 21.5.

By Anatomic Location

- Tissue (liver, spleen, BM sinusoids, soft tissue)—hepatosplenic TCL, subcutaneous panniculitis–like TCL, extranodal NK nasal type
- Aerodigestive tract—extranodal NK/TCL
- Small bowel—enteropathy-associated TCL, HSTL, monomorphic epitheliotropic intestinal T cell lymphoma (MEITL)
- Skin—MF, Sézary, ATLL, AITL, PTLC, ALCL, subcutaneous panniculitis-like T cell lymphoma, lymphomatoid papulosis

TABLE 21.5 ■ T Cell Leukemia and Lymphomas

T Cell Leukemia/ Lymphoma	Phenotype	Virus	Associated Disease	Genetics
T-prolymphocytic leukemia	CD3+, CD4+/CD8– (25% double +, unique)	–	–	inv(14) TCL-1
T-large granular lymphocyte leukemia	CD3+, CD8+	–	Rheumatoid arthritis	STAT3 mutation
Adult T cell leukemia/ lymphoma	CD3+, CD4+, CD8–, CD7–, CD25+ (some 4–/8+; rare 4+/8+)	HTLV– 1	–	–
Aggressive NK leukemia	NK phenotype	EBV	–	–
Angioimmunoblastic T cell lymphoma	CD4+, CD2+, CD7+, CD10+, BCL6+, PD1+, CXCL13+, follicular T cell, cytoplasmic CD3+ (surface negative)	EBV	Polyclonal gammopathy	
Anaplastic large cell lymphoma	CD30+, ALK+/–, CD4+/–, CD8–, CD25+, CD45 variable, CD3–/+ (25%), CD2+, EMA+, CD5+	–	–	t(2;5) ALK, others (NPM1)
NK/T cell lymphoma, nasal type	Most NK phenotype, CD16–	EBV	–	–
Enteropathy-associated T cell lymphoma	CD3+, CD4–, CD8–/+, CD103+, 7+, ab>>gd	–	Celiac disease	–
Hepatosplenic T cell lymphoma	CD3+, CD4–, CD8–/+, gd, CD5–	–	Organ transplant, Crohn's	iso(7q)
Subcutaneous panniculitis-like T cell lymphoma	CD3+, CD8+, ab	–	–	–
Monomorphic epitheliotropic intestinal T cell lymphoma	CD4–, CD8+, CD3+, CD5–, CD56+			
Mycosis fungoides/ Sézary syndrome	CD4+, CD8–, CD3+, CD26–			

- LN—ALCL, AITL, PTCL NOS, ATLL (lymphomatous pattern)
  - Secondary involvement by intestinal T cell lymphoma, hepatosplenic TCL, or MF/SS
  - Most in PB and skin do not go to lymph nodes
- Blood/BM—T-PLL, Sézary, aggressive NK/TCL, ATLL, LGL (T cells and NK cells), NK leukemia (big and atypical or LGL-like, clonal lymphoproliferative disease of NK cells (CLPD-NK)
  - Leukemias usually
  - Secondary involvement by EATL (CD3– and CD5–)

T-Prolymphocytic Leukemia (T-PLL)

- Massive HSM, lymphadenopathy; very high WBC; aggressive!
- Convoluted nuclear envelope/nuclear blebs, cytoplasmic blebs, bigger than lymphs, prominent large nucleolus
- CD2+, surface CD3+, 5+ 7+, TCL1+ in inv(14)
  - 60% = 4+, 8–
  - 25% = 4+, 8+ (also T-ALL)
  - 15% = 4–, 8+
- Inv(14)q(11;q32) +/– chromosome 8 abnormalities *or* t(14;14)
- Poor prognosis

Large Granular Lymphocytic Leukemia (LGLL)

- Can be NK or T cells, defined by CD57 expression
  - sCD3 + → T cells (CD8+) → "T-large granular lymphocytic leukemia"
    - With restricted/clonal TCR
    - Alpha-beta only
  - sCD3– → NK cells (CD16+) → "chronic lymphoproliferative disorder of NK cells"
    - With restricted KIRs
  - Dim CD5, dim CD7
- Diagnostic criteria
  - Increased number (>2000/μL)
    - >0.5 absolute on PB (WBC × % LGL = absolute) or > 5% on BM
  - Chronicity (>6 months)
  - Clonality
    - By *TCR* gene rearrangement or flow cytometry for T cells
    - By KIRS for NK cells
  - No clearly defined cause
- Clinical
  - Indolent/asymptomatic chronic course
  - Cytopenias (which cause the most morbidity/mortality)
    - Usually neutropenia
  - Mild lymphocytosis
  - 50% splenomegaly
  - Up to 30% have rheumatoid arthritis
    - *Be aware of Felty syndrome*
      - *Splenomegaly, rheumatoid arthritis, and neutropenia*
- Normal BM, CD8+ LGLs in sinusoids
  - Reactive lymphoid aggregates are mostly CD4+ and small
- 50% have *STAT3* mutations
- PITFALL
  - LGL expansion can occur after BMT, immunosuppression, or autoimmune

Adult T Cell Leukemia/Lymphoma (ATLL)

- HTLV-1; Africa, Caribbean, Japan
  - Virus also causes tropical spastic paresis
- Variants: acute (most common), lymphomatous, chronic, smoldering
- Skin involvement is frequent

- Hepatosplenomegaly, lytic bone lesions, hypercalcemia (increased RANKL leads to increased osteoclasts)
- Very convoluted nuclear membrane = "flower cell"
- Ample, cleared out cytoplasm
- 2+, 3+, 5+, 7–, 25+, 4+, 8–
  - CD4+ CD25+ cells are T-regulatory cells (Tregs)
  - If Tregs are neoplastic, patient becomes immunocompromised

Mycosis Fungoides/Sézary Syndrome (MF/SS)

- MF = skin only, late dissemination (patch → plaque → tumor)
  - SS = erythroderma + leukemia
  - Early lymph node involvement looks like dermatopathic change
    - Upstaged by small clusters, large clusters, and effacement
- Sparse BM involvement
- Halos, Pautrier microabscesses
- Epidermotropism and exocytosis with spongiosis
- Deeply cleaved and convoluted; cerebriform
- Can be HTLV-1+
- 2+, 3+, 5+, 7–, 25–, 4+, 8–
  - CD4:CD8 is usually > 10

T-PLL, ATLL, MF/SS can all involve skin, have convoluted nuclear membranes, and are mature T cells (EASY TO TEST!). See Table 21.6.

Anaplastic Large-Cell Lymphoma (ALCL)

- CD30+ (membranous with perinuclear dot), CD3+ (can be negative), CD20–
- Hallmark cells (horseshoe nucleus)—T cells with abundant cytoplasm and pleomorphic/horseshoe-nucleus
- Patterns: common, lymphohistiocytic, small cell, Hodgkin-like, composite
- Frequently involves LN and extranodal sites (skin, bone, soft tissues, lung, liver)
- Often high stage with B symptoms
- ALK+
  - t(2;5) = most common *(ALK/NPM)* (nuclear and diffuse cytoplasmic)
  - t(1;2) = second most common (diffuse cytoplasmic, darker on periphery)
- ALK–
  - All strongly CD30+, no small cell variant
  - Poor prognosis
  - 8% have *TP63* mutation, which portends an even poorer prognosis

TABLE 21.6 ■ **Mature T Cell Leukemias with Convoluted Nuclear Membranes and Variable Cutaneous Involvement**

	T-Prolymphocytic Leukemia	Adult T-Cell Leukemia/ Lymphoma	Mycosis Fungoides/ Sezary Syndrome
CD2		+	+
CD7		–	–
CD4/CD8	–/+	+/–	+/–

Breast Implant–Associated ALCL (BIA-ALCL)

- Morphologically and immunophenotypically similar to ALK– ALCL
- CD30+ CD2+ CD4+
- Cytotoxic granule markers are positive (perforin, granzyme, TIA-1)
- Usually indolent, 5% fatal
- Treatment is capsulectomy +/– local radiation
- Most important predictor is mass formation

Primary Cutaneous ALCL

- Primary to skin
- ALK–, but not associated with poor prognosis, 90% 10-year survival rate

Lymphomatoid Papulosis

- Precursor to primary cutaneous ALCL
- Not considered a true neoplasm
- Resolves on own

Angioimmunoblastic T Cell Lymphoma (AITL)

- Morphology
  - Increased arborizing high–endothelial venules (HEVs)
  - Expansion of polytypic B-immunoblasts in background (EBER+, CD20+, CD30+)
    - May eventually get an EBV+ B cell lymphoma without obvious immunosuppression
  - Expanded CD21+ follicular dendritic cell meshworks along HEVs, partial nodal involvement, skips over sinuses
  - Characteristic cytoplasmic clearing with prominent cell borders
- Immunophenotype
  - Positive: CD2, dim surface CD3, cytoplasmic CD3, CD4, CD5
  - A follicular helper T cell lymphoma
  - ICOS+, CXCL13+, PD1+, CD10+, BCL6+
- *RHOA* and *IDH2* mutations

NEW: "Nodal Peripheral T Cell Lymphoma (PTCL) with a T-follicular Helper Phenotype"

Includes angioimmunoblastic and T follicular lymphoma

Peripheral T Cell Lymphoma, Not Otherwise Specified (PTCL-NOS) (Heterogeneous Category)

- Subtype—Leonard (T cells with increased histiocytes)
- Increased HEVs, increased inflammatory cells (especially eosinophils)
- Usually CD4 > CD8, may have dim CD30
- Can have paraneoplastic features

Hepatosplenic T-cell Lymphoma

- Cords and sinuses of spleen, sinusoids of BM and liver
- Iso(7q), immunosuppression
- Gamma-delta T cells with loss of CD5
- CD3+, CD8+, CD2+, CD7+
- Poor prognosis

Enteropathy–Associated T Cell Lymphoma (EATL)

- Small bowel
- Type 1
  - Inflammation and ulceration, intraepithelial lymphs, adjacent mucosal atrophy and crypt hyperplasia
  - CD3+, CD7+, CD5–, CD56–, CD4–, **CD8–, granzyme+**
- Type 2 = "monomorphic epitheliotropic intestinal TCL"
  - No inflammation, more monotonous, no association with celiac
  - Poorer prognosis
  - Gamma-delta T cells
  - CD3+, CD7+, CD5–, CD56–, CD4–, **CD8+, granzyme–**

Extranodal NK/T Cell Lymphoma

- Usually NK cells (T cells are rare); "lethal midline granuloma"
- Geographic necrosis, nasal mass, polymorphous with background eosinophils/neutrophils/plasma cells, increased apoptosis, angiodestructive pattern
- 3+, 7–, 56+, Granzyme B+, perforin+, 5–, EBER+ (in neoplastic cells)
- Asians, southern/central Americans
- CD56+, CD7+, CD94+ (NK cells), CD3+, CD5+, TCR+ (T cells), EBV+
  - There is some difference in treatment if T cells or NK cells
  - Necrosis and perivascular infiltrates with damage to the walls

Aggressive NK/T Cell Leukemia

- Expand BM sinusoids
- Surface CD3–, 2+, 56+, EBER+ (in neoplastic cells)

Adult T Cell Leukemia/Lymphoma (ATLL)

- Flower–shaped nucleus, widespread LN involvement
- HTLV-1 infections (necessary for diagnosis)
- 7–, 2+, 3+, 5+; 4+, 8– (in most)

LYMPHOBLASTIC LEUKEMIA

Overview

- ALL is the most common pediatric malignancy
- Leukemia = >20% blasts in the bone marrow
- B-lineage—bright CD19 (some AML can have dim positivity), CD22, CD79a, CD10
- T-lineage—cytoplasmic CD3, CD7 (2, 4, 8)
- Lymphoblastic leukemia can have abnormal myeloid markers in up to 86%
  - Myeloid—MPO (>3%), CD13, CD33 or two monocytic markers
    - CD14, CD64, CD11c, lysozyme, NSE
- Categorization by morphology (now an outdated classification scheme, but may be used to describe blasts)
  - L1 blasts are small and monomorphic
  - L2 blasts are large and heterogeneous
  - L3 blasts are Burkitt–like with deeply basophilic vacuolated cytoplasm
    - Most turned out to truly be Burkitt lymphoma

B-Lymphoblastic Leukemia/Lymphoma

- Normal B cell precursors (usually in bone marrow) = hematogones (small cells with little to no cytoplasm, smooth and homogeneous chromatin)
- Malignant B cell precursors = lymphoblast
- Clinical
  - Neurofibromatosis type 1, Down syndrome, Bloom syndrome, ataxia telangiectasia
  - Traditionally, clinical trials have defined acute lymphoblastic leukemia as >25% blasts
    - 25% have leukopenia
    - 50% have slightly elevated WBC count (5,000 to 25,000 per microliter)
    - 10% have extremely elevated WBC count (>100,000)
      - t(9;22)
      - t(4;11)
      - T-ALL
- Prognosis
  - Children do better
  - Average 5-year survival—68.1%
  - Favorable factors in children—1 to 10 years, female, WBC <50, CD10+, no blasts in CNS, hyperdiploid, *ETV-RUNX1* translocations, fast response to chemotherapy
- Morphology
  - Can have cytoplasmic granules or vacuoles (PITFALL: granules do not connote myeloid lineage)
    - MPO–
  - May have hand–mirror cells
- Immunophenotype
  - Can lack CD45 (variable)
  - TdT+ (nuclear), CD34+ or variable
  - CD10+ (cytoplasmic)
  - CD19+, CD79a+ (cytoplasmic), CD20–, CD24+, Pax-5+, dim CD22 (surface and cytoplasmic)
- Genetics
  - NOS—no recurrent cytogenetic abnormalities
  - "B-lymphoblastic leukemia/lymphoma with recurrent genetic abnormalities"
    - The good actors
      - t(12;21)(p13;q22) *ETV-RUNX1*
        - Need FISH to identify, typically a cryptic translocation
        - Cryptic = not visible on normal G-banded karyotype
        - CD34+, partial CD20+, CD9–
      - Hyperdiploid—most common
        - More than 50 chromosomes
    - The mediocre actors
      - t(1;19) *TCF3-PBX1*
        - Intermediate to favorable prognosis
        - Pre-B cell phenotype, CD34– and CD9+
        - Alternate translocation t(17;19)—higher risk
      - IgH translocations
        - Bright CD10, may have myeloid markers
    - The bad actors
      - t(9;22) *BCR-ABL1*
        - p190 breakpoint

- Almost all have *IZKF1* deletions (encodes for IKAROS protein)
    - Independent predictor of disease persistence after induction
- Philadelphia–like (or BCR-ABL-like)
    - Genetic changes that involve tyrosine kinases or cytokine receptors so disease acts like Philadelphia chromosome-positive ALL
    - ABL1, ABL2, CRLF2, JAK2
    - Response to TKIs
- *KMT2A* rearrangement (11q23)
    - Especially pre-B ALL
    - Infants, high white count, hepatosplenomegaly, CNS disease
    - CD19+, CD10–, CD24+, CD15+, CD33+, CD65+
    - Do not call mixed lineage if some myeloid markers are present, these need a higher threshold.
    - Rarely can have a "mature B cell" phenotype
- Hypodiploid
    - High hypodiploid = 40 to 45 chromosomes, relatively better prognosis
    - Low hypodiploid = 33 to 39 chromosomes
    - Associated with TP53 mutations
    - Near haploid = 23 to 29 chromosomes, relatively poorer prognosis
    - Associated with *RAS* mutations
- Provisional: iAMP21
    - Associated with chromothripsis (shattering of chromosomes)
    - Amplification of *RUNX1*
    - Older children, low white count, no gender predilection
    - Inferior outcome
    - 2% of all pediatric B-ALL cases

T-lymphoblastic Leukemia/Lymphoma

- Classically has dimorphic population
    - Lymphocyte–like blasts
    - More classic large blasts
- T-ALL with t(4;11) or t(9;22) can have very high WBC (>100,000)
- More frequently presents as lymphoma, typically mediastinal mass

GENETICS

Methods

- Used for definition/diagnosis, classification, prognostic, treatment, monitoring/minimal residual disease testing
- Cytogenetics—larger scale (FISH, chromosome banding, CGH array)
- Molecular—small–scale (sequencing for screening, PCR for targeted, HPLC, SNPs)
- Sensitivities
    - Cytogenetics—5%
    - FISH—1% to 5%
    - NGS—~5% (need around 20% or more tumor in sample)
    - Southern blot—5% to 10%
    - PCR—0.02-5%
- See Table 21.7.
- Can test fresh, frozen, paraffin-embedded, EDTA, ACD
    - Cannot test heparin or decalcified

TABLE 21.7 ■ **Genetic Methods**

Karyotype	Screening
CGH	Large deletions or duplications AML and ALL
FISH	Specific rearrangements (especially promiscuous rearrangements and large gene products) Deletions and duplications
Southern blot, Capillary electrophoresis	Physiologic rearrangements (immunoglobulin or TCR rearrangement) can get false positives if there are a few clones of the same size
SNP, CGH array	Loss of heterozygosity
PCR	Gene mutation with a limited sample Small insertions/deletions/duplications (150–200 base pairs) *Ig* or *TCR* rearrangement SNPs
RT-PCR	Translocations with specific breakpoints *PML-RARA*
Sequencing (NGS)	Multiple mutations/target *CEBPA*

ALL, Acute lymphoblastic leukemia; *AML,* acute myeloid leukemia; *CGH,* comparative genomic hybridization; *FISH.* fluorescent in situ hybridization; *Ig,* immunoglobulin; *NGS,* next–generation sequencing; *PCR,* polymerase chain reaction; *SNP,* single-nucleotide polymorphism; *TCR,* T cell receptor.

- Gene rearrangement testing to assess for clonality (via PCR)
  - Uses
    - If heme neoplasm is suspected and morph/IP testing is inconclusive
    - To evaluate clonality between two lymphoid neoplasms
    - To differ relapse vs. second malignancy
  - Cell lines
    - B cells—immunoglobulin
      - Heavy chain
        - D-J on both chromosomes always
        - V-DJ on first chromosome
        - if it does not work, try the second
      - Light chain
        - First kappa
        - If that does not work, do second kappa
    - T cells—TCR
      - Most T cells are alpha-beta, not gamma-delta
        - Gamma and delta genes are always rearranged first, then alpha and beta. If alpha and beta rearrangement is successful, gamma and delta are deleted
      - Use gamma region as primer though (still present in alpha-beta and rearranged early)
    - NK cells—KIRs
  - Pitfalls
    - Clonality does *not* imply malignancy
      - Can get clonal proliferation during immune response

- CD8+ lymphocytosis, EBV, immunodeficiency, benign cutaneous T cell proliferation (lymphomatoid papulosis)
  - Can get cross-lineage rearrangement
    - Example: immature B neoplasms can rearrange *TCR* genes
  - TCR gamma is structurally simple—may get false positive or oligoclonal results
- In general, negative at diagnosis, use FISH; at follow-up or MRD, use PCR

Diseases

- See Table 21.8.
- Mutations
  - LPL—*MYD88 L265P*
  - CLL/SLL—del13q14 > +12 > del(11q) > del(17q) > del(6q)
  - HCL—*BRAF V600E*
  - DLBCL—*BCL6* aberrations (3q27)
- B-ALL—Ph+ or Ikaros *(IKZF1)* deletion = poor prognosis
  - Children—p190
  - Adults—p190 and p210
- T-ALL—notch gene translocation (and others)
- AML
  - t(15;17), *PML-RARA*—favorable prognosis
  - t(8;21) *RUNX1-RUNXT1*—favorable prognosis
  - *KMT2A* translocations (11q23)—poor prognosis
  - Both *NPM1* and *CEPBA* have a more favorable prognosis if alone
    - *NMP1* is most often associated with a normal karyotype
      - Also CD34– blasts and multilineage dysplasia
  - *NPM1* + *FLT3* is a poorer prognosis
  - *FLT3* alone is the poorest prognosis
  - *FLT3* ITD is defined by allelic ratio (mutant-to-normal)
  - Almost one-half have normal karyotype
  - New
    - *ASXL1*
    - *KIT*—t(8;21), inv(16)—core-binding factor leukemias

TABLE 21.8 ■ Translocations in Mature B- and T-cell Lymphomas

Entity	Translocation	Gene fusion
Mantle cell lymphoma	11;14	CCND1-IGH
Follicular lymphoma	14;18	IGH-BCL2
Marginal zone lymphoma	—	—
Pulmonary > gastric	11;18	API2-MALT1
Skin > salivary gland	14;18	IGH-MALT1
Thyroid > ocular > skin	3;14	IGH-FOXP1
Subset of intestinal and ocular	1;14	BCL10-IGH
Burkitt lymphoma	8;14	MYC-IGH
Anaplastic T cell lymphoma	2;5	ALK-NPM1
Diffuse large B cell lymphoma	—	MYC, BCL2, BCL6

- *RUNX1*
- *TP53*
- MPN—tyrosine kinases!
  - CML—*BCR/ABL1*
  - Eosinophilia—*PDGFA, PDGFB, FGFR1*
  - SM—*c-KIT D806V*
  - PV/ET/PMF—*JAK2*
- Myeloma can have cyclin D1 mutations
- *MYD88* is seen in many LPL cases but is not 100% specific or sensitive
  - Can be seen in DLBCL
- CLL/SLL has somatic hypermutation
  - CD49d and Zap70 are surrogates for somatic hypermutation
- Genetic diseases with increased risk for hematolymphoid neoplasms
  - Ataxia telangiectasia—T-PLL
  - Neurofibromatosis 1—JMML
  - Trisomy 21—TAM, AML, BALL
  - X-linked lymphoproliferative syndrome—hemophagocytic lymphohistiocytosis and Burkitt
  - AIDS—CHL and B cell lymphomas

Epstein–Barr Virus (EBV)-Related Entities

BENIGN

- Infectious mononucleosis (IM)
  - Polyclonal expansion of infected B cells, WBC usually less than 20,000
  - Typically caused by EBV (but you can get similar clinical syndrome from CMV, VZV, HIV, toxoplasma, mumps, HPV, HCV, and adenovirus)
  - Enlarged lymph nodes and fever
  - Numerous large, atypical lymphocytes showing reactive mononucleosis
    - Lymphocytes have abundant, deeply basophilic cytoplasm with cytoplasmic bleb formation or "Ballerina skirt" (vacuolated cytoplasm, scalloped margins, and indentations by the surrounding red blood cells)
    - These are the reactive T cells, not the infected B cells!
- Latent infections
  - Memory B cells
  - No proteins produced (EBV-encoding RNA or EBER is produced) to avoid immune reactions
- Chronic active EBV infection
  - Now in WHO 2016 (revised fourth edition)
  - Commonly misdiagnosed as malignant
  - Intermittent fever, lymphadenopathy, hepatosplenomegaly for >3 months
    - 50% have atypical presentation
  - Mostly children
  - Pancytopenia or lymphocytosis with polyclonal hypergammaglobulinemia
  - Increased anti-EBV IgG and EBV DNA
  - Normally B cells are the infected cells; here it is T and NK cells!
  - EBER+ cells in tissues
  - Monoclonal does not equal malignant!
  - *Systemic form*
    - Poly-, oligo-, or monoclonal T or NK cells

- Presentation
  - IM-like symptoms *or* …
  - Skin rash, uveitis, coronary aneurysm, hepatitis, interstitial pneumonia, CNS involvement, intestinal perforation, myocarditis, hypersensitivity to mosquito bites, vasculitis
- Racial predisposition
- Only therapy is hematopoietic stem cell transplant!
- Fatalities are typically caused by opportunistic infections, hemophagocytic syndrome, or multiorgan failure
- Lymph node
  - Paracortical hyperplasia
  - Follicular hyperplasia
  - Focal necrosis
  - Small epithelioid granulomas
  - Scattered EBER+ cells
  - Does not mimic lymphoma, looks reactive
- Spleen
  - Atrophy of white pulp
  - Congestion of red pulp
  - Erythrophagocytosis
- Liver
  - Looks like viral hepatitis
  - Positive EBER cells for years
- Cutaneous form
  - Hydroa vacciniforme–like lymphoproliferative disorder of childhood
  - Premalignant form
  - CD8+ T cells (rarely NK cells)
  - Not immunosuppressed
  - Papulovesicular eruptions with secondary ulceration and scarring
  - First in sun–exposed areas, then spreads everywhere
  - Nasolabial edema
  - Native Mexican, Central American, Asian
  - Morphology
    - Cells are not atypical
    - Perivascular and adnexal EBER-positive CD8-positive gamma-delta T cells
- Severe mosquito bite allergy
- Japan and Latin America
- High fever, local lymphadenopathy, edema, necrosis
- NK phenotype only, lymphocytosis
- Predisposed to NK/T cell lymphoma

MALIGNANT

- Systemic EBV-positive T cell lymphoma of childhood
- No longer a "lymphoproliferative disorder"
- 15 to 20 years of age
- Fulminant infection after acute EBV infection
- Very aggressive with quick death from hemophagocytosis
- Can have negative antibodies but very high DNA titers
- Spleen and liver infiltrated by reactive/atypical EBER+ CD8+ T cells

- Small depleted lymph nodes
- Always monoclonal
- Aggressive NK/T cell leukemia
  - Neoplastic proliferation of NK cells infected with EBV
  - Asians, young to middle aged
  - Similar to systemic EBV-positive T cell lymphoma of childhood
  - Blood and bone marrow
    - Hard to see on trephine core stained with H&E; use immunostains
  - Lymphadenopathy with lots of leukemic infiltration
- Extranodal NK/T cell lymphoma, nasal type
  - Midline (sinonasal, pharynx, orbit)
  - Destructive angiocentric infiltration, coagulative necrosis
  - Positive for EBER, CD2, CD3 epsilon chain, CD56, CD30
  - 50% outside of nasal cavity, most in GI system and skin
- Primary EBV-positive nodal T- or NK-cell lymphoma
  - Provisionary entity under PTCL NOS
  - Primary nodal, mostly CD8+ CD56− with monoclonal TCR rearrangements
  - Looks like ALCL
  - Every cell expresses EBER, TIA1, and gamma/delta TCR
  - Upregulation of PD-L1

Odds and Ends

- NK/T cells tend to be sinusoidal or interstitial in the bone marrow
- Cold agglutinin seen on PBS = IgM
  - DAT = + poly—IgG + C3
  - Heme malignancy, HIV, EBV, mycoplasma, autoimmune
  - May be clinically significant
- Platelet impedance counters are based on size
  - Bacteria, fungi, cytoplasmic fragments from blasts, cryoglobulins, red cell fragments, schistocytes can all be mistakenly counted as platelets
  - Very large platelets or platelet clumps will not be counted
- LEBR—leukoerythroblastic reaction or leukemoid reaction
  - nRBCs and immature myeloid precursors in peripheral blood (even blasts)
  - Associated with metastases to BM, myelofibrosis of any cause, leukemia, lymphoma, hemolytic anemia, and acute blood loss
- Chromatin gets wrinkled or "mature–appearing" with too much time in EDTA
- Hematolymphoid neoplasms that tend to involve the spleen
  - Splenic marginal zone lymphoma
  - Hairy cell leukemia
  - Large granular lymphocytic leukemia
  - Also others like DLBCL
  - Polyclonal lymphocytosis
  - Middle–aged females
  - Smokers
  - >4 (absolute lymphs)
  - Polyclonal IgM
- Karyotypic changes with small megakaryocytes
  - −5, −5q, inv(3), or translocation involving chromosome 3

- Chemotherapy effects
  - Trephine—gelatinous transformation, hemorrhage, acellular or paucicellular with residual lymphocytes and plasma cells
  - Aspirates—small amounts of dysplasia

Hematopathology Abbreviations

AD	autosomal dominant
AITL	angioimmunoblastic T-cell lymphoma
ALCL	anaplastic large cell lymphoma
ALIP	abnormal localization of immature precursors
ALL	acute lymphoblastic leukemia (T-ALL, B-ALL)
ALPS	autoimmune lymphoproliferative syndrome
AML	acute myeloid leukemia
ANC	absolute neutrophil count
APL	acute promyelocytic leukemia
AR	autosomal recessive
ATLL	adult T-cell leukemia/lymphoma
BCR	B cell receptor, membrane-bound surface immunoglobulin
BL	Burkitt lymphoma
BM	bone marrow
BMT	bone marrow transplant
CBC	complete blood count
CD#	cluster of differentiation (e.g., CD2)
CG	cytogenetics
CGH	comparative genomic hybridization
CHL	classic Hodgkin lymphoma
CLL/SLL	chronic lymphocytic leukemia/small lymphocytic lymphoma
CLPD	chronic lymphoproliferative disease
CML	chronic myeloid leukemia
CMML	chronic myelomonocytic leukemia
CNL	chronic neutrophilic leukemia
CNS	central nervous system
DDx	differential diagnosis
DIC	disseminated intravascular coagulopathy
DLBCL	diffuse large B cell lymphoma
Dx	diagnosis
EATL	enteropathy-associated T cell lymphoma
EBER	Epstein–Barr virus-encoding RNA
ECO	extracutaneous organs
ELP	electrophoresis
EPO	erythropoietin
ET	essential thrombocytosis
FDC	follicular dendritic cell
FH	follicular hyperplasia
FISH	fluorescent in situ hybridization
FL	follicular lymphoma
FSC	forward scatter
GC	germinal center
HCL	hairy cell leukemia

Hct	hematocrit
HEV	high endothelial venule
Hgb/Hb	hemoglobin
HL	Hodgkin lymphoma
HLH	hemophagocytic lymphohistiocytosis
HPLC	high–performance liquid chromatography
HRS cells	Hodgkin/Reed-Sternberg cells
Ig	immunoglobulin
IHC	immunohistochemistry
IP	immunophenotype
ITD	internal tandem duplication
ITP	immune thrombocytopenic purpura
JMML	juvenile myelomonocytic leukemia
KIR	killer immunoglobulin-like receptor
LBL	lymphoblastic lymphoma (T-LBL, B-LBL)
LCH	Langerhans cell histiocytosis
LEBR	leukoerythroblastic blood reaction
LGL	large granular lymphocyte
LGLL	large granular lymphocytic leukemia
LN	lymph node
LPL	lymphoplasmacytic lymphoma
MALT	mucosa–associated lymphoid tissue
MBL	monoclonal B lymphocytosis
MCHC	mean corpuscular hemoglobin concentration
MCL	mantle cell lymphoma
MCV	mean corpuscular volume
MDS	myelodysplastic syndrome
MF	mycosis fungoides
MGUS	monoclonal gammopathy of undetermined significance
MNGC	multinucleated giant cells
MPAL	mixed phenotype acute leukemia
MPN	myeloproliferative neoplasm
MPO	myeloperoxidase
MRD	minimal residual disease
MZL	marginal zone lymphoma
NGS	next–generation sequencing
NLPHL	nodular lymphocyte–predominant Hodgkin lymphoma
NOS	not otherwise specified
nRBC	nucleated red blood cells
NSE	nonspecific esterase
PAS	periodic acid Schiff
PB	peripheral blood
PBS	peripheral blood smear
PC	plasma cell
PCM	plasma cell myeloma, synonymous with multiple myeloma
PCN	plasma cell neoplasm
PCR	polymerase chain reaction
Ph	Philadelphia chromosome (ABL1-BCR)
PLL	prolymphocytic leukemia (T-PLL, B-PLL)
PMBL	primary mediastinal B cell lymphoma

PMF	primary myelofibrosis
PNH	paroxysmal nocturnal hemoglobinuria
POC	point-of-care
PTCL	peripheral T cell lymphoma
PTGC	progressive transformation of germinal centers
PTLD	posttransplant lymphoproliferative disorder
PV	polycythemia vera
RA	rheumatoid arthritis
RBC	red blood cell
RDW	red cell distribution of width
RS	ring sideroblasts
RT-PCR	reverse transcriptase polymerase chain reaction
SD	standard deviation
SFLC	serum free light chains
SLE	systemic lupus erythematosus
SM	systemic mastocytosis
SNP	single nucleotide pleomorphism
SPTCL	subcutaneous panniculitis-like T-cell lymphoma
SS	Sézary syndrome
SSC	side scatter
TCR	T cell receptor
TKI	tyrosine kinase inhibitor
TRAP	tartrate–resistant acid phosphatase
TRMN	therapy-related myeloid neoplasm
WBC	white blood cell

CHAPTER 22

Microbiology

Note

The best way to study for the microbiology portion of your board exams is to (1) understand the basics, (2) memorize some of the classic test fodder, and (3) find new ways to categorize each entity. For example, make a list of each bacterial species by Gram stain and morphology, then reorganize by clinical syndrome, then by vector, and then by best media to culture, and so on.

Basics of Microbiology

- Gram-positive cell walls—thick peptidoglycan with attached teichoic acid polymers
- Gram-negative cell walls—think peptidoglycan layer with outer membrane
- All bacteria like to grow at **37°C** degrees except...
  - *Yersinia enterocolitica* and Pseudomonas at 25° to 30°C
  - *Campylobacter* at 42°C
  - *Listeria*—grows at 37°C but motile at 25°C
    - Can still multiply at 4°C (refrigerator temperature)
- Virulence = infectivity × severity
- Commensal
  - Respiratory tract—*Streptococcus pyogenes, Streptococcus pneumoniae, Staphylococcus aureus, Candida*
  - Gastrointestinal tract—*Lactobacillus, Enterococcus, Bacteroides*
  - Genitourinary tract—*Corynebacterium, Lactobacillus, Bacteroides, Adenovirus, Candida*
  - Skin, ear, eye—*Corynebacterium, Cutibacterium acnes* (formerly *Propionibacterium acnes*), *Candida*
- Pathogenic
  - Blood—coagulase-negative *Staphylococcus, Staphylococcus aureus, Streptococcus pneumoniae, Enterococcus, Bacteroides, Candida,* HIV, HBV, HAV, CMV
  - Central nervous system—*Streptococcus pneumoniae, H. influenzae, Neisseria meningitidis, Streptococcus agalactiae, Listeria,* (others), *Candida,* cryptococcosis, histoplasmosis, coccidiomycosis, enterovirus, HSV, arbovirus, HIV, *Naegleria fowleri*
  - Upper respiratory infection—*Streptococcus pyogenes, Candida,* rhinovirus, coronavirus, HSV, EBV, adenovirus, coxsackie A virus, parainfluenza virus
  - Lower respiratory infection—*Staphylococcus aureus, Streptococcus pneumoniae, H. influenzae, Moraxella, Klebsiella, E coli, Pseudomonas,* (other bacteria), RSV, parainfluenza virus, influenza virus, rhinovirus, adenovirus, PCP, histoplasmosis, blastomycosis, coccidiomycosis, cryptococcosis
  - Ear—*Streptococcus pneumoniae, H. influenzae, Moraxella, P. aeruginosa,* aspergillus, *Candida,* viruses
  - Eye—*Streptococcus pneumoniae, H. influenzae aegyptius, Neisseria gonorrhoeae, Chlamydia trachomatis,* adenovirus, CMV
  - Intestinal—*Campylobacter jejuni, Salmonella,* Shigella, *Vibrio cholerae, E. coli,* giardia, hookworms, strongyloides, rotavirus, norovirus, adenovirus

- Flora inhibits pathogenic microbes by ...
  - Competing for nutrients
  - Competing for host receptors
  - Bacteriocin production
  - Stimulating host immune response
- Virulence factors
  - Attachment—pili, adhesins, biofilms, aggressins (neutralize host response)
  - Motility—flagella and chemotaxis
  - Resistance to serum—lipopolysaccharide (LPS) layer of gram—bacteria
  - Capsules
  - Intracellular residence
  - Enzymes—hyaluronidases, proteases, collagenase, and so on
  - Iron acquisition mechanisms—siderophores, hemolysins
  - Exotoxins
    - A-B toxins (B binds, A is toxic)
    - Membrane–disrupting (pore–forming or phospholipases)
    - Superantigens (activate T cells nonspecifically)
      - Example: toxic shock syndrome
  - Endotoxin—LPS
  - Antigenic variation
- Regulation of virulence
  - Gene amplification or rearrangement
  - Transcriptional regulation (number of transcripts increase)
  - Posttranscriptional regulation (increase gene products)
- Fastidious—can only be grown in complex, very specialized conditions
- Types of respiration/fermentation
  - Aerobic—do not ferment organic substrates
    - May be able to use nitrate, sulfate, or carbonate to live anaerobically (but not anaerobic in standard cultures)
  - Microaerophilic—grow well at low partial pressures of oxygen
  - Strictly anaerobic—oxygen is toxic
  - Facultative anaerobic
    - Bacteria with aerobic and anaerobic capabilities
    - Anaerobes that are aerotolerant
- Inflammatory cells that target specific organisms
  - B cells
    - *Pneumococcus, H. influenzae, Neisseria*
  - T cells
    - *Mycobacterium, Nocardia, Listeria, Salmonella, Legionella*, PCP, *Toxoplasma*
  - Granulocytes
    - Gram-negative rods, Staphylococcus, Corynebacteria, yeast, Aspergillus

Materials and Methods in Infectious Disease/ Microbiology Laboratories

- Gram stain
  - See Table 22.1.
  - Crystal violet—primary stain
  - Iodine—"sets" crystal violet
  - Acetone—decolorizes gram negative

TABLE 22.1 ■ **Gram Stain Morphology**

Gram-positive cocci	Clusters			*Staphylococcus*
	Pairs and short chains			Pyogenic *Streptococcus*
	Long chains			Nonpyogenic *Streptococcus*
	Lancet–shaped diplococci			*Streptococcus pneumoniae*
	Diplococci			*Enterococcus*
Gram-negative cocci	Coffee bean diplococci			*Neisseria*
Gram-positive rods	Short, irregular, pleomorphic		Anaerobic without spores	*Cutibacterium*
			Aerotolerant	*Actinomyces* *Bifidobacteria*
			Aerobic or facultative anaerobic	*Corynebacterium* *Arcanobacterium* *Rothia* *Arthrobacter* *Nonnocardia actinomyces*
	Regular monomorphic	Branching, filamentous	Aerobic or facultative anaerobic	*Nocardia*
			Anaerobic without spores	*Actinomyces israeli*
		Large	Aerobic or facultative anaerobic	*Bacillus*
			Anaerobic without spores	*Clostridium perfringens*
			Anaerobic with spores	Other *Clostridium*
		Small to medium	Aerobic or facultative anaerobic	*Listeria* *Erysipelothrix*
			Aerotolerant	Some lactobacilli
			Anaerobic without spores	*Eubacterium* Some lactobacilli
			Anaerobic with spores	*Clostridium ramosum*

(Continued)

TABLE 22.1 ■ **Gram Stain Morphology** **(Continued)**

Gram-negative rods	Comma–shaped, short	*Vibrio*
	Thin rods (S, seagull, corkscrew)	*Campylobacter*
	Bipolar staining (safety pin)	*Yersinia*
	Invisible	*Legionella*

- Safranin—counter stain
- Nonselective media
  - Sheep blood—bacteria
    - Exceptions: *N. gonorrhoeae, H. influenzae, Legionella*
    - Separate by hemolysis pattern
      - Alpha-hemolysis with a variety of small gray–white colonies most likely represents normal respiratory flora
      - Beta hemolytic with positive oxidase = normal pharyngeal flora *(Neisseria)*
  - Chocolate (hemolyzed blood)—better for *Neisseria* and *H. influenzae* (not for *Legionella*)
  - BCYE—*Legionella*
    - Added cystine, iron, and activated charcoal
  - Mueller–Hinton—antibiotic susceptibility testing
    - *Serratia marcescens*, vancomycin–resistent *Enterococcus* (VRE), *Staphylococcus aureus* (in urine) sensitivities
    - 0.5 McFarland
    - Add 5% sheep blood agar if fastidious
    - Ambient air
  - Thioglycolate broth—allows selection by respiration ability
    - All fluid cultures and sterile site cultures (e.g., joints, CSF) are put in thio broth
      - All colonies are worked up and speciated, even coagulase-negative staphs
  - Brain–heart infusion agar helps isolate fastidious fungi like *Histoplasma*
- Selective media
  - MacConkey—bile salts
    - Only hardy gram-negative rods grow
    - Transparent at first
      - Nonlactose fermenters are clear, fermenters are pink
    - *E. coli*—lactose fermenter = pink
      - MAC with sorbitol (SMAC) is selective for *E. coli* O157:H7
    - *Klebsiella*—lactose fermenter and mucoid
    - *Proteus, Shigella, Salmonella, Citrobacter*—nonlactose fermenter
  - EMB—Abilene—(same)
  - Campy-BAP—antibiotics that *Campylobacter* is resistant to (cephalothin, vanc, trimethoprim, ampho B, poly B)
  - HE (hektoen enteric)—bile salts—best for *Salmonella* and *Shigella*
    - *Enterococcus* speciation
      - *E. faecalis*—lighter gray colonies, smaller alpha hemolytic zone
      - *E. faecium*—darker, larger alpha hemolytic zone
    - Also SS agar, but some strains of *Shigella* will not grow

- Selenite broth is good for *Salmonella*
- TCBS (thiosulfate-citrate-bile salts-sucrose)—*Vibrio*
  - *V. cholerae* ferments sucrose (colonies turn yellow)
- CIN (Cefsulodin-Irgasan-Novobiocin)—*Yersinia*
- CNA (colistin-nalidixic acid)
  - Anaerobic gram-positive *Streptococcus* (can differentiate by pattern of hemolysis)
  - Yeast can grow
  - White, waxy colonies most consistent with coagulase-negative *Staphylococcus* (CoNS)
- Lim—group B *Streptococcus (agalactiae)*
- Regan–Lowe—*Bordetella*
- Thayer–Martin—*Neisseria* from nonsterile sites
- Mannitol/MSA plate—transparent—only for *Staphylococcus aureus*
- Differential media
  - Triple sugar iron (TSI) agar slant
    - Gas production → bubble at butt
    - H_2S production → black (and can assume it is a fermenter)
    - Glucose fermentation
      - Initially color change red → yellow
      - Slant slowly reverts back to red, but the butt remains yellow
    - Lactose/sucrose fermentation
      - Entire tube turns yellow (and stays)
  - MacConkey—only grows gram negative
    - Pink = lactose fermenter
    - Translucent = negative
  - EMB (same as MAC)
    - Purple–black with green sheen = lactose fermenter
    - Translucent = negative
  - HE—Enterics
    - Yellow/orange = lactose/sucrose fermentation
    - Translucent = negative
    - Black = hydrogen sulfide production
  - SS—Enterics
    - Pink/red = lactose fermentation
    - Translucent = negative
    - Black = hydrogen sulfide production
  - TCBS—vibrio
    - Yellow = sucrose fermentation
    - Translucent = negative
    - CIN—*Yersinia*
    - Bull's eye (colorless colony with red center) = mannitol fermentation
    - Translucent = negative
  - Motility
    - Cloudy = positive, translucent = negative
  - Sabouraud dextrose agar (SAB, Sab's agar, Sab's dextrose) for yeast
    - Sab's agar + gentamicin to grow yeast found in mixed plate (yeast and bacteria)
  - Birdseed agar (or caffeic discs)
    - Only *Cryptococcus neoformans* grows BROWN colonies
    - Phenol oxidase → production of melanin
- Yeast—which medium should I choose?
  - CHROMagar → good for *Candida*, greenish (dubliniensis or albicans)

- Sab's agar (without gentamicin if no bacteria present)
- Sheep blood → *Candida glabrata* does *not* grow
- Cream of rice agar is good for morphology, gram stain, MALDI
  - Example: looking for germ tubes with *Candida*
- Dimorphic fungi and molds must be processed in biosafety cabinet (BSC) to prevent release of spores (also known as conidia)
- Tween 80—supplement that induces yeast structure
- Yeast tends to grow well on *Haemophilus influenzae* isolation plate and CNA plate
  - Furry edges/little feet
- Triaging cultures
  - Gram-positive clusters → sheep blood
    - Pairs/chains → sheep and chocolate + vancomycin and optochin
      - *Abiotrophia* needs chocolate plate
  - If blood culture bottle alarms in a continuous monitoring system, but there are no organisms seen (NOS) on gram stain, blind culture onto ...
    - Sheep blood
    - Chocolate
    - Brucella
      - Not looked at until the second day because anaerobes grow slowly
      - Taped, bagged, CO_2-producing packet
    - If bottle alarms 2 × and NOS 2 ×, spin down the sample and use pellet to make ...
      - Sheep blood
      - Chocolate
      - Brucella
      - Thio broth (nonselective, nutrient rich)
      - BCYE (nonselective, nutrient rich)
        - Held for 14 days—*Legionella* grows slowly!
  - Bacterial blood cultures held 5 days, yeast 14 days, "specials" are variable
  - Cell therapy products get 14-day protocol to assess for contamination
  - Transfusion reactions—three bottles!
    - One aerobic
    - One anaerobic
    - One bottle held for 5 days, subbed to sheep blood and chocolate plates, held another 5 days
  - AFB held 42 days
    - If it alarms, then NOS by gram/AFB/modified AFB
      - Sheep blood
      - Chocolate
      - 7H11 (for AFB), held for 4 more weeks
    - If it alarms, then non-AFB bacteria are identified
      - Weekly gram stains and AFB stains
- Obligate intracellular growth (cannot be grown on artificial media)
  - *Chlamydia*
  - *Rickettsia*
- "In broth only" indicates that the inoculum was very small—likely to be a contaminant
  - Gram-positive more likely to be contaminate
    - CoNS, *Bacillus*, *Corynebacterium*
- Save agar slants for 1 month on new organism isolates
  - Except alpha-hemolytic streps, which do not grow well on slants (save plates)

- McFarland suspensions (confirm with Densichek—uses turbidity)
  - Gram negative/gram positive → 0.5 to 0.63
  - "NH/ANC"—*Haemophilus influenzae*, coryne, and so on → 2.7 to 3.3
  - Yeast → 1.8 to 2.2
- Gel electrophoresis for strain relatedness
  - "Indistinguishable" = identical bands
  - "Closely related" = 1 to 3 bands are different
  - "Possibly related" = 4 to 6 bands are different
  - "Different" = >6 bands are different

RAPID TESTING

- Calcium alginate inhibits polymerase chain reaction (PCR)
- Verigene
  - Use nucleic acid detection, 2-hour run time
  - All positive blood cultures are run on the Verigene within 24 hours of alarming
    - Prioritize bloods, run enteric paths when it is quiet
    - Always leave two of the eight machines open in case of positive bloods
  - Susceptibility testing can only be done every 5 days
  - Blood targets
    - Gram positive
      - *Staphylococcus aureus, Staphylococcus epidermidis, Staphylococcus lugdunensis,* "*Staphylococcus* spp."
      - *Streptococcus pneumoniae, S. pyogenes, S. agalactiae, S. anginosus,* "*Streptococcus* spp."
      - *E. faecium, E. faecalis, Listeria*
      - MecA, VanA, VanB
    - *E. coli, Pseudomonas, Citrobacter, Klebsiella Pneumonia, Klebsiella Oxytoca, Proteus, Acinetobacter, Enterobacter*
    - 7 ESBLs (including CXTM)
      - Done on sheep, chocolate, and MAC plates
  - Enteric pathogens
    - *Campylobacter, Salmonella, Shigella, Vibrio,* rotavirus, shiga toxin 1, shiga toxin 2, norovirus, *Yersinia enterocolitica*
    - HE plates as backup
      - Check at 24 hours and 48 hours for growth
- Cepheid infinity—PCR
  - GBS—Lim broth incubation for 16 to 24 hours
    - New confirm test for *Streptococcus pyogenes* rapid test (instead of culture)
    - Reflex to sensitivities on CNA plate
  - *C. difficile*—stool swab
  - MRSA—blood or nasal swab
  - CRE—(carbapenem-resistant)—rectal swab or McFarland suspension from sensitivity desk
  - Flu A, Flu B, RSV—nasopharynx swab
  - Enterovirus—CSF
  - *Trichomonas*—urine
  - GAS

MOLECULAR VIROLOGY

- Cobas AmpliPrep and TaqMan

- Tigris—all herpesviruses
  - CMV target is "highly conserved, nondrug target region of CMV polymerase"
    - Food and Drug Administration approved for EDTA plasma, laboratory–developed tests for urine and bronchoalveolar lavage
  - HBV—not intended for screening or confirmatory—*treatment management*
    - Same for HIV and HCV
  - HCV + → reflex to genotyping (send out test)
    - Target is a highly conserved region of 5' untranslated region
      - Comparable results for genotypes 1 to 6
  - HIV targets are highly conserved regions of HIV-1 *gag* gene and of HIV-1 LTR region
    - HIV-2 is not targeted, only endemic to West Africa
1. Specimen prep to isolate desired DNA/RNA
   a. Use magnetic bead to bind rRNA
   b. Optional number 2 for RNA—reverse transcription to get cDNA
2. Simultaneous amplification and detection (by cleaving dual–labeled oligonucleotides specific to target)
   a. RLU = relative light units
      i. GC glows
      ii. CT flashes

MATRIX–ASSISTED LASER DESORPTION/IONIZATION—TIME OF FLIGHT—MASS SPECTROMETRY (MALDI-TOF MS)

1. Add sample and matrix to chip to let it crystalize
   a. Alpha-cyano-4-hydroxycinnamic acid
   b. Protects and encourages ionization
2. Ionization chamber
   a. Laser at 337 nm (UV nitrogen)
   b. 50 bursts per second
3. TOF mass analyzer (separates)
   a. TOF depends on mass-to-charge ratio
      i. Charge = constant
      ii. Heavier is slower, lighter is faster
   b. Gives mass spectrum, which is unique to each organism
      i. Compare against a library of known spectra
4. Particle detector (electron multiplier)
- Ribosomal proteins are main target of laser
- Peaks between 2,000 and 20,000 Daltons are examined
- Final "score" from binning must be >0.6 (or 60% confidence level)
- Three categories of results
  - Single choice—≥60% match with one organism
  - Low discrimination—1 to 4 significant matches
  - No ID—no significant choice *or* 4 significant choices
- High resolution = better peak separation
- Calibrate with a specific *E. coli* strain
  - *E. coli* quality control is also done at the beginning and end of each run
  - One run = 16 spots. Up to 4 runs per chip
- Yeast needs formic acid before matrix to break down cell walls
- Need at least 100 profiles matched

Bioterrorism

BRUCELLA

- Slow–growing tiny gram-negative coccobacillus (can be confused with *Haemophilus*)
- Serologies are available
- Scant slow growth on blood and chocolate plates
  - Not MacConkey, which is for most gram-negative rods
  - RBM or green malachite green medium agar
- Positive for oxidase, urease, and catalase
- *One of the easiest infections to get in a micro biology lab!*
  - Ingestion or inhalation
    - Unpasteurized milk
  - PRESUME all slow-growing gram–negative *Coccobacilli* are *Brucella* until proven otherwise
  - Symptoms—nonspecific
  - Postexposure prophylaxis = doxycycline and rifampin × 21 days
- *B. melitensis*—goats and sheep
- *M. abortus*—cows
- *B. suis*—pigs
- *B. canis*—dogs

BARTONELLA HENSELAE

- Cat scratch disease
- Diagnosis (Dx)
  - Not culture or gram stain
    - Hard to stain, looks negative
  - Use silver stain (Warthin–Starry) on biopsy or test for serologies and/or DNA
- Ulceration over nodes

BACILLUS ANTHRACIS

- Anthrax
- Clinical
  - Mediastinal X-ray classic findings
  - Ulcerative cutaneous lesions
  - Death by septic shock or pulmonary edema
- Gram-positive *Bacillus* with endospores, has capsule
- *Do not open thio bottles that have a bubbly/gooey growth at the very top—it could be* Bacillus
- Medusa head colonies with comma–like projections
- Mauve capsule with Loeffler's methylene blue
- Can be easily confused with gram-negative rods (colonies look similar, loses gram stain fast, unidentified on MALDI-TOF, catalase+)
  - All bacillus species are catalase+ obligate aerobes (only growth in aerobic bottle and catalase+ → motility test!)
  - Motility test
    - Thio broth at 4 hours incubation
    - NON-MOTILE

- Nonhemolytic, wide–zone lecithinase+, mannitol+, xylose–
- Induce spore production with urea, esculin, and/or TSI slants (48 hours)
  - Spore production = *Bacillus*
- Sheep blood agar (SBA) with vancomycin disk
  - Any inhibition = gram positive, including *Bacillus*
  - Resistant = gram-negative rods are resistant
- Treatment: [ciprofloxacin *or* doxycycline] + [rifampin *or* vancomycin *or* penicillin *or* imipenem *or* clindamycin]

YERSINIA PESTIS

- Bubonic or pneumonic presentation
- Closed safety pin appearance

FRANCISELLA TULARENSIS

- Tularemia
- Clinical
  - Highly infectious—only 10 bacteria needed to cause severe disease
  - Animal handling
  - Types of disease: glandular, systemic, pneumonic, typhoidal
  - Ulcerative granular lesions
  - Treatment: streptomycin, gentamicin, doxycycline
- Sterile MacConkey, faint gram-negative *Coccobacilli*
- Negative for oxidase and catalase
- See Table 22.2.

Bacteria

ALGORITHMS

- See Figs. 22.1 to 22.8.
- See Table 22.1.

TABLE 22.2 ■ *Francisella tularensis* vs. *Yersinia pestis*

Francisella tularensis	Yersinia pestis
Tiny gram-negative coccobacilli	Plump gram-negative bacilli
Intracellular	Safety pin staining
Oxidase negative	
Grows on SAB/choc (not on MAC)	Grows on MAC
SAB, Sabouraud's agar; *MAC,* MacConkey agar.	

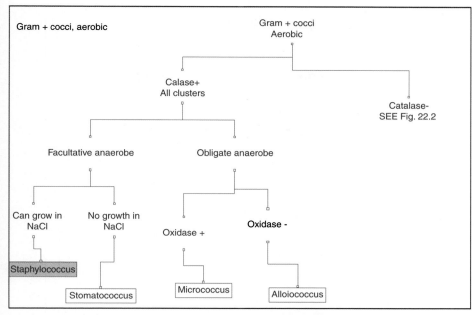

Fig. 22.1 Aerobic gram-positive cocci, catalase positive. *NaCl,* Sodium chloride.

SEPARATED BY METHOD OF METABOLISM

Aerobes

- Microaerophilic
  - *Helicobacter pylori*
    - Shipped on ice, <3-hour transport
    - Campy and blood plates put into a pouch (CO_2 production packet)
    - Tiny (pinpoint) translucent colonies that look like dust
    - Positive for oxidase and urease
    - Purpose of cultures is to find an effective antibiotic in patients with refractory *Helicobacter* gastritis

Anaerobes

- Obligate (*Fusobacterium, Peptostreptococcus*), moderate (*Bacteroides*) (can tolerate 15 to 20 minutes of oxygen), microaerotolerant (can grow in oxygen but grow better without; *Clostridium*)
  - Depends on amount of superoxide dismutase
- Clues: smells bad, near mucosal surfaces, animal or human bite, gas on specimen, previous antibody failure, necrosis/abscess, unique gram stain morphology, no growth on anaerobic plate
- Intrinsically resistant to aminoglycosides and quinolones
- Blood agar plate *(Brucella)*, phenylethyl alcohol agar, *Bacteroides* bile esculin agar, egg yolk agar *(C. difficile)*, THIO broth (anaerobe and aerobe)
- Anaerobes can be flora (which can become pathogenic, more than aerobes)
  - Produce fatty acids and vitamins
  - Oral cavity—*Fusobacterium*
  - Colon—*Bacteroides*

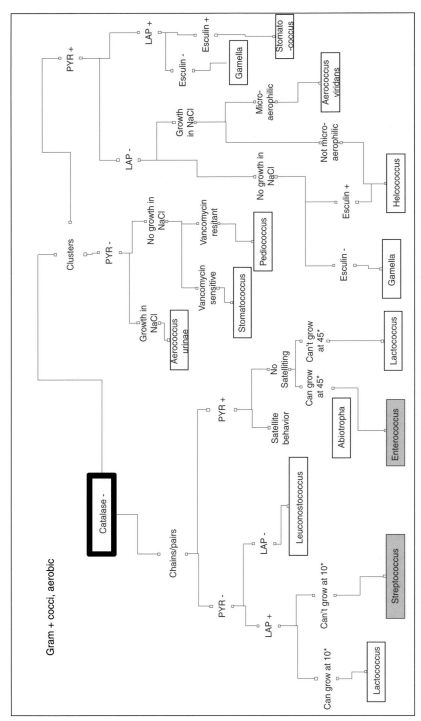

Fig. 22.2 Aerobic gram-positive cocci, catalase negative. *NaCl,* Sodium chloride.

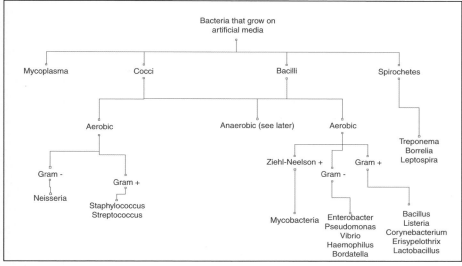

Fig. 22.3 Bacteria that grow on artificial media.

- Anaerobic gram negative causing abdominal infections
  - *Bacteroides*—bile resistant
  - *Prevotella*—bile sensitive, saccharolytic
  - *Porphyromonas*—asaccharolytic
- Obligate anaerobes
  - *Clostridium* (gram-positive cocci)
  - *Bacteroides* (gram-negative cocci)
    - Resistant to colistin, penicillin, kanamycin, and vancomycin
    - Susceptible to erythromycin and rifampin
  - *Fusobacterium* (gram-negative cocci)
    - Halitosis! Smells like bad breath on plate.
    - *Cutibacterium acnes*
    - *Prevotella*
- Cocci
  - Gram positive
    - **Peptostreptococcus*
    - *Peptoniphilus asaccharolyticus*
      - Commensal, can cause opportunistic infections
    - *Finegoldia magna*
    - *Parvimonas micra*
  - Gram negative
    - *Veillonella**
- Rods
  - Gram positive
    - *Actinomyces (israelii)**
      - Aerotolerant
      - "Molar tooth" growth, sulfur granules
      - Gram positive, partially acid fast, modified acid fast (mAF) negative

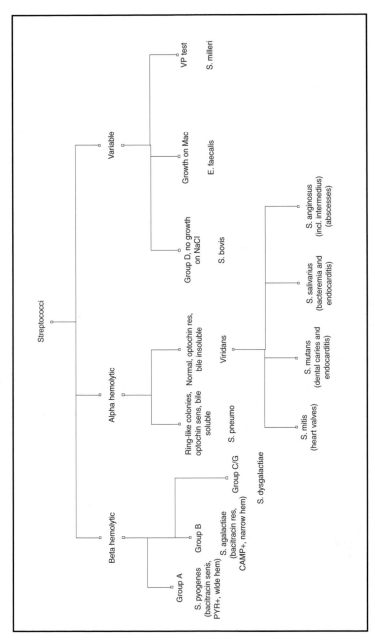

Fig. 22.4 *Streptococci.*

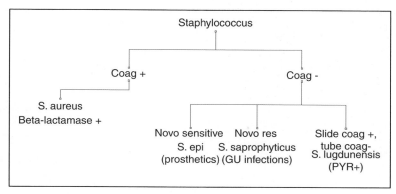

Fig. 22.5 *Staphylococci.*

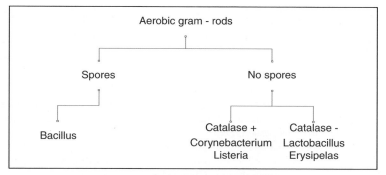

Fig. 22.6 Aerobic gram-negative rods.

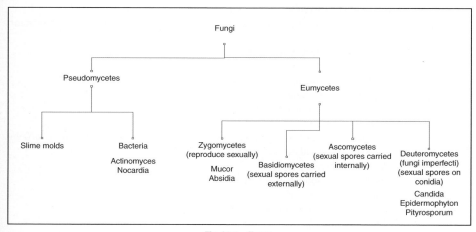

Fig. 22.7 Fungi.

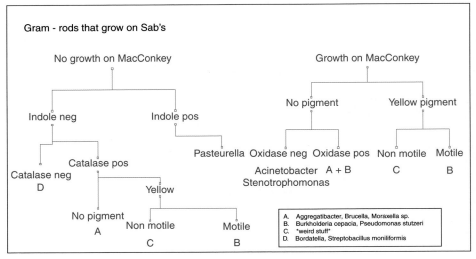

Fig. 22.8   Gram-negative rods that grow on Sabouraud agar.

- Has bacillary and coccoid forms, but usually considered rod
- Risk factors for orofacial actinomyces infection: poor dental hygiene, smoking, diabetes, heavy alcohol use, immunosuppression
- Differential diagnosis (DDx):
  - Nocardia—aerobic, catalase positive, mAF+
  - *Corynebacterium*—club–shaped, aerobic, catalase positive, mAF neg
    - Group and palisade like "Chinese letters"
    - Also called diphtheroids
    - Must confirm pathogenicity (part of normal flora)
- *Cutibacterium acnes**
  - Infections in joint replacements and acne, skin commensal
  - Anaerobic gram-positive rod, kanamycin/vancomycin sensitive, colistin resistant, indole+, catalase+
  - Severe or deep infections need extended cultures (10 to 14 days)
- *Lactobacillus*
- *Clostridium** (Only one to form spores!)
  - Box car, stiff, gram variable rods
    - Really are gram positive but lose stain very early
  - *C. difficile*
    - Produces two toxins (*tcdA* and *tcdB*) → can test for toxin B gene (*tcdB*) by PCR = gold standard but ≥96 hours!
    - NAP1 strain more virulent
    - CCFA plate—fluoresces chartreuse under UV
    - Smells like horse manure
  - *C. botulinum*—gram positive
    - Terminal spore
  - *C. perfringens*
    - Two zones of β-hydrolysis

- Rarely grows spores in vitro (compared with other *Clostridium*)
- Brick–like
- *C. tetani*
  - Thin with terminal spores
- *C. septicum*—swarming growth, blood agar plate shows very thin layer of bacteria
- *C. tertium*
  - Aerotolerant, catalase negative
  - Normal flora, but can be opportunistic
- Gram negative
  - **Bacteroides*
    - *B. fragilis* is resistant to kanamycin, vancomycin, and colistin
  - **Fusobacterium*
    - Lemierre syndrome
      - Pharyngitis, peritonsillar abscess, jugular thrombophlebitis
      - *F. necrophorum > nucleatum*
    - Long, slender, white breadcrumb colonies
    - Oral cavity → brain abscess, chronic sinusitis, osteomyelitis, arthritis, pleuropulmonary
    - Treat with penicillins
  - *Capnocytophaga*
  - **Porphyromonas*
  - **Prevotella*
  - *Campylobacter*

Fermenters

- See Fig. 22.9.

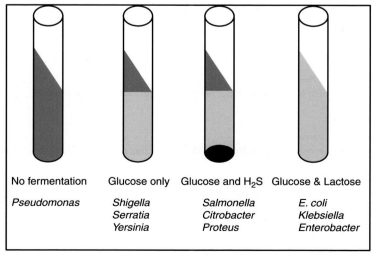

Fig. 22.9 Fermentation studies.

GRAM-POSITIVE COCCI

Streptococcus

- Alpha hemolysis
  - *Streptococcus pneumoniae*
    - "Pneumococcus"
    - Lancet–shaped diplococci on Gram stain
    - Grayish, coin–like or ring–like colony with depressed center
      - "Draughtsman colonies"
    - PYR–, LAP–
    - Optochin sensitive, vancomycin sensitive
    - Pneumonia treated with penicillin G or second- or third-generation cephalosporin
  - Many alpha-hemolytic *Streptococci* are considered normal urogenital flora, but sensitivities are still performed
    - Let clinician decide how to treat
  - *Streptococcus anginosus*
    - Butterscotch smell
    - Can be pleomorphic
  - Alpha-group *Streptococcus* vs. *Enterococcus* on SBA plates
    - Alpha-hemolytic streptococci have large hemolysis zone
      - Exception: VREs are big with large hemolysis zone (usually *E. faecium*)
    - *Enterococcus* will have bigger colonies after 24 hours
- *Beta hemolytic* streptococci categorized by Lancefield groups (depending on cell wall antigens)
  - *S. pyogenes* = group A
    - Patients from care facilities can get GAS bacteremia
    - Fasciitis, pharyngitis, erysipelas, sepsis
  - *S. agalactiae* = group B
    - Chains in certain growth condition
    - May cause neonatal meningitis (screen mother's vaginas for GBS)
  - Group C and group G—weird "group" that may just be *S. dysgalactiae subsp. dysgalactiae*
    - Others are seen in animals (equi, canis, zooepidemicus)
    - *S. dysgalactiae subsp. equisimilis* → pharyngitis in adolescents
- Beta *Streptococcus* hemolysis zones
  - A and C/G—large
    - Can differentiate using serologies against Lancefield antigens for epidemiology and etiology
  - B *(agalactiae)*—small
- *Streptococcus mitis* is glucan negative, *Streptococcus aurelius* is glucan positive

Staphylococcus

- *Staphylococcus aureus*
  - Neon yellow colonies on mannitol/MSA plate (transparent)—*Staphylococcus aureus*
    - Catalase+ (bubbles)
    - Need MALDI-TOF to confirm
  - All *Staphylococcus aureus* from significant sources need to be put on Mueller–Hinton plate with stamper disks
    - Lawn of growth by inoculating in three directions
  - *Staphylococcus aureus*
    - Light yellow/gray (creamy), shiny colonies with *beta hemolysis*
      - *S. lugdunensis* colonies are white

- *Staphylococcal* protein A (spa) is specific for SA
  - SCCmec = genetic element carrying mecA (gene for methicillin resistance) gets inserted into orfX
- Other *Staphylococci*
  - *S. saprophyticus* (see later)
  - *S. epidermidis* (see later)
  - *S. saccharolyticus*
    - Only catalase-negative clinically significant *Staphylococcal* species
    - Prefers anaerobic but will get scant growth in aerobic environments
      - Coagulase negative
- DDx for urinary tract infection caused by *Staphylococcus*
  - *S. saprophyticus*—usually symptomatic, resistant to novobiocin
    - Urease positive, treat with nitrofurantoin
  - *S. epidermidis*—asymptomatic, sensitive to novobiocin
- See Table 22.3.
- *Staphylococcus* and *Micrococcus* are BOTH gram-positive cocci, catalase positive
  - *Staphylococcus* = facultative anaerobe, bacitracin resistant
  - *Micrococcus* = obligate anaerobe

Other Gram-Positive Cocci

- *Aerococcus viridans*
  - Gram-positive cocci in pairs and tetrads
  - Alpha-hemolytic, PYR+, LAP–
  - Vancomycin susceptible

GRAM-NEGATIVE COCCOBACILLI

- *Haemophilus influenzae*
  - Gram-negative *coccobacilli*
  - Anaerobe on sheep blood plate (no growth), can grow aerobically in the presence of hemin (factor X) and NAD (factor V), both are found in hemolyzed blood
    - Grows on chocolate plates (hemolyzed blood), not blood plates
    - Can grow in satellite formation around beta-hemolyzers
    - Sub from *Haemophilus influenzae* isolation plate to chocolate plate
      - *H. influenzae* isolation plate also grows yeast well

TABLE 22.3 ■ *Staphylococcus* Speciation

	Coagulase			
Staphylococcus Species	Slide	Tube	PYR	Ornithine Decarboxylase
S. lugdunensis	+/–	–	+	+
S. aureus	+	+	–	–
S. epidermidis	–	–	–	variable
S. schleiferi	+	–	+	–
S. haemolyticus	–	–	+	–

Slide coagulase negatives should always be confirmed with tube coagulase → S. aureus can have false negatives.

- On rabbit blood agar—can grow, but no hemolysis
- Gray and creamy to colorless, medium-sized monomorphic colonies
- Does not flake off
- Gamma hemolysis (none)
- Type b
  - Sepsis, infant pneumonia, meningitis
  - Now vaccine
- *Haemophilus haemolyticus*
  - Growth with beta-hemolysis on rabbit blood agar
- *Bordetella*
  - See Table 22.4.
  - *B. pertussis*
    - TINY faintly staining gram-negative *coccobacilli*
    - Bordet Gengou agar and Regen–Lowe media are selective
      - Grows in 1 week, then use immunofluorescence
    - Peripheral blood lymphocytosis with butt cells
  - *B. bronchiseptica—coccobacillus/bacillus* that grows on MAC within 24 hours
    - Respiratory pathogen
    - Oxidase positive, urease positive
- *Acinetobacter baumannii*
  - Oxidase negative, nonmotile, gram-negative *coccobacilli*
  - Nonfermenter
  - Colorless on MAC
  - Multidrug resistant
  - Clinical
    - Nosocomial → ventilator-associated pneumonia, bacteremia, wound infections, urinary tract infections, meningitis, ostomy infections
    - Outbreaks in military in Iraq and Afghanistan
    - Can survive for weeks on fomites
  - Biofilm producer, omp38 causes host cell apoptosis
  - Best antibiotics = carbapenem or sulbactam (+ polymyxin B in very resistant infections)
- *Pasteurella*
  - Animal bites
  - *P. multocida* more common than *P. canis*
  - Three clinical presentations
    - Localized, cellulitis and lymphadenopathy
    - Exacerbation of chronic lung disease
    - Systemic (usually in immunocompromised people)

TABLE 22.4 ■ *Bordetella* Speciation

Bordetella Species	Growth on SAB and MAC	Oxidase	Reduces Nitrate	Motile	Urease Production
B. pertussis	–	+	–	–	–
B. parapertussis	+	–	–	–	+*
B. bronchiseptica	+	+	+	+	+**

*in 24 hours.
**in less than 4 hours.
SAB, Sabouraud's agar; MAC, MacConkey agar

- Grows on blood and chocolate (nonhemolytic) but not on MacConkey
- Musty odor
- Treat with penicillin
- *Brucella* and *Tularemia* (see "Bioterrorism" earlier)
- *Prevotella*
  - Anaerobic gram-negative bacilli or *coccobacilli*
  - Indole+, lipase–
  - Resistant to kanamycin and vancomycin
  - Susceptible to colistin
  - Oral flora, female genital tract infections

GRAM-NEGATIVE DIPLOCOCCI

- *Neisseria*
  - Chocolate plates, all oxidase+
  - Ability to ferment sugars
    - See Table 22.5.
  - *N. meningitidis*
  - Ferments glucose and maltose
  - Capsular groups—A, B, C, W-135, X, Y
    - B, C, W-135 cause epidemics in industrialized countries
    - Quadrivalent vaccine against A, C, Y, W-135
  - Prophylaxis for close contacts = rifampin, ciprofloxacin, or ceftriaxone
  - Treatment = penicillin G, cephalosporins, chloramphenicol, rifampin
  - *N. gonorrhoeae*
    - Virulence factors
      - Pili (adhere and phagocytosis)
      - Outer membrane porin protein (phagocytosis)
      - Lipo-oligosaccharide surface protein (tissue damage)
    - Treatment: 1 IM injection of ceftriaxone and 1 oral dose azithromycin
- *Moraxella*
  - Ear infections, lower respiratory infections, normal vaginal flora
  - Will grow on blood plate but not CNA, *waxy* colonies
    - Has hockey–puck sign—if palpated with stick, will slowly move along intact (others will break apart or be sticky)
    - Butyrate esterase = "*Moraxella* disk"
  - Beta-lactamases → resistant to penicillins
  - Nitrate+, oxidase+, asaccharolytic

TABLE 22.5 ■ *Neisseria* Species' Abilities to Ferment Sugar

Sugar	N. meningitidis	N. gonorrhoeae	N. catarrhalis
Glucose	+	+	–
Maltose	+	–	–
Sucrose	–	–	–
Lactose	–	–	–

GRAM-POSITIVE RODS

- *Bacillus*—all are spore-forming gram-positive rods, obligate aerobes that are catalase+
  - Only growth in aerobic bottle and catalase+ → motility test to rule out anthracis)
  - *B. anthracis*—(see "Bioterrorism" earlier)
  - *B. cereus*—beta hemolytic, often in long chains
- *Listeria* monocytogenes
  - Catalase+ and beta-hemolytic
  - CAMP
  - Tumbling motility → umbrella–shaped pattern in semisolid agar
  - Processed food and deli meats
  - Older adults and pregnant women (neonates with fulminant pneumonia)
  - Delicate dented rods
  - Grows at 4°C (refrigerator)
    - Thio broth in refrigerator = "cold enrichment"
    - Other bacteria do not multiply at 4°C
    - Only needed for vaginal and stool samples
    - Sub to CNA plates on day 14 and day 28
- *Corynebacteria* (see later), all listed later are black on tellurite (commensals are gray)
  - Palisade like "logs in a river"
  - See Table 22.6.
- Gram-positive rods "in broth only" needs to be subplated → incubated for 2 days → subbed to *Brucella* plate
- *Lactobacillus*—gram-positive rod, pleomorphic
  - Vancomycin resistant
  - Alpha-hemolytic
  - Makes lactic acid from (ferments) glucose/maltose/sucrose, no urease or nitrate reduction
  - Variable colony morphology
  - Catalase negative
- *Arcanobacterium haemolyticum*—curved gram-positive rod with pointed ends and branching
  - Vancomycin sensitive
  - Beta-hemolytic
  - Produces acetic acid, lactic acid, and succinic acid from glucose
  - May be confused with GAS clinically
    - Facial rash (looks like scarlet fever)

TABLE 22.6 ■ *Corynebacteria* Speciation

Corynebacteria	Features	Glucose	Maltose	Sucrose	Starch	Urea
C. diphtheriae	Volutin granules Chinese letters	+	+	–	+	–
C. hofmannii	Cone–shaped colonies	–	–	–	–	+
C. urealyticum		–	–	–	–	+
C. jeikeium		+	+/–	–	+/–	–

- Isolated from wounds
- On stain looks like *Listeria*
- *Erysipelothrix*—gram variable short rods and long filaments
  - Facultative aerobe, nonmotile, H_2S production
  - Vancomycin–resistant
  - Alpha-hemolytic
  - Produces acetic acid, lactic acid, and succinic acid from glucose
  - Clinical
    - Local (fingers) cellulitis
    - Rarely diffuse cutaneous involvement
    - Very rarely systemic—endocarditis (40% mortality rate), meningitis, and so on
- *Gardnerella vaginalis*—small pleomorphic gram variable *coccobacilli*
  - Vancomycin sensitive
  - Beta hemolytic
  - Produces acetic acid from glucose
- *Weissella*—small short gram-positive rods
  - Vancomycin resistant
  - Alpha hemolytic
  - Produces lactic acid from glucose
- *Vibrio vulnificus*
  - Severe wounds + sea water + warm weather → septicemia
  - Also consumption of raw oysters (more commonly *V. cholerae*)
  - Only *Vibrio* that can ferment lactose
- *Actinomyces* (see "Anaerobics" earlier)
- *Capnocytophaga canimorsus*
  - Gram negative, fastidious
  - Catalase+, oxidase+, indole–
  - Slightly yellow colonies, "gliding" motility causing spread across plate
  - DDx = *Pasteurella* (both from dogs)
    - Opaque/gray, no spreading, mucoid
    - Catalase+, oxidase+, indole+
- *Tropheryma whippelii*—gram-positive rods
  - Whipple disease, can be fatal if untreated
    - Needs long–term antibiotics
  - Can infect almost any organ
  - PAS+ macrophages
- DDx for beaded gram-positive rod morphology, caused by high lipid content in cell walls
  - *Mycobacterium* (do not branch)
  - *Nocardia*
  - *Tsukamurella*
  - *Actinomyces*
  - *Gordonia*
- DDx for bile resistance
  - *Fusobacterium*—sensitive to kanamycin and colistin
  - *Bacteroides fragilis*—resistant to kanamycin and colistin

GRAM-NEGATIVE RODS

- Gram-negative rods must be isolated before doing indole test
  - Mixed cultures can "share" positivity

- Indole+ bacteria break down tryptophan to indole (yellow → red)
  - *E. coli*, Citrobacter, *Haemophilus influenzae*+
  - *Klebsiella* -
- *Streptobacillus moniliformis*
  - "Rat bite fever"
  - "Haverhill fever" when ingested
  - Very pleomorphic gram-negative rod, filamentous
  - Inhibited by SPS (common additive in agar)
  - *Not* biochemically active
- *Legionella* pneumophila—thin, poorly staining
  - BCYE agar because *Legionella* needs cysteine
  - Biochemically not reactive
  - Legionnaires disease
  - Has urine antigen assay
- *Pseudomonas*
  - Mucoid and nonmucoid strains
    - *Pseudomonas stutzeri*—crinkly/crumbly and dry
    - *Pseudomonas aeruginosa*—creamy
      - Green on Mueller-Hinton plate
      - Colorless on MAC
        - Lactose nonfermenters go to oxidase (positive—PA, negative—Acinetobacter)
      - Only species that can grow at 42°C
      - Burn wounds
      - Grape–like odor
  - Oxidase+, motile, does not ferment glucose
  - Confirm using MALDI-TOF
  - *Pseudomonas dermatitis* from hot tub exposure
- *Aeromonas caviae* complex
  - Oxidase+ indole– esculin–
  - Gastroenteritis
  - Looks similar to *V. cholerae* on CIN agar but…
    - Will not grow on TCBS
    - String test
- *Eikenella corrodens*
  - Pleomorphic, can be *coccobacillary*
  - Colonies *pit* the agar and smell like bleach
  - Oral cavity flora, infects wounds associated with closed–fist injury, human bites, and so on
- *Burkholderia cepacia*
  - Transparent copper, dry and wrinkled colonies
  - Slow–growing, nonlactose fermenting, gram-negative rod, weakly oxidase positive
  - CF patients quickly decline and die
    - *Burkholderia* plates saved for 5 days for all CF patients (all others saved for 3)
  - If positive, confirm with (1) gram stain and (2) blood plate with polymyxin B disc (*Burkholderia* is resistant)
    - Resistant to *most* antibiotics
- Other nonfermenting gram-negative rods
  - *Stenotrophomonas maltophilia*
    - Obligate aerobe
    - Motile at room temperature but not at 37°C

- Polar flagella
- Nosocomial infections
- On sheep blood agar: yellow–green to gray, nonhemolytic colonies
- Ammonia smell
- *Eikenella*
- *Flavobacterium*
- *Kingella*

Enterobacteriaceae

- Gram negative, oxidase negative, facultative anaerobes
- *Citrobacter*
  - Indol positive
  - Can use citrate as the only carbon source
    - Koser citrate → blue
- *Enterobacter*
- *Yersinia* (see "bioterrorism")
- Lactose fermenting
  - *E. coli*
    - Lactose–fermenting, oxidase negative, indole positive
    - Beta-hemolytic
    - Fringy
  - *Klebsiella*
    - *K. pneumoniae*
      - Indole neg
    - *K. granulomatosis*—granuloma inguinale, beefy red primary lesion
      - Does not grow in culture
      - Bipolar staining gram-positive rods in macrophages ("Donovan bodies")
- Nonlactose fermenting
  - *Proteus*—Urease+ gram-negative rods
    - *P. vulgaris*
      - Indole+, ODC–
      - Does not swarm
      - Intrinsically resistant to ampicillin
        - Treat with quinolones or Bactrim
    - *P. mirabilis*
      - Indole—(does not need more "i"s), ODC+
      - Swarms with waves
      - Ampicillin sensitive
    - Stinky and mucoid
  - *Salmonella*—BLACK (most) and motile
    - Diarrhea begins → 4 days later: fever, abdominal pain, and hepatosplenomegaly
    - Species
      - *S. typhi*—small amount of H_2S production in TSI → black sliver at top of slant
      - *S. paratyphi* A and B—no H_2S production
      - *S. enteritidis* (and others)—lots of H_2S production
    - Ornithine carboxylase is positive in all except *S. typhi*
  - *Shigella*—colorless and nonmotile
    - All *Shigella* are mannitol+ except S. dysenteriae
    - If shiga-toxin-like 1 and 2 found, but not *Shigella*, STEC (O157:H7 or other)

■ NOTE:

■ *Shigella* and *Salmonella* may appear to be sensitive to gentamicin and first-/second-generation cephalosporins in vitro but are not in vivo (drugs cannot penetrate host cells)

MYCOBACTERIA

■ Aerobic, nonspore forming, nonmotile
■ Nontuberculous mycobacteria are found in rivers, lakes, and so on
  ■ *Mycobacterium tuberculosis* complex = pathogens/colonizers of animals
■ Mycolic acid = long-chain fatty acid that makes mycobacteria acid fast
  ■ *Nocardia* have complex shorter mycolic acid cell walls, so they stain with modified acid–fast stain
  ■ Carbol fuchsin+ heat instead of crystal violet and iodine → methylene blue instead of safranin and decolorize with hydrochloric acid and ethanol instead of ethanol and acetone
■ General laboratory methods
  ■ When trying to grow, process with sodium hydroxide (kill bacteria) and N-acetyl-1-cysteine (liberate mycobacteria)
  ■ VersaTREK and MGIT = automated incubation and recovery
    ■ Can also use high–performance liquid chromatography (HPLC), PCR, or MALDI
  ■ AFB (acid fast bacillus) stain, auramine fluorochrome
  ■ Löwenstein–Jensen (LJ) medium, 4 to 12 weeks for visible growth
  ■ Species that need low temps to grow
    ■ *M. marinum*
    ■ *M. haemophilum*
    ■ *M. chelonae*
    ■ *M. ulcerans*
  ■ *M. fortuitum* can grow on routine agar (MacConkey) within 7 days
  ■ The only tests that can be performed directly on fresh samples
    ■ Fluorochrome stain and nucleic acid amplification test (NAAT)
      ■ Currently NAAT is only available for *M. tuberculosis* (MTb) complex
  ■ Tests that can be performed on bacteria after culture—niacin test, carbol fuchsin stain, DNA probe, HPLC, sequencing
  ■ Can be speciated based on pigment production in the light, light and dark, or neither
    ■ See Table 22.7.

TABLE 22.7 ■ *Mycobacterium* Speciation by Pigment Production

Nonchromogens: No Pigment	Photochromogens: Make Pigment in Light	Scotochromogens: Pigmented in Light and Dark
Tuberculosis	Kansasii	Scrofulaceum
Bovis	Marinum	Avium intracellulare
Ulcerans	Avium intracellulare	Xenopi
Malmoense	Simiae	Fortuitum
Avium intracellulare		
Leprae		
Chelonae		

- Species
  - See Table 22.8 and Fig. 22.10.
  - MTb complex
    - Species
      - *M. tuberculosis*
        - "Breadcrumb" colonies—dry and wrinkled
        - 32° to 36°C
        - Slowly growing
        - Produces niacin!
        - Cording in Middlebrook broth
        - Subtyping *M. tuberculosis* is important
        - Gold standard = RFLD using IS6110

TABLE 22.8 ■ *Mycobacterium* and Sites of Infection

Site	Organisms
Lung	MAC, tuberculosis, kansasii, xenopi, abscessus
Lymph node	MAC, MTb, scrofulaceum, haemophilus
Skin/soft tissue	Fortuitum, chelonae, abscessus, marinum, ulcerans, haemophilum
Gastrointestinal	MTb, MAC

MAC, Mycobacterium avium-intracellulare complex; *MTb, Mycobacterium tuberculosis* complex.

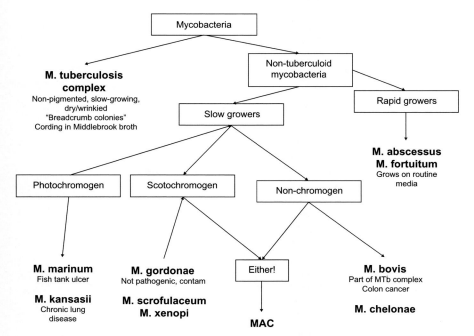

Fig. 22.10 Mycobacterium. *MAC, Mycobacterium avium* complex.

- Mycobacterial interspersed repetitive units/variable # tandem repeat (MIRU-VNTR) typing may be the future
  - *M. bovis*
    - LJ slants with pyruvate instead of glycerol, 36°C, can produce tuberculous disease ("Tb")
      - Cancer in the colon, bovis in the blood
    - Others: *M. microti, M. africanum, M. canetti, M. caprae, M. pinnipedii*
- Standard identification
  - Culture on mycoselective media
  - DNA probes
  - Biochemical tests
- Presentations
  - Classically cavitary lung lesions
  - Miliary spread
  - Hypersensitivity pneumonitis
  - HIV patients with a CD4+ T cell count less than 200 get lung infiltrates, not cavitary lesions
  - Tuberculous pleural effusions
    - Turbid, yellow–green metallic sheen
    - Lymphocytosis with occasional clusters (from fibrin trapping)
    - Rare to no mesothelial cells
    - Dx: AFB stain, culture, PCR, adenine deaminase and interferon
- Normal treatment
  - Isoniazid, rifampin, pyrazinamide, ethambutol
- *M. marinum*
  - Fish tank ulcer
  - Open wound exposed to seawater
  - <35°C
- *M. avium–intracellulare* complex (MAC)
  - "Atypical mycobacteria" (along with *M. kansasii*)
  - Lab features
    - Slow–growing nonchromogen (or scotochromogen)
    - 25° to 44°C
  - Clinical features
    - Disseminated disease in immunocompromised
    - Chronic lung disease
      - Chronic obstructive pulmonary disease with bronchiectasis
      - Hypersensitivity pneumonitis–like syndrome after hot tub exposure
    - Number 1 cause of cervical lymphadenopathy in children
- *M. leprae*
  - Leprosy, 4- to 8-hour incubation
  - Slit skin smears with Ziehl-Neelsen stain
  - Cutaneous leprosy = irregular annular patches
    - Diagnosis (Dx): lepromin skin test (like tuberculin skin test)
    - Therapy: 12 months of rifampicin, dapsone, and clofazimine
- *M. kansasii*
  - Lung disease (mimics classic Tb)
  - Most important photochromogen
- *M. abscessus*
  - Rapid grower

- Group IV—rapid growers of non-Tb mycobacterium (NTM)
  - Citrate–, nitrate–, NaCl+
  - Skin and soft tissue infections, postoperative wounds
- *M. fortuitum*
  - Rapid grower!
  - Fe uptake+, nitrate+
- *M. ulcerans*
  - Mud under stagnant waters
  - Painless lump → ulcer at site of trauma
  - < 30°C
- *M. scrofulaceum*
  - Scotochromogen
  - Cervical LAD in children = scrofula
- *M. gordonae*
  - Nonpathogenic scotochromogen
- *M. haemophilum*
  - Skin nodules in AIDS patients
  - <35°C
  - Needs hemin
    - Use chocolate agar or add ferric ammonium citrate
- *M. malmoense*
  - Scandinavia
  - May take up to 8 weeks to grow
  - Lung disease (classically middle–aged men with previous pneumoconiosis) and cervical lymphadenopathy in children
- *M. xenopi* and *M. simiae*
  - Israel
  - Joint, respiratory, or disseminated infections
  - *M. xenopi* likes it hot (42° to 45°C)
    - Can contaminate water sources
    - Arylsulfatase+
    - No rRNA proves commercially available yet
- *M. chelonae*
  - Slow–growing
    - Rarely fast–growing
    - No Fe uptake–, citrate+, NaCl–
  - Skin and soft tissue
  - 30° to 32°C
  - Surgical implants, catheters
- Treatments
  - High–level isoniazid resistance
    - Mutation in catalase-peroxidase gene (katG) at 315
  - Low–level isoniazid resistance
- Mutation in promoter of *mabA-inhA* gene complex
  - Airborne precautions for pulmonary Tb can be discontinued when
    - At least 3 negative AFB sputum smears AND
    - Diagnosis is made that excludes Tb or
    - Decreased clinical symptoms after 1 week of anti-Tb tx
    - **can add NAAT but not required

WEIRDO BACTERIA

- *Bartonella*
  - Gram negative "coccoid," facultative intracellular parasites
  - Vectors: ticks, fleas, sand flies, mosquitos
  - *B. bacilliformis*—Carrion disease (Oroya fever)
    - In red cells
  - *B. henselae*—cat scratch, bacillary angiomatosis
- *Mycoplasma* and *ureaplasma* are small and cannot be seen on normal gram stains
  - Do not have traditional cell wall
  - "Fried egg" or nipple–like colonies on PPLO agar
- Spirochetes
  - *Treponema pallidum*—syphilis, straight coils
  - *Leptospira*
    - Tightly coiled, hooked spirochetes with flagella for motion
    - Slow–growing obligate aerobe
    - Zoonotic from wild mammal urine
    - Microscopic agglutination test (MAT) checks serologies and requires laboratory to have live organisms to target
  - *Borrelia burgdorferi* (Lyme) or *recurrentis* (relapsing fever)—wavy/loose coils
    - Lyme disease
      - Treat with doxycycline, amoxicillin, or cefuroxime to prevent late complications (acrodermatitis chronica and arthritis)
      - IgG peak at 4 to 6 months
      - NAAT on synovium in Lyme arthritis—50% to 85% sensitive
  - *Rickettsia typhi* and *rickettsii*
    - Cross–react with proteus antigens
  - *Coxiella burnetii*—Q fever
    - Inhalation of aerosolized animal waste
    - Most are asymptomatic, 5% hospitalized
    - Fibrin ring granulomas in the liver
    - Large cell and small cell variants
      - Small cell variant hardier, can survive months to years outside the body
    - Diagnose acute with antibodies against phase 2 antigens
    - Diagnose chronic with antibodies against phase 1 and 2 antigens
    - Treat with doxycycline+ chloroquine
- *Chlamydia*—obligate intracellular (use McCoy cells to grow them)
  - *C. psittaci*—psittacosis, ewe abortions, from parrots
    - Dx: serologies
      - 4 × increase or one IgM ≥1:32
    - 20% fatality in untreated
      - Doxycycline, tetracycline, azithromycin
  - *C. trachomatis*
    - Blindness from strains A to C
    - Sexually transmitted infections from strains D to K
  - *C. pneumoniae*—atypical "walking" pneumonia
    - Can be grown in Hep-2 cells
    - Therapy = macrolides, doxycycline, tetracycline
    - Elementary bodies and reticulate bodies

CLINICAL SYNDROMES

- See Table 22.9.
- Ecthyma gangrenosum
  - Bloody pustules → black necrotic ulcers
  - most common cause = *Pseudomonas aeruginosa*
- Bacterial vaginosis
  - For diagnosis, need three of four
    - Clue cells on vaginal microscopy
    - Positive potassium hydroxide (KOH) amine test
    - Vaginal pH >4.5
    - Fishy, watery discharge
  - Bacterial causes: (all gram negative anaerobic)
    - *Prevotella*—bile sensitive, pigment and saccharolytic
    - *Bacteroides*—bile resistant
    - *Porphyromonas*—pigmented and asaccharolytic
    - *Mobiluncus*
    - *Gardnerella*
- Urinary tract infections
  - For asymptomatic patients, only treat pregnant women and those undergoing GU surgery
  - *E. coli* (UPEC strains)—85%
    - *Staphylococcus saprophyticus* (young, sexually active)
    - *Klebsiella, Enterobacter*
  - Bacterial culture negative → *Ureaplasma, Chlamydia, Mycoplasma*
  - BPH—*Enterococcus*
  - Indwelling catheters or recent antibiotics → *Candida*
  - Hemorrhagic cystitis—adenovirus
    - Especially type II and in BMT recipients
  - Dipstick nitrite is falsely negative with *S. saprophyticus* and *Enterococcus*
- Pneumonia
  - By location/presentation
    - See Table 22.10.
  - By underlying risk factors
    - See Table 22.11.

TABLE 22.9 ■ Unexplained (A) Bacteremia Likely Came from (B)

A	B
Hemolytic streptococcus	Thrombophlebitis of neck or pelvis
S. aureus	Endocarditis Osteomyelitis
Pneumococcus	Pneumonia Osteomyelitis Sinusitis Peritonitis Endocarditis
E. coli	Biliary tract obstruction Liver abscesses Cirrhosis (spontaneous bacterial peritonitis)

TABLE 22.10 ■ Pneumonia by Presentation

Type of Pneumonia	Organisms
Typical or lobar	*Mycoplasma pneumoniae, Chlamydia pneumoniae*
Atypical or walking	*Streptococcus pneumoniae*
Bronchopneumonia	*Haemophilus influenzae*
Necrotizing	*Staphylococcus aureus, Pseudomonas aeruginosa*
Aspiration	*S. pneumoniae, S. aureus, H. influenzae, Enterobacteriaceae, P. aeruginosa*

TABLE 22.11 ■ Pneumonia by Underlying Risk Factor

Host Risk Factors	Organisms
Chronic obstructive pulmonary disease	*Haemophilus influenzae, Moraxella, Legionella*
Alcoholism	Anaerobes, *Streptococcus pneumoniae, Klebsiella pneumoniae*, gram-negative aerobic rods
Neutropenia	Aerobic gram-negative rods
Animal exposure	*Coxiella burnetii*—cattle and cats
	Chlamydophila psittaci—birds
	Cryptococcus neoformans—birds
	Histoplasma—birds (especially pigeons) and bat droppings
	Hantavirus—mouse urine/feces
	Francisella tularensis—rabbits

- *Streptococcus pneumoniae*
  - Most common cause of community–acquired
  - Lobar pneumonia
- *S. aureus*
  - Most common cause of health care–associated pneumonia
  - Necrotizing with cavitation
  - *H. influenzae*
  - Usually nontypable
  - Bronchopneumonia
- *Legionella*
  - Underlying disease + aerosolized particles (construction, hot tubs, air conditioning)
  - "Legionnaires disease"—atypical pneumonia, high fever, hyponatremia, renal dysfunction, diarrhea, neurologic changes
  - "Pontiac fever"—flu–like illness without pneumonia
- *P. aeruginosa, S. marcescens, Acinetobacter*
  - Health care–associated pneumonia and ventilator–associated pneumonia
  - Cystic fibrosis, bronchiectasis, advanced malignancy
- Viral
  - Most common = influenza, respireatory syncytial virus (RSV), parainfluenza, rhino, adenovirus, hantavirus, metapneumovirus, coronavirus, bocavirus

- Hantavirus pulmonary syndrome (HPS)
  - Four corners of New Mexico
  - Sin Nombre virus
  - Deer mouse urine/feces
  - Flu–like → acute respiratory distress syndrome
  - Thrombocytopenia, neutrophilia (no toxic granulation), erythrocytosis, immuno-blastic lymphocytosis
- Parainfluenza—croup
- RSV—bronchiolitis
  - Second most common cause of bronchiolitis—metapneumovirus
- Gastroenteritis
  - Time to symptoms
    - *Bacillus cereus* emetic toxin—1 to 6 hours
    - *B. cereus* diarrheal toxin—10 to 16 hours
    - *Staphylococcal* enterotoxin—1 to 6 hours
    - *Clostridium perfringens* enterotoxin—8 to 16 hours
    - Nontyphoidal *Salmonella*—1 to 3 days
    - *Campylobacter*—2 to 5 days
    - *E. coli* O157:H7—1 to 8 days
  - Viruses (most common cause)
    - Noroviruses (rotavirus, Norwalk–like, enteric adenovirus)
    - Winter, vomiting and diarrhea
  - Bacterial
    - Noninflammatory—watery, no fever
      - *Vibrio cholera*—rice water stool, O1 and O139, shellfish
      - ETEC *E. coli* (cholera–like toxin)—most common cause of travelers' diarrhea
      - *C. perfringens*
      - *S. aureus*—within 8 hours
      - *B. cereus*
    - Inflammatory (dysenteric/bloody)
      - See Table 22.12.
      - Shiga toxin–producing (enterohemorrhagic) *E. coli* (STEC/EHEC)
        - Shiga toxin

TABLE 22.12 ■ **Most Common Bacterial Differential Diagnosis for Bloody Diarrhea**

	Agar	**Key Reactions**	**Transmission**
STEC	SMAC	Sorbitol fermenter	Undercooked beef Spinach
Salmonella	HE	Motile, +H_2S	Meat, poultry Undercooked eggs
Shigella	HE	Nonmotile	Contaminated water
Campylobacter	Charcoal	Microaerophilic curved/ seagull	Undercooked poultry Unpasteurized milk
Yersinia enterocolitica	Cold MAC	Grows at 25°–28°C	Swine and cattle
Vibrio parahaemolyticus	TCBS	Growth on salty media	Seafood (oysters)

HE, Hektoen enteric agar; *MAC,* MacConkey agar; *SMAC,* MacConkey agar with sorbitol; *STEC,* Shiga toxin–producing *E. coli*; *TCBS,* thiosulfate-citrate-bile salts-sucrose agar.

  Undercooked beef or contaminated milk/fruit/vegetables
  O157:H7
  Associated with hemolytic uremic syndrome
Enteroinvasive *E. coli*
  No shiga toxin
Salmonella
  Animal contact or contaminated food
  Bacteremia → seeding of bone, joints, heart, brain, and so on
Shigella
  Only needs very small inoculum (can spread by flies)
Campylobacter jejuni
  Most common cause of bacterial enteritis in the United States
  Chicken or water
  Most common cause of Guillain-Barré
  Reactive arthropathy (HLA-B27)
C. perfringens
  Spores in undercooked food
  Toxins → vomiting and watery diarrhea within 8 hours
C. difficile
  Most common cause of antibiotic-associated diarrhea
  BI/NAP1/O27—deleted *tcdC* gene → ↑ ↑ toxins A and B
  Need to test for toxin, not colonization
Klebsiella—associated with ischemic enteritis
- Parasites
  - *Entamoeba*
  - *Giardia*
  - *Cryptosporidium*
- Endocarditis
  - Native valve
    - Previously normal → **acute**
      - *S. aureus*—left in most, right in IVDA
      - *S. pneumoniae*—concomitant pneumonia and meningitis (Austrian syndrome)
    - Damaged valve → **subacute**
      - *Viridans streptococcus*
      - "Subacute bacterial endocarditis (SBE) with vegetations"
      - *S. bovis* in colorectal cancer
  - Prosthetic valve
    - Very early (≤2 months)—*S. aureus, S. epidermis*, gram-negative rods
    - Early (≤1 year)—*S. epidermis* and *S. aureus*
    - Late—similar to SBE
  - Negative blood cultures (prior antibiotics)
    - Noninfectious—Libman-Sacks, nonbacterial thrombotic (marantic), carcinoid heart syndrome
    - Infectious—*Coxiella, Bartonella, Chlamydia, Legionella, Tropheryma whippeli*, HACEK
      - HACEK = fastidious gram-negative *bacilli/coccobacilli* (aerobic, take ~3 days to grow on chocolate agar)
        - *Haemophilus* (now *Aggregatibacter aphrophilus*)
        - *Aggregatibacter actinomycetemcomitans*
        - *Cardiobacterium*
        - *Eikenella*
        - *Kingella*

- Central nervous system (CNS) infections
  - Encephalitis
    - Arboviruses (mosquito–borne) and HSV1 (necrosis of temporal lobe), HHV6 (most common cause in children), mumps, measles, VZV
    - *Naegleria* (meningoencephalitis), *Acanthamoeba* and *Balamuthia* (granulomatosis)
  - Meningitis
    - Aseptic
      - Most common cause in all ages = enterovirus (summer and fall)
      - HSV2, mumps, HIV, lymphocytic, choriomeningitis virus (LCM, most common cause in winter)
    - Bacterial
      - Neonates
        - GBS, gram-negative aerobic rods (*E. coli, Klebsiella*), *Listeria*
      - Infants → young adults
        - *N. meningitidis*: localized outbreaks, risk for Waterhouse-Friderichsen syndrome
    - Terminal complement deficiency (C5 to C9) ↑ risk
      - Adults—*S. pneumoniae* and *N. meningitidis*
      - Southeast Asia—*Streptococcus suis*
      - AIDS—*S. pneumoniae*, MTb, *Cryptococcus*
      - Tropics—cerebral malaria
- Prosthetic joint infections
  - Early (<3 months)—*S. aureus* and gram-negative rods
  - Delayed (3 to 24 months)—coagulase-negative *Staphylococcus* (CoNS), *C. acnes*
    - Cutoffs
      - Knee—1700 WBCs/mL, 65% neutrophils
      - Hip—4200 WBCs/mL, 80% neutrophils
      - Frozen section—>5 neutrophils/hpf in at least 5 hpfs
- Associations
  - *B. cereus*—cytopenias from hematologic malignancies
  - *Neisseria*—complement deficiencies
  - *Pneumococcus*—plasma cell neoplasms or asplenia
  - Recurrent/persistent *Salmonella*—AIDS
  - *E. coli*—pyelonephritis, biliary tract
  - *Streptococcus pneumoniae*—respiratory tract
  - *N. gonorrhoeae*—salpingitis
  - *B. fragilis*—decubitus ulcers
  - Group C/G *Streptococcus*—endocarditis, malignancy, alcoholism
  - *Corynebacterium*—central lines in cytopenic patient
    - Metallic sheen of colonies
  - *Erysipelothrix*—aortic endocarditis (zoonotic)
  - *Haemophilus influenzae*, mixed—endocarditis
  - *Citrobacter*—gallbladder infection
  - *Aeromonas*—fresh water exposure and wounds
  - *Pasteurella*—cat bites
  - *Vibrio*—raw oysters
  - *Campylobacter fetus*—mycotic aneurysm, thrombophlebitis
  - *Fusobacterium necrophorum*—oral abscess or internal jugular thrombophlebitis
  - *Malassezia*—hyperalimentation
    - Require lipids (sterile olive oil) overlying plate to grow
  - *Clostridium septicum*—malignancy

Fungi

GENERAL

- See Fig. 22.11.
- Blastoconidia
  - Reproduction via new buds
  - *Cryptococcus, Candida glabrata, Malassezia*
- Pseudohyphae
  - Seen in combination with blastoconidia
  - Other *Candida* species, saccharomyces
- Arthroconidia
  - Split up previously existing hyphae into conidia
  - *Trichosporon, Coccidioides* when in mold form
- See Fig. 22.12.

SUPERFICIAL

- Hyphae and/or arthrospores on Sab's agar = fluffy/powdery
- Dematiaceous (melanin–producing) molds
  - Fast growers
    - Transversely septated conidia
      - *Bipolaris, Drechslera, Exserohilum, Helminthosporium, Curvularia*
    - Transversely and longitudinally septated conidia
      - *Alternaria, Ulocladium, Stemphylium*

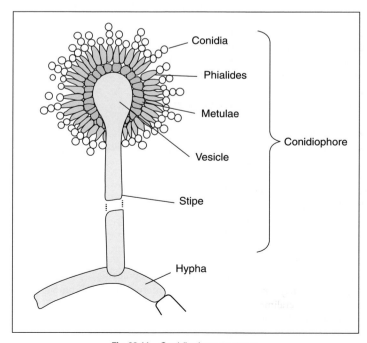

Fig. 22.11   Conidiophore anatomy.

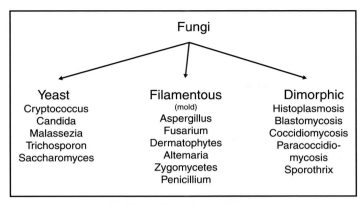

Fig. 22.12 Categorization of fungi.

- Slow growers
  - Early = yeast–like, late = mold–like
    - *Exophiala, Wangiella, Hortaea*
  - Early and late = mold–like
    - *Pseudallescheria boydii/Scedosporium boydii* complex
      - Light bottom (nonmelanized hyphae)
      - Resistant to amphotericin
      - Susceptible to voriconazole
    - *Scedosporium prolificans*
      - Dark bottom
      - Resistant to all antifungals
  - Three types of infection
    - Chromoblastomycosis
    - Mycetoma (also by *Nocardia*)
    - "Other" = phaeohyphomycosis
- Epidermophyton—rough–walled, pyriform macroconidia
- Microsporum—rough–walled, fusiform macroconidia
  - Wood's lamp at 365 nm
    - *Microsporum audouinii, M. canis, T. schoenleinii*—fluoresce
- *Trichophyton*—smooth–walled, cylindrical macroconidia and spiral hyphae
- Sporotrichosis (*Sporothrix*)
  - Dimorphic (yeast in humans)
  - Primary ulcerating nodule at site of injury/inoculation
  - Secondary nodules after lymph drainage
  - Cigar–shaped yeast, conidiophores with rosettes of microconidia
  - "Rose gardener disease"
- *Fusarium*—nonpigmented
  - Canoe–shaped macroconidia
  - Fungal keratitis associated with contaminated contact lens infection; sinusitis, nail infections, septic arthritis
  - Natamycin for several months
- *Penicillium marneffei*
  - Southeast Asia

- Dimorphic, red diffusible pigment
- Tan colonies → blue/green with time
- *Syncephalastrum racemosum*
  - Saprophytic (feeds off decaying plants)
  - Rare cause of systemic/nail infections
  - 45-degree branching, sparse septations
  - Conidia directly attached to vesicle (no intervening phialides)

ENDEMIC

- Coccidiomycosis—Southwest United States (TX, AZ, NM, CA) and Mexico
  - Barrel–shaped arthroconidia
  - Spherules containing endospores
  - Granulomatous cutaneous lesions
  - Sabouraud dextrose agar → glabrous (smooth) mold colonies
  - Disseminated, vertebral, pulmonary
- Histoplasmosis—Mississippi River Valley, Northeast United States, Mexico, Central America
  - Waxy at 37°C on agar (yeast forms)
  - Intracellular yeast
  - Can involve spleen (especially in infants) and lymph nodes
  - Narrow budding
  - Macro- and microconidia at 25°C
  - Calcified lung lesions
- Blastomycosis—endemic area overlaps with histoplasmosis
  - Mold at 25°C (glabrous and waxy) and yeast at 27°C (granular)
    - Darken to tan with age
  - Potassium hydroxide and calcofluor white
  - Broad–based budding
  - One cell conidia on conidiophores (hyphae)
    - "Lollipop" conidia
  - When budding, daughter cell smaller than mother cell
  - Infection—cutaneous, lung, brain, and so on
- Paracoccidioides—"mariner's wheel"

OPPORTUNISTIC

- *Aspergillus*
  - *A. fumigatus*, *A. niger* (black conidia, otitis externa)
  - Clinical—angioinvasive or fungus ball
  - Diagnosis
    - Galactomannan = cell wall component of aspergillus
    - +enzymatic immunoassay of blood helps diagnose invasive aspergillosis
  - Classical conidiophore structure
  - Branched septate hyphae
  - Smokey green colonies with velvety texture
  - Species
    - *A. fumigatus*
      - Conidia on top two-thirds of vesicle
      - Top of plate—blue–gray with white apron
      - Bottom—pale

- *A. flavus*
  - Conidia all the way around vesicle
  - Top of plate—yellow to olive with white apron
  - Bottom—pale
  - Aflatoxin—hepatocellular carcinoma
- *A. niger*
  - Top—dark brown/black
  - Bottom—light
  - Circumferential biseriate (two layers)
    - Like *A. flavus* but two layers
  - Calcium oxalate tissue deposition
- *A. terreus*
  - Top—cinnamon brown
  - Bottom—yellow or orange
  - Arthroconidia like *A. fumigatus* but two layers and longer chains
  - Resistant to amphotericin B
- *Cryptococcus*
  - Sabouraud dextrose agar, wet mount with India ink, calcofluor white, mucicarmine, urease activity
  - YEAST SIZE HAS GREAT VARIATION
  - Brain lesions are classic, but can also get pneumonia
  - Cross–reaction with rheumatoid factor for cryptococcal antigen
  - See Table 22.13.
  - Cryptococcal meningitis in immunosuppressed
    - Low glucose, high WBCs (lymphocytes)
    - Broad–based budding
    - Fontana–Masson and mucicarmine stain capsule
    - Treated with amphotericin
- *Candida*
  - Sab's agar (white), CHROMagar (for speciation)
  - Chlamydoconidia, blastoconidia, pseudohyphae
  - Chronic mucocutaneous infection classically secondary to T cell defects
  - "Loves the kidney"
  - Large gram-positive blastophores
  - See Table 22.14.
  - On CHROMagar:
    - *C. albicans*—blue–green with germ tube formation at 37°C (so does dubliniensis) within 3 hours
      - Other *Candida* species have pseudohyphae directly from blastoconidia
    - *C. tropicalis*—dark blue
    - *C. krusei* and *glabrata*—pink/violet

TABLE 22.13 ■ *Cryptococcal* Speciation

C. neoformans	C. gattii
Most infections in the United States	Mostly tropics
Soil contaminated with bird feces	Soil near eucalyptus trees
Encapsulated, cell walls have melanin, mucoid colonies, never form pseudohyphae	

TABLE 22.14 ■ *Candida* Speciation

C. albicans	C. glabrata
Colonies with feet	No feet on colonies
Green on CHROMagar	No color change on CHROMagar
Germ tubes	No germ tubes
Morphology on Tween: pseudohyphae, clusters of blastoconidia at septations, terminal chlamydospores	Morphology on Tween: just budding yeast
Negative trehalose use	Positive trehalose use
Susceptible to azoles, echinocandins, amphotericin	Resistant to azoles, susceptible to echinocandins and amphotericin
Fast grower	Slow grower

- On cornmeal agar
  - *C. albicans*—chlamydoconidia and regular spherical blastoconidia
  - *C. tropicalis*—randomly placed blastoconidia
  - *C. krusei*—branched pseudohyphae
- *Zygomycetes* (mucormycosis)
  - Systemic, rhinocerebral, pulmonary, other organs
  - Aluminum or iron overload, ketoacidosis, deferoxamine
  - Nonseptate (or pauci-septate) ribbon–like hyphae (broad)
  - "Lid lifters"—grow very fast
  - *Rhizopus*—rhizoids directly opposite sporangiophores
  - *Mucor*
- *Pneumocystis jirovecii* (PCP)
  - AIDS patient with CD4+ <200 cells/mL need prophylaxis (trimethoprim-sulfamethoxazole)
- Using underside of plate for mold identification
  - Top and bottom light—hyaline septate molds (*Aspergillus, Penicillium, Fusarium*)
  - Top and bottom dark—dematiaceous molds (*Alternaria*)
  - Top dark, bottom light—zygomycetes (*Rhizopus, Mucor*)

Parasites

SINGLE–CELL PARASITES = PROTOZOA

- Mucosal
  - Microsporidia (*Enterocytozoon bieneusi*)—diarrhea
    - Obligate intracellular parasite
  - *Entamoeba*
    - Clinical features
      - Prolonged bloody diarrhea in traveler or immigrant
      - Liver abscesses = "anchovy paste–like"
      - Cecal "flask–shaped ulcer"
    - Stool enzymatic immunoassay is best test because microscopy is identical to *E. dispar*, which is not pathogenic
    - In general, cyst looks more complicated than trophozoite

- Species
  - *E. histolytica* trophozoites eat red blood cells; is motile
    - Characteristic "dot in ring" nucleus
  - *Entamoeba coli* (different from *Escherischia coli*) is BIG with up to 8 nuclei in cyst and frayed/inconspicuous chromatoidal bars
  - *E. hartmanni* is tiny (<10 microns)
- *Giardia intestinalis*—diarrhea
  - Cysts in stool, trophozoites in duodenum
  - Falling leaf motility by trophozoites
  - Cysts oval with four nuclei along central bar (axoneme)
    - Same central bar in trophozoite
- *Trichomonas vaginalis*—vaginitis
  - Central axostyle in trophozoite, one nucleus
  - No cyst form
- *Cystoisospora belli*—diarrhea (especially in immunocompromised)
- *Cryptosporidium*—diarrhea (especially in immunocompromised)
  - Oocyst = infective form, contains four sporozoites that invade enterocytes and become trophozoites
- *Cyclospora cayetanensis*—diarrhea
  - Thick–walled oocyst
  - Requires modified acid fast stain or autofluorescence with UV light
- *Balantidium coli* (ciliate)—diarrhea
  - Only ciliated parasite that infects humans
  - Big, round, boring trophozoite
  - Small-ish, plain, round/dome cysts
- *Chilomastix mesnili*—flagellated intestinal protozoan
- *Iodamoeba butschlii*—intestinal amoeba that uses pseudopods
- Blood and tissue
  - *Naegleria fowleri*—swimming pools, meningitis, enters brain through cribriform plate, "brain–eating parasite" in popular media
    - Free–living, 10 to 35 microns
    - Blob–shaped trophozoite
    - Flagellated state resembles giardia
    - Culture on lawn of *E. coli*
    - Do not refrigerate
  - *Trypanosoma*
    - *T. brucei*—African sleeping sickness, tsetse fly
      - Trypomastigotes in blood
    - *T. cruzi*—Chagas disease, reduviid bug
      - Amastigotes in tissues
      - North/Central/South America
      - Clinical
        - Chagoma and Romaña sign (periorbital edema)
        - Myocarditis
        - Destroy Auerbach plexus → dilation of esophagus and colon
      - Therapy = nifurtimox and benznidazole
  - *Leishmania*—sand flies—amastigotes in monocytes/macrophages—"hemoflagellate"
    - Oriental sore (forehead)—*L. tropica*
    - Mucocutaneous leishmaniasis—*L. brasiliensis*
    - Visceral leishmaniasis/kala azar—*L. donovani*

- Organism–laden macrophages accumulate in liver and spleen
- *Plasmodium*
  - General
    - Tropics worldwide
    - Gametocytes are ingested by mosquitoes → *Anopheles* mosquito bite → sporozoites go to the liver to proliferate extracellularly → schizonts (like egg sacs) rupture and release merozoites into blood → merozoites enter RBCs and proliferate more → trophozoite → EITHER schizont or gametocyte
    - Proliferation = schizogony—exoerythrocytic (in liver) or erythrocytic
    - RBCs infected with P. ovale may be oval and fimbriated
    - Children and pregnant women are at the highest risk for death
    - >2% parasitemia is severe
    - Presents in 1 to 4 weeks of inoculation
  - EDTA, thick and thin smears
  - Species
    - See Table 22.15.
    - *P. falciparum*
      - Tertian fever (q48h)
      - Most deadly
      - Cerebral malaria
      - "Blackwater fever"—hemosiderinuria, hemoglobinuria, and renal failure
      - Sequestrates to endothelium
  - Inserts Pfemp (protein) into RBC membrane which adheres to CD36 on endothelium and other RBCs → sludging, hypoxia, ischemia, ring hemorrhage (cerebral malaria)
    - *P. vivax* and *P. ovale*
      - Tertian fever (q48h)
      - Generally mild
      - Can get true relapse after therapy (from merozoites in the liver)
    - *P. malariae*
      - Quartan fever (q72h)
      - Nephrotic syndrome
  - Inherited disorders and effect
    - HbS protects against *P. falciparum*

TABLE 22.15 ■ **Plasmodium Features and Treatment**

	P. falciparum	**P. vivax/ovale**	**P. malariae**
Early trophozoite (ring)	Marginal, headphones, multiple	Schuffner dots	Bird's eye
Late trophozoite	N/A	Schuffner dots	Band
Schizont (merozoites are inside)	N/A	Vivax (12–24 dots) Ovale (6–14 dots)	Rosette around hematin
Gametocyte		Schuffner dots	No Schuffner dots
Treatment	1—chloroquine or hydroxychloroquine 2—mefloquine +/– artesunate, quinine, quinidine, pyrimethamine-sulfadoxine	Chloroquine + primaquine (for killing merozoites/ gametes in liver)	Chloroquine

- Thalassemia, HbC, HbE, ↑HbF thought to protect against malaria
- Duffy negative protects against *P. vivax*
- G6PD deficiency protects against all
- Hereditary ovalocytosis protects against cerebral malaria
- Diagnosis
  - Draw blood right before next anticipated fever
  - Thick smear for screening
  - Need to look at 100 high–power fields
  - Thin smear for speciation
  - 300 high–power fields

- *Toxoplasma gondii*—chorioretinitis and blindness in 60% of in utero infections
  - Can also be in animals like pigs (as intermediate hosts); humans get infection through consumption of raw meat
  - Classically cat urine
  - **B**radyzoites = **b**ig (see later)
    - Seen in chronic infections, always in cysts
  - Tachyzoites = small
    - Seen in acute infections
  - Acute phase lymph node biopsy = clusters of epithelioid histiocytes impinging on germinal centers and paracortical monocytoid B-cell expansion
- *Acanthamoeba* (and *Balamuthia mandrillaris*)
  - Corneal infections associated with contact lens use ("amebic keratitis"), can have CNS spread → "granulomatous amebic encephalitis"
  - Enters at skin or lungs
  - Found in tap water
  - Culture on plate with lawn of *E. coli* to see their tracks
- *Ehrlichia chaffeensis*
  - Monocytes and macrophages as morulae
  - Deer → *Amblyomma* tick → human
- *Anaplasma phagocytophilum*
  - Granulocytes as morulae
  - Vector is the *Ixodes* tick
  - Is immunosuppressive to host (can present like HIV)
- *Babesia*
  - Maltese cross and ring forms
  - Can be outside red blood cells
- For the differential diagnosis of small intracellular organisms, see Table 22.16.

MULTICELLULAR PARASITES = HELMINTHS

- See Fig. 22.13 for ova comparison.

Trematodes = Flukes

- Intestinal
  - *Fasciolopis buski* = giant intestinal fluke
    - Yellow greasy stools
    - Asia (India)
    - Large
  - *Fasciola hepatica* = sheep liver fluke
    - Middle East, smaller

TABLE 22.16 ■ Tiny (<5 microns) Intracellular Organisms

Parasite	Intracellular Form	Extracellular Form	Vector
Leishmania	Histiocytes, amastigotes have small kinetoplast perpendicular to nucleus (black arrow), GMS negative	N/A	Sand fly
Histoplasma (*fungus*)	GMS positive, narrow–based budding, in histiocytes (not amastigote!)	N/A	N/A
Toxoplasma	Bradyzoites in large vesicle, GMS negative	Mostly extracellular curved tachyzoites, some in cyst	N/A
Trypanosoma cruzi	Cardiac muscle = classic, amastigotes with large kinetoplast parallel to nucleus, GMS negative	Large posterior kinetoplast	Reduviid (kissing) bug
Trypanosoma brucei	None	Small posterior kinetoplast with prominent undulating membrane	Tsetse fly

- *Clonorchis sinensis* = Chinese liver fluke
  - Asia, undercooked fish
  - Chronic biliary infection → biliary obstruction → fibrosis → cholangiocarcinoma
  - Therapy = praziquantel
- Blood
  - *Schistosoma*
    - General
      - Bathing/swimming in snail–infested water
      - Fever, skin rash, transverse myelitis
    - Species, see Table 22.17.
      - *S. mansoni*—Africa and South America
      - *S. haematobium*—Africa and Middle East
      - *S. japonicum*—Far East
- Lung
  - *Paragonimus westermani* = lung fluke
    - Snails → crustaceans → human
    - Far East and the Pacific
    - Lung infections and pneumonitis
    - Eggs found in feces, opercular shoulders
    - Therapy with praziquantel

Cestodes = Tapeworms

- Intestinal
  - *Diphyllobothrium latum*—fish tapeworm
    - Longest cestode! (up to 30 feet!!!)
    - Life cycle, see Fig. 22.15.
    - Segments (proglottids) are wider than tall
    - Causes B_{12} deficiency
    - Yellow, elongated scolex (look like labia)

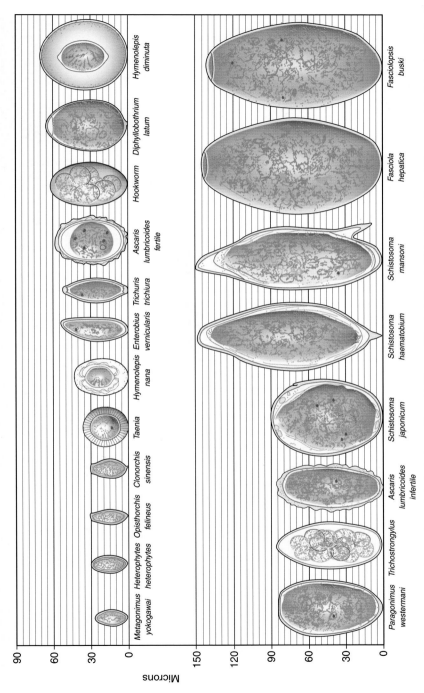

Fig. 22.13 Comparison of ova sizes and morphologic features. (From McPherson RA, et al: Henry's Clinical Diagnosis and Management by Laboratory Methods. 22nd edition. Philadelphia: Elsevier. 1219, 2011.)

TABLE 22.17 ■ *Schistosoma* Speciation

Species	Locale	Disease	Egg
S. mansoni	South America, Africa, Middle East, Caribbean	Cirrhosis, proctitis, colitis	See Fig. 22.14.
S. japonicum	Far East	Cirrhosis	
S. haematobium	Africa, Middle East	Bladder → squamous cell carcinoma	
S. mekongi			Similar to *S. mansoni*
S. intercalatum			Similar to *S. haematobium* but acid–fast

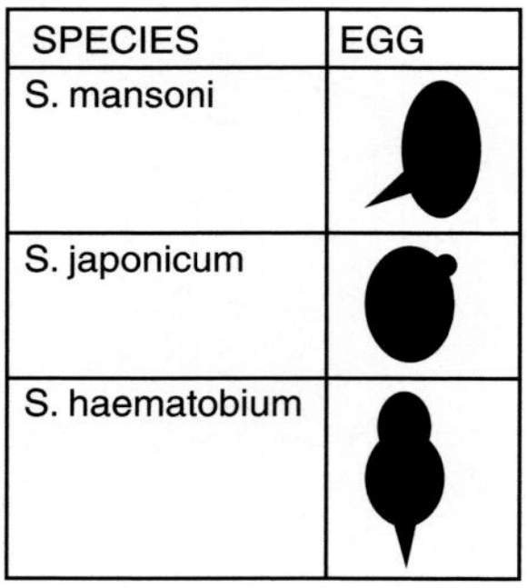

SPECIES	EGG
S. mansoni	
S. japonicum	
S. haematobium	

Fig. 22.14 *Schistosoma* egg morphology.

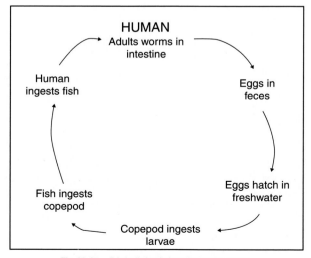

Fig. 22.15 *Diphyllobothrium latum* life cycle.

- Gefilte fish, ceviche, sushi, carpaccio
- *Taenia solium*—pork
  - Scolex = four suckers and many tiny hooklets
  - Proglottid is longer than it is wide
  - <13 uterine branches
  - Found in the United States
  - Intestinal infection from eating encysted larvae
    - → Feces from organism with intestinal infection contaminates soil around produce → ingested → cysticercosis
    - Eggs are not infectious → no cysticercosis
  - Egg: (with three hooklets)
- *Taenia saginata*—beef
  - Same as *T. solium* except....
    - Scolex = four suckers and smooth surface
    - >13 urine branches
    - Not in the United States
- *Hymenolepis nana*
- Tissue
  - *Taenia solium*—Cysticercosis
    - Use steroids with praziquantel to decrease immune response
  - *Echinococcus* (hydatid cysts)—dog tapeworm (near sheep)

Nematodes = Roundworms (filariasis)

- Intestinal
  - *Ascaris lumbricoides*
    - One worm can lay up to 200,000 eggs per day
    - Eggs are bile–stained, 60 microns, thick mammillated shell (grenade)
  - *Enterobius vermicularis*—pinworms
    - Worm has lateral alae
    - Egg is 30 to 50 microns, thin wall
  - Hookworms
    - Can cause iron deficiency
    - Eggs
    - *Ancylostoma duodenale*—teeth
    - *Necator americanus*—cutting plates
    - Treatment—albendazole, mebendazole, pyrantel pamoate
  - *Strongyloides stercoralis*—infection can last decades
    - Eggs not seen in stool, only young (rhabditiform) larvae
    - Hyperinfection can be lethal
    - Versus hookworms—*S. stercoralis* has a shorter buccal cavity, more prominent genital primordium
    - Treatment
      - Uncomplicated—ivermectin, albendazole
      - Hyperinfection—ivermectin/albendazole PLUS broad–spectrum antibiotics
  - *Trichuris trichiura*—whipworm
    - Asymptomatic most commonly
    - Dysentery, rectal prolapse in children
- Blood and tissue
  - Transmitted via mosquito
    - *Wuchereria bancrofti*—elephantiasis

- Tail sheath without nuclei
  - *Wuchereria* is without nuclei in the tip
- Adults found in lymphatics, parasitemia at night
- Vectors: *Culex, Aedes, Anopheles* mosquitoes
- Immunochromatographic card test (ICT)
  - Semiquantitative, point of care, detects circulating antigen
- Africa, South America, Asia, Pacific Islands, Caribbean
- Brugia malayi is very similar to *W. bancrofti*, but has two discontinuous tail nuclei
- *Loa loa*
  - Adults in subcutaneous and conjunctiva (crawl across globe)
    - Leads to blindness
  - Tail sheath with continuous nuclei
    - *Loa loa*'s nuclei "flow-a flow-a" to the tip
  - Diurnal parasitemia
  - West Africa
  - Vector = mango fly (chrysops)
  - Calabar swellings—marked edema when worms are in transit
    - Classically periorbital
  - *W. bancrofti* and *loa loa* have obligate intracellular bacterial symbiotes (*Wolbachia*)
    - If you give antibiotics to kill the bacteria, the worms die
- *Onchocerca volvulus*
  - Diagnosis: skin snips
  - Symptoms caused by immune response
  - Involves skin (craw-craw) and eyes (river blindness)
  - Sub-Saharan Africa
- *Dracunculus medinensis*—guinea worm
- *Trichinella spiralis*
  - Circumorbital edema
  - Can be seen in skeletal muscle, always in 2½ coils
  - Undercooked pork and wild game
    - Will likely see a cyst in the meat
  - Invade muscle because of high oxygen → secrete immunosuppressive products = "muscle nurse cell"
  - CNS manifestations
    - Cerebral artery obstruction
    - Vasculitis
    - Allergic reaction
    - Granulomatous inflammation
  - Europe (especially Romania), Americas, New Zealand
  - Diagnosis: indirect immunofluorescence, latex agglutination (acute), ELISA (IgG antisecretory antigen)
- *Toxocara canis/catis*—dogs and cats
- *Mansonella perstans/ozzardi*
  - Vector = midges (*Culicoides*)
  - Skin, lymphatics, pericardium, peritoneum, pleural cavity
  - No tail sheath
  - Diagnosis: skin snips
- *Dirofilaria immitis* (dog heartworm)
  - Vector: mosquito
  - Subcutaneous or pulmonary granuloma around dead worm

- Dual infections involving parasites
  - *Ascaris lumbricoides* and *Trichuris trichiura*
  - Pinworms and *Dientamoeba fragilis*
  - Babesia, lyme, *Anaplasma phagocytophilum*
  - Leprosy or HTLV-1 and *Strongyloides stercoralis*
- Primary oculocutaneous
  - *Loa loa*—adult worm
  - *Onchocerca*—larva
- Person-to-person spread
  - *Enterobius vermicularis*
  - *Hymenolepis nana*
- Immunodeficient patients
  - T cells
    - Many are common (e.g., *Toxoplasmosis, Cryptosporidium, Cyclospora*)
    - Some severe—*Strongyloides*
  - B cells—*Giardia*
  - Splenectomy—babesiosis

Insects and Ectoparasites

- *Cimex lectularius* = bed bug
  - Macroscopically visible (compared with scabies, which are not)
- Mosquito species
  - *Anopheles* (tan–brown)
    - Malaria
    - Filariasis
    - Alpha- (Venezuelan equine), flavi- (St. Louise encephalitis), and bunyaviruses
  - *Aedes aegypti* (black with white dots)
    - Filariasis
    - Alpha- (chikungunya), flavi- (dengue, yellow fever), and bunyaviruses (Californian encephalitis)
      - *Aedes aegypti* is number 1 vector (not *Anopheles*)
- *Sarcoptes scabiei* = scabies mite
  - Mostly affect wrinkled/thin skin
  - Only skin-to-skin transmission (do not need to disinfect bedding)
- *Amblyomma americanum* = "lone star tick"
  - Red brown
  - Females have white spot on scutum
  - Posterior anal groove
  - Spreads ehrlichiosis and tularemia
- *Ixodes scapularis*
  - Black legged, smallest
  - Anal grove is anterior (points toward head)
  - Can transmit Lyme (Borrelia), Anaplasma, and Babesia
    - Coinfection of 1 or more of the aforementioned AND flavivirus possible (Powassan virus)
- *Dermacentor andersoni* = "Rocky Mountain spotted tick"
  - Females have partial scutum on inferior; soft area can engorge
  - Posterior anal groove
  - Spreads Rocky Mountain spotted fever and tularemia

- Centipede
  - Hundreds of legs, only tropical varieties, produce harmful bites
- Millipede
  - Thousands of legs, cylindrical and segmented body, squirts irritating fluids

VECTORS

- Sandflies
  - Leishmaniasis
  - Oroya fever (bartonellosis)
  - Phlebovirus
- Mosquitos
  - Alpha-, Flavi-, Bunyaviruses
  - Malaria
  - Filariasis
- Black fly—*Onchocerca*
- *Tabanidae—Loa loa* (calabar swelling)
- Tsetse—sleeping sickness (African trypanosoma)
- Reduviid bug—chagas disease (South American trypanosoma)
- Flies
  - Diarrheal illnesses
  - Trachoma
- Lice
  - Typhus
  - Trench fever
  - Relapsing fever
- Fleas
  - Plague
  - Typhus
- Ticks
  - Lyme
  - Relapsing fever
  - Rickettsial
  - Flavi-, Alpha-, Bunyaviruses
  - Babesia
- Mites
  - Scrub typhus
- Water flea
  - Guinea worm
  - *Diphyllobothrium latum*
- Crabs and crayfish—*Paragonimus westermani*

Viruses

- MRC5 cells used for herpes family viral culture
- LLC-MK$_2$—mumps and parainfluenza viral culture
- Viral cytopathic effect and cell culture features (see Table 22.18).

TABLE 22.18 ■ **Viral Cytopathic Effect and Cell Culture Features**

HSV	Ground glass, intranuclear, multinucleate Grows rapidly in any cell type (1–3 days) Sweeping globular cells that start at edge
VZV	(same) Grows poorly in culture and not at all in HEp2/HeLa cells
CMV	Intranuclear (Cowdry A) and intracytoplasmic (Cowdry B), cytomegaly "Owl's eye"—do *not* become multinucleated Only grows in HDF cells → focal plaques in 2 weeks
Adenovirus	Amphophilic or basophilic intranuclear, mature = "smudge cell" HEp2/HeLa is best → grape-like clusters <1 week
Rhinovirus	Focal swollen cells; will not grow in HEp2 or HeLa cells
Influenza/mumps/ parainfluenza	No cytopathic effect Use guinea pig red blood cells to absorb via hemagglutinins
Enterovirus	Angular, teardrop–shaped <1 week
Parvovirus	Nuclear inclusions in erythroblasts in bone marrow (and fetal liver)
Measles	Multinucleated giant cells ("Warthin Finkeldey cells" or reticuloendothelial cells), nuclear and cytoplasmic
RSV	Rare, pink cytoplasmic Syncytial cells in HEp2/HeLa in 2 weeks
Rabies	Negri body: sharply defined eosinophilic cytoplasmic neuronal; found in Purkinje cells in hippocampus and cerebellum
HPV	Koilocytosis
Molluscum	Eosinophilic, large cytoplasmic
JC/BK	Enlarged amphophilic, glassy oligodendroglia or urothelial cells

NONENVELOPED RNA VIRUSES

- *Picornaviridae*–RNA, insensitive to ether (enveloped)
  - Smallest (pico!)
  - *Poliovirus, Coxsackievirus, Rhinovirus, hepatitis A virus*
  - Enteroviruses = polio, coxsackie, ECHO (enteric cytopathic human orphan)
    - Orphan means there is no specific disease association, though it is now associated with meningitis, neonatal infections, rashes
    - Angular
  - Coxsackie
    - A group—hand-foot-mouth, herpangina
    - B group—myalgia, meningitis, myocarditis, pericarditis, pleurodynia (the grippe)
- *Caliciviridae*—RNA, nonenveloped
  - Calyx—cup-shaped depressions on surface
  - Noroviruses, other diarrheal illnesses
- *Rotaviridae*—double-stranded RNA, nonenveloped
  - Double–layer capsid
  - Only group A infects humans
  - Cleaved in GI tract to infectious subviral particles (ISVP)

- G and P surface antigens form serotypes (no cross–immunity)
- Major cause of childhood winter diarrhea
- Rotavirus
  - Does not grow in cell culture
  - Can chronically infect immunosuppressed patients
  - Diagnosis: RT-PCR on stool or emesis
  - Needs low inoculum (as few as 10 virions)
  - Resistant to drying, fecal–oral, contaminated foods
- Vaccines (two oral doses) → decrease hospitalizations by >80%

ENVELOPED RNA VIRUSES

- Envelopes
  - Made of lipid
  - Do not survive long on fomites
  - Lose infectivity if envelope is lost
  - Inactivated by detergents/ether
  - Have glycoprotein spikes that mediate attachment
- Arboviruses
  - *Flaviviridae*
    - Hepatitis C
      - Diagnosis, see Table 22.19.
      - Endpoint of treatment = negative serologies for 24 weeks
      - Genotype 1 is the most common in the United States
        - 1a—60%—more likely to be treatment resistant
        - 1b—10%
    - Yellow fever
      - Extensive midzonal hepatic necrosis without an inflammatory component
    - Dengue fever
    - St. Louis fever
  - *Togaviridae*—Eastern equine, rubella, chikungunya
    - Immunity to rubella wanes
      - Must test for IgG in pregnant women (first trimester congenital disease is commonly fatal)
  - *Bunyaviridae*
    - Nairo
    - Hantavirus
      - Hemorrhagic fever with renal syndrome

TABLE 22.19 ■ **Diagnosis of Hepatitis C**

Stage	Anti-HCV EIA	RIBA	RNA
Very early infection	−	−	+
Current (acute or chronic) infection	+	+	+
False positive	+	−	−
Cleared infection	+	+	−

EIA, Enzyme immunoassay; *HCV*, hepatitis C virus; *RIBA*, recombinant immunoblot assay; *RNA*, ribonucleic acid.

- Mild in northern Europe
- Severe in Far East and Balkans
- Moderate everywhere else
- Hantavirus pulmonary syndrome
  - Caused by "sin nombre" in North/Central/South America
  - 60% mortality!
- *Coronaviridae*—severe acute respiratory syndrome (SARS), Middle East respiratory syndrome (MERS), COVID-19
  - Pleomorphic, helical with glycoprotein (GP) spikes
  - Tends to undergo drastic mutations
- *Rhabdoviridae*—rabies
  - Genus = *Lyssavirus* (Greek for "rage")
  - Vectors in developing world = cats and dogs
    - Vectors in developed world = bats, wolves, coyotes, foxes, raccoons, skunks
  - Enters at neuromuscular junction
  - Fast retrograde axonal transport
- *Retroviridae*—enveloped, cuboidal capsid
  - Linear RNA → DNA → host genome
  - Human immunodeficiency virus (HIV)
    - Use pol gene products—reverse transcriptase, endonuclease, integrase
    - Lentivirus subfamily (slow)
    - Attachment using gp41 and gp120 (encoded by env region)
    - Capsid and matrix encoded by gag region
    - Prenatal screening
      - Test high–risk women in early first trimester and again in third
      - If unknown HIV status and in labor, do rapid test
      - If unknown status and delivered, do rapid test of mother and baby (treatment should start within first 12 hours of life)
    - CD4 counts
      - Undergo daily (diurnal) variation, age difference
      - Monitor every 6 months in stable disease
      - Used in initiating prophylactic therapy
    - VIRAL LOAD is better than CD4 for treatment response and predicts 10-year outcome better
      - CD4 is better for 6-month outcome
      - Combo is better for all!
      - Change > 0.5 log = significant
      - Used for determining when to start HAART
  - Human T-lymphotropic virus-1 (HTLV1)
    - Tropical spastic paresis (myelopathy)
    - Adult T-cell leukemia/lymphoma
      - Thirst, hepatosplenomegaly, jaundice, hypercalcemia, ↑↑ free IL-2 receptor, weight loss
  - Coculture of infected and noninfected peripheral blood mononuclear cells used
- *Arenaviridae*—LCM (lymphocytic choriomeningitis), Lassa virus
  - Has ribosomes that look like grains of sand (*arena* is Latin for sand)
- *Orthomyxoviridae*—Influenza A, B, C
  - H#N#
    - Hemagglutinin—attach to host cell
    - Neuraminidase—release progeny
  - Antigenic drift—season to season

- Shift—dramatic, 10 to 20 years, outbreaks
- Segmented RNA
- *Paramyxoviridae*—parainfluenza, mumps, measles, respiratory syncytial virus (RSV), human metapneumo
  - Nonsegmented RNA
  - Measles—subacute sclerosing panencephalitis (SSPE) occurs in 0.001%
  - RSV—100% infective
    - Recurrence is very common, as we have little immunity to it. Disease severity decreases each episode
- *Filoviridae*—Marburg, Ebola
  - Filamentous

DNA VIRUSES

- Parvovirus—Parvo B19
  - Nonenveloped
- Adenovirus
  - Nonenveloped
  - Respiratory infection with serotypes 1 to 14 and 21
  - Hemorrhagic cystitis—11 and 21
  - Gastroenteritis (in children)—40 and 41
    - Subgenus F
    - No eye or lung symptoms
    - Villous atrophy with crypt hyperplasia
    - Diagnosis: PCR or ELISA
- Papovavirus
  - Nonenveloped, circular dsDNA
  - Papillomavirus (HPV)
    - Epidermodysplasia verruciformis—autosomal recessive, ↓ defense against HPV → "tree boy"
    - HPV-driven squamous cell carcinoma of the head and neck is p16+, favorable prognosis
    - HPV genotypes (see Table 22.20).

TABLE 22.20 ■ Human Papillomavirus (HPV) Genotypes

Lesion	HPV Types
Plantar/common/flat wart	1, 2, 4, 3, 10 (7 in meat/fish handlers)
Oral and laryngeal papilloma	3, 10
Epidermodysplasia verruciformis	2, 3, 10, 5, 8
Genital warts (can go to verrucous carcinoma)	6, 11
Low–grade squamous intraepithelial lesion	6, 11
High–grade squamous intraepithelial lesion	16, 18, 31, 33
Adenocarcinoma in situ or invasive adenocarcinoma	18, 16, 45
Recurrent respiratory papillomatosis (bimodal curve—2–4 years and 20–40 years)	6, 11
Bowenoid papulosis	16, 18
Anogenital squamous cell carcinoma	16, 18

- Polyomaviruses
  - JC and BK
    - Childhood primary infection → latency in epithelium of genitourinary tract and lymphs
    - JC ("Junky Cerebrum") becomes reactivated in AIDS → progressive multifocal leukoencephalopathy (PML, demyelination)
    - BK ("Bad Kidney") reactivates and causes hemorrhagic cystitis or nephropathy, usually in the setting of kidney transplant
  - Merkel cell polyomavirus—dsDNA, nonenveloped icosahedral
    - Clonally integrated and mutated in 80%
    - Normal skin (without clonal integration or mutation) in 15%
    - Associated with chronic lymphocytic leukemia too
  - The -va part of Papova not pathogenic
- Hepadnavirus
  - Hepatitis B
    - Enveloped, dsDNA with one circular strand and one partially circular strand
    - HBsAg—presence >6 months is indicative of chronic Hep B
      - Can be associated with polyarteritis nodosa
    - HBeAg—hepatitis B envelope antigen, indicates highly infectious
      - "HBeAg-negative chronic hepatitis"
        - Circulating DNA
        - Fluctuating liver transaminases
        - Risk for fulminant hepatitis → liver failure
        - Mutations in C or pre-C regions of hepatitis B DNA, adding a stop codon
    - HBeAb does not mean resolved or immune—just means not actively replicating
      - Positive in chronic carriers
    - HBsAb—indicates immunity
    - HBcAb—IgM arises during acute, IgG after acute
    - >10^5 HBV DNA copies = replicative
  - Hepatitis D—DNA, can only infect with hepatitis B
- Human herpes virus (HHV)
  - HHV1 = herpes simplex virus-1 (HSV-1)
    - Becomes dormant in trigeminal nuclei
  - HHV2 = herpes simplex virus-2 (HSV-2)
    - Becomes dormant in sacral ganglia, will not cause encephalitis (only meningitis)
  - HHV3 = varicella zoster virus (VZV)
    - Congenital: mom symptomatic, neonate has dermatomal outbreak
      - Highest risk in third trimester
    - Ramsay Hunt syndrome—reactivation alone geniculate ganglion of facial nerve—otalgia, unilateral palsy, vertigo, hearing loss, and tinnitus
  - HHV4 = Epstein–Barr virus (EBV)
    - Primary infection = infectious mononucleosis
      - See Table 22.21.
    - Enters through pharynx or genitals
    - Enters B cells via C3d receptor (CD21)
    - Atypical lymphocytosis (CD8+ T cells)
    - Latent in B cells (episomally)
    - X-linked lymphoproliferative disease (Duncan disease)
      - Males, *SH2D1A (SAP)* gene
      - Causes overactivation of T/NK cells → fulminant mononucleosis
      - Frequently fatal

TABLE 22.21 ■ **Laboratory Evidence of Epstein-Barr Virus Infection**

Stage	Heterophile antibodies	IgM anti-VCA	IgG anti-VCA	IgG anti-EA	Anti-EBNA
Uninfected	–	–	–	–	–
Early acute	–/+	+	+	–	–
Acute	+/–	+	+	+	–/+
Convalescent	–	–	+	+	+
Remote	–	–	–/+	+	+

EA, Early antigen; *EBNA*, Epstein–Barr nuclear antigen; *VCA*, viral capsid antigen.

- Hepatic necrosis
- Hemophagocytosis
- Agammaglobulinemia
- Aplastic anemia
- B-cell lymphoma
- Burkitt lymphoma—100% caused by EBV in endemic, 25% in sporadic
- Hodgkin lymphoma—Hodgkin/Reed–Sternberg cells EBV+ in 50%
- Primary effusion lymphoma—HHV8—100%, EBV—70%
- Lymphomatoid granulomatosis = systemic angio-destructive lymphoproliferative disease
- Post-transplant lymphoproliferative disorder (>95%)
- Oral hairy leukoplakia—HIV patients (EBV-encoding RNA in situ hybridization may be falsely negative)
- Nasopharyngeal carcinoma—100% EBV-related in Chinese and Inuit, 75% in United States
- Heterophile antibody = strong affinity for bovine red blood cells that are not inhibited by guinea pig kidney antigen absorption
  - Specific but not sensitive—only 40% of children are positive with acute disease
- HHV5 = cytomegalovirus (CMV)
  - Primary disease usually is asymptomatic
  - Infection → IgM → low-avidity IgG → high–avidity IgG → immune
  - Congenital: low birth weight, microcephaly, intracerebral calcifications, hepatospleno-megaly, jaundice, chorioretinitis, thrombocytopenia, petechiae
    - Long–term sensorineural hearing loss
  - Latent in T cells, histiocytes, and endothelial cells
- HHV6 and HHV7 = roseola infantum = sixth disease or exanthem subitum
  - Most roseola cases caused by HHV6
  - Can cause encephalitis
  - Febrile seizures
  - Reactivates in ~50% bone marrow transplant recipients
- HHV8 = Kaposi sarcoma and primary effusion lymphoma
  - Latent in B cells and endothelial cells
  - LANA1+ speckled nuclear immunohistochemistry
- Poxviruses
  - Largest and most complex
  - Lipid envelope but are infectious without it!

TABLE 22.22 ■ **Hepatitis Virus Overview**

Hepatitis	Family	Genetic Material	Route
A	*Picorna-*	RNA	Fecal/oral
B*	*Hepadna-*	DNA	Parenteral
C**	*Flavi-*	RNA	Parenteral
D	*Hepadna-*	DNA	Parenteral
E		RNA	Fecal/oral
G***	*Flavi-*	RNA	Parenteral

*Becomes chronic in 2% to 10% of adults, higher in children
**60%–85% chronicity.
***Not currently known to be pathogenic.

- dsDNA, linear
- *Orthopoxvirus* = smallpox, monkeypox, cowpox viruses
- *Parapoxvirus* = orf virus
- Unclassified = molluscum contagiosum

See Table 22.22 for hepatitis virus overviews.
See Table 22.23 for diagnostic modalities for important viral infections.

Antibiotics

MECHANISMS OF ACTION

1. Damage cell membrane
   a. Polymyxins
   b. Daptomycin
2. Inhibits transcription
   a. Rifampicin
3. Inhibit cell wall synthesis
   a. Cycloserine fosfomycin
   b. Vancomycin
   c. Beta lactams
      i. Penicillins
      ii. Cephalosporins
      iii. Monobactams
4. Damage DNA or ↓ DNA replication
   a. Sulfonamides
      i. Inhibit dihydropteroate synthase
   b. Trimethoprim
      i. Inhibits dihydrofolate reductase
   c. Nalidixic acid
   d. Fluoroquinolones
      i. DNA gyrase
      ii. Example: ciprofloxacin
   e. Metronidazole

TABLE 22.23 ■ **How to Diagnose Viral Infection**

HIV	ELISA (p24 protein within 2–3 weeks) Confirm with Western blot (need two or more: p24, gp41, gp120/160) or PCR	Adenovirus	Serologies (+IgM or 4× ↑ IgG) Antigen testing PCR Histology Culture
HTLV1	ELISAConfirm with Western blot or PCR	Parvovirus	Histology, IHC FISH PCR No culture (not cost-effective)
Rabies	Skin biopsy	Bocavirus	PCR (minor respiratory illness)
Rhino	RT-PCR (better than culture at 32°C)	EBV	Monospot Histology and ISH
RSV	Direct fluorescent antibody test (tests for antigens, DFA) or EIA Culture in HEp2/HeLa PCR	HHV8	FISH PCR IHC for LANA1 Serologies (IFA, ELISA, Western blot)
Mumps	NAT Serology Culture	CMV	Serologies (+IgM or 4× ↑ IgG) pp65 antigen on WBCs by DFA PCR Histology Culture
Para-influenza	Hemadsorption (infected host cells express viral antigens!) after culture Antigen (IF) PCR	VZV	Same as CMV except DFA performed on skin Congenital: neonatal IgM or persistent IgG
Influenza	Culture DFA (30 minutes) NAT/PCR Hemadsorption (hemaglutination) Serology (hemagglutination inhibition)	HSV	Culture (2–3 days, quick!) PCR Tzanck smear (Giemsa stain) Histology
HCV	EIA (serologies) Recombimmunoblot assay (RIBA) RNA PCR		
HBV	SerologiesPCR	HAV	Serologies (IgM anti-HAV)

CMV, Cytomegalovirus; *DFA,* direct fluorescent antibody; *EBV,* Epstein-Barr virus; *EIA,* enzyme immunoassay; *ELISA,* enzyme–linked immunosorbent assay; *FISH,* fluorescent in situ hybridization; *HAV,* hepatitis A virus; *HBV,* hepatitis B virus; *HCV,* hepatitis C virus; *HHV,* human herpesvirus; *HIV,* human immunodeficiency virus; *HSV,* herpes simplex virus; *HTLV,* human T-lymphotropic virus; *IF,* immunofluorescence; *IFA,* indirect fluorescent antibody; *IHC,* immunohistochemistry; *ISH,* in situ hybridization; *NAT,* nucleic acid testing; *PCR,* polymerase chain reaction; *RSV,* respiratory syncytial virus; *RT,* reverse transcriptase; *VZV,* varicella–zoster virus.

5. Inhibit protein synthesis
   a. Aminoglycosides
      i. Tobramycin
      ii. Gentamicin
   b. Tetracyclines
   c. Chloramphenicol
   d. Macrolides
   e. Lincosamides
   f. Oxazolidinones
   g. Fusidic acid
   h. Mupirocin
- Topoisomerase IV is the main antibiotic target for gram-positive bacteria
  - Topoisomerase II (gyrase) is the main target for gram-negative bacteria
  - Quinolones inhibit *both*
- Polypeptide antibiotics = bacitracin, colistin, polymyxin B
  - Interferes with dephosphorylation and recycling of the lipid carrier that transports peptidoglycan (PG) precursors through membrane
- Glycopeptide = vancomycin
  - Stops formation of bridges between PG layers by interacting with the D-Ala-D-Ala termini of pentapeptide side chains
    - Microorganisms can be intrinsically resistant by having D-Ala-D-Ser instead
- Lipopeptide = daptomycin
  - Irreversibly binds to membrane causing depolarization
- Beta-lactams—penicillin and derivatives, cephalosporins, monobactams (aztreonam), and carbapenems (imipenem, meropenem)

MECHANISMS OF RESISTANCE

1. Alternative metabolic pathway
   a. Trimethoprim
   b. Sulfonamides
2. Altered porin
   a. Cephalosporins
3. Altered enzyme binding
   a. Nalidixic acid
   b. Fluoroquinolones
4. Antibiotic pumps
   a. Multiple! Most notable—tetracycline
5. Inhibit antibiotic uptake
   a. Tetracycline
6. Antibiotic-destroying enzyme
   a. Beta-lactams
   b. Penicillins
   c. Cephalosporins
   d. Monobactams
7. Altered cell wall binding sites
   a. Vancomycin
8. Antibiotic–modifying enzymes
   a. Aminoglycosides
   b. Chloramphenicol

TABLE 22.24 ■ Antibiotic Resistance in Gram-Negative Bacteria

	Penicillin	Cephalosporin	Carbapenem	Aztreonam	Beta-Lactamase Inhibitor
CTX-M	+	+			
KPC	+	+			
NDM	+	+	+	+	+
VIM	+	+	+	+	+
IMP	+	+	+		+
OXA	+	+	+		+

- Resistance markers
- Gram negative
  - See Table 22.24.
- Gram positive
  - MecA (methicillin), vanA, vanB (vancomycin)
- Beta lactamase inhibitors
  - Clavulanic acid
  - Sulbactam
  - Tazobactam
- Conjugation—exchanging DNA through sex pilus/bridge
- Transduction—only *Streptococci* and *Neisseria* able to pick up and integrate naked foreign DNA
  - Transduction through bacteriophages performed by *Staphylococcus aureus*
- Carbapenem resistant organisms
  - Gram-negative rods
  - *Acinetobacter*, *Pseudomonas* (green), *Klebsiella* (blue)
  - Meropenem disk
- ESBL (extended spectrum beta-lactamases) done by PCR or culture
  - Inactivates cephalosporins and monobactams
  - Treat ESBL+ infections with carbapenem
- Extended–spectrum beta-lactamases
  - Includes CTXM—cefotaxime (still susceptible to meropenem and amikacin)
- *mecA* gene
- Chemotherapy and antibiotic therapy
  - Affect protein expression of microbes—can cause problems with antigen–based diagnostic tests
  - Affect morphology (more variable)
- MIC—minimum inhibitory concentration—lowest drug level to be bacteriostatic

Odds and Ends

- *Capnocytophaga* (oral flora) and *Eikenella* colonies look the same on the plate
- Testing children for abuse–related sexually transmitted disease
  - NAAT—gonorrhea and chlamydia
  - Serologies—HIV and syphilis
- PYR+ in Group A *Streptococcus (S. pyogenes)*, *Enterococcus*, some CoNS, *Enterobacteriaceae*

- Oxidase+ in *Neisseria, P. aeruginosa, Aeromonas*
  - Negative in *Enterobacteriaceae*
- Hippurate+ in *G. vaginalis, C. jejuni, L. monocytogenes*, and GBS
- Sterilization—kills all microbes
  - Disinfection—kills only pathogenic bacteria
- Sterilization of bacterial spores requires saturated steam at 1 atmosphere pressure for up to 60 minutes

INDEX

Page numbers followed by "*f*" indicate figures, "*t*" indicate tables